Paul Webb
February 1961

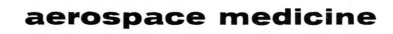

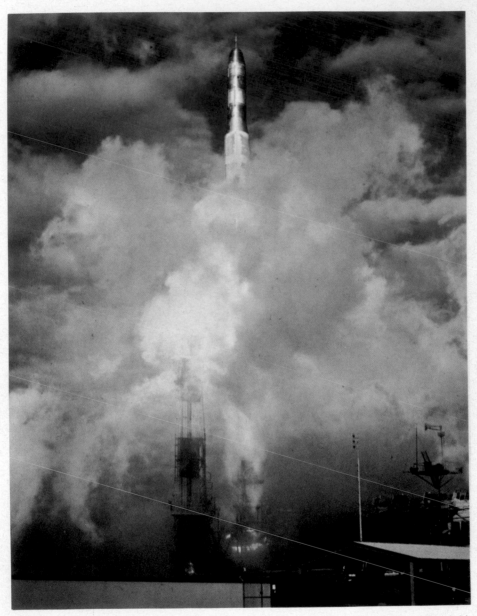

Official U. S. Air Force photo — RCA photo lab.

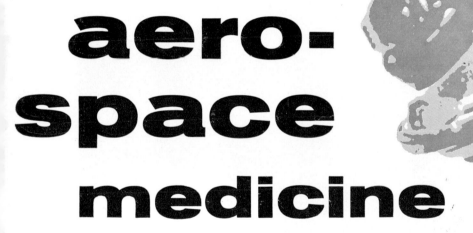

aero-
space
medicine

EDITED BY

Maj. Gen. Harry G. Armstrong, USAF (Ret.)

Formerly, Surgeon General, United States Air Force

 Baltimore 1961

THE WILLIAMS & WILKINS COMPANY

*This textbook is dedicated to the memory of the late
Colonel Harry G. Moseley, a contributing author to this volume,
whose name has been emblazoned on the scroll of those
devoted flight surgeons who have sacrificed their
lives in quest of new scientific knowledge
in the field of aerospace medicine.*

CONTRIBUTORS

MAJ. GEN. HARRY G. ARMSTRONG, USAF
(RET.)
Formerly, Surgeon General, United States
Air Force
(*Chapters 1, 2, 3, 4, 5, 6, 8, 11, 14, 15, 28*)

RICHARD W. BANCROFT, PH.D.
Assistant Chief, Department of Physiology-
Biophysics
USAF School of Aviation Medicine
Randolph Air Force Base, Texas*
(*Chapter 13*)

COL. JOHN E. BOYSEN, USAF (MC)
Deputy Surgeon, Headquarters Air Material
Command
Wright-Patterson Air Force Base, Ohio
(*Chapter 25*)

CAPT. RALPH L. CHRISTY, MC USN
Director, Aviation Medicine Technical Divi-
sion
Bureau of Medicine and Surgery, Navy De-
partment
Washington, D.C.
(*Chapter 16*)

HANS G. CLAMANN, M.D.
Chief, Biophysics Section, Department of
Physiology-Biophysics
USAF School of Aviation Medicine
Randolph Air Force Base, Texas*
(*Chapter 12*)

CAPT. JAMES C. FUELLING, MC USN
Head, Department of Ophthalmology
U. S. Naval School of Aviation Medicine
U. S. Naval Aviation Medical Center

* Relocated at Brooks Air Force Base, Texas, 3
August 1959.

Pensacola, Florida
(*Chapter 21*)

CAPT. CHARLES F. GELL, MC USN
Special Assistant for Medical and Allied
Sciences
Office of Naval Research, Navy Department
Washington, D. C.
(*Chapter 10*)

LAWRENCE E. LAMB, M.D.
Professor and Chief, Department of Internal
Medicine
USAF School of Aviation Medicine
Randolph Air Force Base, Texas*
(*Chapter 22*)

LUDWIG LEDERER, M.D.
Assistant Professor of Medicine,
George Washington University Hospital and
Medical School, and
Medical Director, Capital Airlines, Inc.
Washington National Airport, Washington,
D. C.
(*Chapter 27*)

ULRICH C. LUFT, M.D.
Head, Department of Physiology
The Lovelace Foundation
Albuquerque, New Mexico
(*Chapter 9*)

MAJ. CLARENCE M. McCALL, JR., USAF
(DC)
Head, Periodontology Section, Research
Dentistry Division
USAF School of Aviation Medicine
Randolph Air Force Base, Texas*
(*Chapter 24*)

JOHN C. MEBANE, M.D.
7046 Hollywood Blvd.
Los Angeles 28, California
Formerly: Chief, Department of Neuro-
  psychiatry
USAF School of Aviation Medicine
Randolph Air Force Base, Texas
(*Chapter 23*)

COL. H. G. MOSELEY, USAF (MC)†
Formerly: Chief, Aero Medical Safety Divi-
  sion
Office of the Inspector General, USAF
Norton Air Force Base
San Bernardino, California
(*Chapter 30*)

COL. JAMES B. NUTTALL, USAF (MC)
Chief, Aviation Medicine Division
Office of the Surgeon General, Headquarters,
  USAF
Washington, D.C.
(*Chapter 20*)

HORACE O. PARRACK, PH.D.
Technical Coordinator, R & D Technical
  Areas, Noise and Vibration
Wright Air Development Center
Wright-Patterson Air Force Base, Ohio
(*Chapter 18*)

LT. COL. HUGH W. RANDEL, USAF (MC)
Chief, Department of Preventive Medicine
USAF School of Aviation Medicine
Randolph Air Force Base, Texas*
(*Chapter 29*)

S. B. SELLS, PH.D.
Professor of Psychology
Texas Christian University

† Deceased.

Fort Worth, Texas
Formerly: Chief, Department of Medical
  Psychology
USAF School of Aviation Medicine
Randolph Air Force Base, Texas
(*Chapter 7*)

COL. JOHN P. STAPP, USAF (MC)
Chief, Aero Medical Laboratory
Wright Air Development Center
Wright-Patterson Air Force Base, Ohio
(*Chapter 17*)

BRIG. GEN. BENJAMIN A. STRICKLAND, JR.,
  USAF (MC) Assistant for Bioastronau-
  tics, Headquarters, Air Research and De-
  velopment Command
Andrews Air Force Base, Maryland
(*Chapter 26*)

HUBERTUS STRUGHOLD, M.D.
Advisor for Research and Professor of Space
  Medicine
USAF School of Aviation Medicine
Randolph Air Force Base, Texas*
(*Chapters 31, 32*)

MAJ. LUCIAN SZMYD, USAF (DC)
Head, Oral Surgery Section, Research Den-
  tistry Division
USAF School of Aviation Medicine
Randolph Air Force Base, Texas*
(*Chapter 24*)

PAUL WEBB, M.D.
Chief, Environment Section, Aero Medical
  Laboratory
Wright Air Development Center
Wright-Patterson Air Force Base, Ohio
(*Chapter 19*)

PREFACE

This book is the successor to an earlier book entitled *The Principles and Practice of Aviation Medicine*. The editor and the publisher agreed that *Aerospace Medicine* should appear as a new book and not as a fourth edition of the former work since the two have so little in common. Insofar as the editor is aware *Aerospace Medicine* is the only complete treatise in existence on that subject at the present time. It examines, in detail, the medical problems of both civil and military aviation and astronautics. Appropriate consideration has been given to air travelers as well as to aircrews and among the latter the discussion ranges from the problems of the applicant for a private student pilot's certificate to those of the astronaut in outer space. This great array of diverse subject matter has been arranged into an orderly, logical sequence of 32 chapters within which are 106 tables and 157 figures, many of them appearing in print for the first time. At the end of the book there is both a subject and an author index.

The complexity of aerospace medicine is such that no one person is qualified to speak authoritatively on all its aspects. Accordingly, the highly specialized knowledge and experience of 21 contributing authors has been utilized in this book. Without exception, these contributors have had an extensive background of teaching, research and practical experience. They are nationally or internationally known authorities in their particular fields of endeavor, and possess the happy faculty of being able to express themselves clearly. It is indeed a pleasure for the editor of this volume to have had the cooperation of these distinguished co-authors. He wishes to thank them individually and collectively for the exceptional quality of their presentations.

For medicine to fulfill its function in aviation, a knowledge of aerospace medicine must be acquired and employed by three different groups of individuals. It is the purpose of this textbook to provide a convenient source for this needed information. The three groups referred to consist of the student and practitioner of aerospace medicine, members of the general medical and dental profession and those concerned with the design, construction and operation of aircraft and manned space vehicles. As will be pointed out in the paragraphs to follow, each of these groups has an important part to play in the welfare, comfort, health and safety of those who fly which, in the United States alone, now involves some 1 million airmen and 60 million annual aircraft passengers.

This volume has been written primarily for the use of the student and the practitioner of aerospace medicine. The student will find that this work contains all of the specialized information on the subject that he will require to become fully qualified in this field of knowledge. The first chapter is devoted to historical background material for orientation purposes through which the student can at once become generally familiar with the subject as a whole. This is followed by a logical sequence of chapters dealing with the physical examination for flying, the environmental conditions of flight, the diseases and accidents peculiar to flying, the means of dealing with these various hazards and, finally, two chapters on the medical problems of space flight.

The graduate flight surgeon will find this book to be a handy and useful reference work. It will also serve as a simple means of bringing his knowledge up to date on a subject which has undergone an unprecedented surge of new advances in recent years. The convenience of this can be appreciated when it is realized that the information contained in this volume has been culled from some 1100 scientific journals, periodicals and technical reports, many of which are published in foreign languages.

The second group of individuals requiring a knowledge of aerospace medicine consists of most members of the general medical and dental professions inasmuch as they have a responsibility in this field in the course of their everyday practices. This results from the fact that about nine-tenths of the 1 million airmen and essentially all of the 60 million annual air passengers in this country get their medical advice and treatment from the general medical profession rather than from a flight surgeon and that all of them get their dental care from the general dental profession.

In general medical practice, problems in aerospace medicine may be met in several forms. Any licensed physician may now apply to the Federal Aviation Agency and be appointed an Aviation Medical Examiner if he has the prerequisites. At the present time such designated private practitioners are examining some 250,000 applicants for airmen's medical certificates annually and unless this examination is properly performed and interpreted in terms of flying the consequences can be disastrous. The same thing applies to airmen under treatment by the family physician. In these cases the danger arises when the interrelationships between an illness, convalescence and the taking of drugs by the ambulatory patient and his return to flying is not fully understood.

Another area of responsibility of the general medical profession in aviation concerns advice to patients regarding air travel. Up to the present time the medical profession has been poorly informed concerning this matter and, as a consequence, has adopted a generally negative attitude which in most cases is not in the best interests of the patient. Although it is, of course, true that flying is detrimental to certain types of cases under certain circumstances, the reverse is equally true. The movement of patients by air over long distances may be the means of saving life and limb in emergencies, and in the vast majority of all cases it promotes the health and welfare of the individual concerned when compared to travel by any other means.

All of the information required by the general physician to carry out his responsibilities, in the above-mentioned areas, is contained in this textbook, the major portion of which will be found in the chapters on the physical examination for flying, the aircrew effectiveness chapter and the chapter on aeromedical evacuation. The latter was written with the general medical profession specifically in mind in the hope that the existing misunderstandings and confusion concerning this important matter might be clarified. The profession will also find the chapter on aerial hygiene and sanitation helpful when called upon to give immunizations for overseas travel, by air or other means and also useful medical advice for travelers preparing for a journey to any part of the world. Although they will be mostly of academic interest to the average physician, the two chapters on space medicine at the end of this book will provide fascinating reading concerning the professional aspects of this spectacular new field of science which is currently the leading topic of conversation whenever scientific or world affairs are being discussed.

That all modern physicians should have a thorough knowledge of aerospace medicine, in the areas outlined above, has thus far been ignored or overlooked by all except five of our medical schools. It seems obvious that this situation should be corrected. A failure to do so will result in an ever increasing loss of life, limb and property which might otherwise be saved if the medical profession were trained to carry out its responsibilities in this field which is now a part of everyday practice and is rapidly growing. In the interim the student and practitioner of general medicine must depend on works such as this and their own efforts to acquire the needed information which at best is only a stopgap substitute for the training which should somehow be squeezed into the already crowded courses of our schools of medicine.

The important part that the dental profession plays in the health of airmen and its responsibilities in this regard are dealt with in a separate chapter prepared by dental experts in this field. In addition to describing the role of dentistry in the selection and professional care of airmen this chapter points out the grave dangers that can result from dental operative treatment and the use of drugs in these cases without due regard to their effect on the individual's ability to fly until he has completely recovered.

The third group of individuals who will find this book to be of great value are those concerned with the design, construction, operation and flying of aircraft and space vehicles. Here we are dealing with nonmedical personnel and we are confronted with the problem of the technical language barrier. The best solution to this problem, and the one employed here, is the use of the simplest possible terminology consistent with the professional nature of the subject matter.

The need for designers and builders of aircraft and manned space vehicles to have a knowledge of aerospace medicine is due to the fact that many of the items which provide comfort and safety to aircrews and passengers are built-in features of the craft, such as pressure cabins, safety belts, ventilation, temperature and humidity control. This volume describes in detail the various human requirements which the properly designed and constructed aircraft should provide for. This same information is useful to airline management and other operators of aircraft if their crews and passengers are to be afforded maximum safety and comfort. The designers of manned space vehicles face

a very critical problem in meeting human requirements and the currently available knowledge concerning this is also included.

For well over 20 years crew members of high performance aircraft and air line stewardesses and flight nurses have received extensive training in aviation medicine as a part of their flying training. They are reindoctrinated at intervals of from 1 to 2 years. The reason for this is that many aeromedical problems occur during flight and these are the individuals who must deal with them. Airmen must also have a thorough knowledge of the basic principles of healthful living and the medical pitfalls related to their occupation. All of these various matters are dealt with in detail in this volume and are summarized in chapter 26 entitled "Air Crew Maintenance." Pilots or other crew members of average intelligence will have no difficulty in absorbing this information and it will provide them with a form of insurance which will pay dividends in the form of greatly increased chances of survival.

The editor has received advice and assistance from a number of individuals and agencies and desires to express his appreciation to them. In the Office of the Surgeon General, United States Air Force, Colonel James B. Nuttall, Chief of the Aviation Division, Gertrude B. Dunbar, Librarian and Dr. Mae M. Link of the Historical Affairs Office were most generous with their help, and to each of them, my thanks.

Captain O. W. Chenault, in the Office of the Surgeon General, United States Navy and Lt. Colonel R. B. Austin in the Office of the Surgeon General, United States Army were also consulted on frequent occasions and their assistance is gratefully acknowledged.

Dr. John E. Smith, Acting Civil Air Surgeon of the Federal Aviation Agency was consulted with on numerous occasions and I am especially grateful for the time and effort he expended in this connection.

Two individuals I am most indebted to are Dr. J. W. Heim of the Aero Medical Laboratory, Wright Patterson Air Force

Base, Ohio, and Professor Hubertus Strughold, of the Air Force School of Aviation
Medicine, Randolph Air Force Base, Texas.
From these two friends and co-workers of
long standing I received extensive help in
the planning of this new volume, encouragement to initiate and carry through its preparation and numerous helpful ideas and
suggestions. I should also like to thank
Professor Strughold for allowing me unrestricted use of his extensive lecture notes on
"The Atmosphere" for use in my chapter of
that same name.

Colonel Robert Benford, Editor of both
the *Armed Forces Medical Journal* and *Aerospace Medicine*, provided me with extensive
guidance on matters of editorial policy and
usage as well as assistance in locating numerous items of reference. I am most appreciative of this help and advice and to him
also, my thanks.

Finally I would like to express my sin-
cerest appreciation to those concerned at
the Williams & Wilkins Company and at
the Waverly Press, Inc. for their patience,
understanding and cooperation as well as
for the excellence of their publishing and
printing efforts.

H. G. A.

CONTENTS

1

HISTORICAL

Harry G. Armstrong, M.D.

Aerospace medicine is defined as that specialty of general medicine which concerns itself with the medical problems of aviation. Aerospace medicine is subdivided into the medical problems of flight where spacecraft are employed (aviation medicine) and those peculiar to flight involving the use of aircraft (space medicine). These various problems and their solutions are, of course, the subject of this book and each of them will be discussed in some detail in subsequent chapters. Before considering these problems individually, however, it is believed that those who are not familiar with aerospace medicine will be greatly benefited if they are first given a general orientation and, accordingly, this present chapter will be devoted to that purpose.

It is proposed to accomplish this orientation by briefly reviewing the general history of aviation and aerospace medicine followed by a summary of their recent status using the situation in the United States as an example. By making this information available at the outset the reader will be able to develop an initial general knowledge of the subject as a whole which in turn will make subsequent discussions of the various disease entities and individual problems easier to comprehend.

The depicting of angels as having wings was no doubt based originally on the ancient concept that flight was a heavenly attribute beyond the attainment of mortal man, and that flying, along with everlasting life, was man's supreme spiritual reward. In spite of this, few such seemingly impossible ideas so stubbornly persisted in the human mind as the desire to fly. It is quite probable that long before the dawn of recorded history individuals made attempts to emulate the birds soaring over their heads, for the earliest legends tell us of characters who flew.

The most familiar legend is the one from ancient Greece concerning Daedalus and his son Icarus who attempted to escape imprisonment on Crete by fashioning wings and fixing them to their shoulders with wax. Icarus, in his youthful zest, flew too close to the sun and the intense heat caused the melting of the wax which held his wings in place. He fell to his death in the sea and thus attained the doubtful honor of being the first to die in a flying accident. Meanwhile, the more conservative father who chose to fly at a moderate altitude made good his escape and landed safely on the island of Sicily.

In the latter part of the 13th century, the English philosopher Roger Bacon in his *Opus Majestus* looked down through the years and saw flight as a distinct possibility. "It is entirely possible," he wrote, "that a device for flying shall be made such that a man sitting in the middle of it and turning a crank shall cause artificial wings to beat the air after the manner of a bird's flight." Leonardo da Vinci (1452–1515), the Italian engineer, architect, anatomist, sculptor and painter is famous for his study of the flight of birds, his models of helicopter-type aircraft which flew, and his drawings of conventional-type aircraft that in many respects were very similar in appearance to those in use today.

THE BALLOON

In 1782 Joseph and Jacques Montgolfier, the sons of a wealthy paper manufacturer of Annonay, France, discovered that if they held a paper bag inverted over a fire until it was filled with smoke it would ascend to the ceiling of their room. Encouraged by this they constructed a balloon over 90 feet in circumference. Made of linen, lined with paper and inflated by the hot air from a fire of chopped straw, this balloon made its first flight on 5 June 1783. Within a few months another ascent was made at Versailles, France, before Louis XVI and his court and for the first time passengers were carried. These passengers, a sheep, a cock, and a duck rose to an altitude of 1500 feet and then returned to earth unharmed. The date was 19 September 1783.

A month later arrangements were made to send a condemned criminal aloft with the stipulation that if he returned to earth alive he was to be given his freedom. A French apothecary from Metz, Pilâtre de Rozier, hearing of this protested that the honor of being the first to fly should not go to a criminal and insisted that he himself be allowed to make the attempt. His first flight took place on 15 October 1783, in a captive balloon, and de Rozier with the Marquis d'Arlandes as a passenger next successfully undertook the first free balloon flight on 21 November 1783.

On 23 November 1784, and again on 7 January 1785, balloon flights of special interest were made by an American physician by the name of Jeffries. Dr. John Jeffries was born in Boston, Massachusetts, on 5 February 1744, and after graduation from Harvard College studied medicine in England where he received his M.D. degree in 1769. He practiced medicine for a time in Boston after which he again returned to England where he became interested in making balloon flights as a means of studying the properties of the upper atmosphere. Accordingly, arrangements were made with the French balloonist M. Blanchard.

On their first flight Jeffries carried a thermometer, a barometer, a hydrometer, an electrometer and six small glass-stoppered vials filled with distilled water. During the hour and 21 minutes of the flight it was noted that the hydrometer fluctuated whereas the electrometer showed no change. The temperature change was from $+51°$ to $+28.5°$ F. and the barometric pressure decreased from 30 to 21.25 inches of mercury. This latter represents an altitude of approximately 9250 feet above the starting point. The vials of water were emptied one by one and samples of the upper air collected for analysis. During the flight Jeffries dropped a written message to a friend, a Mr. Arodi Thayer. This note is now in the Snell Museum of Physics at Amherst College and is the first piece of mail carried by air. The second flight of Jeffries and Blanchard was across the English Channel from Dover, England, to near Calais, France. In 1786 Jeffries wrote a book describing his experiences.

Altogether, Dr. Jeffries has a remarkable record of accomplishments in aeronautics to his credit. He was the first American to fly and the first to publish a book on aeronautics (1). He was the first to study scientifically the composition of the upper air, the first to carry air mail and the first to make an aerial over water crossing. To honor this famous American physician the Institute of Aeronautical Sciences, in 1940, established the John Jeffries Award which is presented each year to the physician who makes the greatest contribution to aviation in the field of medicine.

Shortly after the middle of the 19th century several ascents by Coxwell and Glaisher were sponsored by the British Association for the Advancement of Science on behalf of the latter who made a total of 28 flights. James Glaisher collected air for analysis at different heights; observed the temperature, pressure and electricity of the air; determined the dew point; measured the oxygen of the atmosphere; made experiments on sound; and closely observed his own and his companion's physical reactions (2). On 5 September 1862, a flight was made to an altitude of 29,000 feet at which point Glaisher became unconscious from lack of oxygen. Coxwell was so nearly overcome that he lost the use of his arms but had the presence of mind to grasp the balloon relief valve rope in his

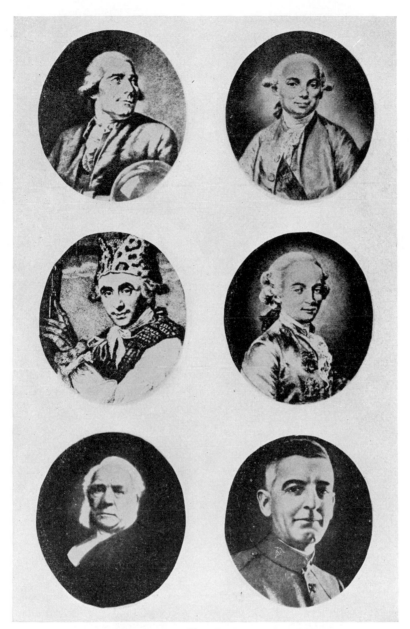

FIG. 1

Joseph-Michel Montgolfier (1740–1810)   Jacques-Etienne Montgolfier (1745–1799)
John Jeffries (1744–1819)   Jean-François Pilatre de Rozier (1756–1785)
James Glaisher (1809–1903)   Theodore Charles Lyster (1875–1933)

teeth which caused the balloon to begin its descent.

In 1874 two balloonists, Sivel and Crocé-Spinelli, came to Paul Bert's physiology laboratory in Paris to subject themselves to very low barometric pressures in his low pressure chamber in preparation for some future high altitude flights. In this experiment they went to a pressure of 304 mm. of mercury which corresponds to an altitude of about 23,000 feet. Here, for the first time, they learned of the use of oxygen to prevent the effects of hypoxia. On 22 March 1874, Sivel and Crocé-Spinelli made their first high altitude flight and almost reached the same altitude pressure as they had in the altitude chamber. They took along bags of oxygen furnished them by Paul Bert. One mixture consisted of 40 per cent oxygen and 60 per cent nitrogen, and the other of 70 per cent oxygen and 30 per cent nitrogen. The former was used at the lower altitudes and the latter after they reached 18,000 feet.

On 15 April 1875, Tissandier (3) joined Crocé-Spinelli and Sivel in another ascent to high altitude which was to end in disaster. They carried with them on this flight three 150-liter bags of 72 per cent oxygen which Bert warned them by letter were of insufficient capacity. Unfortunately, Bert's letter arrived too late and their plan to use the oxygen only at the last moment was a fatal

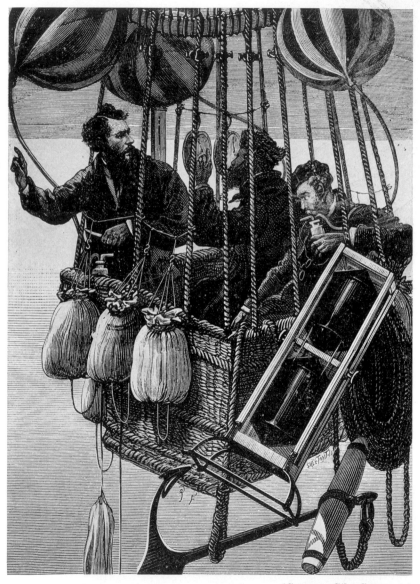

(Courtesy Ciba Symposia)

FIG. 2. The famous flight of Tissandier and his two companions, Sivel and Crocé-Spinelli in 1875. Sivel is dropping ballast, Tissandier reading the barometer and Crocé-Spinelli holding his oxygen respirator.

decision. When they finally felt themselves being overcome they were paralyzed and unable to grasp the oxygen tubes. The balloon ascended to 28,820 feet and then descended of its own accord during which all three occupants of the balloon became unconscious. Only Tissandier survived. Upon landing he found that his companions were dead.

PAUL BERT

Paul Bert (1833–1886) obtained his M.D. degree in 1863, and in 1869 was appointed Bernard's successor to the chair of physiology at the Faculté des Sciences in Paris. At about this time Bert became interested in the effects of changes in barometric pressures through his close friendship with Jourdanet who had studied this matter during the latter's extensive mountain travels in Mexico. A little later Bert became acquainted with Tissandier, Sivel and Crocé-Spinelli, and through them became interested in the problems of flying. Finally he interested himself in the problems of caisson disease, and about 1870 began experimental studies in these three areas.

During the following 8 years Bert carried out 670 separate experiments, and in 1878 published his famous *La Pression Barometrique* (4), a book of 1178 pages and 89 text figures. Altogether this volume is a masterly presentation of research recorded in an orderly, clear, concise and logical manner which anyone would do well to utilize as a model for any similar task.

It is not practical to even outline the extensive research of Bert in a work of this type, and the serious student is urged to consult the original or the English translation (4) which is available. From this one will learn how Bert related the air, its component gases, the barometric pressure, the blood gases and their partial pressures to the effects of caisson work, mountain travel and high altitude flight. Paul Bert did all of these things and emerged from his laboratory with the answers to the many questions he had

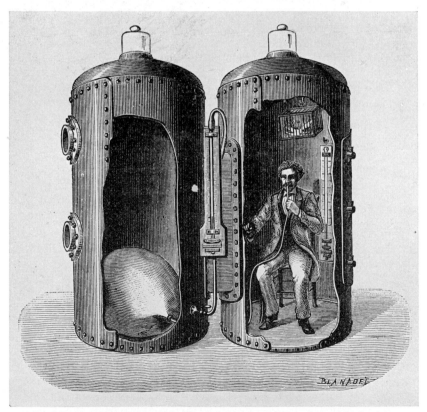

FIG. 3. Paul Bert (1878) in his altitude chamber breathing air enriched with oxygen

set out to study with one exception. Bert did not find that gas bubbles were formed in the blood as a result of a decrease of atmospheric pressure below 1 atmosphere. He carried out a few experiments on this question but drew conclusions based on inadequate evidence. It is curious to note that the *Lancet* of 20 November 1886, in reporting Bert's death did not even mention *La Pression Barometrique* and it was over 50 years later that this work became famous.

THE AIRPLANE

In 1840 George Peacock of England demonstrated a man lifting kite, and, 2 years later, Stringfellow and Henson built a model airplane similar in appearance to our early monoplanes. This machine had a wingspan of 10 feet and was powered by a single cylinder steam engine. This was the first self propelled, power driven, heavier than air machine to sustain itself in the air. Beginning in 1891 Dr. Samuel Langley in the United States developed steam driven models one of which flew a distance of 4200 feet in 1896. A full sized Langley plane was tested on 7 October and again on 8 December 1903, but each time crashed on being launched.

Meanwhile, the theory of flight was being studied by Wilbur and Orville Wright at Dayton, Ohio, and by 1900 they were flying gliders. In 1903 they completed an airplane and power plant of their own design and shipped it to Kitty Hawk, North Carolina. There, on 14 December, their first attempt to fly resulted in a crash, but on 17 December 1903, Orville Wright took off and flew a distance of 120 feet in 12 seconds. The seemingly impossible had been accomplished.

In 1908 the Wrights opened negotiations with various governments, and on 10 February of that year the United States Army signed a contract with them for its first airplane. Soon afterward several nations in Europe also bought aircraft for military use and by the time World War I began all of the major powers had small air services. The aircraft engines of that time developed up to 200 horsepower and the better planes could climb to about 13,000 feet carrying two people. Flights of 600 miles had been covered without landing and planes had remained aloft for as long as 21 hours. By the end of

1913 the altitude record for airplanes stood at 20,010 feet and the speed record was 126 miles per hour. However, planes were not yet reliable and their only use in the first part of World War I was for reconnaissance.

It is a historical fact that the first meeting of two hostile aircraft in that conflict resulted in nothing more than an exchange of greetings between the pilots. This soon changed, however, and aerial combat began with weapons consisting of bricks, pistols, rifles, and finally machine guns. Later, bombs were carried and dropped on enemy targets. Aerial photography was developed and also aircraft radio. Toward the end of the war the Germans had equipped at least some of their aviators with parachutes and all the warring nations had developed oxygen equipment. Meanwhile, rapid improvements in airplanes and engines were made because of the urgency of the war, and by 1918 the speed record had increased to 162 miles per hour and the altitude record to 31,390 feet.

Following World War I the great surplus of war planes hampered the development of new and better ones in all countries, and for a number of years aviation was at a low ebb. Some of the war planes were used to equip the postwar Air Forces and the surplus was sold to civilian users. Most of this surplus went to ex-service pilots, and the next 8 years were noted principally for the barnstorming tours of these aerial gypsies.

Gradually, however, aircraft development began again and the airplane came to be used more and more for commercial purposes. In 1927 Lindbergh made his epic solo nonstop flight from New York to Paris and the world became air minded almost overnight. In the United States, by 1927, 30 airmail contracts were held by various private airline operators and some of the mail planes which were flying back and forth across the continent began to carry passengers. In this same year Pan American Airways was formed and subsequently extended its routes to all parts of the world. From 1930 on, the new aircraft developed for the military services and the demand for larger faster commercial planes resulted in an increase in size, weight, speed and maneuverability of airplanes to a remarkable degree. By 1939 aircraft engines were developing three times the horsepower that they had had only a few years previously. Operating speeds had changed from 100 to 200 miles per hour and military fighter aircraft were attaining speeds in excess of 375 miles per hour. Commercial airlines were carrying thousands of tons of mail, freight and express, and their annual passenger list passed the million mark in 1937.

The Origins of Aviation Medicine

The first scientific paper on aviation medicine, following the invention of the airplane, was published in 1907 and the second in 1910. The latter was actually a series of papers which were later translated from French to English and published as a book in the United States under the title, *Air Sickness* (5). During 1911 there were 11 papers published on various medical aspects of flying; in 1912 there were five; in 1913 seven and in 1914 seven. Thus, when World War I began, which was 11 years after the Wright brothers' first flight, the world's literature devoted to the medical aspects of aviation consisted of 31 papers and one small book.

However, there was considerably more medical interest developing in this field than one might suspect from a review of the literature of that period, for on 2 February 1912, the United States War Department had published its first instructions concerning the physical examination of candidates for aviation duty. This was followed in a few months by similar instructions issued by the United States Navy. Even before this, in 1910, minimum standards for military pilots had been drawn up in Germany. In France the first official circular with reference to the medical examination of aviators appeared in 1912 but was not put into effect until 1914. The Royal Flying Corps was established in England in 1912 and medical regulations soon followed. In Italy and in most of the other major nations of the world there were similar developments during this same period.

Inasmuch as the development of aviation medicine into a well organized science during the period of World War I occurred more or less simultaneously and along parallel lines in the major countries involved in that conflict, this development will be reviewed in detail only as it occurred in the United States.

General Theodore Charles Lyster, Medical Corps, United States Army (1875–1933) is acknowledged as being the father of aviation medicine in America. He was on duty in the office of the Surgeon General of the Army just prior to World War I and was one of the first to appreciate the medical problems of flying. In september 1917 General Lyster became the first Chief Surgeon, Aviation Section, Signal Corps, United States Army, in which capacity he guided the development of American aviation medicine during the period of World War I. In general, this development concerned itself with the selection of pilots, aviation medical research and the formation of a special medical service for air units.

In 1916 Lyster, assisted by Colonel William H. Wilmer and Colonel I. H. Jones, devised a completely new record sheet, established new standards and wrote new regulations for the physical examination of pilots. These were issued in May 1917 in time for use during the war period during which over 100,000 applicants were processed at examining centers located throughout the United States.

The physical standards, established for pilots by Lyster and his co-workers in 1916, were based largely on empirical grounds and they felt it necessary that this whole question be given further study. At the same time the appalling death rate among flying cadets at the training centers in the United States and among the allies in France from aircraft accidents indicated the need for an extensive research program. Accordingly, an Aviation Medical Research Board was appointed on 18 October 1917. The powers delegated to this board were:

1. To investigate all conditions which affect the efficiency of pilots.

2. To institute and carry out such experiments and tests as will determine the ability of pilots to fly at high altitudes.

3. To carry out experiments and tests to provide suitable apparatus for the supply of oxygen to pilots at high altitudes.

4. To act as a standing medical board for the consideration of all matters relating to the physical fitness of pilots.

The first act of this board was to establish a research laboratory at Hazelhurst Field, Mineola, Long Island, which opened early in January 1918. One of the major items of experimental equipment in this new laboratory was a low pressure chamber. This was used extensively in studying the effects of lack of oxygen at high altitudes and to classify pilots in accordance with their altitude tolerance inasmuch as aircraft had not then been fitted with oxygen equipment. The other principal field of study was the physical standards for flying.

The original examination required no psychologic or psychiatric evaluation and the neurologic system was given only perfunctory attention. This latter was corrected, and by 1923 Longacre had developed a comprehensive personality study to be used in selecting candidates for flying training.

In 1920 Schneider (6) described a cardiovascular rating which he had developed to measure physical fatigue and efficiency. This became a part of the flying examination until 1943 when it was abandoned as being unreliable.

The Otology Department of the research laboratory carried out a great amount of work on the relationship between the vestibular function of the ear and flying. As a part of this work deaf-mutes, tabetics, professional dancers and cats were studied as to their reactions to accelerations, and altogether a great amount of excellent data was collected. Unfortunately, in applying this knowledge to the problem of flying the importance of the ear was exaggerated. For example, a test was developed in which candidates were whirled on a piano stool. If they vomited—which in most cases was a perfectly normal reaction—they were rejected. The Barany chair was soon substituted for the piano stool in the routine testing of the vestibular apparatus, but this too finally fell into disuse except for individuals in whom definite pathology was suspected.

The work of the research laboratory in ophthalmology consisted principally of studies to determine the relationships between various functions of the eye and the piloting of aircraft. Studies were carried out in relation to color vision, visual acuity, eye muscle

balance, fields of vision and depth perception under normal conditions and under conditions simulating high altitudes. The work on depth perception resulted eventually in the development of the Howard-Dolman depth perception apparatus.

In addition to the research referred to above a great amount of other work was carried on and this is described in the *Air Service Medical* (7) published in 1918 and is recommended reading to those interested in a detailed account of the World War I research work of that laboratory.

The Air Service Medical Research Laboratory was the first of its kind to be established and its contributions to aviation and to aviation medicine are incalculable in relation to the saving of lives and equipment. Of equal importance is the fact that this institution was the medium through which aviation medicine in all its ramifications was placed on a sound scientific basis in America.

CARE OF THE FLYER

When an American Medical Mission departed for Europe in October 1917 to study aviation medicine in England, France and Italy, those concerned were quite satisfied that everything possible had been done to provide a superior medical service for American flyers. When this mission visited the American air squadrons in France, however, it was at once recognized that this idea was far from correct. The pilots were losing weight, their physical condition was poor and their morale was low. Flying accident rates were high and the fatalities from crashes were three times those resulting from enemy action. There was one crash per 241 hours and one fatality per 721 hours flown. In addition, many of the flyers were suffering from conditions associated with flying which were not recognized or understood by the medical officers assigned to the squadrons inasmuch as the latter had had no training in aviation medicine. To make the situation worse a flyer was not permitted to see a medical officer without the express permission of his commanding officer.

This state of affairs made it apparent to the mission that something very important had been overlooked. When word was received in the United States of the conditions in France, General Lyster made plans for medical officers to be trained in aviation medicine. For the training of these officers a school, known as the School for Flight Surgeons, was established. This school was not ready to open until May 1919, and long before that date 34 officers and 15 enlisted men had been detached from the Air Service Medical Research Laboratory at Hazelhurst Field and sent to Issoudun, France.

In a remarkably short time after the arrival of this group, flying accidents and deaths were markedly reduced and commanding officers were more than pleased to give full credit to the work of these trained flight surgeons for this improvement. As soon as they could be trained other flight surgeons were assigned to flying fields in the United States. By the end of the war a complete medical service for the air service was organized and functioning. This service combined the selection, the classification and the maintenance of the flyer and those trained in this work were considered specialists.

Although these developments were taking place in the United States similar research was being conducted by the other major powers of the world. In addition, they carried out considerable work on the development of oxygen equipment, goggles, safety belts and flying clothing. In several of the countries a separate Medical Service was created to serve the Air Forces concerned and the assigned medical officers were given special training in Aviation Medicine.

POST-WORLD WAR I AVIATION MEDICINE

For 10 years following the end of World War I aviation medicine almost ceased to exist as a living science and was kept from utter decay only by the efforts of a few individuals who had the foresight to realize that aviation and aviation medicine were more than a transient necessity of World War I.

Although it is true that for the first year or 2 after that war there were a number of papers published on aviation medicine, these were almost entirely devoted to reporting the results of observations and investigations made during the war period. This applies generally also to the three books on the subject which appeared at about that time.

These were *Medical Examination of Airmen* by Maublanc and Ratié (8), *Fisiologia ed Aviazione* by Herlitzka (9) and *Aviation Medicine* by Bauer (10).

Of the few advances made in aviation medicine during this postwar period, two are of special significance and were as follows. Mashburn (11, 12) developed a serial reaction time machine to measure an individual's aptitude for flying training. This was by far the most effective method developed up to that time and, of even greater significance, it is the most accurate single measure of this trait today. The other great advance of this period was the work of Myers (13) on the physiology of blind flying. This latter work was not published until 1936 but it was applied, beginning in 1924, in the development and use of blind flying instruments and has been one of the greatest contributions of medicine to the technical advancement of aviation. Both of the individuals mentioned above were associated with the School of Aviation Medicine during the time their work was accomplished and it was this school alone in the United States that survived the neglect of that period.

The revival of aviation medicine in the United States following World War I was a direct result of the eventual expansion of aviation, both commercially and in the military services, and also to the increased performance of the newer aircraft. One of the first evidences of this revival was the establishment of a medical section in the Bureau of Air Commerce, of the Department of Commerce, when the latter was established in 1926. This Bureau required all civil aviators to pass a prescribed physical examination before being granted a license to fly and, for the first time in the United States, there existed a need for civilian flight surgeons. These flight surgeons, although few in number, were determined to advance their profession and, accordingly, formed the Aero Medical Association in 1929 which, in March 1930, began the publication of an official journal, the *Journal of Aviation Medicine*.

The first medical director of the aeronautics branch of the Bureau of Air Commerce was Dr. Louis H. Bauer who resigned his commission in the regular Army to accept this new position. For the previous 6 years

Dr. (Lt. Col.) Bauer had been commandant of the Army School of Aviation Medicine and, it will be recalled, wrote the first text book on aviation medicine in America in 1926. The founding of the Aero Medical Association and it's *Journal* were both first suggested by Dr. Bauer and came into being only through his personal efforts and leadership. He was the first president of the Association, editor of the *Journal* for 25 years and in many other ways contributed to the advancement of aviation medicine.

Dr. Bauer resigned from the Bureau of Air Commerce in 1930 to enter private practice. In 1952 he became the president of the American Medical Association, and from 1948 to the present has served as the Secretary-General of the World Medical Association. These great honors and responsibilities in other fields, however, did not lessen Dr. Bauer's interest in aviation medicine and his efforts in its behalf continued unabated.

A second important sign of aviation medicine revival occurred in 1934 when the Aero Medical Research Laboratory was established at Wright Field, Dayton, Ohio. Prior to this time, medical efforts had been directed principally to selecting flyers who could tolerate the stresses inherent in flight. As a result of increased performance of the newer aircraft it became apparent that this should be supplemented by studies concerning the effects of high performance flight on the human organism and methods of neutralizing or eliminating those factors which were detrimental to the efficiency, health or safety of flying personnel.

The need for this new laboratory was first recognized by Major Malcolm C. Grow and it was through his efforts as air surgeon in the Office of the Chief of the Army Air Corps in Washington that its establishment was approved. This was but one of the many great contributions of this officer who retired from the service in 1949 after having attained the grade of major general and serving as the first Surgeon General of the United States Air Force.

The third important development of this period was the establishment in 1939 of the United States Navy School of Aviation Medicine at the Naval Air Station, Pensacola, Florida, with Captain Frederick Ceres as its first commanding officer. This institution contained excellent facilities for research as well as for teaching and its establishment at that particular time was in response to a need generated by the marked increase in aviation in the Navy during the preceding decade.

The last important element in this chain of events that will be mentioned here was the establishment by several of the aircraft manufacturers and the commercial air lines of their own medical departments. Although the primary responsibility of these medical departments was to examine and provide aeromedical supervision of the flight personnel of the companies concerned they often provided other important services as well. One of these was to provide consultant services to aircraft manufacturers as to the medical aspects of aircraft design as regards safety and comfort. The other was an airline program aimed at protecting the health and promoting the safety and comfort of those traveling on the airline concerned.

WORLD WAR II

With the onset of World War II the previous activities in aviation medicine, in all of the nations involved, were greatly expanded and intensified. It was soon learned that many of the known problems had not been adequately solved and a great variety of new problems began to manifest themselves. Most of the existing oxygen systems, flying clothing and other items of protective flying equipment were found to be inefficient, inadequate or both. Plans, procedures and equipment for air rescue, survival and air evacuation on a large scale had to be developed. Frostbite at high altitude became a matter of major concern as did burns from aircraft catching on fire in combat and after crashes.

Streamlined methods of selecting trainees for the thousands of aircrews needed for the war effort became urgent as well as better means of selecting individuals for the different type aircraft and the various crew positions. Emotional breakdown as a result of fear of flying or combat also became a major consideration. The temporary loss of vision or consciousness from high speed turns during dogfights was of vital concern and demanded renewed attention. Bullet proof clothing was found to be highly effective against low velocity missiles and was used by U. S. Air Force bomber crews.

All this was complicated by the advent of new and faster aircraft and the necessity for flying most combat missions at maximum speed and altitude. Near the end of the war this particular problem was compounded by the advent of jet airplanes with a performance that greatly exceeded anything that had previously been even imagined.

As is usual in war, medicine made great strides forward and aviation medicine was in the forefront of this advance. That this is so is evidenced by the fact that when all of the work of this period was documented after the war, the bibliography of aviation medicine had grown to more than 15,000 articles which had appeared in some 1100 different medical journals and, in addition, there were in existence about 150 books and monographs on the subject.

Following World War II, aviation medicine did not fade into insignificance as it had after the first world war but, on the contrary, gained in stature and importance. One reason for this was the phenomenal growth of civil aviation and the other the fact that the air arm had emerged from World War II as the acknowledged first line

of a nation's military defense. Added to this was the further development of jet aircraft which greatly increased the complexity of the medical problems to be dealt with in civil as well as in military flying. This latter was of such magnitude that the human element was recognized as potentially the future limiting factor in aircraft performance and the real possibility that air superiority in any future war might well be gained by that nation which was best able to solve the growing difficulties in this area.

THE WAR IN KOREA

The war in Korea was the first in which jet aircraft were utilized in combat on a fairly large scale and served to emphasize the medical problems of extremely high altitude and high speed flight and the problems associated with bail-out using the ejection seat under those conditions. It was also during this war that helicopters were first used in large numbers near and behind the enemy lines for rescue and air evacuation and that conventional aircraft were used to evacuate large masses of wounded from the forward areas in short periods of time and later to evacuate wounded over distances equal to half the circumference of the globe.

From the viewpoint of new technical medical problems, the events of the Korean War

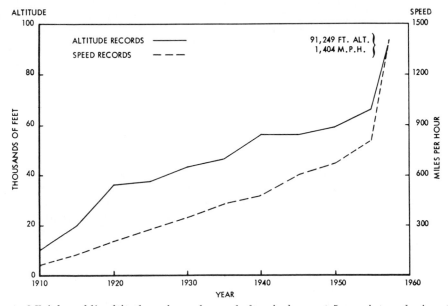

FIG. 4. Official world's altitude and speed records for airplanes at 5 year intervals since 1910

were overshadowed by the concurrent development of new experimental rocket propelled aircraft. These new types not only broke the sound barrier and all unofficial speed and altitude records but introduced the problem of the heat barrier and many other difficult problems of a medical nature.

By 1955, 2 years after the end of the Korean War, aviation and aviation medicine had again assumed a typical peacetime pattern and a brief resumé of their status during that year will conclude this historical review. More recent developments will, of course, be considered in subsequent chapters and those interested in a more detailed history than that presented up to this point are referred to the first two chapters of this author's *Principles and Practice of Aviation Medicine* (14) and Benford's *Doctors in the Sky* (15).

CIVIL AVIATION—1955

The student of aviation medicine will be interested in acquiring a general knowledge of aviation as regards its scope and composition and how it is organized. Accordingly, some of the more important facts and figures concerning this will next be presented. In all cases the data will be that from the United States and for the calendar year 1955 unless otherwise indicated.

For the year under discussion, the manufacture of aircraft and its ancillary equipment required a labor force of some three quarters of a million men. On this basis the aircraft manufacturing industry was second only to the automobile industry in size. Inasmuch as the manufacture of aircraft involved a considerable amount of research and development with respect to aircrew and passenger safety and comfort, this segment of the industries' effort was of interest and concern to aviation medicine. Aircraft manufacturing also involved a considerable amount of flying of experimental aircraft, the flight testing of production models and general flying for business purposes by the companies concerned.

As far as civil flying itself was concerned, all civil aviation was subject to federal regulations which were carried out by two agencies, the Civil Aeronautics Administration (CAA) and the Civil Aeronautic Board (CAB). The CAB, an independent 5-man panel, prescribed the civil air regulations which dealt with the competency of airmen, airworthiness of aircraft and air traffic control. It issued certificates permitting persons to engage in air transportation as a business and was concerned with the economic regulation of air carriers. It investigated accidents in air transportation and compiled accident reports and statistics.

The CAA was a Bureau of the Department of Commerce with the Administrator of Civil Aeronautic exercising his functions under the direction and supervision of the Secretary of Commerce. The CAA constructed and operated the vast system of civil airways and acquired, established, operated and maintained air navigation facilities along the airways and at landing areas. It made provision for the control and protection of air traffic moving in air commerce. It acted in an advisory way in the design and construction of airports and administered the federal aid airport program. It also promoted safety through the certification of of airmen, aircraft and air agencies, such as flight and ground schools, and checked the design, structure and performance of new planes to insure the safety of the flying public.

In the continental limits of the United States there were 6839 civilian and military airports. Many of the former were not only utilized for scheduled airline traffic but also served as a base of operations for aircraft sales, flying training schools, air charter services, agricultural dusting and spraying services, aircraft maintenance, repair and overhaul facilities or furnished a base of operations for commercial, business and private aircraft.

The larger public airports were linked together by 80,185 miles of federal airways operated by the Civil Aeronautics Administration. These airways were designated lanes through the airspace along which aircraft were guided in moving from airport to airport. To provide the navigational guidance and to control the movement of air traffic the airways system consisted of an integrated pattern of radio signal stations, beacon lights, a weather reporting system, intermediate landing fields, instrument approach systems, radar facilities, air route traffic

TABLE 1

United States Airline Revenue Passenger Traffic, 1945 to 1970*

Year	Total	Domestic	International
1945	7,051,810	6,576,252	475,558
1950	19,019,158	17,343,681	1,700,000
1955	41,623,000	38,223,000	3,400 000
1960†	72,200,000	66,000,000	6,200,000
1965†	101,900,000	93,000 000	8,900,000
1970†	129,500,000	118,000,000	11,500,000

* Source: CAA.

† CAA estimate.

control centers and air route traffic control towers.

Civil flying was divided into commercial air carriers and general aviation, and these in turn further subdivided into various types. We will first consider the commercial air carriers.

Commercial Air Carriers

In 1955 there were 12 domestic trunk lines most of which operated high density traffic routes between the principal traffic centers of the United States and another 14 domestic local service lines which operated routes of lesser traffic between the smaller traffic centers and between these centers and the large cities. The 19 international and overseas lines included all United States flag air carriers operating between the United States and foreign countries, other than Canada, whereas the 18 territorial lines operated in the United States island possessions in the Pacific and the Caribbean and the Alaskan lines operated between the United States and Alaska and within Alaska. The three helicopter airmail lines and the five all cargo lines were utilized for the purposes indicated by their titles. The former operated between the downtown post offices of large cities and their adjacent airports. The latter carried cargo only and were not permitted to carry mail or passengers.

The total number of aircraft operated by the scheduled airlines at the end of 1955 was 1773 and the pilots and copilots utilized to operate this equipment numbered 10,846. The total employees of the airlines amounted to 127,000. During the calendar year 1955 the scheduled airlines carried over 275 mil-

lion ton-miles of freight, 142 million ton-miles of U. S. mail and 51 million ton-miles of express. The greater part of their service, however, was devoted to the carrying of passengers, and for the year they transported some 41,623,000 individuals. The actual growth of this traffic since 1945 and an estimate of its future growth up to 1970, is shown in table 1. Although the number of air carriers listed above total 72, there were only 56 different certified airlines in operation which is explained by the fact that some of the latter provided two or more types of service.

In addition to the scheduled airlines, there was a diversified group of noncertified air carriers in operation consisting of 53 transport carriers, 1589 air taxi operators, 153 Alaska pilot owners and 62 air freight forwarders.

General Aviation

The second principal type of civil flying, referred to as general aviation, included everything not already discussed under civil air transport operations. It will probably come as a surprise to the reader to learn that in many respects general aviation overshadowed airline operations. Table 2 shows the four types of general flying and the hours flown by each during 1955. It will be noted that business flying accounted for 45.9 per cent of the total. Some 18,570 aircraft were used primarily for business purposes and another 16,000 were used part time. A high proportion of the large multiengine types of aircraft employed in business flying were owned by large corporations for the transportation of their personnel whereas smaller aircraft were used by farmers, ranchers, physicians, contractors and a host of others in carrying on their occupations. Flying for

TABLE 2

General Aviation; Hours Flown by Types, 1955

Type	Hours Flown	Per Cent
Business	4,300,000	45.9
Pleasure	1,975,000	21.0
Commercial	1,829,000	19.5
Instructional	1,275,000	13.6
Total	9,379,000	100.0

pleasure or recreation employed principally the small single engine aircraft that were easy to fly and economical to own and operate.

Commercial flying included a great number of things such as passenger and cargo carrying for hire, patrolling, surveying, aircraft testing, experimental flying, ferrying and aerial dusting, spraying, seeding, fertilizing and pest control.

The average number of students undergoing flying training during the year was about 80,000. This instruction was available at 991 different airports most of which also conducted ground school courses. The great majority of the ratings sought were for student pilot or private pilot licenses which together accounted for some 60,000 of the total, whereas, at the other end of the scale airline transport students, for example, numbered 860. One other type of general flying will also be mentioned here because of its particular interest to aviation medicine. This was the existence of several hundred civil aircraft available and equipped for air evacuation on a charter basis.

If we combine the data for the commercial air carriers and general aviation we get the totals shown in table 3. This table gives not only the figures for 1955 but also for the two preceding decades, at 5 year intervals, in order to demonstrate the marked growth of civil aviation during that period of time. Inasmuch as all certified aircraft and airmen are not necessarily actively engaged in flying at any given period of time the number of active aircraft and airmen were substantially less than the number certified.

MILITARY AVIATION—1955

The total strength of the military forces in the United States over the past 50 years has fluctuated widely resulting principally from changes in the international situation and the occurrence of wars. This same thing may be said concerning the aviation components of these forces but up until 1947 the ratio of air strength to surface strength in both the Army and Navy showed a fairly constant and continuous increase. This pattern was interrupted when the Army Air Forces were removed from Army control and reconstituted as the Department of the Air Force by the National Security Act of 1947.

Although this reorganization markedly reduced the air strength of the Army, it did not eliminate it inasmuch as the Army still had a requirement for light aircraft and helicopters as organic equipment in many of its combat and service units. As an example, the Army Medical Service required such aircraft as a part of its field equipment in order to provide aeromedical support for Army troops within the combat zone. By this means, selected cases could be quickly flown from the front lines to their field hospitals or between such hospitals or to a link-up point with the Military Air Transport Service of the Air Force for movement further to the rear.

The total number of aircraft and flying personnel in the Army Reserve forces, the Army National Guard, as well as in the regular Army itself during 1955 is shown in table 4. For these three combined, the totals were: aircraft, 4184; pilots, 6112; and other aircrew members, something in excess of 509.

TABLE 3

United States Certified Civil Aircraft and Airmen, 1935 to 1955

As of 1 January	Number of Civil Aircraft	Certified Airplane Pilots				Other Certified Airmen†	Annual Student Pilot Issuance
		Total	Airline transport	Commercial	Private		
1935	8,322	13,949	676	7,484	5,789	9,013	14,572
1940	13,772	33,706	1,197	11,677	20,832	11,337	110,938
1945	27,919	183,383	3,046	68,449	111,888	41,155	77,188
1950	92,622	525,174	9,025	187,769	328,380	94,219	44,591
1955	92,067	613,695	13,341	201,411	398,913	118,327	44,354

* Source: modified from CAA.

† Includes glider pilots, mechanics, parachute riggers and ground instructors.

In contrast to the Army, the National Security Act of 1947 initially had no effect on Naval Aviation. In 1948, however, the Naval Air Transport Service was merged with the Air Transport Command of the Air Force to form the Military Air Transport Service operated by the Air Force. In that same year, the Joint Chiefs of Staff directed that all military patients of all three services who were to be transported over long distances would be moved routinely by air, unless medically contraindicated, and this responsibility was also assigned to the Air Force.

In 1955 the Navy had 17 carrier air groups, 19 carrier antisubmarine squadrons and 48 other squadrons. The Marine Corps had three air wings to provide tactical air support to its three ground divisions. For that year the number of aircraft, pilots and other aircrew for the various components of the Navy and the Marine Corps is shown in table 4. The totals for these various naval components combined were: aircraft, 15,950; pilots, 28,843; and other aircrew something in excess of 25,933.

When the United States Air Force was established as a separate service in 1947, it had a total active duty military strength of 305,827 personnel and had 38 wings. By 1955 its total personnel strength had increased to 959,946 and its number of wings to 121. At this same time the Air National Guard had 27 and the Air Reserves 24 wings. The number of aircraft and flying personnel for these various components of the Air Force is given in table 4. The totals for these components combined were: aircraft, 26,400; pilots, 64,087; and other aircrew, 52,982.

AVIATION MEDICINE—1955

One index of the work load in aviation medicine during 1955 can be arrived at by determining the total number of flying personnel of all categories for that year.

About 50 per cent of all military pilots also hold concurrent civil pilot ratings so that to arrive at a fairly accurate total of flying personnel in the United States in 1955 from the tabulations in the foregoing paragraphs, we must subtract 49,551 pilots to correct for this duplication. After having made this adjustment, the total number of

TABLE 4

United States Military Aircraft and Airmen, 1955

Service	Aircraft Inventory	Pilots	Other Aircrew
Army	3,539	4,902	509
Army Reserve	0*	400	NA†
Army National Guard	645	810	NA
Navy	9,660	17,507	23,588
Marines	3,161	4,386	2,167
Naval Air Reserve	1,600	6,000	NA
Marine Air Reserve	1,529	950	178
Air Force	23,694	56,847	51,477
Air Force Reserve	763	4,177	1,163
Air National Guard	1,943	3,123	342
Total	46,534	99,102	79,424+

* Regular Army aircraft utilized for training.
† NA = not available.

flying personnel of all categories was approximately 860,997, consisting of 663,246 pilots and 197,751 other aircrew. To this must be added some 85,000 to 90,000 military and civil aviation trainees, an unknown number of applicants who took but failed their physical examinations and those additional aircrew on whom, it will be recalled, strength figures were not available. Thus, the grand total of all known airmen was 950,000 and it is estimated that the actual total was about 1 million. Other responsibilities of aviation medicine for the period being discussed included teaching, research, aeromedical evacuation and a concern for the comfort and safety of the 41 million passengers carried by the commercial airlines.

To accomplish these various tasks the CAA had approximately 1800 designated examiners, the Army 30 flight surgeons, the Navy 297 and the Air Force 814 for a total of 2941. In addition, there were 1507 flight surgeons with the Reserves and National Guard units of the three military services and perhaps another 100 trained flight surgeons with the airlines, aircraft manufacturers and in civil medical institutions for a grand total of 3546.

The United States Navy and the Air Force Schools of Aviation Medicine were the two such schools regularly conducting basic courses in aviation medicine whereas postgraduate training in aviation medicine, of 1 year's duration, was regularly conducted by the Schools of Public Health at Johns Hopkins and at Harvard Universities. In 1947 the CAA established an aeromedical research laboratory in Oklahoma City which was transferred to the campus of Ohio State University at Columbus in 1955 as a first step in an effort to create a civil institute of aviation medicine for teaching and research. During these same years, the Navy and Air Force established a number of additional aeromedical research laboratories and hundreds of research projects were being carried out in civil medical institutions, most of which were supported by military contracts.

The Council on Medical Education and Hospitals of the American Medical Association approved board certification in aviation medicine on 8 February 1953, after an agreement had been reached on an affiliation of the interim board of aviation medicine with the American Board of Preventive Medicine. Under this agreement, the American Board of Preventive Medicine was made up of representatives from these two specialties and issued separate certification to the successful candidates in the two fields. The original requirements for board certification in aviation medicine, announced by this board in 1953, specified the following qualifications as a minimum:

1. Successful completion (after internship) of at least 2 academic years of graduate study in preventive medicine and aviation medicine, 1 year of which graduate study shall be in a school of public health accredited for the purpose of such graduate study by the American Public Health Association and 1 year of which shall be in a school of aviation medicine accredited for the purpose of such graduate study by the Council on Medical Education and Hospitals of the American Medical Association; or training and study deemed by the Board to be substantially equivalent to such graduate study.

2. Residency (after internship) of at least 2 years of supervised experience in aviation medical practice, which includes planned instruction, observation and active participation in a comprehensive, organized program of aviation medicine, 1 year of which may be an approved clinical residency in a field directly related to aviation medicine.

3. A period (after internship) of not less than 2 years, in addition to 1 and 2 above, of special training in or teaching or practice of aviation medicine.

4. Limitation of practice to full time teaching, research or practice of aviation medicine.

5. Regular and frequent participation in aerial flight.

The Aero Medical Association, following World War II, became an international society with a worldwide membership. The Airline Medical Directors Association was organized on 13 May 1944, and included in its membership the medical directors and staff physicians of the world's commercial airlines. The Airline Medical Examiners Association was formed in 1947 by a group of those physicians designated by the Civil Aeronautics Authority to conduct periodic physical examinations of airline pilots. This association later changed its name to the Civil Aviation Medical Association.

The Space Medicine Association was organized in 1951 as a branch of the Aero Medical Association by members of the latter who were especially interested in the problem of flight in the outer fringes of, or beyond, the earth's atmosphere. Even earlier than this, in 1949, a department of space medicine had been established at the Air Force School of Aviation Medicine and the tremendous advances made in this new field of science are described in detail in the last two chapters of this book.

REFERENCES

(1) JEFFRIES, J.: A Narrative of the Two Aerial Voyages of Doctor Jeffries with Mons. Blanchard; with Meterological Observations and Remarks. London, J. Robson, 1786.

(2) GLAISHER, J., ET AL.: Travels in the Air, (2nd Ed) London, Richard Bently and Son, 1871.

(3) TISSANDIER, G.: Le Voyage à Grande Hauteur du Ballon "Le Zenith." Nature, Paris, 3: 337–344, 1875.

(4) BERT, P.: La Pression Barometrique; Recherches de Physiologie Experimentale. Paris, G. Masson et Cie., 1878. (English translation by HITCHCOCK, M. A., AND HITCHCOCK, F. A.: Barometric Pressure. Columbus, Ohio, College Book Co., 1943).

(5) CRUCHET, R., AND MOULINIER, R.: Air Sickness. New York, William Wood and Co., 1920.

(6) SCHNEIDER, E. C.: A cardiovascular rating as a measure of physical fatigue and efficiency. J. A. M. A., 74: 1507–1510, 1920.

(7) ANON: Air Service Medical. Washington, Government Printing Office, 1919.

(8) MAUBLANC, P., AND RATIÉ, V.: Medical Examination of Airmen. New York, William Wood and Co., 1921.

(9) HERLITZKA, A.: Fisiologia ed Aviazione. Bologna, N. Zanichelli, 1923.

(10) BAUER, L. H.: Aviation Medicine. Baltimore, The Williams & Wilkins Co., 1926.

(11) MASHBURN, N. C.: The complex coordinator as a performance test in the selection of military flying personnel. J. Aviation Med., 5: 145–154, 1934.

(12) MASHBURN, N. C.: Mashburn automatic serial action apparatus for detecting flying aptitude. J. Aviation Med., 5: 155–160, 1934.

(13) MYERS, D. A.: The medical contribution to the development of blind flying. The Army Medical Bulletin, War Department, Washington, 36: 18–37, 1936.

(14) ARMSTRONG, II. G.: Principles and Practice of Aviation Medicine. (3rd Ed) Baltimore, Williams & Wilkens Co., 1952.

(15) BENFORD, R. J.: Doctors in the Sky. Springfield, Illinois, Charles C Thomas, 1955.

2

GENERAL PHYSICAL EXAMINATION

Harry G. Armstrong, M.D.

The physical examination for flying is not only one of the major functions of aviation medicine but it is also one of the most important inasmuch as it is based primarily on considerations of safety. The Army, Navy and Air Force each issue regulations governing the conduct of the examinations for their flying personnel whereas the Federal Aviation Agency (FAA) issues instructions concerning the examination of civil airmen. In addition, commercial agencies, such as the airlines, may issue their own regulations which set a higher standard than that required by the FAA.

Within each of the agencies mentioned above, there are different types of examinations for flying personnel depending on several factors. In the Air Force, for example, the applicant for flying training must meet the most rigid standards which are designated Class I. Among trained airmen there are in addition Classes IA, II and III, the latter applying to those not in primary control of the aircraft such as the flight engineer.

It would be quite impractical to describe each of these different examinations in a work of this type but this problem can be solved in a generally satisfactory manner based on the following considerations. The procedures used by all of the different agencies and for all of their various examinations are basically the same. Thus, the dif-

ferences in the examinations are a matter of scope, of standards to be met or both. As a consequence anyone who learns how to perform the examination with the highest standards can accomplish any of the lesser examinations by merely omitting procedures not required and applying the lower standards specified by the regulations of the agency concerned.

Accordingly, the physical examination for flying to be described in this and the four chapters to follow will be patterned after that prescribed for candidates for military flying training in this country. A further discussion having to do specifically with civil flying examinations will be found in Chapter 27.

PRELIMINARY CONSIDERATIONS

In order properly to conduct the examination of a candidate for flying training there are certain important considerations to be borne in mind with reference to space and equipment. With regard to the amount of space required five rooms should be available as an absolute minimum. These should consist of an office; eye examination room; ear, nose and throat room; general physical examination room; and laboratory. These rooms should insure strict privacy, be free from noise and disturbing influences, be well ventilated, have proper artificial lighting and, except for the eye room, should have good natural lighting.

The eye room must be at least 25 feet long and 7 feet wide to accommodate properly the necessary equipment. The doors and windows of this room should be capable of being readily covered to exclude all light. This is difficult to do in the case of outside windows and it is usually preferable to omit windows entirely from the eye room and to provide ventilation indirectly. An especially important feature is that the interior of the room be painted with a coating that will not in any degree reflect light. If this is not done a great deal of confusion will result during certain tests involving the use of the spot light.

The ear, nose and throat room should be adequate in size to accommodate the equipment required in the examination and allow freedom of movement for the examiner and examinee. This room should be soundproofed to give accurate results in hearing tests and also to serve as a place of absolute quiet for the examination of heart and lungs.

The general examining room should be large, well lighted and have a considerable amount of free floor space in addition to the space required for equipment. A toilet immediately adjacent to this room is desirable.

A diagnostic laboratory must be available for carrying out routine procedures and also for any special tests required.

The equipment for the examination of candidates for flying training is rather extensive, should be of good quality and manufactured by a reliable concern. It should be kept clean and in good repair, and those instruments likely to get out of adjustment should be checked frequently for accuracy.

Having made provision for adequate space and equipment the actual examination can be conducted in a most efficient and thorough manner only if certain general principles are kept in mind. The examination is time consuming at best and requires infinite care and patience. The time required, however, can be kept at a minimum if a routine for the examination is worked out so that there is no lost motion and also such that those systems of the body which are most likely to show disqualifying defects are examined first. The exact procedure to be followed will

vary somewhat depending on developments immediately following the examiners first contact with the applicant.

Where possible the examination should be arranged for several days in advance and adequate time allowed for it on the appointed day. The candidate should be instructed to appear in a rested condition after a full night's sleep. If no opportunity to contact the examinee prior to the actual time of the examination has occurred this question should be determined at once. If the candidate has lost sleep, traveled a long distance in the preceding 18 hours or is fatigued for any reason he should be told to rest for 24 hours and present himself again for examination. If he is found free from fatigue he should then be questioned concerning the presence or absence of any acute infectious conditions. The presence of any such infection or a history of a recent operation or illness from which the candidate has not had time fully to recover should cause him to be examined at a later date.

Assuming that the candidate is free from all of the conditions mentioned above the next step is to make a rapid informal general inspection of the individual to determine if possible whether or not he has any manifest condition which probably will be found disqualifying. For example, an examinee who enters the examination room with a noticeable limp should have that condition investigated immediately to determine its cause. Likewise, overweight or underweight individuals, those with manifest squint or with other similar obvious defects should have those conditions checked at once, and if disqualifying there is no need for the examination to continue. Thus, a great deal of time and useless effort can be saved for everyone concerned.

In the absence of obvious defects in a candidate the next step is to secure a detailed medical history which may lead directly to the discovery of disqualifying defects. When the actual examination is begun it is advisable to adopt a procedure which will allow those systems of the body most likely to disclose defects to be done first. In order to accomplish this the following sequence is suggested: eye (except refraction and ophthalmoscopic examination);

cardiovascular system; ear, nose and throat; general physical; neurologic; refraction and ophthalmoscopic examination of the eye; and personality study.

The reader is not to gain the impression that the sole purpose of the examiner is to disqualify the examinee. On the contrary, it is to the interest of all concerned to qualify every candidate who can meet the requirements and every effort should be made to attain this objective. However, it seems obvious that nothing is to be gained by postponing the search for likely disqualifying defects, and to do so only consumes needless time and effort for both the examiner and examinee without accomplishing any useful purpose.

As stated above the detection of a disqualifying defect is normally sufficient to terminate the examination but there is an important exception to this general rule. If a disqualifying defect is found which is of a temporary or remedial nature the examination should always be completed or carried on until a permanently disqualifying defect is found. If this is not done a candidate may spend considerable time and money having his defect corrected only to learn, upon reexamination, that he has other disqualifying defects.

Having adopted an examination procedure which is both efficient and timesaving it is to be remembered that this alone is not sufficient to assure accurate results. In the examination of candidates for flying training there are certain considerations which must be observed if their rights and interests are to be properly guarded. As mentioned above the examinee should not be allowed to appear for the examination in a fatigued state or when suffering from an illness or when he has not had time to fully recover from a previous illness. Of extreme importance is the initial meeting between the examiner and the candidate. The latter usually appears for examination with a good deal of misgiving. He normally is worried about the tests which he believes are unduly severe and is concerned as to his success or failure. The first duty of the examiner then is to gain the confidence of the candidate. No examination should ever be begun until an informal talk has been had and the examinee put at ease

insofar as that is possible. This can best be accomplished by demonstrating an interest in him as an individual and in his success. The assurance that the examination is not strenuous but simply thorough and that the object of the examination is to pass him if possible and not fail him will in most cases change a tense individual into one who is more nearly his normal self.

Through the examination there should be an air of unhurried calm and there must never be any evidence of impatience on the part of the examiner. A casual conversation carried on throughout the course of the examination will do much to maintain a friendly attitude and divert the mind of the applicant from himself. This will also serve as a valuable means of gaining an insight into the personality of the individual. The rooms should be quiet and strict privacy prevail. When it becomes necessary for the candidate to undress care should be exercised that he does not become chilled and, in any event, the period of exposure should be as short as is consistent with a thorough examination.

In candidates where borderline findings are noted or conditions are encountered whose significance is not fully understood these should be given careful study until a definite decision can be reached. This is important for two reasons. First, if the condition is in fact not disqualifying it is an injustice to the candidate to reject him and thus bar him from his chosen occupation. On the other hand, if a disqualifying defect is overlooked by carelessness of the examiner, by subterfuge on the part of the examinee, or if a favorable decision is rendered upon insufficient information, a whole series of most unfortunate events may ensue.

All examiners should realize that, just as in a serious illness, the life of the examinee may depend on a careful, thorough examination. Most of the standards for flying are based on considerations of safety and a pilot who is allowed to train or fly with a disqualifying defect is usually an undue hazard to himself, to others and to property. There is yet another reason why all defects should be detected on the original examination in all fairness to the candidate. This is that any disqualifying defect will be detected on subsequent examinations and, if serious enough to cause the flyer to be grounded, will work an untold hardship on him. It means that the time and money which he has spent during training has been wasted and, in addition, he has been prevented during that time from pursuing another occupation. It should be remembered that to reject a man on an original examination is only a disappointment but that the grounding of a flyer after he has been trained is a calamity. To avoid the difficulties mentioned above it should be a fixed rule in all doubtful cases to re-examine the candidate on several different occasions and to use every possible diagnostic procedure to reach a definite decision.

Having taken every precaution to protect the interests of the examinee it is also necessary that the examiner be prepared to protect his own interests and the interests of those to whom he is responsible. In rejecting an applicant for flying training it is to be remembered that the reasons for rejecting him must be capable of being adequately substantiated and defended not only to the satisfaction of the candidate himself but also for the benefit of anyone else who may be interested. For this reason alone it is necessary that the examiner keep an open-minded attitude at all times. Clashes of personality, it should be remembered, may be the fault of the examiner as well as that of the examinee. Especially to be avoided is the utilization of insignificant pet aversions as an over-all yardstick in the estimation of an applicant's personality or flying adaptability.

Whereas the great majority of candidates for flying training are inherently honest there are a sufficient number who are not to make this a formidable problem and it is necessary to use every precaution in all cases in order not to be deceived. Whenever possible the examination should be conducted by objective methods. In cases where the subjective method is the only means available questions should always be of the affirmative and never of the negative type. Thus, ask "how often do you have headaches?" Not, "do you ever have headaches?" During the personality study, it is difficult to check up on statements of the applicant concerning his past experiences and candidates are more apt to give an answer that they believe is favorable rather than one that is correct.

Finally, before proceeding with the actual examination, a careful past medical history must be obtained. The securing of this history differs in no way from the methods in use in general clinical practice but there are certain conditions which are of special importance in aviation. Among the more important of those to be specifically inquired about are:

Malaria
Uncinariasis
Tuberculosis
Deficiency diseases
Rheumatic fever
Cellulitis and osteomyelitis
Malignant diseases
Scarlet fever
Hemophilia and purpura
Leukemia
Pernicious anemia
Diabetes
Endocrine disturbances
Chronic metallic poisoning
Syphilis
Hay fever
Asthma
Epilepsy
Actinomycosis
Leprosy
Aplastic anemia
Hemolytic icteroanemia (hemolytic jaundice)
Splenic anemia
Polycythemia vera
Sickle cell anemia
Motion sickness

All of the above conditions should be considered disqualifying except as follows:

An isolated instance of motion sickness without emotional involvement may be considered qualifying. In the case of a history of malaria, it may be considered qualifying provided there have been no symptoms for at least 6 months during which time no antimalarial drugs have been taken, the red cells are normal in number and structure, the blood hemoglobin is at least 12 grams and a thick smear is negative for parasites. A candidate may be qualified with a history of syphilis if documentary proof is available that the individual concerned has been clinically cured with no evidence of recurrence for a period of 2 years subsequent to treatment, careful examination shows no evidence of syphilitic lesions and examination of the spinal fluid shows a negative serologic test for syphilis, and the cell count and protein content are within normal limits.

Having given due consideration to proper space and equipment, the candidate's general health and condition, the interests of the candidate and examiner and having obtained a good medical history of the applicant the examiner is now prepared to begin the actual physical examination itself. Throughout the examination the various systems of the body will be dealt with under four headings as follows:

1. *Underlying principles:* (a) Concerning the relationship between flying and the system of the body being examined. Certain bodily attributes and conditions may be of vital importance in aviation even though they have no adverse effect on health or are unimportant in other occupations. Where this exists it will be pointed out; and (b) concerning the technical procedures utilized in the examination.

2. *Procedure to be followed:* Technical procedures not normally used in general practice will be described in some detail. Ordinary procedures will not be described except as necessary to insure uniformity of findings among different examiners. Where an examiner cannot reach a firm decision in a case, outside laboratory or clinical consultant aid should be utilized and, if necessary, the examinee hospitalized for a few days observation.

3. *Special precautions:* Will list those omissions or errors which have been found to be the most common cause of unsatisfactory results in conducting the examination.

4. *Interpretation of results:* Will list those conditions which should be considered disqualifying for candidates for flying training who aspire to qualify as an airline or military pilot.

The General Physical Examination

UNDERLYING PRINCIPLES. The structural systems of the body must be intact and all joints have a complete range of normal motion. To determine this the candidate should be examined in a well lighted room with all of his clothing removed. This part of the examination is a good illustration of the fact that considerations other than flying

per se must be taken into account. The limitations on height, for example, are related to the limited space available in most high performance aircraft cockpits whereas structural defects of the body are disqualifying in part, because of the fact that they interfere with the wearing of flying equipment.

The limitation on the age of candidates is generally an administrative matter and trainees are usually limited to those between the ages of 19 and 29.

Height

The height of candidates for flying training in high performance aircraft is important because of the fact that the cockpits of such aircraft are usually designed to accommodate only average sized individuals. The extremely tall individual is not only cramped for head and leg room but the controls are improperly placed for his hands. The short individual has difficulty reaching the rudder bar, the controls are placed too far away for convenience and, if he is of slight build, he has difficulty managing a heavy airplane.

Candidates who are 72 or more inches tall should also have their sitting height measured inasmuch as certain "long waisted" individuals will not have adequate head clearance under the cockpit canopy even though they are within the standing height limits.

Weight

Underweight candidates should not only be considered from the viewpoint of their ability to manage a heavy airplane but also from the standpoint of general health. Obesity should also be regarded as possibly leading eventually to health complications. It may interfere with normal activity as well as cause crowding in the cockpit and thus interfere with control of the aircraft.

Height-Weight Measurements

The height should be determined by means of a measuring rod with the candidate's shoes removed and the weight should be determined on a beam type scale of known accuracy with the candidate completely stripped.

The sitting height should be measured with the candidate seated with his back

TABLE 5

Weight Table*

Height in Inches	18 to 20			21 to 25			26 to 30†			31 to 35		36 to 40		41 and Over	
	Mini-mum	Stand-ard	Maxi-mum	Mini-mum	Stand-ard	Maxi-mum	Mini-mum	Stand-ard	Maxi-mum	Stand-ard	Maxi-mum	Stan-dard	Maxi-mum	Stand-ard	Maxi-mum
60	105	117	146	108	120	150	110	122	153	125	157	128	160	131	164
61	107	119	149	110	122	153	112	124	155	127	159	130	163	133	166
62	109	121	151	112	124	155	113	126	158	129	161	132	165	135	169
63	111	124	155	113	126	158	115	128	160	131	164	134	168	137	171
64‡	113	127	159	115	128	160	118	131	164	134	168	137	171	140	175
65	115	130	163	119	132	165	121	135	169	138	173	141	176	144	180
66	117	133	166	122	136	170	125	139	174	142	178	145	181	148	185
67	121	137	171	126	140	175	129	143	179	146	183	149	186	152	190
68	125	141	176	130	144	180	132	147	184	150	188	153	191	156	195
69	129	145	181	133	148	185	136	151	189	154	193	157	196	160	200
70	133	149	186	137	152	190	139	155	194	158	198	161	201	164	205
71	137	153	191	140	156	195	143	159	199	162	203	165	206	168	210
72	141	157	196	145	161	201	148	164	205	167	209	170	213	173	216
73	145	161	201	149	166	208	152	169	211	172	215	175	219	178	223
74	149	165	206	154	171	214	157	174	218	177	221	180	225	183	229
75	153	169	211	158	176	220	161	179	224	182	228	185	231	188	235
76	157	173	216	163	181	226	166	184	230	187	234	190	238	193	241

* Source: modified from Air Force Manual 160-1 (3).

† The standard weight for each height for the age group 26 to 30 is the ideal one to be maintained thereafter. For age groups after this the minimum allowance should be that for the age group 26 to 30.

‡ Minimum height for mature adults.

against a wall and his thighs exactly parallel with the floor. The distance to be measured is from the seat to a measuring rod, which is also exactly parallel with the floor, that is on a level with the top of the candidate's head.

INTERPRETATION OF FINDINGS. Applicants should conform to the standards shown in table 5. A height of less than 64 inches (in the mature individual) or more than 76 inches should disqualify as well as a weight below or above those indicated in the table. For younger candidates allowance may be made as to the minimum height and weight for anticipated growth. A sitting height of over 38 inches should disqualify.

Bones, Joints and Muscles

PROCEDURE. The applicant should be put through a series of movements, described below, which will bring into action the various joints and muscles of the body. This purpose is best accomplished by requiring the applicant to follow the movements as made by the examiner or an assistant.

Extend and flex each finger separately;

bring the tips of the thumbs to the base of the little fingers; close the hands, with the thumbs covering the fingers; extend and flex the hands on the wrists; rotate the hands so that the fingernails will first be up and then down; move the hands from side to side. Extend the arms and forearms fully to the front and rotate them at the shoulders; flex the forearms on the arms sharply, striking the shoulders with the fists. Extend the arms at right angles to the body; place the thumbs on the points of the shoulders; raise and lower the arms, bringing them sharply to the sides at each motion. Swing the right arm in a circle rapidly from the shoulder, first to the front and then to the rear; swing the left arm in the same manner.

Extend one leg, lifting the heel from the floor, and move all the toes freely; move the foot up and down and from side to side, bending the ankle joint, the knee being kept rigid; bend the knee freely; kick forcibly backward and forward; throw the leg out to the side as far as possible, keeping the body squarely to the front; repeat all these movements with the other foot and leg; strike the breast first with one knee and then with the other; stand upon the toes of both feet; squat sharply several times; kneel upon both knees at the same time (if the man comes down on one knee after the other there is reason to suspect infirmity).

Have the examinee stand erect, present his back to the examiner, and then hold up to view the sole of each foot; leap directly up, striking the buttocks with both heels at the same time; hop the length of the room on the ball of first one foot and then the other; make a standing jump as far as possible and repeat it several times; run the length of the room several times.

INTERPRETATION OF FINDINGS. Although the exercises prescribed may cause some breathlessness and accelerated throbbing of the blood vessels they should not cause manifest exhaustion or great distress in a healthy man. Lack of ability to perform any of these exercises indicates some defect or deformity that should be investigated further.

The following conditions should disqualify:

1. Any deformity which prevents the proper functioning of any part to a degree interfering with normal efficiency.
2. Inability to perform any of the above exercises as the result of causes listed under the section entitled "Extremities" at the end of this chapter.
3. Evidences of physical characteristics of congenital asthenia. The physical characteristics of congenital asthenia are slender bones, a weak, ill developed thorax, nephroptosis, gastroptosis, constipation, the "drop" heart, with its peculiar attenuation, and weak and easily fatigued musculature.

Skin

PROCEDURE. The skin will be inspected for eruptions and for signs of anemia, jaundice and other symptoms of disease, for hypodermic and other scars and for pediculi. As a general rule, applicants extensively infested with vermin and filthy in person and clothing should be rejected as probably being unsuited by reason of habits, character or mental deficiency.

INTERPRETATION OF FINDINGS. The following conditions should disqualify:

1. Eczema of long standing or rebellious to treatment.
2. Chronic impetigo, pemphigus, lupus or sycosis.
3. Actinomycosis, dermatitis herpetiformis or mycosis fungoides.
4. Extensive psoriasis or ichthyosis.
5. Acne upon face or neck which is so pronounced as to amount to positive deformity.
6. Elephantiasis.
7. Pediculosis or scabies.
8. Carbuncle.
9. Ulcerations of the skin not amenable to treatment, those of long standing or of considerable extent or of syphilitic or malignant origin.
10. Extensive, deep or adherent scars that interfere with muscular movements, with the wearing of equipment or that show a tendency to break down and ulcerate.
11. Naevi and other erectile tumors if extensive, disfiguring or exposed to constant pressure.
12. Chronic trichophytosis or other chronic fungous infections which have not been amenable to treatment.
13. Chronic urticaria or chronic angioneurotic edema.
14. Exfoliating dermatitis; severe chronic seborrheic dermatitis.
15. Chronic lichen planus; dermatitis factitia; scleroderma.
16. Pilonidal cyst, if evidenced by the presence of a tumor mass or a discharging sinus or if there is a history of inflammation or discharging sinus.
17. Filariasis; trypanosomiasis; schistosomiasis.

Head

PROCEDURE. The head will be carefully inspected for stigmata of degeneration. The scalp will be examined for pediculi. Every portion of the cranium will be palpated for evidence of former injury, depression from any cause and for other deformity.

INTERPRETATION OF FINDINGS. The following conditions should disqualify:

1. Tinea in any form.
2. All tumors which are of sufficient size to interfere with the wearing of headgear.

3. Imperfect ossification of the cranial bones or persistence of the anterior fontanelles.

4. Extensive cicatrices, especially adherent scars that show a tendency to break down and ulcerate.

5. Depressed fractures or depressions or loss of bony substance of the skull, unless the defect is slight and will cause no future trouble.

6. Monstrosity of the head, hydrocephalus or microcephalus.

7. Hernia of the brain.

8. Deformities of the skull of any degree associated with evidence of disease of the brain, spinal cord or peripheral nerves.

Face

PROCEDURE. The face will be examined by inspection and, if necessary, by palpation.

INTERPRETATION OF FINDINGS. The following conditions should disqualify:

1. Unsightly deformities, such as large birthmarks, large hairy moles, extensive cicatrices, mutilations caused by injuries or surgical operations, tumors, ulcerations, fistulas, atrophy of a part of the face or lack of symmetrical development.

2. Persistent neuralgia, tic doloreux or paralyses of central nervous origin.

3. Loss of the nose, malformation or deformities thereof that interfere with speech or breathing; extensive ulcerations.

4. Ununited fractures of the maxillary bones, deformities of either maxillary bone interfering with mastication or speech, extensive exostosis, caries, necrosis or osseous cysts.

5. Chronic arthritis of the temporomaxillary articulation, badly reduced or recurrent dislocations of this joint or ankylosis, complete or partial.

Mouth, Larynx, Trachea and Esophagus

PROCEDURE. These parts will be examined by inspection and palpation. When considered necessary roentgenograms will be made.

INTERPRETATION OF FINDINGS. The following conditions should disqualify:

1. Harelip, loss of the whole or a large part of either lip, unsightly mutilations of the lips from wounds, burns or disease.

2. Malformation, partial loss, atrophy or hypertrophy of the tongue, split or bifid tongue or adhesions of the tongue to the sides of the mouth, provided these conditions interfere with mastication, speech or swallowing or appear to be progressive.

3. Malignant tumors of the tongue or benign tumors that interfere with its functions.

4. Marked stomatitis, ulcerations or severe leukoplakia.

5. Ranula if at all extensive or salivary fistula.

6. Perforation or extensive loss of substance or ulceration of the hard or soft palate, extensive adhesions of the soft palate to the pharynx or paralysis of the soft palate.

7. Chronic laryngitis from any cause.

8. Paralysis of the vocal cords or aphonia.

9. Tracheostomy, until 3 months have elapsed without sequelae.

10. Stricture or pronounced dilation of the esophagus.

11. Recurrent calculi of salivary glands or ducts.

12. Loss of taste and/or paresthesias.

13. Any lesion of the nasopharynx causing nasal obstruction.

14. Adenoids which encroach upon the torus of the Eustachian tube or obstruct the nasal airways.

15. Any congenital or acquired lesion of the nasopharynx or Eustachian tubes which interfere with the functions of these structures.

16. History of recurrent hoarseness or laryngeal pain.

17. History of recurrent aphonia or a single attack if the cause was such as to make subsequent attacks possible.

18. History of tracheotomy caused by tuberculosis, angioneurotic edema or tumor.

19. Any surgical procedure until recovery is complete and the part is functionally normal.

20. Any infectious lesion until recovery is complete and the part is functionally normal.

21. Any acquired or congenital lesion which interferes with the function of the larynx.

Teeth

The teeth and related structures should be examined by a dentist in accordance with the procedures presented in detail in Chapter 24 which also lists the findings which should be considered as disqualifying.

Neck

PROCEDURE. The neck will be examined by inspection and palpation. Cervical adenitis must be given careful consideration with a view to determining its cause. The presence of adenitis should always be borne in mind as a possible symptom of syphilis.

INTERPRETATION OF FINDINGS. The following conditions should disqualify:

1. Cervical adenitis of other than benign origin, including cancer, Hodgkin's disease, leukemia, tuberculosis, syphilis etc.

2. Adherent and disfiguring scars from disease, injuries or burns.

3. Extensive or progressive goiter interfering with breathing or with the wearing of clothing.

4. Exophthalmic goiter or myxedema.

5. Thyroid enlargement from any cause associated with toxic symptoms.

6. Benign tumors or cysts which are so large as to interfere with the wearing of equipment.

7. Torticollis; cervical rib.

8. Congenital cysts of branchial cleft origin or those developing from the remains of a thyroglossal duct, with or without fistulous tracts.

Spine

PROCEDURE. The spine should be examined by inspection and palpation. The mobility should be observed while the applicant is performing exercises. When necessary, roentgenograms should be made.

INTERPRETATION OF FINDINGS. The following conditions should disqualify:

1. Lateral deviation of the spine from the normal midline of more than 1 inch (scoliosis).

2. Curvature of the spine of any degree in which function is interfered with or in which there is noticeable deformity when the applicant is dressed (scoliosis, kyphosis or lordosis).

3. Fractures or dislocations of the vertebrae.

4. Vertebral caries (Plott's disease).

5. Abscess of the spinal column or its vicinity.

6. Osteoarthritis of the spinal column, partial or complete.

7. Fracture of the coccyx.

8. Spondylolisthesis, herniated nucleus pulposus or history of operation.

9. A history of disabling episode of back pain, especially when associated with significant objective findings.

Chest and Lungs

UNDERLYING PRINCIPLES. The chest contains the vital organs of circulation and respiration; it is, therefore, essential that it be well developed and justly proportioned to the other body measurements. Any marked deviation in form, either a flattening of the chest or more especially a persistence of the round or infantile type, is an element of weakness. Abnormal development, such as pigeon breast, funnel chest or rachitic chest, is also to be regarded with suspicion as such conditions usually coincide with a somewhat enfeebled constitution and a predisposition to disease of the lungs. Hence, any anomaly in the shape of the chest must be given careful consideration, especially in connection with the results found in the examination of the contained organs and of other parts of the body.

PROCEDURE. The lungs should be examined by inspection, palpation, percussion and auscultation of the chest. A roentgenogram of the lungs should be made on all candidates routinely. In the inspection and interrogation of applicants the following points should lead to a suspicion of pulmonary tuberculosis: apparent undue prominence of the clavicle on one side, caused by a deepening of the hollow above and a flattening of the space beneath; a wasting of the muscles of the shoulder girdle on one side, as evidenced by apparent excessive prominence of the shoulder and scapula; and a history of recent loss of weight, especially if associated with long and severe cough and night sweats. In suspected cases observation, with complete record of temperature, pulse and respiration, may be of assistance. As pleurisy, with or without effusion, is a very frequent indication of early tuberculosis, examiners should examine with the greatest care applicants who have apparently recovered from this disease. Distinction must be made between active and inactive pulmonary tuberculosis. In this connection conservatism must be exercised in the interpretation of physical signs over the apices of the lungs.

Each applicant should be required to exhale his breath, cough and immediately breathe in. The chest should be auscultated during this process. All men who show moist sounds during cough or during respiration should be classed as doubtful cases. All cases should be also classed as doubtful in which there is well marked dullness on percussion, well marked increased transmission of voice, harsh respiration and well marked prolonged expiration, even though there be no rales present. Men underweight or with sunken or deformed chests should be considered with special care, and if the conditions are marked should be classed as doubtful, even though definite signs of tuberculosis are not detected. Doubtful cases, even in the absence of a positive diagnosis, should normally be rejected.

PRECAUTIONS. The following signs should not be regarded as evidence of pulmonary disease in the absence of other signs in the same portion of the lungs:

1. Slightly harsh breathing or slightly prolonged expiration over the right apex above the clavicle anteriorly and the third dorsal vertebra posteriorly. The same signs at the extreme apex on the left side.

2. Same signs in second interspace, right, anteriorly near sternum (proximity of right main bronchus).

3. Increased vocal resonance or slightly harsh breathing immediately below center of left clavicle.

4. Fine crepitations over sternum heard when stethoscope touches the edge of that bone.

5. Clicks heard during strong respiration or after cough in the vicinity of the sternocostal articulations.

6. The so-called atelectatic rales at the apex during the first inspiration which follows a deeper breath than usual or a cough.

7. Sounds resembling rales at base of lung (marginal sounds), especially marked in right axilla, limited to inspiration.

8. Similar sounds heard at apex of heart on cough (lingula).

9. Slightly prolonged expiration at left base posteriorly.

10. Very slight harshness of respiratory sounds with prolonged expiration in the lower paravertebral regions of both lungs posteriorly, most marked at the angle of the scapula, disappearing a short distance above that point, equal on both sides or slightly more marked at the angle on one side, more frequently the left.

INTERPRETATION OF FINDINGS. The following conditions should disqualify:

1. A history of clinical tuberculosis which exceeds minimal extent; tuberculosis of minimal extent clinically active within the preceding 5 years; known tuberculous pleurisy with effusion and pleurisy with effusion of unknown origin within the preceding 5 years.

2. Active tuberculosis, including pleurisy with effusion which is to be considered of tuberculous origin if no other cause can be proved.

3. Reinfection type of pulmonary tuberculosis of any degree.

4. Inactive pulmonary tuberculosis except: scarred fibroid or fibrocalcific tuberculous lesions of the lungs not associated with symptoms of clinical activity within the preceding 5 years and represented in roentgenograms as a sharply demarcated, strandlike or small, well defined, nodular shadow not exceeding a total area of 4 sq. cm., after serial observation of roentgenograms has demonstrated stability for a period of not less than 1 year; residual calcified lesions of primary tuberculosis in the pulmonary parenchyma or hilum lymph nodes, provided the size, number and character of such lesions suggest that the possibility of reactivation is unlikely.

5. Spontaneous pneumothorax, history of spontaneous pneumothorax, within the last 3 years or history of repeated spontaneous pneumothorax.

6. Empyema; residual sacculation or unhealed sinuses of the chest wall following operations for empyema.

7. Chronic bronchitis if more than mild or if mild and does not respond to therapy or the cessation of smoking.

8. Bronchiectasis.

9. Asthma of any degree or a history of asthma, except a history of childhood asthma with a trustworthy history of freedom from symptoms since the 12th birthday.

10. Bullous or generalized pulmonary emphysema.

11. Cystic disease of the lung.

12. Silicosis, as represented in the roentgenogram by strandlike and nodular shadows; other forms of severe pulmonary fibrosis including sarcoidosis.

13. Abscess of the lung.

14. Coccidioidomycosis, unless healed with no evidence of cavitation or other residuals.

15. Foreign body in the lung, exceeding 1 cm. in diameter or any foreign body with evidence of surrounding pulmonary reaction; foreign body in a bronchus.

16. Chronic adhesive pleuritis of such extent as to interfere with respiratory function or obscure a lung field in roentgenograms.

17. History of pneumonectomy or lobectomy for any cause.

18. Atypical or other type of pneumonia until a final physical examination shows recovery without disqualifying sequelae.

19. Tumor, benign or malignant, of the trachea, bronchi, lungs, pleura or mediastinum.

20. Congenital malformations or acquired deformities which result in reducing the chest capacity and diminishing the cardiac or respiratory functions to such degree as to interfere with vigorous physical exertion or that produce disfigurement when the applicant is dressed.

21. Pronounced contraction of the chest wall following pleurisy or empyema.

22. Deformities of the chest or scapulae sufficient to interfere with the wearing of flying equipment.

23. Absence or faulty development of the clavicle.

24. Old fracture of the clavicle, if there is much deformity or interference with the wearing of flying equipment; ununited fractures; or partial or complete dislocation of either end of the clavicle.

25. Suppurative periostitis, osteomyelitis, caries or necrosis of the ribs, sternum, clavicles, scapulae, vertebrae or other bones.

26. Old fractures of the ribs with faulty union, which interfere with function.

27. Malignant tumors of the breast or chest wall and benign tumors which interfere with the wearing of equipment.

28. Unhealed sinuses of the chest wall.

29. Scars of old operations for empyema, unless the examiner is assured that the respiratory function is entirely normal.

Endocrine System

INTERPRETATION OF FINDINGS. The following conditions should be considered disqualifying: diabetes mellitus or insipidus; renal glycosuria; acromegaly; gigantism; myxedema; cretinism; Addison's disease; and Simmond's disease.

Abdomen and Viscera

PROCEDURE. The abdomen should be examined by inspection, palpation and percussion. When indicated, roentgen ray examinations and laboratory tests should be made. Examination for inguinal, femoral and ventral hernia should be made by both inspection and palpation.

Applicants who are from regions in which uncinariasis or malaria is prevalent and who present symptoms of anemia or enlargement of the spleen should be placed under observation for these diseases (examination of feces and blood). This applies also to the dysenteries, especially the entamebic form.

INTERPRETATION OF FINDINGS. The following conditions should disqualify:

1. Wounds, injuries, cicatrices or muscular ruptures of the abdominal walls sufficient to interfere with function.

2. Fistulas from visceral or bony lesions or following operation.

3. Hernia of any variety other than small umbilical.

4. Tumors of the abdominal walls.

5. Scar pain.

6. Chronic diseases of the stomach and intestines.

7. History of gastroenterostomy, gastric resection, resection of peptic ulcer, partial resection of the intestines or operation for relief of intestinal adhesions.

8. Blood in the feces unless shown to be the result of unimportant causes.

9. Ptosis of the stomach or intestines.

10. Chronic appendicitis.

11. Chronic diseases of the liver, gall bladder, pancreas or spleen.

12. Chronic peritonitis or peritoneal adhesions.

13. Chronic enlargement of the liver.

14. Chronic enlargement of the spleen or history of splenectomy for reason other than trauma.

15. Jaundice.

16. Marked engorgement of superficial abdominal vessels.

17. Uncinariasis.

Pelvis and Rectum

PROCEDURE. The pelvis should be examined by inspection and if necessary by palpation. To inspect the anal region the applicant is directed to bend forward from the hips and to draw apart the buttocks with both hands. Digital examination of the rectum and proctoscopy should be used if necessary.

INTERPRETATION OF FINDINGS. The following conditions should disqualify:

1. Malformation and deformities of the pelvis sufficient to interfere with function.

2. Disease of the sacro-iliac or lumbo-sacral joints.

3. Urinary fistula.

4. Stricture or prolapse of the rectum.

5. Fistula *in ano* or ischiorectal abscess.

6. Fissure of the anus or pruritis ani.

7. External hemorrhoids sufficient in size to produce symptoms. Internal hemorrhoids, if large, if they hemorrhage or if they protrude intermittently or constantly.

Genitourinary System

PROCEDURE. The genitourinary organs should be examined by inspection and palpation. Evidence of venereal disease or malformation should be searched for. The glans penis and corona should be exposed and the penis stripped. Both sides of the scrotum should be palpated, as should also the inguinal glands. When necessary, further examination by the roentgen ray, by urethral instrumentation and by laboratory methods should be conducted.

Urinalysis, including tests for albumin, specific gravity and sugar and a microscopic examination of the sediment should be made in the case of all candidates, the urine being voided in the presence of one of the examiners.

The term "albuminuria" should not ordinarily be used as a cause for rejection, nor does its presence alone justify a diagnosis of nephritis. When albumin or casts are found in the urine the applicant should be retained under observation and daily complete examinations of the urine made for at least 5 days, unless the presence of albumin and casts is associated with enlargement of the left heart, high blood pressure or other evidence of cardiovascular disturbance to such a degree that a diagnosis of chronic nephritis may be made immediately. When albumin is constantly or intermittently present the underlying pathologic conditions should be determined and stated as the cause for rejection, but if albuminuria is present daily during a period of 6 days it should be regarded as reason for rejection, even if the origin cannot be determined.

When the specific gravity of the specimen first examined is abnormally low further observation of the applicant and repeated complete urinary examinations are indicated.

If glucose if found in the urine at the first examination, further observation is indicated, including an estimation of the 24-hour amount of urine and the employment of more than one test to demonstrate the possible existence of diabetes. When considered necessary blood sugar estimations should also be made.

The Wassermann test should be required on all candidates. Whenever a double plus reaction is obtained another specimen should be examined after a lapse of 2 weeks.

INTERPRETATION OF FINDINGS. The following conditions should disqualify:

1. Acute or chronic nephritis, and diabetes mellitus or insipidus.

2. Blood, pus or albumin in the urine, if persistent.

3. Floating kidney, hydronephrosis, pyronephrosis, pyelitis, tumors of the kidney or absence of one kidney.

4. Acute or chronic cystitis.

5. Vesical calculi, tumors of the bladder, incontinence of urine, enuresis or retention of urine.

6. Hypertrophy or abscess of the prostate gland or chronic prostatitis.

7. Varicocele, if large and painful, or hydrocele if large.

8. Pronounced atrophy of both testicles or loss of both.

9. Undescended testicle when the organ is in the inguinal canal or when outside the

canal and lying against the pubic bone; infantile genital organs.

10. Chronic orchitis or epididymitis.

11. Syphilis in any stage.

12. Gonoccocus infections, acute or chronic (including gonorrheal arthritis), chancroids or buboes.

13. A substantiated history of bilateral renal calculi or of repeated attacks of renal or ureteral colic. Examinees with a history of one attack are acceptable, provided the calculus has passed and the roentgenogram shows no evidence of concretion in the kidneys, ureter or bladder, the excretory urography reveals no congenital or acquired anomaly and the renal function is normal.

EXTREMITIES

PROCEDURE. The extremities will be carefully examined for deformities, old fractures and dislocations, amputations, partially flexed or ankylosed joints, impaired functions of any degree, varicose veins and edema. The feet will be especially examined for flat foot, corns, ingrowing nails, bunions, deformed or missing toes, hyperidrosis, bromidrosis and clubfoot. When any degree of flat foot is found, the strength of the feet should be ascertained by requiring the applicant to hop on the toes of each foot for a number of times and by requiring him to alight on the toes while jumping up and down with both feet.

INTERPRETATION OF FINDINGS. The following conditions should disqualify:

1. All anomalies in the number, the form, the proportion and the movements of the extremities which produce noticeable deformity or interfere with function.

2. Atrophy of the muscles of any part, if progressive or if sufficient to interfere with function.

3. Benign tumors if sufficiently large to interfere with function.

4. Ununited fractures, fractures with shortening or callous formation sufficient to interfere with function, old dislocations unreduced or partially reduced, complete or partial ankylosis of a joint or relaxed articular ligaments permitting of frequent voluntary or involuntary displacement.

5. Reduced dislocations or united fractures with incomplete restoration of function.

6. Resection of a joint or amputation of any portion of a limb, except fingers or toes as specified below.

7. Excessive curvature of a long bone or extensive, deep or adherent scars interfering with motion.

8. Severe sprains.

9. Diseases of the bones or joints.

10. Chronic synovitis, or floating cartilage or other internal derangement in a joint.

11. Varicose veins in an extremity when they cover a large area or are markedly tortuous or much dilated or are associated with edema, varicocele or hemorrhoids, or are accompanied by subjective symptoms.

12. Varices of any kind situated in the leg below the knee if associated with varicose ulcers or scars from old ulcerations.

13. Chronic edema of a limb.

14. Chronic and obstinate neuralgias, particularly sciatica.

15. Deviation of the normal axis of the forearm to such a degree as to interfere with the proper execution of the prescribed exercise.

16. Adherent or united fingers (web fingers).

17. Permanent flexion or extension of one or more fingers as well as irremediable loss of motion of these parts.

18. Total loss of either thumb.

19. Mutilation of either thumb to such an extent as to produce material loss of flexion or strength of the member.

20. Loss of more than one phalanx of the right index finger.

21. Loss of the terminal and middle phalanges of any two fingers on the same hand.

22. Entire loss of any finger except the little finger of either hand or the ring finger of left hand.

23. Perceptible lameness or limping.

24. Knock-knee when the gait is clumsy or ungainly or when subjective symptoms of weakness are present.

25. Bowlegs if so marked as to produce noticeable deformity when the applicant is dressed.

26. Clubfoot unless the defect is so slight as to produce no symptoms during vigorous exercise.

27. Pes cavus if extreme and causing symptoms.

28. Flat foot when accompanied with symptoms of weak foot or when the foot is weak on test. Pronounced cases of flat foot attended with decided eversion of the foot and marked bulging of the inner border, resulting from inward rotation of the astragalus, should disqualify regardless of the presence or absence of subjective symptoms.

29. Loss of either great toe or loss of any two toes on the same foot.

30. Webbing of all the toes.

31. Over-riding or superposition of any of the toes to such a degree as will produce pain when wearing the shoe.

32. Ingrowing toe nails when marked or painful.

33. Hallux valgus when sufficiently marked to interfere with locomotion or when accompanied with a painful bunion.

34. Bunions sufficiently pronounced to interfere with function.

35. Hammer toes when existing to such a degree as to interfere with function when wearing the shoe.

36. Corns or callous on the sole of the foot when they are tender or painful.

37. Hyperidrosis when present to a marked degree.

38. Habitually sodden feet with blistered skin.

REFERENCES

(1) Standards of Medical Examination for Flying; Army Regulations No. 40-110 (Sept. 1956, reprint). Washington, D. C., Government Printing Office, 1952.

(2) Manual of the Medical Department, U. S. Navy (NAVMED P-117), Chapter 15, Physical examinations, Section V, Aviation (Feb. 1958, reprint). Washington, D. C., Government Printing Office, 1952.

(3) Medical Examination, Air Force Manual 160-1 (Aug. 1957, reprint). Washington, D. C., Government Printing Office, 1953.

3

EYE EXAMINATION

Harry G. Armstrong, M.D.

It is quite obvious that a normal optic system is one of the primary requisites for safety in flying. This is not limited to visual acuity but includes such things as color vision and depth perception as well as some nine other optic functions each of which must be measured by the examiner. Most of these measurements require the use of equipment and procedures that the average physician is unfamiliar with and, accordingly, the eye examination is usually the most difficult for the student of aviation medicine to master. For that reason the procedures to be followed will be described in more detail for the eye than for the other systems of the body.

The equipment and methods to be discussed below will be the traditional ones that have been in general use for a number of years. However, it should be noted that there is an alternate method of measuring distant vision, heterophoria, near vision and depth perception through the use of fairly recently developed equipment referred to as a "machine vision tester" which is shown in figure 5. If this equipment is available it should be employed in accordance with the instructions accompanying the instrument and the corresponding conventional tests may then be eliminated.

VISUAL ACUITY

UNDERLYING PRINCIPLES. Visual acuity is the ability of the eye to appreciate form. The usual method by which visual acuity is measured is by utilizing the visual angle.

By visual angle is meant the minimum angle formed by the intersection of two axial rays crossing at the nodal point of the eye when two points are seen as being separate and distinct. Thus, two points at a distance may be so close together that the rays of light from them pass through the optical center of the dioptric system of the eye and both fall on a single cone of the retina. Inasmuch as the stimulation of a single cone gives but a single image in consciousness the two points mentioned above are thus seen as a single point. If the two points are far enough apart, however, separate cones are stimulated and two separate images are formed.

In the case of a normal eye where the retinal images are clear and distinct two points appear separate when the visual angle formed by the crossing of the two axial rays is a minimum angle of 1 minute. In the ametropic eye, inasmuch as the retinal images are blurred and indistinct, a visual angle of more than 1 minute is required to distinguish two separate points and the greater the ametropia the greater the visual angle required to discriminate them.

By far the simplest and the most frequently used method of measuring the visual angle and, hence, visual acuity is by means of Snellen test letters. Each Snellen test letter is formed such that at a given distance from the eye each stroke of the letter subtends an angle of 1 minute and the letter as a whole an angle of 5 minutes (fig. 6). The shape of the letter is such that it can be placed in a square. There are nor-

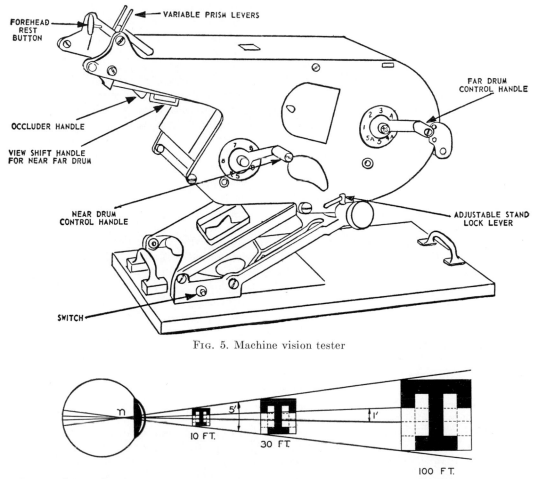

FIG. 5. Machine vision tester

FIG. 6. Schematic representation of the manner in which Snellen test letters are formed. The axial rays form an angle of 5 minutes and the distance from the eye determines the size of the letters.

mally at least eight rows of test letters on each Snellen chart the size of the letters in each row getting progressively smaller from above downward. The top row of letters is of such a size that at 200 feet distance from the eye each stroke of the letters subtends an angle of 1 minute. Each stroke of the lower rows of letters also subtends this angle if the eye is at 100, 70, 50, 40, 30, 20 and 15 feet from the chart respectively.

Inasmuch as the visual acuity test is normally conducted at 20 feet (6 meters) distance from the chart the normal eye should read the line second from the bottom. and this is recorded as 20/20. If the bottom line can be read at 20 feet distance this should be recorded as 20/15. Where all of the 20/30 line can be read and three letters

of the 20/20 line this is recorded as 20/30 + 3. A visual acuity of 20/20 is generally considered as normal although there are many people who can read 20/15 without difficulty.

Factors which tend to lower visual acuity are errors of refraction, the size of the pupil, the amount of illumination and pathologic changes in the eye or optic tract.

PROCEDURE. In conducting the examination for visual acuity the candidate is seated in the eye room exactly 20 feet (6 meters) from the Snellen test chart. One eye of the candidate is covered by a blank card 6 by 9 cm. in size. The room is darkened, the chart exposed to the illumination of two 100 watt daylight Mazda lamps and the candidate required to read the chart from above downward as far as possible. The smallest line of letters that can be read measures the visual acuity of the eye being tested. The blank card is then shifted so that the other eye is exposed and the above procedure repeated.

PRECAUTIONS. Every effort should be made that no opportunity is given for a candidate to memorize a chart either through his own efforts or through an accomplice. Examinees awaiting their visual acuity test should not be permitted a view of the test charts or allowed to hear them repeated by another candidate. In case of doubt extra charts with different lettering should be available. During the test the candidate should not be allowed to squint but made to read with his eyes open in their natural position. Care should be exercised that no miotic has been used to improve the vision of myopics by producing pin-point pupils.

INTERPRETATION OF FINDINGS. A visual acuity in either eye of less than 20/20 should disqualify.

DEPTH PERCEPTION

UNDERLYING PRINCIPLES. Depth perception may be defined as the ability to appreciate or discriminate the third dimension, to judge distance and to orient oneself in relation to other objects within the visual field. It is evident that this faculty is required to a high degree in aviation because upon it depends the ability of pilots to avoid obstacles, to land properly and to fly in formation with other aircraft.

There are eight separate factors concerned in depth perception four of which are inherent in, and are a basic part of, the physical function of the individual and four which are an adjunctive group independent of the individual and common to all persons. The first group of factors consists of:

1. Physiologic diplopia
2. Accommodation
3. Convergence
4. Binocular parallax

Physiologic diplopia is the ability to recognize differences in distance between two objects within the visual field based on the fact that all objects in the field closer or farther away than the object fixed gives rise to diplopia (figs. 7, 8 and 9). When the normal eyes fix any object the image of that object falls upon the maculae of both retinas and is projected outward to where the visual lines cross and that marks the location of the object. If at the same time there is a second object in the visual field but closer to the eyes than the object fixed the image of the near object will fall on the temporal side of the macula of both eyes. Then the image from the right eye is projected to the left of the near object and the image from the left eye will be projected to the right of the near

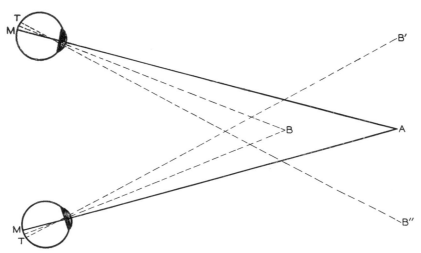

FIG. 7. Physiologic diplopia. Eyes fixing far object. *A*, the far object; *B*, the near object; *M-M*, maculae; *T-T*, temporal sides of retinas. Eyes are fixing the far object *A* and image falls upon the maculae at *M-M*. Image of *B'* the near object, falls upon the temporal sides of the maculae at *T-T* and is projected to *B'* with the right eye and to *B''* with the left eye thus inducing crossed diplopia.

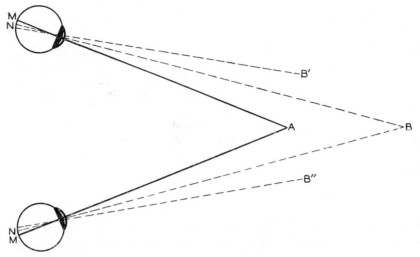

FIG. 8. Physiologic diplopia. Eyes fixing near object. *A*, the near object; *B*, the far object; *M-M*, maculae; *N-N*, the nasal sides of the maculae. Eyes are fixing the near object *A* and image falls upon the maculae at *M-M*. Image of *B*, the far object, falls upon the nasal sides of the maculae at *N-N* and is projected to *B″* with the right eye and to *B′* with the left eye thus inducing homonymous diplopia.

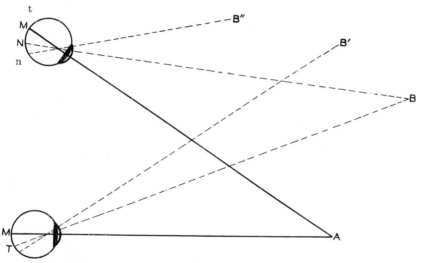

FIG. 9. Physiologic diplopia. Objects arranged similar to those in testing apparatus. *A*, the near rod; *B*, the far rod; *M-M*, maculae; *t*, temporal side of retina, *n*, nasal side of retina. Eyes have fixed the near rod *A* and image falls upon the maculae at *M-M*. Image of the far rod *B* falls upon the temporal side of the right macula and upon the nasal side of the left, but the image falls upon the retina of the left eye at a greater distance from the macula than in the right eye. Therefore, the image of *B* is projected to *B′* with the right eye and to *B″* with the left eye thus inducing homonymous diplopia with the left eye and crossed diplopia with the right.

object and bilateral crossed diplopia results. Conversely, when the eyes fix on an object and a second object is farther away and in the visual field the image of the latter falls on the nasal side of the maculae of both retinas. Here the image of the far object is projected to the right from the right eye and to the left from the left eye and bilateral homonymous diplopia results. In either instance the diplopia is not recognized as such in consciousness but is interpreted in terms of distance nearer or farther away than the object fixed. When an object is equidistant from the eyes as the one being fixed the image of the former falls on symmetrical points of the retinas, the images are fused and projected to the same point in space and diplopia does not occur. Thus, the recognition of distance of objects is determined in part by the presence or absence of physiologic diplopia, whether the diplopia is crossed or homonymous and the degree of diplopia. This factor is present with binocular single vision only.

Accomodation is the faculty of increasing the dioptric power of the lens and is the factor that enables the normal eye to focus near objects at less than infinity (for practical purposes 20 feet or 6 meters) on the retina to form a clear image.

If for any reason there is failure of accommodation the images of objects at less than 20 feet (6 meters) on the retinas are blurred and, thus, visual acuity and depth perception are interfered with. However, inasmuch as this factor operates only for distances of less than 20 feet it is of little importance in aviation for aviators are seldom called upon to judge such small distances. This factor operates with both monocular and binocular single vision.

Convergence is the ability of the two eyes to fix on an object at a distance less than infinity. The closer the object the greater the amount of convergence required for bilateral fixation. Failure of convergence causes a blurring of vision or a pathologic diplopia with a resultant decrease in depth perception. This factor operates with binocular single vision only.

Binocular parallax is the impression of relief or solidity given to an object by the slightly different view of it which is obtained by the fact that the right eye sees a little more of the right side of the object and the left eye a little more of the left side of the object. This produces two slightly different retinal images which when fused lose this difference in consciousness and is interpreted in terms of relief and depth.

The amount of difference in the retinal images on the retinas of the two eyes depends on the distance of the object from the eyes and on the amount of convergence necessary to fix the object. The difference between the angles formed when the two eyes fix on a distant object and on a near object is called the binocular parallactic angle and our conception of the difference between the distance of objects is in part determined by this angle. This angle is diagrammatically illustrated in figures 10 and 11. This factor operates with binocular single vision only.

The second or adjunctive group of factors which are important in depth perception consists of:
1. Size of the retinal image
2. Motion parallax
3. Terrestrial association
4. Aerial perspective

The size of the retinal image varies inversely as the distance of an object from the eye. Therefore, the closer an object is to the eye the larger the retinal image and the further away the smaller the image. Thus, the size of the retinal image is a measure of the distance of an object from the eye but it has been found that this factor operating alone is quite inaccurate. This factor operates with both monocular and binocular single vision.

Motion parallax is based on the same general phenomena seen in binocular parallax but differs in that the former depends on motion of the observer or of the object being observed. It also differs in that it operates with monocular as well as binocular single vision. This is possible inasmuch as in monocular vision a motion of the observer or the object gives different views of the object either to the right or the left, above or below and these different images on the retinas are interpreted in consciousness in terms of distance.

Terrestrial association and *aerial perspective* are both acquired characteristics which develop with training and experience and depend on an association of ideas. In the former, linear perspective, overlapping contours, light reflections and shadows are utilized in the judgment of distance. In aerial perspective the same factors apply but objects when seen from above have an entirely different appearance than from the ground. Both of these factors operate with single and with binocular single vision.

Factors which may produce poor depth perception are inequality of vision, insufficiency of convergence, accommodation asthenopia and heterophoria.

With reference to inequality of visual

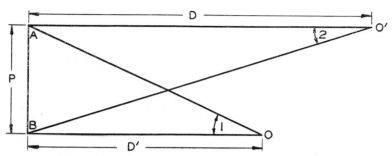

FIG. 10. Binocular parallax (after Howard). Two objects O and O' located at unequal distances from eyes A and B. D' distance to near object, O. P, the interpupillary distance, A-B. D, distance to far object, O'. D minus D' equals difference in distance or the depth difference. Angle one minus angle two equals the binocular parallactic angle.

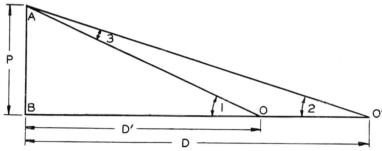

FIG. 11. Binocular parallax (after Howard). A more diagrammatic illustration of binocular parallax. Consider one eye B and the two objects O and O' in a straight line. P, the interpupillary distance A-B. D', the shorter distance B-O. D, the longer distance B-O'. D minus D' equals the depth difference. Let angle one equal AOB, the angle of convergence upon the near object and angle two equal $AO'B$, the angle of convergence upon the far object, and angle three equal angle OAO', then angle one minus angle two equals angle three, which is the binocular parallactic angle represented by the depth difference D minus D'.

acuity it has been found to affect depth perception more than an equivalent amount of equal defective visual acuity. Thus, a man with 20/20 vision in one eye and 20/40 in the other will normally have much poorer depth perception than if he had 20/30 bilaterally. This seems to be caused by the fact that the greater the inequality of vision the closer binocular depth perception approaches monocular depth perception because of a tendency in the former to lose physiologic diplopia and binocular parallax and, hence, the perception of relief and solidity.

In devising a test for depth perception it is important that only those factors which are inherent in the individual and which operate at distances greater than 20 feet be considered. In order to do this all of the external or artificial aids such as motion parallax, terrestrial association and aerial perspective must be eliminated from the test. When this

is accomplished we can then establish the inherent ability of the candidate to judge distance and, with this as a basis, he can learn to utilize all of the adjunctive factors. After one becomes an experienced flyer it is possible to lose many of the basic factors and still fly well as has been demonstrated in the case of one eyed pilots. For candidates, however, good inherent depth perception must be demonstrated.

For the actual measurement of depth perception all external factors are eliminated as well as those operating at less than 20 feet and the following factors only are allowed to operate in the test:

1. Size of the retinal image
2. Physiologic diplopia
3. Binocular parallax
4. Convergence

The Howard-Dolman apparatus (fig. 12) is normally used to measure the above factors and, hence, the inherent depth percep-

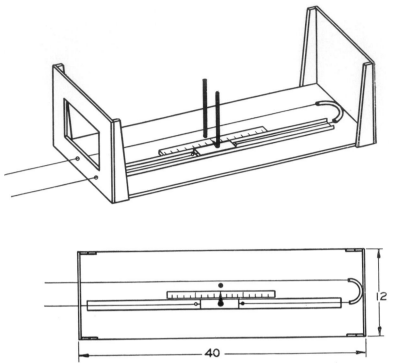

FIG. 12. Side and top views of the Howard-Dolman depth perception apparatus

tion. This apparatus consists of a box 40 inches long and 12 inches wide, open at the sides and top. The end nearest the examinee has an opening 7¼ by 5 inches through which can be viewed two black vertical rods 64 mm. apart laterally against a white background. One of these rods is mounted stationary at the center of the floor of the box while the other can be moved forward and back in a groove by means of cords held in the examinee's hands. A small millimeter scale on the floor of the box is marked off to measure the horizontal distance between the rods.

PROCEDURE. The examinee is seated facing the depth perception apparatus and at exactly 20 feet (6 meters) distance. The movable rod is placed at various distances off center and the candidate is required, by means of the cords, to place it as nearly as he can judge opposite the stationary rod or such that both are equidistant from him. This is repeated several times, the rods being widely separated after each trial. The result of each attempt is read directly off the millimeter scale, the results of all the trials

averaged and the average depth perception recorded.

PRECAUTIONS. Uniform overhead illumination without shadows should be provided. The candidate should be straight in line with the box so that when the rods are on zero they are each equidistant from him. He should not be allowed to move his head or body during the test and, thus, utilize motion parallax or to pull the movable rod the length of the box and, thus, be able to estimate its midpoint.

The examiner should not give any indication by word, act, or facial expression as to when the movable rod is at or near zero or the extent of any error. He should remove the cords from the examinee's hands between each trial to prevent his judging the movement of the rod by the length of cord that passes through his hand during each setting.

INTERPRETATION OF FINDINGS. A depth perception error of more than 30 mm. should disqualify.

Alternate Method

If the Verhoeff depth perception apparatus is available it may be substituted for the

Howard-Dolman test. The former is a binocular test and shows, with each exposure, the relative position of three vertical rods. One or two positions are shown at close range to the examinee to demonstrate clearly that one rod is always closer or farther than the other two with the further explanation that the size of the rods is not a clue to the relative distances. Eight different rod relations are possible by showing four and then reversing the instrument for four more. All eight positions should be used in this examination.

The device should be kept centered on a frontal plane normal to the subject's binocular vision midline. To avoid helpful extraneous cues the examiner must hold the device steady and not rotate it on its vertical axis. Moreover, the examinee must not be permitted to move his head. The target window should not be exposed while the device is being placed in position or while the sets are changed. A convenient method of manipulation is to grasp the device over the target window with the left hand, place the desired set into position with the right hand, then grasp the device below with the right hand and expose the target window by moving the left hand up or down. Thus, while the target window is exposed, the device is supported by both hands of the examiner.

The examinee should answer each of the eight presentations correctly. If an error is made on the first run, two more runs should be made and the examinee must report eight out of eight correctly on both trials. If this is not done, the examinee should be failed.

Near Vision

PROCEDURE. Any of the standard near vision acuity test charts may be used to measure near vision. Each eye is tested separately and the examinee required to read the smallest print possible with the results recorded as a fraction, if the Snellen English linear chart is used. Equivalents for the other various commonly used methods are shown in table 6.

INTERPRETATION OF FINDINGS. A near vision acuity of less than 20/20 on the Snellen test chart, or the equivalent on other standards charts, should disqualify.

TABLE 6
Near Vision Test Card Equivalents

Snellen English	Snellen Metric	Jaeger
	M	
20/20	0.50	J-1
20/25	0.62	J-2
20/30	0.75	J-4
20/40	1.00	J-6
20/50	1.25	J-8
20/70	1.75	J-12
20/100	2.25	J-14
20/200		

Intraocular Tension

Intraocular tension should be tested for by palpation. If an abnormal tension is found it should disqualify. Inasmuch as a positive finding suggests ocular pathology the examinee should be referred to an opthalmologist for diagnosis and treatment.

Ocular Movements

General Considerations

In selecting candidates for flying training, it is necessary to determine whether or not there is any abnormality in the motility of the eye. In order to accomplish this five separate tests are used but before discussing them each in detail certain general considerations will be reviewed.

In flying, bodily movements are normally very restricted and a wide range of vision can be obtained only by turning the head and eyes. However, it is not only necessary for clear vision that an object be in the visual field but that both eyes be capable of fixing the object so that the retinal image falls on the fovea of each eye. In order for this to be accomplished the two eyes must be parallel in all positions when looking at an object at infinity and convergent when looking at an object at less than infinity. The amount of convergence in the latter case will depend of course on the nearness of the object.

It has been found in most cases that one eye first fixes an object and the other then arranges itself in proper relation to the first to give binocular fixation. The first is called the sighting eye and the second the nonsighting eye. In right handed people the right eye is usually the sighting eye and in left handed people the left eye is usually the sighting eye. In pathologic diplopia the sighting eye is always the one that fixes the object looked at and the nonsighting eye is the one that deviates.

Each eye is equipped with six external muscles which rotate the eye ball about its center to an average maximum of 33° upward, 47° upward and inward, 50° inward, 47° inward and downward, 57° downward, 47° downward and outward and 45° outward.

In binocular vision when the two eyes fix on an object at infinity the visual lines of the two eyes are parallel and this relationship is maintained by the fusion center in the brain whose nervous regulation normally assures binocular fixation. When for any reason the action of the fusion center is weakened or destroyed the two eyes will remain parallel only if the muscles of the two eyes are perfectly balanced. In all other cases there will be a diplopia. The amount and type of diplopia depends on which muscles of the eyes are weak or which are overacting. None of the movements of the eye are dependent on any one muscle alone but on a principal muscle and a synergist, each of which may have a primary and a secondary action and its action opposed by one or more antagonists. The external muscles of the eye,

their actions and their synergists are given in table 7.

There are two general types of diplopia. One is latent and occurs only when the fusion center is weakened or abolished and the other is manifest and occurs when the fusion center is presumably functioning.

The terminology applied to these conditions is as follows:

I. ORTHOPHORIA. Normal binocular balance.
II. HETEROPHORIA. A latent imbalance or tendency toward deviation of the two visual lines from parallel. It includes the following:
  a. Esophoria. A latent deviation of the visual lines inward.
  b. Exophoria. A latent deviation of the visual lines outward.
  c. Hyperphoria. A latent deviation of the visual lines of *one* eye above that of the other. It is designated as right or left.
  d. Hypophoria. A latent deviation of the visual lines of one eye below that of the other. Designated as right or left.
  e. Double hyperphoria. A latent elevation of both visual lines.
  f. Double hypophoria. A latent lowering of both visual lines.
  g. Cyclophoria. A latent deviation of the globe about its anteroposterior axis, *i. e.,* an *intorsion* (rotation of the upper portion of the cornea about the anteroposterior axis of the globe nasally or inward) or an *extorsion* (outward rotation) necessarily designated as right or left.

TABLE 7

Primary and Subsidiary Actions and Synergists of the Individual Ocular Muscles

(Peter)

Muscle	Primary Action	Subsidiary Action	Synergist
Internal rectus	Internal rotation	None	Superior rectus Inferior rectus
External rectus	External rotation	None	Superior oblique Inferior oblique
Superior rectus	Elevation	Internal rotation Intorsion	Inferior oblique Internal rectus
Inferior rectus	Depression	Internal rotation Extorsion	Superior oblique Internal rectus
Superior oblique	Intorsion	Depression External rotation	Inferior rectus External rectus
Inferior oblique	Extorsion	Elevation External rotation	Superior rectus External rectus

III. HETEROTROPIA. A manifest deviation of the visual lines.
  a. *Esotropia*. A manifest deviation of the visual lines inward—a convergent squint.
  b. *Exotropia*. A manifest deviation of the visual lines outward—a divergent squint.
  c. *Hypertropia*. A manifest deviation of one visual line above the other—right or left.
  d. *Hypotropia*. A manifest deviation of one visual line below the other—right or left.
  e. *Cyclotropia*. A manifest deviation about the anteroposterior axis.

Other diagnostic terms used in connection with defective ocular movements are:
  1. *Hyperkinesis*. Excessive action of an individual muscle.
  2. *Hypokinesis*. Deficient action of an individual muscle.

Heterophoria at 6 Meters

UNDERLYING PRINCIPLES. Heterotropia is disqualifying for aviation, and where it exists it is usually (but not always) immediately apparent on inspection of the eyes. Heterophoria being latent must be made manifest and, inasmuch as a certain degree of heterophoria is acceptable in aviation, its extent and type must be determined. This can be accomplished by weakening or abolishing the action of the fusion center and then measuring the resultant deviation of the two eyes. This is done by the use of a multiple Maddox rod and a rotary prism mounted in a phorometer trial frame (fig. 13).

The multiple Maddox rod is a series of sections of glass rods superimposed with their axes parallel and in the same plane and mounted in a black opaque frame. If a small point of light is looked at through this rod the light is refracted such that the point of light appears as a streak or line of light at right angles to the long axis of the rod.

A rotary prism is two prisms of equal value mounted superimposed and arranged to rotate in opposite directions by turning a milled thumbscrew. With this arrangement any prismatic effect from zero to the sum of the values of the two prisms may be obtained. The base of this prism may be placed in any position.

If one should look at a spot of light with a Maddox rod before one eye and with the other eye uncovered the light would appear as two entirely different objects, *i.e.*, a line of light to the eye looking through the Maddox rod and a point of light to the uncovered eye. This effect tends to abolish or weaken the action of the fusion center and any latent deviation of the eyes then becomes manifest.

The amount of this deviation can be measured by means of the rotary prism. In order to do this a multiple Maddox rod and a rotary prism are both placed before one eye while the other eye is left uncovered as before. Looking at the spot of light at 6 meters distance the streak of light will usually be seen either to the right or to the left of the spot of light. By rotating the prism the

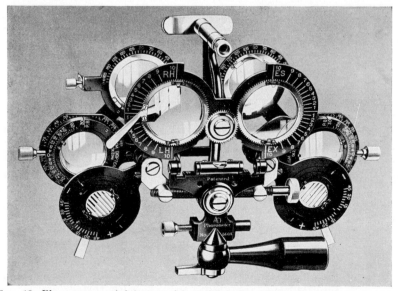

FIG. 13. Phorometer trial frame with multiple Maddox rods and rotary prisms

streak of light will appear to move laterally and when it has been placed so that it passes exactly through the spot of light the amount of heterophoria may then be read directly from the prism scale which is graduated in prism diopters. The term prism diopter is used as the measure of strength of a prism and one prism diopter is that which will deviate a beam of light 1 cm. at 1 meter distance and equals 34.37 minutes.

If the eyes are perfectly balanced the scale should read zero when the streak and spot are superimposed. With the prism set at zero when the nonsighting eye tends to deviate inward the image of the streak of light falls on the nasal side of the retina and is projected out to the temporal side and will be seen to the left of the spotlight when the left eye is the nonsighting eye and to the right side of the spotlight when the right eye is the nonsighting eye (homonymous diplopia).

Inasmuch as rays of light passing through a prism are refracted or bent toward its base the prism correction in these cases will be prism base out and the light rays entering the eye will be shifted away from the nasal side of the deviating eye until it strikes the fovea when the streak of light and the spot of light will appear superimposed while the eye remains deviated and stationary.

When the nonsighting eye deviates outward the reverse of the above occurs. In the nonsighting eye the streak of light falls to the temporal side of the retina, the image is projected outward to the nasal side (crossed diplopia), and the correcting prism will be base in.

For measuring vertical deviations of the eye (hyperphoria) the same procedure is repeated except that the rotary prism is turned with the adjusting thumbscrew pointing laterally and the Maddox rod turned with its long axis vertical. In this case the streak of light appears horizontal and appears to move up and down with rotations of the rotary prism.

The term hyperphoria is always applied to the eye that deviates upward. Thus, if the left eye is the nonsighting eye and a deviation is found corrected by prism base down there is said to be hyperphoria of the left eye while if the prism is base up, there is said to be hyperphoria of the right eye.

PROCEDURE. For this and the succeeding test—the Maddox rod test at 33 cm.—the candidate is first required to demonstrate which of his two eyes is the sighting eye. This is accomplished by having the examinee gaze at a spotlight at 6 meters distance and while looking directly at the light he grasps a 5 by 7 inch white card having a 1.5 cm. round hole in its center and raises it at arm length until the light is seen through the hole. The eye which sees the light through the hole is the sighting eye. Having determined the sighting eye the candidate is seated before the phorometer trial frame and at 6 meters distance from the spotlight. Carefully adjust the phorometer frame so that the cells are spaced properly for his two eyes and place the multiple Maddox rod with its axis horizontal before the nonsighting eye. The Risley rotary prism is also swung in place before the nonsighting eye with the thumbscrew pointing upward and set on or near the zero reading.

The procedure and the manipulation of the prism which he himself is required to do is then carefully explained to the examinee. When all is in readiness the room is darkened and the spotlight turned on. The candidate is next instructed to look with both eyes through the phorometer trial frame and asked if he sees a spot of light and a vertical line of light. If the answer is in the negative the preceding procedure should be rechecked. If the answer is in the affirmative he should then be instructed to turn the thumbscrew one way or the other until the line of light passes exactly through the spot of light. While this is being done a small card is passed up and down in front of the nonfixing eye by the examiner in order alternately to cover and uncover the spotlight to further weaken fusion.

When the candidate has the line of light through the spot of light the examiner reads from the scale on the prism the amount of latent deviation and whether it is esophoria or exophoria.

The next step is to test for vertical deviation (hyperphoria) of the eyes. This is done exactly as described above for lateral deviations except that here the rotary prism is turned with the thumbscrew pointing laterally and the Maddox rod with its long axis vertical. With this arrangement the streak of light is horizontal and moves up or down when the prism is rotated. When the candidate has placed the streak of light through the spot of light the amount of deviation is again read directly from the prism scale. To determine which eye shows hyperphoria it is to be remembered that base down prism shows that the nonsighting eye deviates upward and base up prism that the sighting eye deviates upward.

PRECAUTIONS. The room should be perfectly dark and the walls free from light reflections which may be seen through the prism and cause confusion. The candidate should place his head against the head rest on the trial frame and hold it perfectly still during the test. The Maddox rod and the rotary prism must always be placed before the nonsighting eye and the light before that eye interrupted frequently if accurate results are to be obtained.

INTREPRETATION OF FINDINGS. An esophoria of more than 10 diopters, exophoria of more than 5 diopters or a hyperphoria of more than 1 diopter should disqualify.

The Maddox Rod Test at 33 cm.

UNDERLYING PRINCIPLES. This test is based on the same general considerations as those described above for the Maddox rod test at 6 meters. The difference is that at 33 cm. the test will uncover any latent deviation at reading distance. It may give some information also as to the existence of refractive errors, insufficiency of convergence and reduction of fusion control.

PROCEDURE. The same as that described above for the Maddox rod test at 6 meters except that the spotlight is at 33 cm. distance and the test for hyperphoria is omitted.

PRECAUTIONS. Same as for the 6 meter test.

INTERPRETATION OF FINDINGS. Exophoria of 4 diopters may be considered normal. An exophoria of more than 12 diopters should disqualify.

Power of Divergence

UNDERLYING PRINCIPLES. Prism divergence is a measure of the ability of the eyes to abduct. A low prism divergence indicates an underaction of the external recti or an overaction of the internal recti or both. The amount of abduction is measured by means

of the rotary prism at 6 meters distance from a spotlight. The method by which this is accomplished is as follows:

With the prism set at zero before the nonsighting eye and with the thumbscrew in the up position the spotlight is fixed by both eyes. If the prism is then rotated slowly base in the ray of light is refracted toward the base of the prism. When this occurs the image of the light ray shifts to the nasal side of the fovea of the nonsighting eye and in order to maintain binocular single vision that eye must rotate outward. Inasmuch as the fusion center is functioning the eye continues to rotate outward as the prism is rotated until the limit of divergence is reached when the eye swings back parallel to the sighting eye and diplopia results. The onset of diplopia marks the limit of prism divergence and, hence, the power of abduction.

PROCEDURE. The examinee is seated before the phorometer trial frame with the prism set at zero before one eye and at 6 meters distant from the spotlight. If the examinee sees two spotlights when the prism is set at zero he has diplopia and cannot be tested. If he sees but a single spotlight the examiner then turns the prism slowly and steadily by means of the thumbscrew base in until the candidate announces that he sees two lights. The number of prism diopters of divergence is then read directly from the prism scale.

PRECAUTIONS. This test is very fatiguing to the eyes and should not be repeated more than twice at any one sitting.

INTERPRETATION OF FINDINGS. When an esophoria at 6 meters exists the diverging power in prism diopters should equal or exceed the esophoria in prism diopters.

Prism divergence of more than 15 or less than 3 prism diopters should disqualify without further evidence.

Power of Convergence

UNDERLYING PRINCIPLES. Adduction of the eyes is not measured in the same way as abduction because accommodation plays an important part in convergence. A reliable and satisfactory method is to determine the point of convergence (fig. 14).

The point of convergence is the nearest point directly in front of, and closest to, the center of rotation of the eyes to which the two eyes can fix an object without diplopia.

Inasmuch as the center of rotation of the eyes is 13.5 mm. back of the cornea the near point is computed from that point as a base line.

PROCEDURE. The candidate is placed facing a window and the end of a prince rule is placed edge up at the side of his nose 11½ mm. out from the anterior surface of his cornea. Hold a white headed pin in the midline and just above the edge of the rule 33 cm. distant from his eyes and ask the candidate to gaze intently at it. The pin is then moved steadily and slowly toward the eyes until they are no longer able to converge and one eye swings outward. Note the distance of the pin from the end of the rule toward the eyes and to this add 26 mm. (distance from end of rule to center of rotation of eye). This total gives the distance from the base line of the eyes to the near point of convergence.

PRECAUTIONS. The point of convergence should be determined two or three times and the average result used. It is to be noted, however, that too frequent testing is fatiguing and gives erroneous results. Both eyes should converge on the test object at the beginning of the test and the onset of diplopia should be determined by the examiner and not left to the statement of the examinee. The test object should be moved toward the eyes at a moderate steady speed.

INTERPRETATION OF FINDINGS. A point of convergence which exceeds 70 mm. should disqualify.

Associated Parallel Movements

The associated parallel movements of the eyes may be tested either by means of the tangent curtain or by means of the red lens.

Tangent Curtain Test

UNDERLYING PRINCIPLES. In addition to latent and manifest deviations of the eyes there is another type of motility defect which must be tested for. This is underaction or overaction, a paresis or paralysis of the external ocular muscles. This defect is normally apparent when the eyes are rotated so as to bring all of the ocular muscles into play. A defective muscle is detected by noting whether or not one eye lags or overshoots.

In order to accurately determine the muscle or muscles involved and the amount of impairment a tangent curtain (fig. 15) is normally employed. A tangent curtain consists of a cloth panel 60 by 72 inches, white on one side and black on the other and mounted on a rigid frame. The white side of the curtain is marked off in 2 inch squares, each square amounting to a deviation of 5° at 75 cm. distance. From a point midway between the sides of the curtain and 30

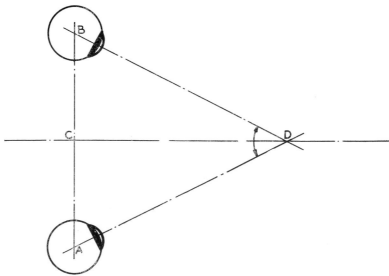

FIG. 14. The power of convergence. Where the point *D* is the nearest point on which the two eyes can fix an object without diplopia, the measure of the point of convergence is the distance *CD*.

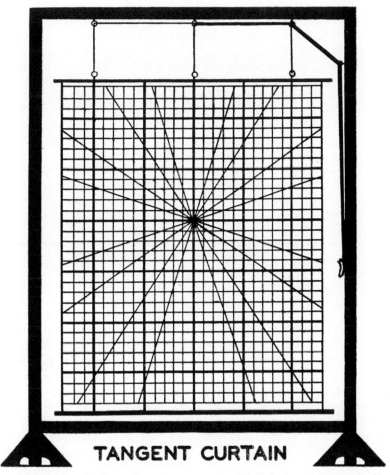

FIG. 15. Tangent curtain. Each small square represents 5° deviation at 75 cm. Radiating lines are placed at angles of 15°.

inches down from the top, radiating lines pass out at angles of 15°.

PROCEDURE. The examinee stands near a window where good illumination falls on both eyes. The examiner holds a white headed pin about 33 cm. directly in front of the examinee's eyes and directs him to look at it steadily. Nystagmus in the primary position is to be noted at this stage of the test. The examinee is then instructed to hold his head still and watch the pin as it is moved slowly to his right. The pin is not carried beyond the field of binocular fixation, but is held motionless for a moment near the lateral limit of the field. Each eye is inspected to discover any failure in fixing the pin. The lagging or overaction of either eye is noted. The pin is then carried slowly to the extreme left, up and to the left, straight up, up and

to the right, down and to the right, straight down and down and to the left. The lagging of either eye in any one of these eight cardinal directions is caused by underaction of at least one of the extrinsic ocular muscles. It may indicate a paresis or a complete paralysis. This underaction is recorded by stating which eye lags and in which direction the lagging is observed. In the same way any overshooting of either eye is recorded by stating which eye is involved and in which direction.

If any underaction or overaction is revealed by this test the final diagnosis is made or verified on the tangent curtain by means of a small electric light or candle and a red glass. From the associated parallel movement test and the plotting of diplopia on the tangent curtain a diagnosis of the individual muscle or muscles involved is readily made.

To use the tangent curtain place the examinee comfortably seated 75 cm. from the black side of the tangent curtain with a red glass in front of his right eye. A black pin is placed in the center of the curtain; the head is so adjusted that when the eyes are directed at the center pin they are on a level with it and looking straight ahead. A small electric light is then carried over the curtain in the six cardinal directions of the muscles' actions and, in addition thereto, straight up and down. The point where diplopia occurs in each meridian is noted by thrusting in a black pin at the point of the light itself and a light colored pin at the site of the other image. This latter is evidently the false image, and if it is red it is known that the left eye is fixing and if it is white that the right eye is fixing. In the great majority of cases the examinee fixes with the eye not covered by the red glass.

Whether the diplopia is crossed or homonymous is evidenced by the side on which the red image appears in relation to the eye before which the red glass is placed.

PRECAUTIONS. The head must be held erect and steady and only the eyes are to follow the electric light bulb. The eyes must be on a level with the center pin and directly in front of it.

INTERPRETATION OF FINDINGS. The examinee should be disqualified if the underaction or overaction of any of the extrinsic ocular muscles produce diplopia except in the extreme positions. A small separation of the images may be disregarded. Nystagmus should disqualify if it is demonstrated except in extreme positions.

Red Lens Test

UNDERLYING PRINCIPLES. To check the associated parallel movements of the eyes without the use of the tangent curtain the red lens test may be substituted.

PROCEDURE. The examinee is seated in the dark room and a spectacle trial frame is adjusted in place with a red lens in one of the cells. A tangent screen is placed 30 inches from the examinee's eyes and a point of light is then moved laterally from the center of the screen in the six cardinal directions, right, left, up and to the right, up and to the left, down and to the right and down and to the left. The examinee is instructed to follow the light with his eyes without moving his head and to report either a change in the color of the light (suppression), or a doubling of the light (diplopia). Change in the color of the light should be demonstrated at the beginning of the test by use of the occluder, showing that it may be either red, white or pink. To avoid the danger of a routine negative response, a 5 diopter prism placed base up or base down before one eye will produce diplopia which should be reported by the examinee. This prism may be alternated with a plano lens of the same size in order to confuse the examinee. If diplopia or suppression develops when no prism is being used, the point on the screen at which this occurs is noted and recorded.

PRECAUTIONS. The head of the examinee must remain fixed while the light is being moved with no tilting or rotation of the face being permitted.

INTERPRETATION OF FINDINGS. Diplopia within 20 inches in any meridian should disqualify.

INSPECTION OF THE EYE

UNDERLYING PRINCIPLES. Inspection of the eye is entirely objective in nature. It involves an examination of the external and internal structures of the eyes and their adnexa. A part of the examination is conducted in daylight and part in the dark room. The various structures to be examined are:

The eyelids
Lacrimal apparatus
Conjunctiva
The globe
The sclera
The cornea
The iris and anterior chamber
The lens and vitreous

Each of the structures should be inspected in turn and any defect classified as temporary or permanent. In case a temporary defect is noted the candidate should be advised to have it corrected and allowed to return at a later date.

PROCEDURE. *Examination of the eyelids* should be conducted in good daylight. The following conditions should be noted:

Ptosis	Entropion
Blepharitis	Ectropion
Trichiasis	Chalazion

Examination of the lacrimal apparatus should disclose defects in the excretory portion such as improper drainage of the lacrimal sac, stenosis of the canaliculi and displacement of the puncta. In case of doubt a lacrimal syringe should be used to determine the patency of the system.

Examination of the conjunctiva should include both the palpebral and bulbar portions. The lower palpebral conjunctiva and the lower fornix can be readily exposed by placing a finger just below the edge of the lower lid and exerting traction downward while the examinee is told to look up.

The upper palpebral conjunctiva and upper fornix can be readily exposed by the following procedure: Take an ordinary applicator and place one end of it horizontally across the upper lid at the level of the upper margin of the tarsus. Direct the examinee to gaze downward and grasping the cilia gently evert the lid by pulling the cilia in a rotary direction downward, then outward and upward, while at the same time the applicator is pressed gently backward against the lid to act as a fulcrum. The applicator is left in place during this phase of the examination and is moved laterally back and forth to help expose the superior fornix. The abnormal conditions to be looked for are:

Pterygium	Chemosis
Pinguecula	Xerosis
Concretions	Cysts
Ecchymosis	Tumors
Hyperemia	Conjunctivitis

If pterygium is found it should be determined whether it is a true or false pterygium and differentiated from pinguecula. Any encroachment in the cornea should be noted and also whether it is progressive or nonprogressive.

Conjunctival and ciliary injection may be distinguished by the following differential points:

Conjunctival Injection

1. Derived from posterior conjunctival vessels
2. Accompanies diseases of the conjunctiva
3. More or less mucopurulent or purulent discharge
4. Most marked in fornix conjunctivae
5. Fades as it approaches the cornea
6. Bright, brick red color
7. Composed of a network of coarse tortuous vessels, anastomosing freely and placed superficially so that the meshes are easily recognized

Ciliary Injection

1. Derived from anterior ciliary vessels
2. Accompanies diseases of the cornea, iris and ciliary body
3. Often lacrimation, but no conjunctival discharge
4. Most marked immediately around the cornea; hence, called "circumcorneal"
5. Fades toward the fornix
6. Pink or lilac color
7. Composed of small, straight vessels, placed deeply, so that individual vessels cannot be recognized easily but are seen indistinctly as fine straight lines radiating from the cornea

The examination of the globe at this point should include an inspection of the bulbar conjunctiva, the position of the globe within the orbit, the presence of exophthalmus or enophthalmus and deformities or deviations of the globe itself. The tension of the globe should be estimated by palpation to detect glaucoma.

Examination of the sclera should reveal any evidence of scleritis, episcleritis or staphylomota.

In examining the cornea special illumination and magnification is desirable. This can best be carried out in a dark room. The examinee is seated with a lamp located two feet above and to one side of his head. The examiner then uses a strong convex spherical lens to concentrate the light rays on the examinee's eye. By the use of a second similar lens held between the eye of the examiner and the eye being examined an enlarged image may be obtained. Other means of getting good illumination or magnification is by the use of the binocular loupe which gives a true stereoscopic effect as well as magnification and the hand slit lamp which gives a good illumination through the transparent structures.

Defects to be looked for in the cornea are:

Abrasions	Leukoma
Depressions	Pannus
Ulcers	Interstitial keratitis
Nebula	Degenerative changes
Macula	Anterior synechiae

The importance of an opacity of the cornea depends to a great extent on its location centrally (where vision is interfered with) or peripherally and also whether or not there is a deformity of the curvature of the cornea causing astigmatism.

An examination of the iris should include the anterior chamber which may contain foreign material such as blood or pus. The color and texture of the iris should be noted and if "muddy" with irregular contracted pupil indicates the presence of iritis. Posterior synechia and persistent pupillary membranes should be noted.

Examination of the pupils should include a test for their reaction to light and accommodation. To test the reaction to light, the examinee should stand facing a good source of illumination. Both eyes are then shaded by the examiner's hands and one eye exposed to the light and the reaction noted (direct reaction). The other eye is tested for direct reaction, then each eye for consensual reaction. This latter is accomplished by shading both eyes, then exposing one eye to the light and noting the reaction of the shaded eye.

The reaction to accommodation is tested by observing whether or not the pupils contract when the gaze is suddenly shifted from an object in the distance to an object about 10 cm. away. Pupils that react to accommodation but not to light are known as Argyll Robertson pupils and are commonly found in syphilis of the central nervous system.

Unusually small pupils may be caused by central nervous system diseases, use of drugs locally or internally, a past iritis or syphilis.

Unusually large pupils may be caused by the use of drugs locally or internally, complete optic atrophy, glaucoma, cervical sympathetic irritation or trauma.

The examination of the lens and vitreous should not be done until the pupil has been dilated with a mydriatic in preparation for refraction. At that time the slit lamp, oblique illumination and the ophthalmoscope should be used in the dark room. When this is done opacities of the lens or lens capsule as a result of an old iritis or an existing cataract should be looked for. The vitreous should be viewed for the purpose of detecting any floating opacities which may sometimes be brought into view by having the candidate turn his head quickly back and forth just before the examination.

PRECAUTIONS. The examination must be done in a regular routine manner so that no phase of it is overlooked. Care must be exercised in determining defects which are correctable and those that are permanently disqualifying.

INTERPRETATION OF FINDINGS. Distinction should be made between defects considered as being of a temporary or of a permanent nature and notation made as to interference with function. A small chalazion, which is nonirritating and does not interfere with the normal function of the lid, may be disregarded. A hordeolum should be considered as a temporary disqualifying condition but the possibility of error of refraction being an etiologic factor should be considered. Corneal opacities which in no way interfere with vision may be disregarded. An inactive pterygium that does not encroach more than 1 mm. upon the cornea is of no significance but one that is definitely progressive, as evidenced by marked vascularity and thick elevated head, should temporarily disqualify and its removal is indicated even though it barely encroaches on the cornea. Any evident increase or decrease in intraocular tension should disqualify. Actual nystagmus should disqualify but nystagmoid movements which are noted only at extreme limits of the normal ocular movements are of no significance and must be differentiated from a true nystagmus. Any defect, disease or abnormality that actually materially interferes with the normal ocular function should disqualify. Evidence of past or present iritis should be given particular attention as frequently the etiologic factor may be found to be of rheumatic, syphilitic or focal infectious origin.

CENTRAL COLOR VISION

UNDERLYING PRINCIPLES. The term "color blind" is applied to those whose color perception is different from normal and in general more limited. Color blindness may be complete or incomplete, congenital or acquired. Acquired color blindness is rare and inasmuch as it is a complication of a grave intoxication or a serious ocular or neurologic disorder it need not concern us here. Congenital color blindness exists in about 8.5 to 10 per cent of the male adults in the United States and to a marked degree in 3.5 per cent.

For aviation all except minor degrees of color blindness should disqualify because of the necessity of:

1. The recognition of various luminous signals such as field boundary lights, obstruction lights, navigating lights and rocket signals. Distinctive colors are employed to signify various vital conditions and prompt comprehension of their portent is essential for efficient flying.

2. The recognition of colored flags and other daytime signaling devices.

3. Discriminating between varying conditions of terrain by the colors thereof in cases of forced landings.

Color blindness has been classified by Ishihara as follows:

I. Total color blindness (achromatopsia)
  A. Complete
  B. Incomplete
II. Red-green blindness (Daltonism)
  A. Red blindness (protanopsia)
    1. Complete
    2. Incomplete
  B. Green blindness (deuteranopsia)
    1. Complete
    2. Incomplete

Color perception is a sensation and depends on the vibration rate and length of light waves striking the retina. Normal color vision exists only around the fovea and as the periphery of the eye is approached color vision is gradually lost.

The Ishihara or the American Optical Company pseudoisochromatic abridged plates are among the most convenient to use in routine examinations. The test can be given quite rapidly and a permanent record of the result can be made on a mimeographed sheet by filling in the numbers as called by the examinee opposite the proper plate designation. The plates should be exhibited in irregular order and the plate designation should always be concelaed from the examinee. The test is now quite well known and the possibility that a poor color sense may be fortified by an excellent memory should be kept in mind. Much time is often saved if the examinee is told at the beginning of the test that he will be shown a series of colored plates some of which bear numerals, others which do not, and that he is not to waste time in looking for numerals that he does not see.

PROCEDURE. The demonstration plate is first shown to the applicant, so that he understands the test and then all of the remaining plates are shown at about 2 second intervals. The plates should be at right angles to the applicant's line of sight and 30 inches distant. He should not be permitted to trace the patterns with his finger or touch the test plates.

PRECAUTIONS. Care should be taken that the plates are neither soiled nor faded. A plea of color ignorance is never valid as it is not a factor in this type of test.

INTERPRETATION OF FINDINGS. More than five errors on the American Optical Company's abridged 14 plate test or its equivalent with other test sets should disqualify.

ACCOMMODATION

UNDERLYING PRINCIPLES. Accommodation is the process of increasing the dioptric power of the lens of the eye. In the normal human eye rays of light coming from infinity (for practical purposes 20 feet or 6 meters) are focused on the retina. Rays of light coming from a point closer than 20 feet are not parallel as they are from infinity but divergent and tend to come to a focus behind the retina and produce a blurred image. In order that divergent rays may be brought to a focus on the retina it is necessary that the dioptric system of the eye be increased and this is accomplished by contraction of the ciliary muscles which in turn causes an increased convexity, especially of the anterior surface, of the crystalline lens. This change in the dioptric system of the eye is accompanied by a convergence of the two eyes and a contraction of the pupils.

In the normal eye the amplitude of accommodation is the difference between the dioptric power of the eye when accommodation is completely relaxed and when it is exerted to its utmost. The amplitude of accommodation depends on the difference of the far point and the near point at which an object can be distinctly seen but it is customary to convert this distance into its dioptric equivalent which is the reciprocal of the focal distance in meters. Thus, in an emmetropic eye the far point is located at infinity and the dioptric value is zero. If the

TABLE 8

Accommodative Power—Minimum for Age

Age	Diopters	Age	Diopters
18	8.6	32	5.1
19	8.4	33	4.9
20	8.1	34	4.6
21	7.9	35	4.3
22	7.7	36	4.0
23	7.5	37	3.7
24	7.2	38	3.4
25	6.9	39	3.1
26	6.7	40	2.8
27	6.5	41	2.4
28	6.2	42	2.0
29	6.0	43	1.5
30	5.7	44	1.0
31	5.4	45	0.6

near point is at 10 cm. ($10/100$ meters) then the accommodation of the eye is 10 diopters.

Factors which may affect accommodation are:

Oculomotor paralysis	General debility
Iridiocyclitis	Atropine
Glaucoma	Homatropine
Ciliary spasm	Cocaine

PROCEDURE. Accommodation is measured by a Prince rule and an accommodation card. The zero point on the rule should be placed 15 mm. from the cornea. The rule is held horizontally and extends directly to the front, edge up. The card of test letters is held not more than 5 cm. in front of the examinee's right eye. His left is screened from sight of the letters by the flat side of the rule. The card of test letters is now carried slowly away from the eye and the examinee instructed to begin reading the letters aloud as soon as they become legible. The card is halted the instant that he begins to read the letters correctly and the point on the rule opposite the card is read off in diopters. This is the measure of accommodation of the right eye. To test the left eye the rule is changed to the left side of the nose and the above procedure repeated using a different line of letters. If a Prince rule is not available, diopter values can be computed by dividing the near point in inches into 40 or in centimeters into 100.

PRECAUTIONS. Care must be taken that the examinee is seated with his back to a window and the card is illuminated by good daylight.

The letters on the test card are read aloud. The same line of letters is not used for testing both eyes. The size of the letters on the card should be that of Jaeger type no. 1 (Snellen 0.5 or 50 cm.) and the Jaeger card may be used as test letters, provided the Jaeger no. 1 type only is used. The card is first held within 5 cm. from the eye and slowly carried away from it.

INTERPRETATION OF FINDINGS. A near point of accommodation less than the minimum for age as shown in table 8 should disqualify.

FIELD OF VISION

UNDERLYING PRINCIPLES. Normal visual acuity is well defined only in the foveal region. However, vision in the peripheral portion of the retina is of great importance especially in aviation and its function must be determined in all cases. Peripheral vision differs from central vision in two principal respects. In ordinary light central vision is the most acute whereas in low illumination peripheral vision is the most acute. The peripheral portion of the retina is remarkably sensitive to moving objects which acts as a valuable protective device in all forms of locomotion. In addition to perception of form the periphery of the retina is sensitive to color to a decreasing extent from the fovea outward.

PROCEDURE. The confrontation test is employed based upon a comparison of the monocular fields of vision of examiner and examinee, which, assuming their facial conformations to be alike, should be similar. The examiner faces the examinee at a distance of 2 feet with their heads on the same horizontal level. Each holds his head normally erect. The examinee closes his left eye with gentle pressure of the little finger and fixes his right eye upon the examiner's left eye. The latter closes his right eye and fixes his left upon the examinee's open eye. This fixation is continued throughout the test of the examinee's right eye. The examiner holds a plain white 1 cm. sphere on a wire handle overhead and in a plane midway between the two. He lowers the sphere until it is seen by the examinee. Assuming similar brow conformation, the examiner and the examinee should see the sphere simultaneously. The superotemporal, superonasal, nasal, inferonasal and inferior limits of the field of vision are similarly compared. To estimate the examinee's temporal and inferotemporal limits of vision, the sphere is held behind the plane of the examinee's eye and brought forward until visible; in these meridians the visual field normally extends to 90° or more. A similar technique is used to test the left eye.

If on the confrontation test the field of vision appears to be constricted to a degree not attributable to prominent nose or brow or if for any other reason the examiner suspects a visual field defect, a more exact perimetric study is made, employing the perimeter and tangent screen.

The average normal field for form is approximately as follows: temporally, 90° or more; supertemporally, 62°; superiorly, 52°; superonasally, 55°; nasally, 60°; inferonasally, 50°; inferiorly, 70°; and inferotemporally, 85°.

PRECAUTIONS. The test object should be attached to a slender black rod of such length that the examiner's hand is not seen by the examinee during the actual test. The eye being examined must not be permitted to shift fixation. Good illumination of the test object is essential and it should be kept clean and free from discoloration.

INTERPRETATION OF FINDINGS. The following should disqualify:

1. Contraction of the field for form of 15° or more in any meridian unless the contraction is the result of the anatomical conformation of the examinee's face.

2. Any demonstrable scotoma other than physiologic.

REFRACTION

UNDERLYING PRINCIPLES. Refraction of the eyes is done to determine whether they are emmetropic or ametropic and if the latter the kind and degree of ametropia. Inasmuch as many ametropic eyes may have normal visual acuity because of the action of the muscles of accommodation these muscles must be paralyzed and the eye tested in a state of rest.

PROCEDURE. The candidate is first examined for glaucoma. If the eyes are free from glaucoma the candidate is placed in a darkened room and one drop of 4 per cent homatropine instilled into each eye every 5 minutes until three drops have been instilled in each eye then wait for 1 hour. For the refraction the examinee is seated at 1 meter's distance from the examiner in a dark room and instructed to look at the forehead of the examiner. Refraction of each eye is then done as described below and the results verified by the use of the Snellen test charts.

Rays of light from a mirror are reflected into the eye being examined and as the mirror is tilted back and forth the direction of movement of the light as seen in the pupillary area is noted. Either a plane or concave mirror may be used but with a concave mirror all movements of the spot of light will be in a direction opposite to those when the plane mirror is used. The plane mirror is more commonly used and, henceforth, any further reference to the retinoscope will be to one with a plane mirror.

The simple retinoscope is a small circular mirror with a hole through the center or, instead, of a hole a minute portion of the "quicksilver" may be removed at the center through which the examiner observes the reflex in the eye of the patient. A handle is attached to one margin of the mirror. This retinoscope is used in conjunction with a source of light placed alongside the examinee. The light should be screened as with an opaque chimney which has an opening approximately 1 cm. in diameter on the side facing the examiner.

The electric retinoscope has its own source of illumination placed below the mirror which is set at an angle that reflects the rays of light at a right angle, *i.e.*, when the retinoscope is held vertically the rays of light pass forward from the mirror in a horizontal plane.

The purpose of retinoscopy is to neutralize as nearly as possible the movement of the illuminated area within the examinee's pupil by the interposition of suitable lenses. The illuminated area is called the "shadow" and when it has no movement with movements of the retinoscope, that is, neither "with" nor "against" it, is an indication that the emergent rays of light from the eye of the examinee are brought to a focus at the eye of the examiner. The lens which accomplishes this neutralization of movement is the lens which will correct the examinee's vision for the distance at which the retinoscope is used.

It is impractical to attempt retinoscopy at a distance of 6 meters. One meter is a convenient working distance and is the distance at which the retinoscope is ordinarily used. In addition, it is simpler to make the deduction for a working distance of 1 meter which is the focal distance of a lens of 1 diopter. Therefore, a correction of 1 diopter deduction must be made for the correction for infinity.

With the retinoscope held in this manner the examiner will obtain a reflection from the pupillary area of the examinee's eye which will vary in its appearance depending on the amount of illumination used and the refractive error. The periphery of the so-called "shadow" is to be ignored and only the central point noted. If it is circular it is an indication that there is no great difference in the two principal meridians and very little, if any, cylinder will be required in the correction. A band shaped reflex or "shadow" is indicative of a cylinder being required and the position of the band indicates the axis. Next, the retinoscope is gently tilted back and forth not more than 2 or 3 mm. or the reflex will be lost. The most common two principal meridians are at 90° and 180° but they may be at any axis and they are always at right angles to one another. The two axes are indicated by the direction in which the shadow moves when the mirror is tilted. If the mirror is tilted in the vertical meridian and the shadow slides off toward 45° we know that the two principal meridians are at 45° and 135°. The examiner notes the form of the illuminated area, its direction of movement in the different meridians, and the rate of movement. If the mirror is tilted vertically it is rotated about its horizontal axis and if it is tilted laterally it is rotated about its vertical axis. The axis about which the mirror is tilted indicates the axis of the cylinder required.

A movement of the illuminated area with the movement of the retinoscope indicates hyperopia, emmetropia or myopia of less than 1 diopter and a "with" movement is neutralized by a plus lens. A movement "against" the movement of the retinoscope indicates a myopia greater than 1 diopter. An "against" movement is neutralized by a minus lens. Spheres are used to neutralize the movement in the two principal meridians.

The exact point of neutralization is difficult to obtain and, consequently, the point of reversal is recorded. The weakest sphere that causes a reversal of the movement is recorded as the end point. Where a movement "against" is found it may be overcorrected by a minus lens that is obviously too high thus giving a movement "with," and then plus lenses added until the first movement against is noted. The value of the combination of the two lenses is noted and recorded.

From the findings that have been determined by retinoscopy the examiner has the data necessary for the subjective check. If the cycloplegic is complete and the retinoscopy done carefully the correction for infinity found by retinoscopy should obtain an acuity of 20/20 or better, *i.e.*, with accommodation paralyzed. There are several factors that necessitate a subjective test immediately after retinoscopy particularly the exact determination of axis of a cylinder as well as strengths of both sphere and cylinder. In the subjective examination the formula will be found to be somewhat less as to spherical value (less plus or more minus). The addition of a minus 1.00 sphere to the findings at 1 meter corrects for infinity; with the Snellen test types at 6 meters there must be brought into play either $\frac{1}{6}$ diopter of accommodation or $\frac{1}{6}$ diopter added to the formula. Consequently when the patient is fully corrected for a distance of 6 meters he may be slightly overcorrected for infinity. A $\frac{1}{4}$ diopter sphere is usually subtracted from the trial lens for 6 meters distance for actual correction for infinity.

A subjective examination should follow retinoscopy immediately. This is of particular value where there is a cylindrical correction and both the strength and axis of the cylinder should be checked carefully. Each eye should be checked separately of course. In checking the axis of the cylinders it is shifted quickly from one side to the other (about 15° to 20°) from that found by retinoscopy and the degree of rotation gradually decreased until maximum vision is obtained. The position of the axis of a cylinder may be confirmed by employing a stronger cylinder than that found by retinoscopy. This naturally will result in some blurring of vision but is of value as the axis may be shifted back and forth until all vertical lines appear as vertical to the patient and then the stronger cylinder may be replaced by one of the strength as found by retinoscopy.

PRECAUTIONS. Failure to allow accommodation to completely relax is a frequent cause of error.

INTERPRETATION OF FINDINGS. Hyperopia greater than 1.75 diopters in any meridian; myopia greater than 0.25 diopter in any meridian; or astigmatism greater than 0.75 diopter in any meridian should disqualify.

OPHTHALMOSCOPIC EXAMINATION

UNDERLYING PRINCIPLES. The ophthalmoscopic examination is conducted to detect any congenital or pathologic abnormality in the media, iris, disc, blood vessels or retina of the eye. This is accomplished by the use of an ophthalmoscope through which the examiner may obtain a view of the interior structures of the eye.

The essential features of an ophthalmoscope consist of a plane or concave mirror with a small aperture in its center. Rays from a source of light are reflected by the mirror through the pupil being examined. Various strength lenses may be rotated before the aperture in order to give a clear image to the examiner.

PROCEDURE. The ophthalmoscopic examination is accomplished more thoroughly through a widely dilated pupil and with the accommodation of the examinee relaxed. The reasons are quite obvious. In the examination of applicants the ophthalmoscopic examination should follow refraction routinely while the pupil is still widely dilated and accommodation paralyzed. The examiner should wear his own correction for error of refraction when using the ophthalmoscope. The ophthalmoscope should be used in a darkened room.

In the examination of the media the examiner standing or sitting on the right side of the examinee when examining the right eye holding the ophthalmoscope in his right hand before his right eye (in a manner similar to the retinoscope) approaches the examinee until the details of the iris pattern are seen

through the aperture. The pupillary area will appear as a dull red reflex. Where an opacity exists (in cornea, anterior chamber, lens or vitreous) it will appear dark against the red background—a bit darker than it actually is as it is seen partially by reflected light. The approximate location of the opacity may be determined by having the examinee shift his visual axis slightly from the right to the left or up and down; if the opacity is anterior to the pupillary plane it will move "with" the eye movement, if it is posterior to the pupillary plane it will move "against" the movement of the eye. The strength of the lens before the aperture may be increased or decreased as desired but with any change in the lens strength the position of the ophthalmoscope before the eye must be altered, *i.e.*, brought closer to the eye with a stronger and farther away with a weaker lens. The self illuminating types of ophthalmoscopes are usually equipped with a rheostat which controls the amount of illumination and faint and diffuse opacities may be seen more easily with illumination reduced. The examiner should always use his right eye in examining the right eye and left when examining the left eye of the examinee.

After the media has been inspected the fundus may be examined by the indirect method. The indirect method of ophthalmoscopy is not employed as frequently as it should be in many instances. It should be remembered that it has several distinct advantages, a greater portion of the fundus is seen at one time than by the direct method and it is particularly applicable in high degrees of ametropia and where there exist slight opacities in the media. A plus 4 to 8 diopter lens is rotated before the aperture of the ophthalmoscope and a plus 18 diopter lens (from the trial lens case) is held before the examinee's eye with the other hand. The examinee is directed to look directly forward. The plus 18 lens held between the thumb and forefinger of the examiner is held before the eye being observed and steadied by the other fingers resting against the examinee's forehead. The examiner then approaches the examinee until a view of the fundus is obtained. By shifting the position of the plus 18 lens the details may be brought more clearly into focus. Various portions of the

TABLE 9

Summary of Disqualifying Eye Measurements

Measurement	Disqualifying Finding
1. Inspection or cover test	Heterotropia
2. Visual acuity	Less than 20/20
3. Near vision	Less than 20/20
4. Depth perception	More than 30 mm. average error on Howard-Dolman or less than eight out of eight trials on Verhoeff
5. Heterophoria—6 meters	More than 10 diopters of exophoria, 5 diopters of exophoria, or 1 diopter of hyperphoria
6. Heterophoria—33 cm.	Exophoria of more than 12 diopters
7. Intraocular tension	Abnormal
8. Power of divergence	More than 15 or less than 3 diopters
9. Power of convergence	More than 70 mm.
10. Color vision	More than five errors in 14 plate test
11. Accommodation	Less than minimum for age, (see table 8)
12. Field of vision	More than 15° contraction or demonstrable scotomata
13. Red lens test	Diplopia or suppression less than 20 inches from center
14. Refraction (total in any one meridian)	More than 1.75 diopters hyperopia, 0.25 diopters myopia, or 0.75 diopters astigmatism
15. Night vision	Below normal

fundus may be brought into view by having the examinee shift his visual axis. The indirect method gives a magnification of three to five diameters and the image of the fundus is always seen inverted. It is to be remembered that the room must be darkened.

In the direct method of using the ophthalmoscope the examiner holds the instrument as near the examinee's eye as possible, using right eye for right eye and left for left. The strength of the lens to be used in the aperture will depend upon the dioptric power of the eye being examined and the ability of the examiner to relax his own accommodation (taking for granted he is wearing his correction for ametropia). If the examinee is emmetropic and the examiner can voluntarily relax his accommodation no lens will be required in the aperture. As a rule the beginner will have some difficulty in learning to relax his accommodation and at first will prefer to use a weak concave lens in the aperture. He should learn to use the ophthalmoscope with both eyes open and, in examining the fundus, should imagine that he is looking at a picture some distance away in order to relax his accommodation. In exploring the fundus the position of the ophthalmoscope may be shifted and the position of the examinee's visual axis changed to bring into

view different portions. By the direct method of ophthalmoscopy a magnification of about 14 diameters is obtained and the image is upright.

In the examination of the fundus by the direct method a change in the dioptric strength of the lens in the aperture of the ophthalmoscope of 3 diopters represents an approximate difference in depth of 1 mm. For example, with no lens in the aperture the level of the outer portion of the disc is clearly seen but the bottom of the physiologic cup is blurred; if a minus 3 diopter sphere in the aperture gives a sharp definition of the bottom of the cup we may conclude that it is 1 mm. below the level of the disc itself.

PRECAUTIONS. This examination should not be done until refraction is completed.

INTERPRETATION OF FINDINGS. Any abnormality that materially interferes with the normal ocular function should disqualify. Pathologic conditions of the retina and choroid are most frequently indicative of extraocular or systemic disease. Particular attention should be paid to the ophthalmoscopic examination of individuals past mid-life, where arteriosclerosis may be suspected or where there is a history of rheumatic or focal infections. Any abnormality found should be classified and described accurately and, where possible, substantiated by subjective findings (visual field defects, reduction in visual acuity, etc.). Lenticular opacities should be described as to appearance, location and interference with function.

NIGHT VISION

If there is a history of poor night vision or reason to suspect such a deficiency based on the family history, fundus changes or the applicant's behavior in dim light during the examination then the examinee's night vision should be measured by a night vision tester.

INTERPRETATION OF FINDINGS. A finding of night blindness should disqualify.

REFERENCES

(1) Standards of Medical Examination for Flying; Army Regulations No. 40-110 (Sept. 1956, reprint). Washington, D. C., Government Printing Office, 1952.
(2) Manual of the Medical Department, U. S. Navy (NAVMED P-117), Chapter 15, Physical examinations, Section V, Aviation (Feb. 1958, reprint). Washington, D. C., Government Printing Office, 1952.
(3) Medical Examination; Air Force Manual 160-1 (Aug. 1957, reprint). Washington, D. C., Government Printing Office, 1953.

4

CARDIOVASCULAR EXAMINATION

Harry G. Armstrong, M.D.

UNDERLYING PRINCIPLES. In aviation the cardiovascular system is important in relation to the maintenance of an adequate tissue metabolism in order that the different organs of the body may operate continuously at a high level of efficiency. Of special importance is the maintenance of an adequate cerebral circulation for the support of consciousness for it should be quite evident that those who are subject to such things as fainting without adequate cause, even in the absence of cardiovascular diseases, should be rejected for flying.

At the present time an electrocardiogram is not routinely required on the original examination for flying but becomes a part of the annual physical examination of most career pilots at age 35 to 40. It is believed by many authorities in aviation medicine that an electrocardiogram should be required on all original examinations for two reasons: one is that mild coronary and other heart disease is much more frequent in young men than formerly realized and which otherwise remained undetected; the second reason is that it is often extremely difficult to properly interpret an electrocardiogram in a trained pilot where there is only a moderate degree of deviation from the normal and there is no way of knowing whether this represents a cardiac defect or whether it is a normal finding in that individual.

Rhythms of the Heart. A sinus arrhythmia,

which is caused by vagal sensitivity, results in a waxing and waning of the heart rate with respiration and its presence can be ignored. It can be identified by having the examinee hold his breath which abolishes the arrhythmia.

Premature contractions are common. Following a normal beat, there will be another less loud beat ahead of time and usually with only one heart sound. This is followed by a pause, then the heart beats normally again. If the wrist is palpated the beat fails to come through at all or is felt very faintly. In the absence of other signs of cardiac disease they are of no significance. Acceleration of the heart rate will usually cause them to disappear. As the heart slows again they reappear. It is only when they are very frequent that they may be confused with any other arrhythmia.

Heart block or partial heart block may be found occasionally. In the absence of a graphic record partial heart block may be determined by listening with the stethoscope and feeling the radial artery at the same time. Not only is there an occasional beat missed at the wrist but there is no sound over the heart. In partial block the rate is usually slow, 40 to 50, and the dropped beat occurs at fairly regular intervals. In complete block the rate is very slow, 30 to 40, although the rhythm is regular.

Auricular fibrillation is an irregular irregularity made worse by exercise. The pulse is irregular both as to rate and volume. The ventricular rate may or may not exceed the pulse rate. The pulse rate may be slow particularly when the heart is under the effect of digitalis so the rate itself does not rule out fibrillation. Where a fibrillating heart is beating at a normal rate it is hard to detect the presence of fibrillation unless the examiner is accustomed to musical rhythm. If the applicant is exercised so as to speed up the heart rate the fibrillation is more easily detected.

Notation should be made as to the character of the pulse, whether or not equal on the two sides, whether of the Corrigan type such as is found in aortic insufficiency and, of course, as to its rhythm, volume and rate.

Vasomotor instability is indicated by a rapid pulse which accelerates unduly on change of posture or after exercise and is slow to return to normal. Other symptoms are breathlessness on slight exertion, headaches, lassitude, constipation, relaxed peripheral circulation, increased psychomotor tension and tremors.

Many candidates who are being examined for the first time are found to have pulse rates well over 100 without any evidence of cardiac disease. Such tachycardia should, of course, be regarded with suspicion but if careful examination brings out no signs of heart disease wait until the examination is practically complete and after frequent reassurance take the pulse again. Frequently it will be found to have slowed down. The rate following exercise is important and also the rapidity with which it returns to the pre-exercise rate. Some candidates should be requested to return the following day. Bearing in mind that the cardiac examiner is also the neuropsychiatrist these tachycardias must be considered as evidence of an emotional instability. Cyanosis, sweating, poor exercise response, tremor and other nervous signs accompanying a tachycardia should be considered disqualifying.

PROCEDURE. The heart should be examined by inspection, palpation, percussion, auscultation and when necessary by mensuration, the roentgen ray and the electrocardiograph.

Inspection. For this and the following steps in the examination of the heart the applicant should be stripped to the waist and have good natural daylight falling on his chest. From above downward, the candidate should be observed for: color of skin and mucous membrane; arcus senilis; pulsations of neck vessels; enlargement of the thyroid gland; pulsations in the suprasternal notches and in the intercostal spaces; deformities of the chest wall; precordial impulse; and pulsations in the hepatic, abdominal or dorsal region.

Palpation. Palpate first for the detection of thrills over the carotids (aortic stenosis), thyroid gland (exophthalmic goiter), suprasternal notch (aneurysm), apex of heart (mitral stenosis) and at the base (aortic stenosis). Use palms of hands in palpating and use light pressure as hard pressure may obliterate a thrill. To locate the maximum cardiac impulse have the applicant stoop and throw his shoulders slightly forward thus bringing the heart into the closest possible relation with the chest wall. Palpate both radials at the same time for equality in rate and volume. Run the finger along the artery to note any changes in its walls. Place the palm of one hand over the heart and fingers of the other over the radial to see if all ventricular contractions are transmitted. Palpate to determine the degree of tension or compressibility of the pulse, the finger nearest the patient's hand compressing the artery and preventing any impulse reaching the middle or palpating finger from the deep palmar arch. The middle finger is the palpating finger and the third is to make gradually increasing pressure upon the artery to obliterate the pulse wave and estimate its volume. The dorsalis pedis and posterior tibial arteries of both feet should also be palpated. In estimating pulse rates, the excitement of undergoing a physical examination must be considered. A rate of 50 or below should excite suspicion of heart block and be made the subject of further investigation. Rates of 90 or over should be investigated with a view to the exclusion of heart lesions, hyperthyroidism and nervous instability.

Percussion. Light mediate percussion should be used. The right and left cardiac borders as well as the diameter of the transverse arch may be determined by percussion. In doubtful cases where it is important to determine the actual cardiac boundaries roentgenograms should be taken and also cardiac mensuration done.

Mensuration. If there is any evidence that the heart is enlarged, this question should be investigated by fluoroscopy or teleoroentgenography. Films taken for the study of the lungs are not suitable for a cardiac estimation of heart size and for the latter purpose the film should be taken at a distance of 2 meters. The total transverse diameter of the heart is the most useful in estimating cardiac size and this should not exceed the normal by more than 10 per cent except in short, thick-set men a slightly greater figure may be regarded as normal provided no other signs of cardiovascular disease are present.

Even though an electrocardiogram is not required routinely, one should always be obtained on those examinees who do not respond satisfactorily to exercise, present a history of cardiac symptoms, have a sitting pulse under 50 or present any other suggestions of cardiac abnormality.

Auscultation. In auscultating the heart, the examiner should bear in mind the four points where the normal sounds of the heart are heard with maximum intensity, *viz.*:

1. Aortic area, second interspace to right of sternum. Here the second sound is distinct.
2. Tricuspid area at the junction of the fifth rib with the sternum. Here the first sound is distinct.
3. Pulmonic area, second interspace to left of sternum. Here the second sound is most distinct.
4. Mitral area, fifth interspace to left of sternum. Here the first sound is most clearly heard.

In doubtful cases the examiner should make inquiry into the use of alcohol or tobacco, overindulgence in athletics, habitual use of coal tar derivatives or narcotic drugs. He should also ascertain whether the applicant has had any of the following diseases: scarlet fever, chorea, diphtheria, measles, rheumatic fever, tonsillitis, influenza, typhoid fever, syphilis, gonorrhea, tuberculosis, chronic focal infections, etc.

Examination After Exercise. Examiners will use judgment and discretion in applying the exercise test to those who present evidence of incompetency of the heart. An exercise test is required in order to determine the efficiency of the heart muscle. Have the applicant hop 100 times on one foot, clearing the floor about 1 inch at each hop or engage in an equivalent exercise. Take pulse rate before exercise, immediately after completion of test and 2 minutes later. A heart muscle may be said to be efficient if the pulse rate taken 2 minutes after the above exercise approximates the initial rate.

Example of normal response:

Before exercise, 80

Immediately after, 120

Two minutes after, 84

Immediately after the exercise auscultation should be repeated with particular reference to the detection of murmurs previously inaudible.

In an otherwise normal heart a slight to moderate pulmonary systolic murmur, louder in the recumbent position and on expiration and largely or entirely abolished by deep inspiration, is the most common of all murmurs and may be considered physiologic. A faint systolic murmur localized at the aortic area without thrill and followed by a normal second sound may be considered normal but any aortic systolic murmur of moderate or greater intensity suggests disease and demands further study. A loud systolic murmur, usually with thrill, best heard at the left of the sternum in the third and fourth spaces, suggests a congenital ventricular septal defect. A faint systolic murmur at the apex, varying in intensity with forced respiration, heard less well in the erect position than when recumbent and unattended by cardiac enlargement or other evidence of heart disease, may be considered physiologic. However, a moderate to loud apical systolic murmur which persists in all phases of respiration and body positions and is intensified by exercise is evidence of abnormality of the heart. Any diastolic murmur heard over any portion of the cardiac area is evidence of disease. The presystolic or midiastolic murmur of mitral stenosis may be confined to a small area at, or just within, the cardiac apex and may be heard only in the recumbent position. It is heard best in the left lateral decubitus and is accentuated by exercise. A slight aortic diastolic murmur, on the other hand, may be heard only along the left sternal border with the patient erect or leaning slightly forward. This murmur is heard best at the end of forced expiration with the Bowles stethoscopic chest piece. Frequently, interpretation must be based on cumulative evidence or a number of relatively slight deviations from the normal. Note should be made of the degree of dyspnea and other symptoms of circulatory failure such as cyanosis.

Blood Pressure. The blood pressure is best obtained by using a standard mercurial manometer. The point at which the sound disappears is not the measure of diastolic pressure and the practice of using this method is inaccurate. Serious error may also be introduced in the blood pressure readings from the following sources:

1. Taking the blood pressure or pulse rate within 5 minutes after the person has assumed the position in which the blood pressure is taken.
2. When the individual is not completely relaxed physically.
3. Psychic disturbances produce extreme variations especially in the systolic readings and pulse rates.
4. Prolonged compression of the arm band may cause stasis of blood in the limb.
5. The bell of the stethoscope may be tilted, not directly over the brachial artery or applied with too much pressure.
6. The brachial artery may be abnormally small.
7. Considerable adiposity or edema of the limb prevents accurate reading.
8. Contraction of the muscles of the limb produces errors.
9. Contraction of the muscular wall of the brachial artery may produce an error of as much as 30 mm. of mercury in adults.

In addition to taking the pulse and blood pressure in the seated position and after exercise, the examinee should be given an orthostatic tolerance test. He should first be required to lie recumbent for 5 minutes after which his reclining pulse rate and blood pressure are taken. He is then required to stand for 3 minutes and his pulse rate and blood pressure again recorded. Abnormal findings on this test are to be rechecked morning and afternoon daily for 3 consecutive days before a final decision is reached. If there is a history of fainting the sensitivity of each carotid sinus will be tested separately with the subject in a sitting position.

INTERPRETATION OF FINDINGS. The following conditions should be considered disqualifying:

1. All valvular diseases of the heart.
2. Transverse heart diameter 10 per cent greater than that predicated by the Ungerleider-Clark formula.
3. A heart rate of 100 or over, when persistent after repeated examination in the recumbent position.
4. A heart rate of 50 or under, if the history, physical examination or an electrocardiogram shows the presence of A-V heart block or other evidence of heart disease.
5. Hypertension evidenced by an average systolic blood pressure of 150 mm. of mercury or more or an average diastolic blood pressure of 90 mm. or more if the candidate is over 35 years of age and an average systolic blood pressure of 140 mm. or more, or an average diastolic blood pressure of 90 mm. or more if the candidate is 35 years of age or under.
6. Arterial hypotension, when the systolic blood pressure is persistently less than 100 mm. of mercury in the sitting or standing position, unless a complete evaluation shows no cardiovascular or other abnormality.
7. Pericarditis, endocarditis, myocarditis or myocardial insufficiency.
8. Coronary heart disease including angina pectoris.
9. Congenital disease or deformity of the heart or great vessels.
10. Thrombophlebitis or chronic venous insufficiency resulting from thrombophlebitis of one or more extremities if there is a persistence of the thrombus or any evidence of circulatory obstruction.
11. Varicose veins if severe in degree or if symptomatic.
12. Other abnormalities of the peripheral vascular system including Raynaud's disease, thromboangitis obliterans and erythromelalgia.
13. Aneurysm.
14. Arteriosclerosis disproportionate to age.

15. Arrhythmia except sinus arrhythmia and occasional extrasystoles.

16. Evidence of vasomotor instability or neurocirculatory asthenia, if persistent on examination on at least 3 successive days.

17. Electrocardiographic evidence of paroxysmal tachycardia, auricular fibrillation, auricular flutter, incomplete A-V block with or without dropped beats, complete A-V block, bundle branch block and recent or remote coronary occlusion.

18. Unsatisfactory orthostatic tolerance test indicated by a pulse rate increase to more than 120 beats per minute (orthostatic tachycardia), blood pressure fall to values less than 90 mm. systolic or 60 mm. diastolic (orthostatic hypotension) or a display of faintness or syncope (orthostatic syncope).

19. Vasomotor instability indicated by a slowing of the pulse, fall in blood pressure or alteration in cerebral circulation resulting in fainting or syncope owing to digital pressure on either carotid sinus.

20. Inadequate arterial blood supply to any limb.

21. Arteritis of any artery.

22. Intermittent claudication if confirmed by peripheral vascular tests.

23. A history of paroxysmal tachycardia or paroxysmal circus rhythm (auricular fibrillation, auricular flutter) unless there has been a single brief attack attributable to a temporary cause, such as a generalized infection.

24. A history of rheumatic fever or chorea or recurrent migrating polyarthritis, chorea, carditis or other manifestations indicating rheumatic fever within 5 years.

25. Questionable or borderline cardiac findings. Unusual findings of any degree in the cardiovascular examination require a complete cardiac survey prior to final determination.

REFERENCES

(1) Standards of Medical Examination for Flying; Army Regulations No. 40-110 (Sept. 1956, reprint). Washington, D. C., Government Printing Office, 1952.

(2) Manual of the Medical Department, U. S. Navy (NAVMED P-117), Chapter 15, Physical examinations, Section V, Aviation (Feb. 1958, reprint). Washington, D. C.: Government Printing Office, 1952.

(3) Medical Examination. Air Force Manual 160-1 (Aug. 1957, reprint). Washington, D. C.: Government Printing Office, 1953.

5

EAR, NOSE AND THROAT EXAMINATION

Harry G. Armstrong, M.D.

In aviation the ear, nose and throat present certain problems which do not ordinarily occur in other occupations. For this reason these structures must not only be normal, in the ordinary sense of the word, but must exhibit certain favorable characteristics in order to avoid difficulty in flying. The special requirements and the method of examination of each of these systems will be discussed in order.

The Ear

UNDERLYING PRINCIPLES. The ear possesses two different functions, that of hearing and of equilibration. In the early days of aviation hearing acuity was of no particular value as long as it was sufficient to detect alterations in the sound of the motor. Inasmuch as the sound levels of the motors were of a high order no difficulty was experienced even in those individuals with a marked loss of hearing. Today, however, the almost universal use of aircraft radio makes it imperative that all pilots be essentially normal in this respect. A further consideration is the fact that many persons can hear the spoken or whispered voice but are deaf for tones which may be identical with certain radio signals. For this reason it is necessary that the hearing be tested not only by the voice but also by means of a good audiometer which covers a wide range of tones.

The principles upon which audiometers are designed and the methods of operation vary with the type of instrument used and this will not be discussed here. The important thing to be remembered is that inaccurate results will be obtained unless a properly standardized instrument is used.

Like those of hearing, our ideas of equilibration have changed radically from the early days of aviation. During World War I great emphasis was placed on turning tests and at one time those with normal reactions were rejected for training. At the present time two exactly opposite conditions are desirable with reference to the sensitivity of the vestibular mechanism. As an aid to spatial orientation in ordinary flying a sensitive vestibular mechanism is desirable. On the other hand in acrobatics, in rough air or during blind flight a relatively nonsensitive vestibular mechanism is desirable to prevent the occurrence of air sickness and vertigo. It has been adequately demonstrated in the latter situations that the ear not only fails to properly orient the pilot in space but that it invariably gives a false sensation leading to disorientation. Inasmuch as no vestibular apparatus can be both sensitive and nonsensitive at the same time it is necessary to accept the average normal as the best compromise.

In addition to the two functions of the ear mentioned above there is a third factor of importance in the examination of the ear based on an anatomical peculiarity. The middle ear is an air filled cavity communicating with the outside atmosphere through the eustachian tube, a potential tube, which opens at the posterior wall of the pharynx. This tube is normally closed except during swallowing or other similar physiologic acts. If, for any reason, this tube cannot be readily opened during a change in altitude either a relative vacuum or pressure with reference to the outside atmospheric pressure will develop in the middle ear leading to discomfort or pain and possibly temporary loss of hearing.

PROCEDURE. For examination of the external ear the candidate is seated with a source of light about 2 feet above and back of his head. The examiner inserts an ear speculum into the external auditory canal and notes the presence of wax or other obstructions. If wax is present it should be removed by an ear spud if external to the bend of the canal and by syringing with a soda solution if internal to the bend of the canal. The external canal is then examined throughout. Any permanent blocking of the canal or any diseased condition should be noted.

The tympanic membrane is then examined and the presence of the following looked for:

    Perforation
    Inflammation
    Healed scars
    Mastoidectomy
    Chronic otitis media
    Acute otitis media (in past 6 months)
    Retraction of drum membrane
    Thickening and dullness of drum membrane

The hearing should be tested both by the whispered voice and by the audiometer. Each ear should be tested separately. For the whispered voice test the examinee should be placed 15 feet from the examiner with the ear being tested facing the examiner. An assistant should occlude the ear not being tested by pressing the tragus firmly against the meatus. The examinee should be directed to repeat promptly the words heard. The examiner should use a whispered voice with the lungs in a state of complete exhalation to assure uniform output and the whisper should be plainly audible to the assistant. If the examinee cannot hear the words at 15 feet, the examiner should approach, foot by foot, using the same volume of whispered sound until the words are repeated correctly.

Include words in which vowel sounds predominate and words in which consonants predominate. The vowels represent for the most part low frequency. By using the numerals two and four as low frequency words and six and seven as high frequency words, for example, the examiner can judge the examinee's acuity throughout the conversational frequency range. Other words rich in low frequency sound are: door, floor, large, provide, Toledo, wear, murmur, under, mild, normal and eye. The ability to differentiate between such similar words as the following is a good test of high frequency perception: chess, chest, guess, guest, bathinet, bassinet, you, youth, true and truth. A variety of test words should be used until the examinee's auditory acuity is evident. Acuity of hearing should be expressed as a fraction; the numerator should be the distance in feet at which the whispered words are detected by the examinee and the denominator should be 15. Thus 15/15 indicates normal hearing and 10/15 indicates that the examinee hears at 10 feet what an individual with normal acuity would hear at 15 feet.

The audiometer is used to determine a candidate's ability to perceive pure tones over a wide frequency range. For each ear separately, thresholds should be determined for frequencies at 256 c.p.s., 512 c.p.s., 1024 c.p.s., 2048 c.p.s., 4096 c.p.s. and 8192 c.p.s. (Some audiometers use a round number progression: 250, 500, 1000, etc.)

Audiometer tests must be made under as quiet conditions as can be found because the norms for these instruments are based on tests conducted in quiet. A sound treated room should be used if available. Otherwise, a separate room should be used and the noise level should be considered sufficiently low if a person with known normal hearing can perceive each frequency at the zero level.

At each frequency, for each ear, the tone should be presented first at a level of 25 to 30 decibels as read on the hearing-loss dial. This intensity is sufficient to give a clear but not too loud signal for a normal ear. If the examinee indicates perception by pressing the signal button the tone is immediately interrupted. The hearing-loss dial is then turned to a 10 or 15 decibel lower level and the interrupter is released. If the examinee indicates perception the tone is again interrupted and presented at a lower level. At the level where the examinee no longer responds the tone is presented two or three times in quick succession. If he then perceives, that reading on the hearing-loss dial is recorded as the threshold. If the examinee does not respond the tone is interrupted and the intensity is raised by 5-decibel steps until perception again is indicated. The threshold is the point at which tone is just heard as it is raised from below the perceptible level. Minus values should be recorded as well as plus and zero values.

If the examinee does not hear a tone at the initial intensity level (25 or 30 decibels) the tone should be raised in steps of no more than 10 decibels either until it is perceived or until the maximum intensity for the audiometer is reached. If the examiner discovers impairment for one frequency he should not assume that the succeeding frequency also will be impaired. The next tone should be presented first at a normal intensity level. These precautions are required to prevent the presentation of painfully loud tones. Many persons who have a hearing impairment have also a very rapid recruitment of hearing, that is, once the tone is heard it becomes loud very rapidly as intensity is raised above the threshold.

EUSTACHIAN TUBE PATENCY. A drum membrane with normal light reflex and which is not retracted can be interpreted as indicating patency of the eustachian tube on the corresponding side. However, this should be verified in all cases by Valsalva's test or by the Politzer technique. In the former, with the tympanic membrane in view of the examiner, the examinee holds his nostrils closed with the finger of one hand. shuts his lips tightly and expires forcefully. Positive pressure is produced in the nasopharynx and causes air to enter the middle ear cavity if the Eustachian tube is patent. The examiner is able to note an increased convexity of the tympanic membrane, especially in Shrapnell's area and in the posterior superior quadrant of the drum.

Politzer's technique consists of placing one earpiece of the auscultation tube in the external auditory canal of the examinee and the other in the external auditory canal of the examiner. The tip of a Politzer bag is fitted with a nasal adapter which is seated in one anterior naris. The other side of the nose is closed firmly with a finger and as the examinee swallows or says "K," the Politzer bag is compressed. If the Eustachian tube is open, air will be heard to rush up the tube. An easier method, which does away with the need of synchronizing the compression of the Politzer bag with the examinee's closure of the nasopharynx, is that of "constant pressure inflation." Air under pressure of 1 p.s.i. is fed into one side of the nose through a nasal tip. The other side of the nose is occluded and the examinee swallows at will. The results are apparent from the sounds coming to the examiner through the ausculation tube or from observation of the ear drum.

EQUILIBRATION. *Self Balancing Test.* The applicant stands erect, without shoes, with heels and toes touching. He then flexes one knee backward to a right angle, being careful not to support it against the other leg (the leg will not be bent at the hip) and then closes his eyes and endeavors to maintain this position for 15 seconds. He will keep the foot still on which he is standing and not hop or move it about. The test is then repeated on the other foot. The applicant should be instructed that this is an equilibration test. There is no objection to his assisting balance by moving the bended leg back and forth or moving his arms. The finding "steady" will be reported when he remains stationary without moving appreciably; "fairly steady," when he moves slightly either the bended leg or his arms; "unsteady" when he manifestly has marked difficulty in maintaining his balance and "failed" when he is unable to maintain his position for 15 seconds one out of three trials on each foot.

In questionable cases based on the self balancing, Romberg or gait tests, or if there is any suggestion that the examinee is susceptible to motion sickness, he should be given the caloric test for vestibular function or, if the equipment is available, the Barany Chair Test.

Barany Chair Test. The examinee is seated in the chair and the pulse and blood pressure are taken. They are to be taken again as soon as the turning tests are completed. The candidates head is placed against the headrest at a forward angle of 30°. The examinee is then asked to fix his eyes on a distant point and the chair turned slowly from side to side in order to note whether or not spontaneous nystagmus is present. Then turn the examinee to the right, eyes closed, 10 times in exactly 20 seconds. The instant the chair is stopped click the stop watch; examinee opens his eyes and looks straight ahead at some distant point. There should occur a horizontal nystagmus to the left of 26 seconds' duration. Examinee then closes his eyes and is turned to the left; there should occur a horizontal nystagmus to the right of 26 seconds' duration. When practicable it is best to have one observer note the nystagmus rate and another the pulse and blood pressure.

PRECAUTIONS. In testing the hearing, it is to be remembered that in the presence of any extraneous noise that it is this noise level that is being measured and not the examinee's hearing.

INTERPRETATION OF FINDINGS. The following should disqualify:

1. Simple mastoidectomy until recovery is complete and the ear is functionally normal.

2. Radical mastoidectomy and modified radical mastoidectomy.

3. Any infectious process of the ear, including external otitis, until completely healed.

4. Deformities of the pinna if associated with tenderness which may be distracting when constant pressure is exerted, for instance, by head phones or helmet.

5. Postauricular fistula.

6. Atresia of the external auditory canal which prevents an adequate view of the tympanic membrane or effective therapeutic access to the entire auditory canal.

7. Perforation of the tympanic membrane.

8. Scars or calcareous plaques which involve more than 50 per cent of the pars tensa when associated with loss of auditory acuity or with immobility of the tympanic membrane.

9. Marked retraction of the tympanic membrane if mobility is limited or if associated with occlusion of the Eustachian tube.

10. Abnormal labyrinthine functions as evidenced by: (a) failure in all three balancing trials on either foot; (b) a nystagmus of less than 5 or more than 34 seconds duration after rotation or a variation in the two directions of more than 5 seconds; or (c) a marked increase in systolic pressure or fall in diastolic pressure after rotation.

11. Recurrent or persistent tinnitus.

12. History of attacks of vertigo with or without nausea, vomiting, deafness and tinnitus.

13. Any disease of the ear with subjective or objective evidence of residuals interfering with the auditory or vestibular functions.

14. Failure to pass the whispered voice test at 15 feet; more than a 15 decibel loss of hearing in either ear on the audiometer at frequencies of 256, 512, 1024 and 2048 or a loss greater than an average of 40 decibels for both ears at frequencies of 4096 and 8192; that is, a total for the four readings of more than 160.

THE NOSE AND SINUSES

UNDERLYING PRINCIPLES. Airplane pilots must have good ventilation of the lungs at all times and it is essential that there be no obstruction of the nasal passages. The nasal accessory sinuses, like the middle ear, are air filled cavities within the bony skull. They drain directly into the nose and, during changes of altitude, air must be free to enter or leave these cavities in order to avoid a relative vacuum or pressure developing in them.

Before examining the nose and sinuses inquiry should be made regarding a history of nasal obstructions, frequency of colds, sinusitis, allergic rhinitis, injuries, neoplasma, operations or a defective sense of smell. If a history of recurrent sinusitis or nasal allergy is obtained the sinuses should be studied by roentgen ray and, if indicated, skin tests and a cytologic study of the nasal secretions should be accomplished.

PROCEDURE. The candidate is seated before the examiner and the latter inspects each nasal passage with the aid of a nasal speculum and a source of good light. The following conditions should be looked for: acute or chronic infections, deviation of the nasal septum, polyps, tumors or other conditions causing irritation or obstruction. A perforated nasal septum should arouse a suspicion of syphilitic infection.

Following the examination of the nose proper the antrums and the frontal sinuses should be viewed in the dark room by transillumination for evidence of acute or chronic inflammation.

INTERPRETATION OF FINDINGS. The following findings should disqualify:

1. Allergic, hypertrophic or atrophic rhinitis.
2. Nasal polyps.
3. Anosmia, parosmia and paresthesia.
4. Deviation of nasal septum or septal spurs which result in 50 per cent or more obstruction of either airway or which interfere with drainage of the sinuses on either side.
5. Perforation of the nasal septum unless small, asymptomatic and the result of trauma.
6. Submucous resection until recovery is complete and the nose is functionally normal.
7. Any congenital or acquired lesion which interferes with the functions of the nose.

THE THROAT

UNDERLYING PRINCIPLES. The throat is important in aviation principally because the adenoids and tonsils may act as sources of obstruction or focal infections and because of the pharyngeal opening of the eustachian tubes which may be obstructed.

The tonsils if normal in size and not infected may be disregarded. If infected or hypertrophied to the extent that they encroach on the lumen of the throat they should be removed and the candidate reexamined at a later date.

Adenoids should not be present in amounts sufficient to obstruct nasal breathing in any degree or to have caused habitual mouth breathing.

The pharyngeal orifices of the eustachian tubes should be inspected to determine whether or not they are obstructed by tumors, growths, scar tissue, inflammatory processes or tonsillar tissue.

PROCEDURE. The candidate is seated in front of the examiner and by means of a tongue depressor and a good light a general inspection of the throat is made. A tonsillar pillar retractor is then used to pull the anterior pillars forward and laterally in order that the tonsils can be more fully exposed. Attempts should be made to express material from the tonsillar crypts by gentle pressure on the tonsil with a blunt instrument or a good tongue blade. Care should be taken that debris is not confused with pus.

To inspect the pharyngeal openings of the eustachian tubes a small pharyngeal mirror is placed just back of the soft palate where the openings can be seen high up and laterally on the posterior pharyngeal wall.

INTERPRETATION OF FINDINGS. Diseased or hypertrophied tonsils should be temporarily disqualifying until removed.

Adenoid tissue sufficient to cause mouth breathing or any degree of obstruction should disqualify.

Chronic inflammation or obstruction of the pharyngeal openings of the eustachian tubes should disqualify.

REFERENCES

(1) Standards of Medical Examination for Flying; Army Regulations No. 40-110 (Sept. 1956, reprint). Washington, D. C., Government Printing Office, 1952.
(2) Manual of the Medical Department, U. S. Navy (NAVMED P-117), Chapter 15, Physical examinations, Section V, Aviation (Feb. 1958, reprint). Washington, D. C.: Government Printing Office, 1952.
(3) Medical Examination. Air Force Manual 160-1 (Aug. 1957, reprint). Washington, D. C.: Government Printing Office, 1953.

6

NEUROPSYCHIC EXAMINATION

Harry G. Armstrong, M.D.

UNDERLYING PRINCIPLES. The neurologic examination in aviation generally follows the procedures used in clinical practice but in the former much greater significance is attached to such things as the sense of balance and neurocirculatory stability. The psychiatric examination is not only concerned with the presence or absence of frank or incipient psychoses or psychoneuroses but also with the question of the examinees probable tolerance to the stresses inherent in flying. In addition, personality traits must be evaluated in relation to the individuals probable success in flying training and performance in the air. This evaluation consists of a careful survey of the candidate's heredity, past personal history, past emotional experiences, temperment, volition and intelligence.

Although the neuropsychic examination should be conducted as a separate phase of the whole proceedings a great deal can be accomplished if the examinee is kept under close observation from the moment he enters the examiner's office. During the time the other systems of the body are being evaluated an alert examiner will frequently uncover neurologic defects and he is also afforded an excellent opportunity to do a personality and psychiatric evaluation which will be as least as fruitful as the conventional psychiatric interview which is normally not done until the rest of the examination has been completed.

As an aid to examiners in conducting this portion of the examination, there is outlined below the abnormal neuropsychic conditions that should be watched for, with a very brief reminder of some of the more prominent signs and symptoms that may appear in each instance. For a more thorough review of the diagnosis of neurologic and psychiatric entities, standard textbooks on these subjects should be consulted.

RÉSUMÉ OF COMMON ABNORMAL CONDITIONS. 1. *Anatomical Stigmata of Degeneration.* Cranial abnormalities in outline, capacity or dimensions; excessive development of the occipital protuberance and ridges, the frontal eminences and the mastoid processes; reduction of the facial angle; asymmetrical facial development; lower jaw disproportionately large and prognathic; hard palate sharply vaulted; dental arches narrowed or angular; teeth defective or misplaced; ears disproportionate in size or malformed; extreme refractive anomalies and strabismus; deviation of the nose; septal deformities; harelip; cleft palate; remnants of branchial clefts; spina bifida; sacral growths of hair; deep sternal furrows and concavities; disproportion between thorax and abdomen; upper and lower limbs disproportioned to each other or to the trunk; abnormality in size of hands or feet; tendency to left sided overdevelopment; deformities of the fingers; syndactyly; excessive length or shortness of the

66

fingers, undersize of the ring and little fingers; genitalia undeveloped; hyposadipas; epispadias; scrotal fissure; albinism; melanism; multiple naevi; defective development of hair and nails. The degenerate physique as a whole is often marked by diminished stature and inferior vigor; males may present the general body conformation of the opposite sex with sloping narrow shoulders, broad hips, excessive pectoral and pubic adipose deposits, with lack of masculine hirsute and muscular marking.

2. *Functional Stigmata of Degeneration.* Defective mental qualitites; moral delinquencies such as wilfulness, deceitfulness, indecency; stammering; urinary incontinence; regurgitation and rechewing of food; color blindness; perverted tastes and cravings leading to alcoholism and drug habits; sexual perversion.

3. *Chronic Alcoholism.* Suffused eyes; prominent superficial blood vessels of the nose and cheek; flabby, bloated face, reddened aspect of the face; red or pale purplish discoloration of mucous membrane of the pharynx and soft palate; muscular tremor of the protruded tongue end extended fingers; tremulous handwriting.

4. *Drug Habit.* Peculiar pallor and dryness of the skin; needle marks and scars on skin of arms and thighs; in opium users, contracted pupils; in users of cocaine, widely dilated pupils.

5. *Schizophrenia (Dementia Praecox).* Indifference, apathy, withdrawal from environment; ideas of reference and persecution; feelings that the mind is being tampered with or that thought is being controlled by hypnotic, spiritualistic or other mysterious agencies; hallucinations of hearing; bodily hallucinations, frequently of electrical or sexual character; meaningless smiles; in general, inappropriate emotional reaction and lack of connectedness in conversation. There may be sudden emotional or motor outbursts. The history of family life and of school, vocational and personal career will usually show erratic and more or less irrational conduct.

6. *Manic-depressive Insanity.* Mild depression, with or without feeling of inadequacy or mild manic states with exhilaration, tion, talkativeness and overactivity.

7 *Paresis (General Paralysis).* The diagnosis of paresis may be made when at the examination of the applicant a majority of the following signs and symptoms are demonstrated: Argyll-Robertson pupil or pupils; facial tremor; speech defect in test phrases and in the slurring or distortion of words in conversation; writing defects, consisting of omissions and the distortion of words; apathetic, depressed or euphoric mood. These applicants may show memory loss or discrepancies in relating facts of life; the knee jerks may be plus, minus or normal.

8. *Tabes Dorsalis (Locomotor Ataxia).* The diagnosis of this disease should be made when at the examination of the applicant several of the following signs and symptoms are present: Argyll-Robertson pupil or pupils; absent knee jerk; Romberg sign; ataxia of hands or legs (especially when the eyes are closed); hypotonia, anesthetic areas of the skin. The history of locomotor ataxia is usually that of slow progression, of failing sexual power and of pains in the legs or back which are often described as rheumatic.

9. *Cerebrospinal Syphilis.* The prominent diagnostic signs and symptoms are headaches, varying deep and superficial reflexes, pupillary changes, ptosis, ocular palsies, facial paresis. The mental state is normal, dull or apathetic. Comparative motor weakness may occur on one side of the body or in one extremity.

10. *Multiple Sclerosis.* The diagnosis of this disease rests upon the following signs and symptoms: intention tremor, nystagmus, absent abdominal reflexes, increased tendon reflexes and scanning speech. In cases of this kind the history obtained is not characteristic but sometimes there may be a history of urinary disturbance.

11. *Paraplegia.* The diagnosis of paraplegia from whatever cause will rest upon weakness of the lower extremities associated with lost or increased knee jerk. Babinski reflex, disturbances of the sphincters of the rectum and bladder and sometimes a girdle sensation. Sensory disturbance of the skin may or may not be present. Muscle sensibility may be diminished.

12. *Syringomyelia.* Syringomyelia is usually evidenced by more or less loss of power and atrophy of groups of muscles of one or more extremities with disturbance of the sen-

sations of the skin, more especially in the form of analgesias and diminution of the temperature sense. If in the upper dorsal cord, it is often associated with stooped shoulder posture; if in the lower dorsal, with weakness in one or both lower extremities.

13. *Muscular Atrophies and Dystrophies.* The signs and symptoms of muscular atrophies and dystrophies are atrophy of the small muscles of the hand and of the muscle groups of the shoulder, associated with fibrillary twitchings. The history of these defects rarely furnishes reliable data although it will usually be found that the applicant has shown evidences of awkwardness. There is never a history of pain in the affected muscles.

14. *Multiple Neuritis.* The chief manifestations are more or less pain in the course of the affected nerves, with tenderness over the trunks of the nerves and of the muscles supplied by them; lessened muscular power of varying degrees; more or less atrophy of muscles, with or without contraction; and evidences of trophic changes of the skin. The deep and superficial reflexes may be diminished or absent; the sphincters are not involved. A history of recent infectious disease or of exposure to poisons such as alcohol, lead or arsenic is of importance.

15. *Pathologic Personality Types.* There is a large group of individuals, who, though not necessarily suffering from epileptic, psychotic or psychoneurotic symptoms, alcoholic or drug addiction or feeble mindedness, in the strict sense of the term, are nevertheless incapable of attaining a satisfactory adjustment to the average environment of civilized society. This group is very heterogeneous, yet there is much evidence, in family and personal histories and in clinical manifestations to show that the various conditions comprised in it are in some way related to one another and to other neuropathic conditions. A study of the individual's past life readily shows a psychopathic make-up, if one exists. The types are: (a) inadequate personality, (b) paranoid personality, (c) schizoid personality, (d) cyclothymic personality, (e) antisocial and asocial personalities, and (f) sexual psychopathy.

15. *Psychoneuroses.* These conditions being functional, often with no objective signs, may escape notice. Such individuals show emotional disturbances, have hypochondriac complaints, undue fatigability and general nervous instability. The history of these conditions and of interference with progress in civil life is important.

16. *Epilepsy.* History of dizziness (without definite cause), many severe headaches and undue muscular tiring in early morning are often the result of epilepsy. Unexplained scars on tongue, chin or face give reason to suspect epilepsy. Epileptics often refer to seizures as "fainting fits" or "spells of dizziness."

17. *Head Injuries.* History of severe head injuries must be fully investigated and persistent symptoms referable to trauma should be carefully considered. Change in disposition or shifting occupational history, following accident, should be regarded as disqualifying.

18. *Peripheral Nerve Injuries.* These conditions are manifested by history of injury with localized motor or sensory disturbances. Any such case with an incomplete regeneration is a poor risk.

19. *Endocrinopathies.* Functional disturbances of ductless glands are very important in the production of neuropsychiatric conditions. The applicant should be closely observed for goiter, exophthalmos, tremors, tachycardia, acromegaly, myxedema, cretinism, smooth glossy skin, brittle nails, absent or unnatural hair distribution, faulty skeletal development, infantile or hypertrophied genitals, scanty and downy beard, female figure and vasomotor disturbances.

PERSONALITY TRAITS. In table 10 are given the personality traits which experience has shown to be favorable and those unfavorable for success in flying.

It is not expected that any candidate will exhibit all the best qualities to the exclusion of all the poor ones, but the preponderance toward a favorble or unfavorable, satisfactory or unsatisfactory, efficient or inefficient type, will lead to an estimation of the personality of the examinee.

PROCEDURE. The candidate should be subjected to a thorough, careful neuropsychic examination with special attention being given to the following points:

Neurologic. 1. Pupils. Carefully observe

TABLE 10
Personality Traits

Favorable	Unfavorable
1. Youth	Increased age
2. Single	Marriage, if wife opposes flying
3. Good family history	Poor family history (tuberculosis, nervous and mental diseases, etc.)
4. Few and only minor diseases—especially those with few complications and sequelae	Numerous and severe diseases of childhood—especially nervous diseases and defects. Severe infections in adult life and nervous or mental breakdowns
5. No operations, or serious injuries, or serious stresses	Operations—which may have left permanent impairment
6. High school and college education with good scholarship throughout	Inadequate education with poor scholarship
7. Unusual ability in athletics	Little or no athletic training
8. Evidence of manual dexterity, good at billiards, tennis, sailing, golf, violin, piano, horseback riding	No evidence of manual dexterity
9. Active, successful civil life	Sedentary civil occupation with poor or moderate success
10. Liking for normal amusements—no evidence of excesses and dissipations	No interest in amusements
11. Extreme moderation in use, or complete abstinence from tobacco and alcohol	Excesses in tobacco, alcohol and sexual life
12. Good appetite and digestion	Poor appetite and digestion
13. Normal sleep and absence of dreams, normal sexual tendencies	Insomnia and frequent unpleasant or terrifying dreams, especially of an occupational type, abnormal sexual tendencies or perversions
14. Good, active, sympathetic cooperation of family in all that pertains to flying	Anxiety concerning, or active opposition to flying, on part of family, especially mother and wife
15. Normal reactions throughout physical examination and satisfactory physical examination	Unsatisfactory physical examination
16. Personality showing: Temperament: cheerful, stable, self reliant, aggressive, modest, frank, fond of people, satisfied, punctilious, serious, good cooperation in work and in examination, good sportsmanship, moderate tension, enthusiastic, adaptable Intelligence: precise, penetrating, sharp, alert, resourceful Volition: energetic, quick, deliberate or moderately impulsive, controlled, good tenacity of purpose	Personality showing: Temperament: Depressed, unstable, submissive, pacific, vain, withholding, secretive, loquacious, likes to be alone, hypercritical of conditions, careless, frivolous, poor cooperation, irritable, poor sportsmanship (under adverse circumstances querulous and complaining), exceedingly high tension, lost enthusiasm Intelligence: Vague, superficial, dull, hesitant, without initiative, untrained Volition: Sluggish, slow, recklessly impulsive, restless, poor tenacity of purpose

size, equality or inequality and outline. As to size, whether normal, miotic or mydriatic; in comparison whether equal or unequal; and as to outline, whether round, or if otherwise, whether the result of disease or operation. Reaction to light and accommodation to be observed with utmost care; particularly whether the reaction to light is normal, slowed, diminished or lost. Any pupillary abnormalities to be interpreted as significant for leutic infection and requiring clinical as well as serologic proof of the absence of such infection.

2. Station. a. Romberg. Examinee to

stand with knees pressed back, arms hanging loosely, eyes closed and inner margins of feet in apposition. Interpretation of abnormalities to be clearly stated. b. Modified Romberg. The examinee stands with one foot in front of the other, heel touching toe, arms hanging loosely, eyes closed. The normal may exhibit slight unsteadiness. This test is particularly useful in connection with interpretation of unsteadiness on the self-balancing test.

3. Gait. To be carefully observed as examinee with eyes open walks forward and backward along chalk line or crack in floor, and repeats with eyes closed; walks in circle with eyes open and repeats with eyes closed; walks heel to toe with eyes open and repeats with eyes closed. Interpretation of abnormalities to be clearly stated.

4. Deep Tendon Reflexes. Classified as absent (0); diminished (−); normal (+); hyperactive (++); exaggerated (+++); unequal. Care should be exercised in making these distinctions. Reflexes should not be recorded as absent or diminished without using the so-called re-enforcement aids in the test. Mere briskness does not necessarily express hyperactivity. Abnormalities are to be interpreted as significant for neurocirculatory asthenia, psychoneurotic disorders, lues, organic diseases of the cord, etc.; the genesis, therefore, to be clearly established.

5. Tic. Note part or parts affected and as to degree, whether or not tending to incapacitate or make conspicuous. The presence of tics may be associated with other evidences of nervous instability.

6. Tremor. Note whether fibrillary, fine or coarse, part or parts affected and whether of the intention or continuous type. Standing with hands outstretched and fingers separated and slightly flexed, a marked tremor of the fingers may be indicative of some functional nervous disturbance and a pronounced tremor, if associated with marked unsteadiness in the self balancing test, should be disqualifying. In the case of marked tremor look also for other evidences of nervous instability and evidences of thyroid disease. Slight or fine tremors may be disregarded.

7. Other Motor Disturbances. If abnormalities are observed, note type, part or parts affected, cause and degree of functional disability.

8. Psychomotor Tension. To be interpreted in terms of ability or inability to voluntarily relax. The examinee rests his forearm, with utmost relaxation, in palm of examiner's hand. With the unexpected removal of the examiner's supporting hand, examinee's arm does or does not drop naturally to his side. Increased tension may be present in organic nervous disease and may be indicative of psychoneurotic coloring.

9. Peripheral Circulation. Examine for flushing, mottling and cyanosis of face, trunk and extremities. Question concerning the presence of localized sweating (axillae and palms) and cold extremities. Cold blue hands may be indicative of neurocirculatory asthenia, constitutional psychopathic inferiority or dementia praecox types.

Psychic. 1. Procedure in Making Personality Studies. There must be quiet, privacy and care that the surroundings make for such relaxation and intimacy as will win the complete confidence of the subject and secure full cooperation. The examiner must be on the alert and the subject at ease, never being permitted to feel that his innermost self is under minutest scrutiny and his entire life history and ancestry under review. It must be borne in mind that while the scheme itself is formal, it concerns an investigation which must be conducted informally. Interrogations should be in the accusative, rather than in the indicative form; that is, "How much do you drink?" Not, "Do you ever use liquor?"

2. Family History. Inquire for psychotic and psychoneurotic manifestations in the record, and if such be found, examine carefully for degenerative modifications expressing transmitted taint. However, if the candidate be found normal, then the isolated occurrence of mental disturbances in ancestors will be deemed negligible; the examiner should not overvalue the influence of direct heredity but duly weight all considerations pertinent to the situation.

3. Personal History. The personal history should be searched on the points mentioned below in order to develop and complete the balance of the examination. The infantile period should be searched for evidences of retardation, and particular study made of the factors which obtained during the formative years and determined the personality trend.

To this end study should be made of the family life, play life, sex life, school and college life, trends of thought, athletic tendencies, degree of manual dexterity, personal and family attitude toward flying, reactions concerning the ordinary stresses of life and particularly the probable reactions under the special stresses incident to flying.

The moderate use of tobacco and alcohol is permissible but excessive use requires examination for deleterious effects and determination of significance as a nervous habit or as an indication of nervous instability. Not only drug addiction but the habitual use of medicines for ailments, either mild or severe, fancied or real, should be considered as a very undesirable trait.

A most searching investigation should be made of an examinee's life record, not only for a history of epileptic seizures, either major or minor, but also for those equivalents establishing an epileptic background. Of these latter enuresis, headaches, dizziness, fainting, stammering, somnambulism, pavor nocturnus and migraine are particularly to be considered significant. An occasional mild headache can be deemed negligible but frequent or migraine types should be considered as a definite bar to aviation.

A history of dizziness or fainting is important, or not, depending on whether there is a reasonable explanation for their occurrence. For example, fainting from severe pain following a serious injury or dizziness from excessive whirling is normal and not pathologic.

If stammering has been found to have existed in the candidate during childhood but has been overcome and does not show during anger or excitement it may be disregarded except that such a history calls for a searching examination of the entire life history for related factors which together may furnish proof of a psychopathic constitution.

Somnambulism, pavor nocturnus and insomnia are definite evidence of a temporary or permanent deeply seated functional nervous disturbance and should be considered as evidence of unfitness for flying training.

The candidate's memory should closely approximate a hypothetical norm and knowledge concerning it will develop as the examination proceeds. Defects of memory may be uncovered. Periods of amnesia are most apt to follow injuries, particularly head injuries and certain illnesses. Given a history of these the examiner should search carefully for a history of complete amnesia or "islets of memory."

Temperament is a complex factor very difficult of definition; however, it should be considered as the fundamental and prevailing life mood peculiar to the individual's personality as to irritability and apathy, elation and depression. Concerning phobias, care should be exercised in differentiating between mere aversion and dislike and morbid unreasonable fear or dread. When the latter motivates conduct in directions interpreted as odd and peculiar it expresses fundamental instability. Anxiety trends, deeply seated worries, irritability and apathy or elation and depression require careful study with a view to determining whether they are within the range of normal or are abnormal.

Sensory disturbances are founded on either a hysterical or organic basis and if there is any appreciable interference with function the type and amount should be determined.

In the study of the candidate a review should be made of his total experience. Every candidate will be found to have met with situation difficulties requiring solution. The extent and type of these difficulties will, of course, vary with the individual. The manner in which he has met worries, handled conflicts and sublimated complexes is an indication of the degree to which he can adjust himself to his environment.

Predetermination of anyone's ability to qualify as a pilot is difficult. The study of his adjustment to reality will aid in the assessment of his probable adaptability for aeronautics. The physical examination and personality study should establish a fitness, stability and endowment making for probable successful training and performance in the air. The assessment of his adaptability should be expressed as satisfactory or unsatisfactory. If the latter, the reasons therefore should be clearly stated. No one individual will show all favorable traits and no unfavorable ones but a preponderance of one or the other should determine qualification or disqualification. Such a determination in the Military Services is referred to as an adaptability rating for military aeronautics

(ARMA) and is based on a perfect score of 200 with 160 as the minimum for a satisfactory rating.

INTERPRETATION OF FINDINGS. The following conditions should disqualify.

Neurologic.

1. Neurosyphilis of any form (general paresis, tabes dorsalis or meningovascular syphilis).

2. Degeneration disorders (multiple sclerosis, encephalomyelitis, cerebellar and Friedreich's ataxia, athetoses, Huntington's chorea, muscular atrophies, dystrophies of any type and cerebral arteriosclerosis).

3. Residuals of poliomyelitis, meningitis, abscesses, paralysis agitans, postencephalitic syndromes and Sydenham's chorea.

4. Paroxysmal convulsive disorders and disturbances of consciousness (grand mal, petit mal, psychomotor attacks, syncope and narcolepsy).

5. Migraine.

6. Tics, spasmodic torticollis, spasms, brain and spinal cord tumors, cerebrovascular disease, congenital malformations, including spina bifida if associated with neurologic manifestations, meningocele and Meniere's disease.

7. A history of nonsyphilitic meningitis or meningismus unless it occurred at least 1 year before the examination and the examinee has been without residuals or sequelae for the period beginning 1 month following recovery from the acute phase of the disease.

8. A history of encephalitis accompanying acute exanthemata unless it occurred at least 10 years before the examination and the examinee has been without residuals or sequelae for the period beginning 6 months following recovery from the acute phase of the disease.

9. Atrophy of an isolated muscle or muscle group, unless: (a) slight; (b) nonprogressive; (c) does not interfere with prolonged normal function in any practical manner as determined by careful history and examination; or (d) had its onset at least 5 years before the examination.

10. A history of polyneuritis unless nonincapacitating without present symptoms and unless it occurred at least 5 years prior to the examination.

11. Isolated neuritis which occurred within the 5 years preceding the examination unless the cause is definitely determined and found to be no basis for future concern and examination reveals no, or only minimal, residuals considered inconsequential.

12. Poliomyelitis unless it occurred 1 year prior to the date of the examination and shows no residuals. Residuals will be evaluated as in 9 above.

13. Craniocerebral injury that produces loss of consciousness, amnesia, focal neurologic signs, fracture or penetration of the skull, prolonged headache, change in personality or combinations thereof with: (a) unconsciousness unless shorter than 2 hours in duration and, if multiple, episodes shorter than 2 hours combined duration; (b) amnesia unless shorter than 4 hours in duration; (c) focal neurologic signs, such as paralysis, weakness, disturbance of sensation or convulsive seizure; (d) post-traumatic headaches unless shorter than 3 months in duration; (e) change in personality or deterioration of intellect; (f) depressed fracture or absence of bony substance of the skull; (g) craniotomy. Examinees with a history of a single brief period of unconsciousness or amnesia (less than 15 minutes) as a result of head injury are acceptable but circumstances may indicate need for a complete neurologic survey or delay of 1 year from the time of the accident to permit questionable sequelae to develop or to recede. Subjects with unconsciousness or amnesia of more than 15 minutes duration should not be accepted within a year of the injury and then only after a detailed neurologic study.

14. A history of fractured skull, unless unaccompanied by disqualifying signs as listed above for craniocerebral injury and unless without sequelae for 1 year with negative physical and laboratory data at the time of the examination.

15. Any other current organic disease of the central or peripheral nervous system or definite history thereof.

Psychic.

1. A psychoses of any type of any degree or a history thereof.

2. Anxiety, dissociative, phobic, conversion, somatization, obsessive—compulsive, hypochrondrical or neurotic depressive reac-

tions of sufficient degree to materially motivate or influence general behavior.

3. Pathologic or psychopathic personalities.

4. Chronic alcoholism or drug addiction.

5. Psychoneurotic disorders.

6. Major abnormalities of mood.

7. Below normal intelligence.

8. Schizoid personality.

9. Two or more instances of major psychoses in the immediate family.

10. Two or more instances of somnambulism after the age of 10 years or somnambulism within the year preceding the examination.

11. Severe, repeated pavor nocturnus persistent up to the time of examination.

12. Severe or prolonged insomnia.

13. Repeated enuresis past the age of 10 years.

14. Tic, severe habit spasm or marked mannerism.

15. Stammering or stuttering which has its onset after the age of 10 years or persists beyond the age of 10 years.

16. Epilepsy or convulsions of any type other than during acute febrile illnesses of childhood.

17. Migraine or migrainous type of head-ache if it occurs repeatedly and is of sufficient intensity to incapacitate the examinee temporarily for his usual pursuits or to require regular medication.

18. Psychogenic amnesia.

19. Fainting, except when (a) caused by pain following a severe injury; (b) during convalescence from an acute infection or severe illness; or (c) from severe loss of blood. Failure to maintain the stream of consciousness for unknown reasons or for such reasons as minor trauma or epilepsy is regarded as incompatible with qualification for flying duty.

20. Vasomotor instability.

21. History of attempted suicide.

REFERENCES

(1) Standards of Medical Examination for Flying; Army Regulations No. 40-110 (Sept. 1956, reprint). Washington, D. C., Government Printing Office, 1952.

(2) Manual of the Medical Department, U. S. Navy (NAVMED P-117), Chapter 15, Physical examinations, Section V, Aviation (Feb. 1958, reprint). Washington, D. C., Government Printing Office, 1952.

(3) Medical Examination; Air Force Manual 160-1 (Aug. 1957, reprint). Washington, D. C., Government Printing Office, 1953.

7

PSYCHOLOGIC METHODS
OF AIRCREW SELECTION

S. B. Sells, Ph.D.

Psychologic test batteries for selection and classification of aircrew personnel are used routinely today by most military and civilian aviation organizations. For the most part the content and basic pattern of such tests is essentially the same as those developed during World War II by the Aviation Psychology Program of the U. S. Army Air Forces (1). The research and development which produced these tests has had a profound influence, not only on the personnel administration of military and civil aviation, but also on the scientific approach to personnel selection in industry.

A detailed understanding of the psychologic basis for selection of pilots, observers and other members of the aircrew is useful to the flight surgeon and airline medical director. As the famous physician, Sir William Osler, once remarked, "It is important not only to know what disease the patient has, but also what patient has the disease." In this respect the patterns of abilities, interests and temperament traits which uniquely characterize men capable of completing flight training and whose careers primarily involve flying, give invaluable insights concerning them to the physicians responsible for their health and maintenance. Knowledge of the capabilities and limitations of the selection program and understanding of the implications of various patterns of scores on the various tests further enables

the physician to apply this general background to the individual case.

It is desirable that the flight surgeon or medical director be sophisticated and knowledgeable about the psychologic selection of aircrew personnel. Physical and psychologic selection are integral and interrelated aspects of assessment of the whole man and should be administered as an integrated total program. This policy is followed by the U. S. Navy and also by several airlines which have placed responsibility for the total aircrew selection program in the Medical Department and by several organizations which have made other comparable arrangements. In the U. S. Air Force physical standards and selection are under medical auspices but the operation of the total selection program is under the direction of Personnel and is administered by the Training Command.

This discussion of psychologic methods of aircrew selection is addressed to physicians, military and civilian, who are responsible for maintaining the effectiveness of flying personnel. It covers the content of aircrew selection batteries and the relevance of various components to flying success. In order to provide a meaningful context for these topics, some general principles of the nature and purposes of selection and classification are first outlined. The treatment includes the impact of jet and high performance aircraft on selection and looks ahead briefly to the era of rocket engines and space craft.

Nature and Purpose of Selection

The Relation of Selection to Over-all Personnel Management. Personnel selection is an important phase of organizational staffing, which is in turn a major function of personnel management. The total staffing function consists of a number of interrelated phases which are the responsibility of management and operating officials. These include the establishment of personnel requirements; the definition of various jobs in terms of duties to be performed, level of responsibility and pay scales; recruiting, selecting, hiring, training and assigning of personnel to utilizing units for duty. Physicians and psychologists may participate in most of these phases by performing research, consulting, and in the case of selection, by administering and evaluating examinations. In some cases psychologists have been attached to the medical service, in others to personnel management and in still others have functioned independently.

The net result of the staffing process is to determine the qualifications of personnel employed and, therefore, the potentiality for success of individual members and, indirectly, of the total organization. However, successful performance is only partly accounted for by selection and other phases of staffing. It depends also on the adequacy of utilization of personnel. This involves the nature of the work environment provided and is reflected in the equipment, work space, work schedules, communication of information, provision of job satisfactions and other aspects defined by the terms group dynamics, management and leadership. Utilization thus determines the extent to which the potentiality acquired through staffing may be realized in action.

Selection Instruments and Selection Standards. The particular task of selection is to assess the qualifications of candidates for specified jobs or job categories with reference to established standards of acceptance. Selection tests, prerequisites and nontest predictors (e.g., education, marital status, age, height, weight, absence of police record, etc.) are used to measure (or assess) candidates in terms of their relative prognosis for job success. Selection standards are qualifying scores on tests and other predictors. Standards are set by administrative authorities, usually with reference to three considerations: (1) minimum qualification level to perform the job safely, proficiently and (if desired) for a minimum period of time without impairment; (2) the number of employees required at the time; and (3) the number of applicants available from whom to select. Standards, therefore, tend to fluctuate with supply and demand and have even been set aside on occasion for administrative (staffing) reasons.

Utility of Selection Depends on Validity. The utility of a selection program depends on the accuracy with which it predicts job success. Tests which predict measures of success accurately are valid. The higher the validity of predictors, the more accurately can standards based on them be set. Predictors which fail to differentiate successful from unsuccessful performance have no value in selection. The history of aircrew selection has witnessed the abandonment of many promising and "authoritative" tests which proved to be worthless for selection when evaluated on the basis of predictive validity.

Some Common Misconceptions About the Functions of Selection. Although the purpose of selection is to contribute to individual and group performance effectiveness, selection is not a universal panacea for all organizational problems, as some persons imagine. A few of the more common misconceptions are reviewed in the hope that exposure may speed their correction:

1. *That Selection (Staffing) and Leadership (Utilization) are Alternative Approaches to Achievement of Organizational Effectiveness.* In fact they are complementary functions. Before attempting to solve a problem by raising selection standards it should be ascertained that substandard performance is the result of personnel shortcomings and not environmental difficulties. For example, a high failure rate in pilot training might reflect poor aptitude among students, which may be remediable by selection. However, it might also reflect other factors, such as unrest caused by rumors of curtailment of the training program; and if so, would require quite different corrective action.

Another example is taken from Fitts and Jones' study in which "confusion of two controls" was reported as one of the most frequent errors made by airline and military pilots (2). This is a problem which could be greatly reduced by application of well established principles of cockpit design and arrangement. Such errors may well reflect confusion resulting from pilots having to alternate frequently between different aircraft with different arrangements of controls, as well as from individual variations in alertness and attention.

The most effective personnel management policy, of course, is to obtain the highest qualifications of personnel through optimal staffing (including selection) and then to strive for the utmost of their potential performance through a thorough program of effective utilization. Such a thorough program includes human engineering of equipment as well as the "enlightened self interest" of effective leadership and management.

2. *That the Best Organization is Made Up of the "Best Men."* The problem here concerns the definition of "best," which is ambiguous. Experience has taught that people can be "overplaced" as well as "underplaced." The latter difficulty is more common inasmuch as inadequate ability to perform is more readily observed. However, highly trained, intelligent persons often become bored with work that is too "easy," unchallenging or uninteresting for them and this may result in poor performance, behavior problems and even resignation. The following observation by McFarland (3) with reference to this problem in selection of airline pilots is relevant:

"While no cutoff point for the higher levels of intelligence has been formulated or even proposed, serious attention should be given to this question since it has been found that individuals with very high IQ's are apt to be poor at routine work. Several follow-up case studies of pilots . . . revealed that very superior mental ability, particularly when coupled with very strong nonaviation interests, tended to result in the resignation of a pilot in order to enter professional fields. Since the tests should predict not only success but also occupational stability, an upper limit of intelligence might also be desirable" (p. 61).

As a general principle in personnel selection "best" means "best fit" and not necessarily "having the highest score." Hence, the most effective personnel placement would be to put "round pegs in round holes;" that is, to assign individuals to jobs whose patterns of abilities and interests are compatible with the demands of the jobs. This implies that for routine and less demanding jobs, individuals who would be considered best fit would be those whose scores and qualifications are in line with the mediocrity required.

The concept of best fit actually implies a pattern of abilities determined by job requirements. Such patterns will be seen to vary in the importance attributed to various component factors, even within the relatively homogeneous family of jobs constituting an aircrew. Effective selection and placement (staffing) contribute to the broader goals of conservation of manpower and elimination of waste by enabling the optimal utilization of all available talents.

3. *That as Long as Selection Tests are Valid, Selection Will be Successful.* Validity is, of course, a basic requirement. But valid selection tests will be successful only if other necessary conditions are met. These include the recruitment of a sufficient number of qualified applicants and maintenance of all required conditions of testing and processing of results. But above all, it is necessary that the standards employed be high enough to reject unqualified applicants. If standards are relaxed, for instance, because of manpower requirements, as has happened at times in selection of military aircrew after World War II, the increased attrition rate and poor quality of trainees should not be assessed against the validity of the selection battery.

NECESSARY CONDITIONS FOR SUCCESSFUL SELECTION. Even when it is determined that a selection program is necessary to assure required qualifications of personnel, certain basic conditions must exist. First, the specific qualifications relevant to job success must be identified; and second, tests and other predictors must be developed and validated to measure these qualifications. Research methods for the development of a selection program, including job analysis, measurement of performance, test development and validation are discussed below. It is also necessary that the job relevant characteristics exist in varying amounts among the population available for testing and that part of that population be qualified. This point illustrates the dependence of selection on other phases of the staffing process, particularly pay scales, recruiting and employment policies. The results achieved with a selection program are usually greatest when (1) validity is high, (2) standards reflect reasonable levels of qualification, (3) the number of applicants exceeds the number of employees required and (4) a sufficient proportion of the applicants is qualified. However, even if the number of applicants is low, there may still be an advantage in testing to identify those whose qualifications are below minimum standards.

LOGISTICS OF SELECTION. In general, the number of qualified applicants will tend to vary inversely with the stringency of selection standards, *i.e.*, the higher the standards the fewer the qualified applicants available. Consequently, when standards are raised there must be an increased number of applicants available for screening to obtain any desired number of selectees. At the same time the number of rejections will be greater. However, with higher standards the proportion of successful selectees also tends to increase, in relation to the validity of the battery. The administrative and economic consequences of these relationships are important and must be taken into consideration in adopting or revising standards. As a rule, higher entrance standards imply lower training attrition and training costs and better performance, but they require a greater supply of qualified candidates and higher costs of recruiting, testing and administration of the selection program. The personnel administrator must weigh the costs consequent to each decision concerning standards against the expected results in operation effectiveness. Figure 16 illustrates these principles in terms of three standards of acceptance of pilot candidates in the United States Air Force.

SELECTION AND CLASSIFICATION. In the foregoing discussion the term selection has been used in a general sense (as in common usage) to describe the methods of assessing the qualifications of applicants for particular categories of jobs. A distinction has for some time been recognized among selection re-

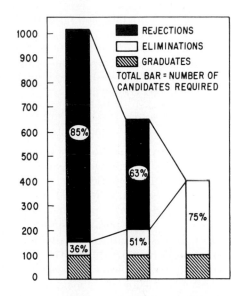

	STANDARD 1	STANDARD 2	STANDARD 3
CANDIDATES REQ.	1020	553	397
REJECTION RATE	85%	63%	0
ATTRITION RATE	36%	51%	75%
NO. OF GRADUATES	100	100	100

FIG. 16. Comparison of three standards for pilot candidates on U. S. Air Force aircrew selection battery. The chart illustrates that higher entrance standards provide lower training costs (reduced attrition rates) but require more qualified candidates (and higher rejection rates) to obtain the same number of graduates.

search workers between single purpose and multipurpose assessment of applicants. According to this convention, single-purpose assessment is called selection and involves only a decision to accept or reject. Multipurpose assessment, which is called classification, involves selective placement (3, p. 406) of persons employed to the particular job category, among several alternatives, for which each individual is best qualified and for which vacancies exist.

Classification is most likely to be employed in large organizations, such as military services, which train their own personnel. Military air services, for example, have usually selected aircrew candidates by means of a preliminary general qualification test and then classified the tentatively qualified group by a classification test battery which gives separate aptitude scores for pilot and observer training. These scores are consulted in connection with physical examination results and other data in making assignments to training. Candidates failing to qualify for any specialty assignment may also be rejected at this second hurdle. On the other hand, airlines which employ pilots and other crew members who are already trained, select for each category separately.

Military and Civilian Problems of Aircrew Selection

Military and civilian aviation have many similarities, but also some differences which have implications in selection. Although the fundamental characteristics of aircraft and duties of flight crews are inherently alike, the nature of the operations and criteria of performance are significantly dissimilar.

The most obvious differences can be observed in the typical missions and flight operations. Airline missions involve transportation of passengers (and freight) with primary emphasis on safety, first and service, second. Service implies regularity and dependability of schedules, speed and comfort. Military missions require attainment of military objectives and particularly combat objectives above all other considerations. Although military air services have achieved a magnificent safety record, safety must be subordinated to the military mission when a critical situation requires a choice. High performance military aircraft often allow lower error tolerances in critical maneuvers and some maneuvers and combat missions are inherently dangerous. As a result, the successful military airman may differ significantly from the successful airline pilot in his attitudes about flying (involving motivational and temperamental characteristics) and possibly in certain aspects of ability.

Inasmuch as military air operations are diverse and include support missions, such as transport of passengers and cargo, administrative flights and extensive training as well as purely combat type flying, these differences are less extreme in practice than in the abstract. Nevertheless, they should be and are reflected in selection practices, although not necessarily in formal testing procedures. To some extent the airlines have been able to give weight to transport and multiengine preferences and experience in relation to these factors.

This point introduces another major difference between the military and civilian selection problems, namely that military air services have traditionally selected trainees, whereas civilian companies select trained airmen. Military services have always been required to teach men to fly in order to staff their crews and until recently military training was the principal source of civilian airmen as well. Selection, in these circumstances, has necessarily been oriented to the assessment of basic aptitudes predictive of success in learning how to fly in a military school. The military air services were forced by the nature of the problem to pioneer in development of selection and classification tests and procedures. On the other hand, airlines and other civilian employers of airmen have often been able to select their personnel on the basis of demonstrated flight experience.

Since World War II, however, a number of airlines have found it profitable to use selection tests patterned on the military aircrew tests to select their aircrew personnel. Minimum experience qualifications may be adequate to meet the requirements of safety, but are obviously inadequate to assess other relevant qualifications important to the company. For example, McFarland (3) reported that one airline had a turnover of 10 per cent of its copilots in 1 year. This was extremely costly because of the expensive flight checks and training in company procedures given to new personnel. Apparently this turnover was a reflection of shortcomings in the men employed, inasmuch as the problem was reduced after a selection program was adopted. The content and capabilities of representative selection batteries for military and civilian aircrew are presented below.

According to Dr. John C. Flanagan, whose A.I.R. (American Institute of Research) Stanine Tests for pilot selection are currently used by a number of airlines and aircraft companies, the airlines have been showing an increased interest in assessment of attitudes of flight crew candidates. "They are now realizing that the crew serves an important public relations function, and would like to use more sensitive procedures for picking men likely to enhance passenger good will" (4).

Basic Issues in the Design of a Selection Test Battery

The flight surgeon or medical director may be called on by top management to advise on significant decisions, such as the relative merits of alternative selection programs, evaluation of the results of an on-going selection program or standards to adopt in a selection program. The information in this section provides necessary background concerning the logic and procedures followed in the design of selection programs generally. These have been developed with reference to psychologic selection programs but are equally applicable to physical selection. This discussion will be useful to the medical officer in clarifying psychologic selection issues involving psychometric concepts. It will also facilitate constructive communication between physicians and psychologists working together on selection problems.

Basic Decisions—Purposes and Goals. When it has been decided that a selection program is needed, the first step should be to specify the purposes of selection and the goals to be accomplished. To the extent that such specification is concrete and explicit all subsequent considerations will be expedited. Thus, if the objective is principally a matter of obtaining personnel capable of improved performance, consideration involving retention or accidents would receive relatively less weight than if they were focal. Clarification of purposes is essential to every phase of development of a selection program and also to its evaluation. Unless one understands what a particular program is intended to accomplish it is meaningless to attempt to evaluate it.

Three basic purposes of aircrew selection have been implicit in military and civilian aviation in addition to others specific to particular situations (5). These basic purposes are (1) safety, to select personnel potentially free of physical and mental characteristics which might compromise their ability to fly safely; (2) longevity, to screen latent or chronic physical or mental conditions which might later progress to the point of disqualifying the candidate (closely associated with this is the problem of retention which in selection implies long-term career motivation); and (3) proficiency, to identify characteristics related to development and maintenance of performance proficiency.

These purposes are interrelated to some extent, but have significant areas of independence. For example, safety and proficiency are related in that poor proficiency may be unsafe as well. On the other hand, a proficient pilot might have tendencies to take undue risks which threaten safety. Another example, crossing physical and psychologic qualifications, is that of a highly experienced, proficient pilot who has an unsafe physical history, such as a coronary infarction. The independent aspects of these purposes furnish guidance for the breadth of content of the selection program. They also help define successful performance in terms of independent multiple criteria; in relation to all three purposes, the successful pilot must have a satisfactory safety record, remain effective on the job for a satisfactory period of time, and perform his duties with satisfactory proficiency. There are no scientific rules for what is satisfactory, however, and this is another problem requiring a decision by top management. This point is developed below in the discussion of criteria.

In addition to the general, basic purposes of aircrew selection, a particular organization may have specific purposes of its own. For example, most military air services have structured their aircrew positions so that pilots, observers and certain other crew members are officers. Although this may not be intrinsic to the flying duties, it is intrinsic to the job as constituted and must, therefore, be included in the statement of purposes and reflected both in the content of the selection battery (prediction) and in the measurement of performance on the job (criteria). Similarly, if an airline desires that its flight crews have specific qualifications, such as appearance, courtesy to passengers or any others, these must be considered in planning the selection program.

A specific purpose will usually be focal in circumstances involving the revision of an existing selection program. If it were found, for instance, that under existing operational conditions flight crews are performing satisfactorily in all respects except that an excessive number are resigning after a short period of service, it might be decided to try to select personnel who are more likely to remain on the job longer. Such a decision should, of course, be made only after remedial utilization efforts (*e.g.*, pay, work schedules, promotion policies, etc.) have been considered. Accomplishment of the special purpose of the revision is the central point of interest in evaluation of results in such cases.

FORMAL CHARACTERISTICS OF PREDICTORS. Every test or measure that enters into the total assessment of an applicant in selection is a predictor of successful performance. The processes of identification, development and validation of predictors are, therefore, fundamental to the selection program. Before outlining these processes, the following necessary characteristics of useful predictors should be understood: (1) relevance to successful performance, (2) discreteness and (3) measureability.

Relevance implies that an aptitude, trait or particular qualification assessed in an applicant contributes in some degree to successful performance. The usual measure of relevance is the validity coefficient or correlation of the predictor with a criterion of performance. In general, the greater the contribution and, hence, the more relevant a predictor the higher will be the validity coefficient. In developing a selection battery potentially relevant predictors may be tentatively identified by techniques of job analysis discussed below.

Discreteness (or separateness) is related to the scope and extensiveness of coverage of relevant functions in the predictor battery. Predictors which are highly correlated with each other overlap in coverage and are redundant in relation to the criterion. The rule to obtain maximum efficiency in a predictor battery is, therefore, to choose predictors which have highest correlations with the criterion and minimum correlations with each other. Thus, in reviewing the experimental validity results for a number of proposed predictors, the first test chosen for a selection battery would be the one with the highest validity. The next one chosen, however, should not only have the next highest validity, but also the lowest correlation with the first, and so on. An important implication of this rule is that frequently the addition of a discrete test with only

minimal validity is of greater value to the total validity of a test battery than the addition of a highly valid but redundant test. The discrete test contributes something new, whereas the redundant test duplicates measures already included.

Discreteness and validity need to be understood in relation to the complex nature of the criterion of flying success. The total performance is made up of the contributions of many different discrete functions. Each one, by itself accounts for only a small part of the total variance and usually has a low validity coefficient. In fact most of the individual tests in aircrew selection batteries have validity coefficients between 0.2 and 0.4 or even lower. However, by combining a number of significantly, but marginally valid tests into a battery, the composite score of the battery may attain practical predictive power. Multivariate statistical methods, such as the multiple regression equation commonly used to combine tests into a battery composite, assign weights to the component tests essentially in proportion to their validity and discreteness.

Measureability is extremely important inasmuch as it is essential that the selection measures reflect the performance of the applicant reliably. Informal methods of observation often result in impressions which reflect the biases, opinions or transitory fluctuations of the examiner and involve considerable error. To the extent that predictor scores are unreliable (that is, not reproducable) they introduce errors of prediction and lower validity. One of the most serious limitations of the selection interview is its dependence on subjective factors in the interviewer. Properly constructed tests assure greater consistency and reliability by reason of their objectivity and standardization.

In addition to these considerations, it is practically desirable to insure that predictor tests are as consistent as possible with administrative limitations of time, cost and space, special equipment and special personnel required. Selection tests should also be screened by responsible officials to insure in advance of their adoption that there is nothing in their content which might compromise public relations with the general public or employees. When problems of purely administrative or public relations nature are suspected, it becomes necessary for the operating officials and personnel scientists to consult on possible consequences of the inclusion or exclusion of the particular material.

DETERMINATION OF PREDICTORS—JOB ANALYSIS. Various techniques of job analysis have for years been used to discover and identify the significant, relevant components of jobs as a basis for developing predictors. A common principle of job analysis in selection is to make the description in terms of meaningful and testable characteristics of people rather than in terms of technologic or administrative aspects of the job. For example, it is important to know that success in the pilot's job depends on the individual's sense of timing, visual-motor coordination, quickness in perceiving and reacting, judgment, ability to anticipate future situations and to visualize mechanical movements. These characteristics describe the pilot and can be measured by tests of complex reaction time, tracking, psychomotor coordination, perceptual judgment, mechanical principles, intelligence and the like. On the other hand, description in terms of phases of flight, various maneuvers and similar technical breakdowns require further analysis before they can be used for planning predictors. Job analyses which develop the required characteristics of the worker in terms of aptitudes, abilities and various traits that contribute to job success are valuable guides in deciding on predictors to be tried out for a selection battery.

A wide range of sources of information have been employed in job analyses of aircrew positions for selection test development (1, 3, 6–8). Among these are (1) analyses of syllabuses, training manuals, personnel files, accident reports and other documents describing how the job is taught, the characteristics of people who perform it well and of those who are unsuccessful at it and the various personnel characteristics that are associated with accidents and other difficulties; (2) interviews with and surveys of experienced, successful and unsuccessful performers; (3) direct observation of performance, using precoded recording schedules and time sampling methods; (4) tape recordings of communications; (5) motion picture records of eye and body movements, time and motion studies of cockpit duties; (6) objective recording of control movements and forces, using flight analyzer equipment; and (7) survey studies of near accidents and near accident incident reports. A number of psychologists have gone through pilot and observer training at various times in order to acquire more intimate knowledge of the requirements of these jobs. Although opinions vary as to the value of such experience it is doubtful that there would be serious objections to it in any new situation before extensive knowledge is accumulated.

From a wide range of studies using the types of information enumerated present knowledge of the job requirements of military and civilian (airline) aircrew positions is comprehensive. It is well established, for instance, that the most critical phase of the pilot's job involves the skills incident to establishing and maintaining a proper angle of glide on the landing approach. These include sense of timing and coordination, perceptual judgment, anticipation and reasoning ability. However, consideration of the total job involves other factors, as shown in Table 11, which is based on a study of airline pilots by Gordon (7).

Studies of requirements of aircrew jobs have made it clear that the relative impor-

TABLE 11

Traits and Characteristics Differentiating Good and Poor Pilots in Terms of Per Cent of Respondents Mentioning Each Category*

	Safe vs. Unsafe	Good vs. Poor	Successful vs. Eliminated Pilot Trainees
	per cent	per cent	per cent
Ability to think and learn	23	14	25
Lack of nervous behavior	10	30	10
Ability to get along with others	—	12	11
Attitude and interest	17	8	9
Attention and alertness	16	7	6
Industry and effort	2	2	6
Initiative, forcefulness and aggressiveness	—	1	6
Other	31	32	28

* Based on Gordon (7) and McFarland (3, table 2.5).

tance of various characteristics to job suc- cess depends on a number of factors. One is the stage of development of proficiency at which a job is studied. Studies focused on training, in which the emphasis is on learn- ing, developing skills and passing the course, attribute greater importance to aptitude and skill factors than those focused on post- training performance, which reflect greater importance for personality and temperament factors, such as emotional control, dependa- bility and working effectively with associ- ates. A second influencing factor is the type of mission, which accounts for wide differ- ences between military and civilian flying and between combat and noncombat flying. Still another involves the types of equipment flown, which accounts for variations among fighter, bomber and transport flying and more recently has introduced new problems in jet and rocket aircraft. Closely associated with type of equipment, and to a lesser ex- tent type of mission, are factors of altitude, speed and duration of flight, which have implications for both physical and psycho- logic selection.

Initial selection of trainees in military aviation must take the requirements of the training situation into consideration as well as those of all types of subsequent flying experience, inasmuch as military aircrew training cannot be differentiated except with regard to pilot, observer and other basic positions. To the extent that civilian opera- tors can tailor their selection programs to particular types of missions and equipment, the efficiency of their selection programs may be increased.

JOB REQUIREMENTS FOR PILOT. The Army Air Forces' comprehensive studies of the job requirements for pilots, navigators, bombardiers and other aircrew positions are still a basic source of information after over 15 years (1, 6, 8–13). These studies place judgment, which implies principally intelli- gence, alertness, attention, foresight, plan- ning ahead and anticipation at the top of the list of critical requirements for pilots in all situations. Other specific characteristics considered generally important for pilots were memory, visualization of flight course, estimation of speed and distance, division of attention, speed of decision and action and emotional control.

The following characteristics were found to have critical importance in combat flying, although they were not conspicuous in relation to training: dependability, leader- ship, motivation, attitudes and accuracy of orientation. Faulty progress in the develop- ment of techniques was a critical factor in training eliminations, but does not, as ex- pected, appear in combat studies.

Interesting differences were reported be- tween bomber and fighter pilots in these same studies. In training and in combat, division of attention and estimation of speed and distance were rated as more important for single engine, fighter pilots than for bomber pilots. Accuracy of orientation was not rated high in training, nor in combat for bomber pilots but was considered important for fighter pilots in combat. This factor has recently received increased attention from the standpoint of vestibular sensitivity in single engine, fighter type jet aircraft as a result of the suspicion that disorientation induced by head movements during turns at high speed is responsible for a number of "unexplained" jet accidents. The traits of dependability, devotion to duty, cooperation and ability to work in a team were rated as important for both fighter and bomber pilots. In addition, the bomber pilot (and also the transport pilot) must act as the aircraft commander and must fulfill certain further requirements demanded by this position. He is in a position of leadership and must instill his crew with confidence in him and his decisions and create a team with disci- pline and cooperation. The single occupant of a fighter must have greater self confidence and alertness than is required in multiplace aircraft.

Because of the overwhelming importance attributed to judgment, the following quo- tation from Guilford (8) is instructive to those who attempt to relate the results of job analysis to test construction (predictor development):

"Of all traits, judgment stands out as being most persistent and universal. This is not the place to define judgment or to break it down psy- chologically. In the minds of aviation observers it undoubtedly means a great variety of things. At best it signified good or bad decisions (where 'good' and 'bad' mean that the result turned out well or did not turn out well, or that the decision was or was not what the observer would have done under similar circumstances). However this may be, the frequent mention of judgment for the pilot, and for other aircrew personnel as well, was a persistent challenge to break it down to manageable components and to devise tests for it" (p. 11).

Job requirements for airline pilots were summarized by McFarland on the basis of studies by Gordon (7) and Van Lennep *et al.* (14) in addition to his own. The following tabulation summarizes, in logical order, the principal components of the position of Captain (3). With the exception of the personality and attitude items in paragraph 4, this description shows considerable similarity to that of the military pilot, above.

"1. Mental ability, mechanical comprehension and judgment:
   a. Adequate intelligence to acquire the necessary information relating to aeroequipment, principles of flight, instrument flying, navigation and meteorology.
   b. Capacity for giving an accurate account of what has occurred during flight and for remembering details in checking or monitoring the instruments and controls and the ability to report impartially the necessary information regarding difficulties encountered in flight.
   c. A good 'technical feeling' for the ordinary working of the machine and its deviations, including the ability to comprehend mechanical principles and to visualize mechanical movements, the attitude of the airplane, and the flight path of the aircraft through space.
   d. Ability to plan a flight beforehand in order to minimize the element of surprise or panic, to reason logically in anticipation of difficulties, and to use good judgment in practical situations.
2. Alertness, observational ability, motor skill, and technique:
   a. Capacity for obtaining information from instruments quickly and accurately and for interpreting this information effectively in relation to the attitude of the plane and flight path of the aircraft.
   b. Ability to recognize landmarks from maps or photographs and to orient oneself with reference to fixed positions in space.
   c. Ability to perceive a situation correctly, to decide quickly on the appropriate responses, and to make correct movements in the proper sequence.
   d. Adequate motor skill for making smooth and precise movements in the handling of the controls with a high degree of coordination and technique.
3. Emotional control, presence of mind, and perseverance:
   a. Ability to maintain a high degree of emotional control in order to make appropriate responses in adverse or unusual situations.

   b. Presence of mind in case of emergency in order to react in a quick and mechanically correct manner.
   c. Capacity for endurance or perseverance in the presence of adverse operating situations.
   d. Ability to maintain genuine self-confidence and control without fear of physical harm while taking necessary risks.
4. Interest and attitude, character, and leadership:
   a. Possession of a basic interest in airline piloting as a career with incidents from personal history as evidence for it.
   b. Attitude of cooperativeness and willingness to take the responsibility of an airline pilot representing the crew and the company at home and abroad.
   c. Administrative exactitude in organizing, planning, and executing the details of the flight plan and the management of the aircraft.
   d. Ability to handle the crew and passengers with authority and tact during routine as well as under difficult operating conditions." (Table 2.6.)

JOB REQUIREMENTS FOR NAVIGATOR-OBSERVER. Although equipment and conditions of flight have undergone constant changes, the navigator of a multiplace bomber or transport aircraft has traditionally been regarded as the "intellectual" member of the crew. The nature of his work demands principally an interest in numerical operations and facility (speed and accuracy) in making calculations. To perform effectively he must habitually display foresight and planning ability, avoiding problems in most cases by anticipation and good planning. His functions demand the ability to think abstractly and to understand abstract concepts.

In addition to these qualifications, the job analyses of military navigators in training and in combat (11) have emphasized a number of other significant traits. Neatness and accuracy in work habits are essential to successful performance; many navigational failures were found to be based on seemingly trivial errors such as a student's misreading his own log entries or making simple errors of addition or multiplication. Other needed abilities include thoroughness in work, ability to analyze one's own errors, to exercise good judgment, to concentrate on navigational problems for long periods of time and sufficient manual skill to manipulate instruments such as a drift meter, pelorus or astrocompass.

The navigator must be confident enough to perform accurately under stress and to display coolness and deliberation to his fellow crew members. However, this behavior must be based on knowledge of his own ability and systematic habits of self criticism rather than overconfidence and bluster. He must also avoid self distrust which may be displayed by excessive checking and undermines the confidence and morale of fellow crew members, especially in critical circumstances such as combat, long over water flights and bad weather. Although command is the responsibility of the pilots, military navigator-observers are officers and in both military and civil aviation, the navigator is usually third in command of the crew.

Speed and accuracy of arithmetic computation ranked high for navigators in combat as well as in training and motor coordination ranked low in both. The characteristics that were most relevant to navigational success in training were: judgment, visualization of spatial relations (which is essential to orientation in flight), reasoning, ability to learn abstract concepts, neatness and orderliness in work habits. Orientation was ranked highest in combat. For the navigator orientation implies ability to maintain awareness of position in flight and to correct for factors affecting it, particularly under the stress of adverse conditions. Hence, as might be expected, emotional control and dependability, which rank low in training, are among the most important attributes of successful combat navigators.

In the era of the B-25, B-17, B-24 and B-29 aircraft, navigators and bombardiers had different functions. But as automation entered the cockpit with computers, radar bombing systems and other electronic aids, the navigator position gradually absorbed the functions of the separate and independent bombardier. Today a new and more versatile military aircraft observer has emerged who can perform the duties of navigator, radar observer and bombardier.

Some of the requirements for the separate bombardier position are applicable to the present day observer. These are division of attention, the ability to keep up with a variety of simultaneous detailed activities,

the ability to remember a serial order of events and the coordination (two hand) and perceptual skill to judge accurately minute changes of rate of movement and drift synchronously. Bombardier duties involve intense task loading as a characteristic stress. On the bomb run a complex series of reactions must be made rapidly and in sequence and the bombardier must be alert to changes and make rapid corrections. Even when much of the job is taken over by computing devices he is an integral part of a man-machine complex.

DEVELOPING TRENDS IN AIRCREW REQUIREMENTS. The aircrew position of flight engineer was created in heavy four-engine aircraft such as the B-29, DC-6 and Constellation to control the complex power plant in flight. More recent propeller driven transports, such as the DC-7 and multiengine jet aircraft, such as the B-47, B-52, 707 and DC-8, do not have a flight engineer's console. With the transition to all jet operation, the military flight engineer has become obsolete. Airlines, however, have continued to maintain three man flight crews on multiengine domestic flights (navigators are used on overseas flights primarily) and there has been a tendency to require the third man to be qualified as a pilot even though he is called flight engineer.

Flanagan (4) regards the role of the "third man" in the jet airliner cockpit as a transitional problem awaiting policy decisions by airline managements which will define his duties. "The airlines seem to feel that the flight engineer should be checked out as a pilot to spell the others during very high altitude flight, to handle special emergencies, and so on. But not everyone shares this point of view. Some good research seems to be needed on the critical requirements for flight engineers in jet aircraft."

Despite the increased speed and altitude, and the changes in flight profiles associated with higher performance characteristics of jet aircraft, no substantial changes in the basic job requirements for pilot or observer have yet been recorded which have caused changes in existing aircrew psychologic selection test content or standards (15). Although all jet training *ab initio* is still relatively new and the situation must be monitored carefully for a number of years, drastic changes in aptitude requirements are not expected for jet aircraft. The selection problems for rocket craft and space travel are quite different, as pointed out recently by Sells and Berry (16), because they will draw initially from a pool of seasoned, experienced, high performance jet pilot volunteers. Basic requirements which are significant in initial aircrew selection will have been optimally satisfied in these applicants and selection will concentrate on the additional requirements for the new jobs, which are still largely in the talking stage.

TEST DEVELOPMENT. Preparation of experimental selection tests and nontest predictors proceeds with the insights obtained from job analysis, guided by the statement of purposes and definition of successful performance. Although it had generally been found that work-sample tests, which sample realistically the actual performance of a job, have maximum validity with the criteria they simulate, such tests have not been widely used in aircrew selection. This principle had held for single tests and with relatively simple jobs, but for jobs as complex as pilot or navigator work sampling must simulate segments of the job and it was found that such tests were highly correlated with each other. The result was that the validity of the composite of a number of tests was not much higher than the single highest validity coefficient in the group.

The practice followed by the Army Air Forces Aviation Psychology Program (6, 8), which resulted in the excellent composite validities obtained for the aircrew batteries, was to construct tests of independent traits, which were largely uncorrelated with each other and at the same time considered relevant to job success on the basis of the job analyses. Once these traits have been defined and tests devised to measure them, they can be weighted differentially for different job specialties (for classification) and the relative weights rather than the specific tests can be changed as the nature of the criterion changes.

At the time of development of the aircrew tests in World War II this approach was limited by lack of knowledge of basic human traits and tests tailored to their measurement. With the use of factor analysis techniques, which were then relatively new, this

TABLE 12

*Relative Importance of Principal Ability Factors of Wartime Aircrew Battery for Four Composite Predictor Scores**

Factor	Bombardier Composite	Navigator Composite	Pilot Composite	Officer Quality
	per cent	*per cent*	*per cent*	*per cent*
Verbal		17		50
Perceptual	22	10	08	
Numerical	23	45		
Spatial relations	34		07	11
Mechanical experience	12		14	18
Psychomotor coordination	07		53	
Pilot interest			14	
General reasoning		14		23
Mathematical background		12		

* Based on Guilford (8, table 28.13).

program contributed greatly to the knowledge of the organization of human abilities into independent traits. This basic research is probably the explanation both of the success of the program and of the amazing durability of the test battery over the years.

Table 12, based on the original report of Guilford (8), shows the relative importance of the nine principal factors in the wartime aircrew battery for bombardier, navigator and pilot specialties and for a measure of officer quality. It will be noted that these results provide striking confirmation of the job analyses discussed earlier.

The present aircrew selection batteries are composed principally of paper and pencil and apparatus tests of abilities. Two of the tests in the original aircrew battery of the Army Air Forces could be considered as measures of interest as well. However, the measurement of personality, character and dynamic traits, such as interests and attitudes (which are intrinsic to motivation), has not reached the level of stability and validity of ability measurement. This area is still the subject of intensive basic research and development. It is apparent that the most important further advances in aircrew selection yet to be made are in this area (17–19).

CRITERION MEASURES OF SUCCESSFUL PERFORMANCE. It is a truism that prediction of performance on any job cannot be better than the accuracy with which that performance can be measured. Measurement of performance of pilots, navigators and other members of the aircrew has been difficult and unrewarding and this has seriously limited the efficiency of selection programs.

The approach to measurement of performance depends on the definition and structure of the job which should ordinarily be the source of the statement of the purposes of selection. In this respect it is apparent that performance measurement is not simply a matter of finding reliable units of performance; the dimensions of the job which must be measured and the definition of the whole job are subject to top policy. However, top management does not always accept its responsibility to make such policies explicit and, in practice, it is frequently necessary to extract a formulation of the policy from job descriptions, correspondence, interviews and job surveys. When the technology of a job is in transition, as in the case of jet airliners, a period of experience may be needed before decisions can be made, with proportionate ambiguity in the interim.

However, even when purposes are explicit, the collection of evidence embodying them in measurement of performance remains a major problem. For a complex job such as pilot, military or civilian, the problem involves not only obtaining reliable quantitative measures expressing each major purpose, but also putting these relatively independent and sometimes contradictory measures together into an integrated over-all measure of total performance.

Inasmuch as most of the important dimensions of aircrew performance success to be predicted occur after completion of flight training and must be measured over a period of time on the job, the measurement of these dimensions involves time and depends on the adequacy of personnel records maintained. It would greatly facilitate the application of selection and other scientific methods to personnel management if record systems were adapted to research requirements which could be accomplished with minimal cost.

The records required for evaluation of safety in job performance should include documents concerning accidents in which the individual was a participant, near accident incidents and reports of inspections and supervisory ratings concerning compliance with regulations regarding flight procedures, equipment use and maintenance and the like. Inasmuch as aircraft, missions and conditions of flight vary in susceptibility to accidents and, hence, determine the degree of exposure of the individual to hazard (20), exposure must be measured in any meaningful analysis of accidents in relation to safety. The development of adequate criteria expressing the purpose of safety can thus be seen to be a formidable research task, but one very much worth doing (21).

Records required for evaluation of longevity on the job involve the individual's personnel file, including medical records. Particular importance must be attached to grounding actions for various reasons and voluntary withdrawal by an individual. Inasmuch as longevity of service for any desired minimum period must be measured with reference to minimum satisfactory standards of safety and proficiency, these must also be defined. Records could be filed and arranged with appropriate notations to facilitate extraction of the required information. However, most military and civilian record systems make such effort unduly expensive, time consuming and sometimes forbidding.

The measurement of proficiency on the job is one of the most baffling tasks yet contemplated. Ideally such measures should reflect the actual performance of the job, 365 days each year, and not be confined to a proficiency check flight or test given on one or a few occasions. In addition, flight proficiency of one member of a flight crew, for example the aircraft commander, is always a function of the coordinated proficiency of other members, such as the copilot, navigator-observer, bombardier-observer and flight engineer. As a result measurement of individual proficiency may also require measurement of the performance of the crew as a whole. Most of the readily available objective measures in the flight situation, such as accuracy of meeting the estimated time of arrival on scheduled flights, success in destroying targets, circular error in bombing and the like, are subject to too many uncontrolled extenuating variable factors and are too unreliable to be useful as criterion measures.

The difficulties and expense of serious efforts at direct, objective measurement are apparent and the attempts to employ indirect measures can well be understood. One of the most widely used procedures is that of ratings of over-all performance by supervisory check pilots, commanding officers and also by peers (22, 23). Supervisors, both in military and civilian operations, make use of check flight procedures (24), standardization boards and proficiency competitions (as in the U. S. Air Force Strategic Air Command), but their ratings can most profitably be used over uniform periods of time. Another promising procedure for rating proficiency over

time, which embraces a broader definition of the job and includes general conduct as an officer as well as flight performance, was developed by Trites and Kubala (25). They extracted a series of items from personnel records, including rate of promotional advancement, schools attended, qualifications earned, types of job assignments held and conditions of grounding or separation, as shown in table 13. This measure was predictable for a group of pilots from training records and also from psychologic tests administered prior to training.

In the development of a new test battery, particularly under the pressure of wartime demands, and to a similar degree in any new situation even when the exigencies of a war

TABLE 13

Criterion Weighting System of Trites and Kubala (25)

Form 66: Officer's, Warrant Officer's and Flight Officer's Qualification Record

(This is an official record containing a variety of biographic data and a chronologic history of an individual's military career. Information is first recorded on the form after commissioning. All accomplishments, awards, changes of duty, and so on, are posted subsequently.)

Weighting System

(Weights in parentheses after each item)

Military Schools. Air War College (+3); Air Command and Staff School (+3); instructor's school or language school (+2); administration and personnel school (+1); two or more schools of other types except those listed with zero weight (+1); squadron officers' course, USAFI, technical courses, combat crew training, gunnery school, transition training, and psychological warfare (0).

Decorations. Congressional Medal of Honor (+10); Distinguished Service Cross, Silver Star (+4); Distinguished Flying Cross, Distinguished Service Medal (+3); Bronze Star, Soldiers' Medal, Legion of Merit (+2); Airman's Medal, Commendation Ribbon (+1); Purple Heart (0).

Promotions and Rank. First lieutenant in 4 months or captain in 18 months after commissioning (+3); general officer (+3); first lieutenant in 5 to 8 months or captain in 19 to 24 months after commissioning (+2); lieutenant colonel or colonel (+2); first lieutenant in 9 to 12 months after commissioning (+1); captain or major (+1); first lieutenant in 13 to 18 months after commissioning (0); first lieutenant in 20 to 25 months after commissioning (−1); first lieutenant in 26 to 30 months after commissioning (−2); 30 months or more without becoming a first lieutenant (−3).

Airplane Qualifications and Ratings. Command pilot (+3); 4 or more aircraft qualifications (+2)*; senior pilot or pilot with two additional ratings (+2); 2 to 3 aircraft qualifications (+1); pilot with one additional rating (+1); best qualified aircraft in accident hazard group I (+1); only one aircraft qualification and/or pilots' rating only (0).

Command Positions. Air Force or air division commander (+4); wing or squadron commander (+3); flight commander, engineering officer, operations officer, armament officer, communications officer, director of personnel (+2); aircraft commander in multiengine (+1); material and supply officer, administration and personnel officer, adjutant (+1).

Disposition. Released after 60 or more months of service (+2); released after 48 to 60 months of service (+1); killed or missing in action (+1); released after 36 to 48 months of service (0); released or resigned after 24 to 36 months of service (−1); discharged for convenience of government (−1); resigned after 12 to 24 months of service (−2); summary court martial or letter of reprimand (−2); resigned after less than 12 months of service (−3); suspended from flying for fear of flying (−3); suspended from flying for psychogenic causes or at own request (−3); discharge other than honorable (−3); general court martial or dishonorable discharge (−3 to −5).

---

* All scoring is cumulative except number of aircraft qualifications.

are absent, the elapse of years while waiting for criterion data to mature is a frustrating problem. Unfortunately, there is no short-cut in time, but in many practical situations time is not available. The Army Air Forces Aviation Psychology Program faced this problem realistically and resigned the war-time luxury of post-training criteria. In order to get the job done when needed, a decision was made to use graduation *versus* elimination in training (pass-fail) as the basic criterion for test validation. During the early years of the war, pass-fail in primary training was used, making criteria available in all cases within 6 months and frequently earlier. However, despite its convenience, objectivity and importance as a necessary first hurdle in a flying career, pass-fail, even when reasons for failure are analyzed from faculty board records, is at best a primitive measure of flying success and one of imperfect reliability.

The differences between training and combat requirements of aircrew jobs, discussed earlier, imply that a test battery tailored to training requirements may omit characteristics that are important in later performance. Generalizing from job analysis information and other available research, the present writer (17, 18) proposed that personality and motivational factors have minimal importance in the training (pass-fail) criterion and assume increasing importance throughout subsequent stages of the flying career. Impressive evidence supporting this generalization was obtained by Kubala (26). These considerations reinforce the observation made earlier that the most important further advances in aircrew selection yet to be made are in the area of assessment of personality, character and dynamic traits of applicants.

The cost of extracting follow-up data from existing records, which are usually ill suited for such use and the time involved in waiting for the information to mature have apparently been an effective deterrent to systematic collection and use in long term validation studies of post-training criteria. One research program which has devoted considerable effort to such follow-up studies was concerned principally with personality and motivational predictors; in this program (19) the results have more than justified the effort.

EXPERIMENTAL DESIGN FOR VALIDATION OF A SELECTION TEST BATTERY. The design of an experiment to determine the validity of predictors is an important part of the development of a selection program. Several principles are fundamental to effective experimental design, as follows:

1. It is essential that the candidates tested be representative of those to whom the final selection battery is to be applied. For this reason it is preferable to administer the experimental tests to candidates, under simulated operational selection conditions, than to administer them to employees whose performance standing is already known. The former procedure is longitudinal and requires waiting for criterion data to develop but is less likely to be complicated by extraneous factors which may be involved in the performances of experienced employees.

2. Although in many cases only small numbers of cases are available for testing, experience has shown that effective results in selection research should be based on samples of at least 1000 cases. If attrition rates are high and follow-up studies are to be attempted the size of sample should be appropriately increased.

3. All persons tested in the experimental sample should be employed regardless of test scores. This practice has two implications: first, it will insure an unbiased comparison between predictors and criteria, covering the full range of talent measured by the tests; and second, it will help fulfill the basic experimental condition that the criterion outcome be determined entirely by the candidates' performance and in no manner by their performance on the tests. In general, it is desirable that the experimental tests be withheld from all personnel connected with the operating program and that criterion data be compiled by persons who have no knowledge of the test scores.

4. Validity is commonly expressed in terms of a correlation coefficient between the experimental predictor (test) and a criterion measure. The correlation coefficient is a statistical index of relationship or covariation. It ranges from $+1.00$ (indicating perfect positive covariation) through zero (or no relationship) to -1.00 (perfect negative covariation). In positive correlation both the predictor and criterion scores are associated

in the same direction, that is, when one tends to be high the other is high, etc. In negative correlation, they covary in opposite directions. Positive correlation is illustrated by the relationship between height and weight. Negative correlation is illustrated by the relationship between neurotic tendency and adjustment. Zero correlation or random relationship is represented by the relations between height, weight, hair color or somatotype and flying success.

A simple way to understand the magnitude of relationship indicated by a correlation coefficient is to square it. The square of the correlation coefficient (written as r^2) represents the proportion of common variance among two variables. Thus a correlation of $+1.00$ or -1.00 signifies 100 per cent of common variance and implies that 100 per cent of the variation in the predictor is accounted for by the variation in the criterion and *vice versa*; the sign of the correlation coefficient indicates the direction of the relationship. Table 14 shows how rapidly the per cent of common variance (r^2) falls off as the correlation coefficient (r) is reduced from 1.00 to zero. It is apparent that correlations below 0.40 represent only very tenuous relationships, in which less than 10 per cent of criterion variance is accounted for by the predictor, whereas correlations of 0.70, which are often considered high, express common variance of less than 50 per cent.

A distinction must also be made between the statistical significance of a correlation coefficient and its practical significance. The statistical significance indicates the confidence with which a given correlation can be accepted as a true relationship. The practical significance of the magnitude of a correlation is that it is an index of the accuracy with which one variable can be predicted from knowledge of the other. Statistical significance increases with the number of cases on which a correlation is based. It is usually calculated in terms of the standard error of the coefficient which varies inversely with the size of the sample. In general, a coefficient which is three times as large as its standard error is significant; if it is about two times as large it is marginally significant. Inasmuch as selection research deals commonly with validity coefficients of low magnitude (between 0.2 and 0.4 and even lower),

TABLE 14

The Percentage Fall of Common Variance (r^2) as the Correlation Coefficient (r) is Reduced from 1.00 to zero

r	r^2	r	r^2
1.00	1.00	0.40	0.16
0.90	0.81	0.30	0.09
0.80	0.64	0.20	0.04
0.70	0.49	0.10	0.01
0.60	0.36	0.00	0.00
0.50	0.25		

it is necessary to work with large samples to evaluate accurately the statistical significance of experimental predictors.

5. Cross Validation. Even experienced personnel psychologists have often been at a loss to explain how a promising test may show encouragingly high validity in one sample and then "wash out" in others. A conservative convention is to require additional evidence, or "replication" of the study on one or more independent samples, before accepting validity results (8, 27). The term cross validation is a special form of experimental replication used when scoring keys are developed for test items according to their discrimination of "high" and "low" criterion groups. Inasmuch as such keys tend to maximize any chance variations in the samples from which they were derived, they must be validated on independent, new samples. The cross validation procedure is to use two (or more) samples, keying the test separately on each sample. Then the keys developed on each sample are validated on the other sample. If they agree, it has usually been found that the average of the two cross validated keys has higher validity than either one alone.

6. Assembling a Test Battery. The basic principle of a test battery which covers the widest range of independent, criterion relevant measures, has already been discussed. Additional considerations of importance, which have been mentioned, concern the compliance with administrative considerations of time, equipment and personnel required for the operation of a selection program and the public relations aspects. Straightforward techniques of multivariate statistical analysis have been widely used in

test battery construction and standardization.

As mentioned above, tests in a classification battery may be combined by differential weighting into a number of different score composites to predict different criteria. The weights, reflecting validity and discreteness, may vary from zero to any amount. However, most recently adopted weighting procedures favor conservative weighting, such as 0, 1 and 2 to reflect all necessary degrees of importance. The present military aircrew classification batteries employ composites primarily for pilot and observer specialties, but use these in conjunction with an aptitude for officer status score of officer quality, which is principally a measure of general intelligence.

Another convention which has been widely adopted in the standardization of selection tests is the use of a transformation scale for individual tests and for the composite scores. The most popular scale is the 9 point *stanine scale* developed by the Army Air Force program. The term stanine is a contraction of the longer expression "standard score on a nine point scale" and means literally *sta(ndard) nine*. This transformation assumes that the variables are distributed in the normal, bell shaped form, and assigns scores according to the proportion of the total distribution achieving in each segment, as shown in table 15. This distribution has a mean of 5 and a standard deviation of 2.

Validation follow-up studies, carried beyond the period of training, can be conducted only on those who successfully complete training and consequently must omit the failures (and rejectees, if any applicants are rejected in the experimental sample). The result of this circumstance is a reduction of the range of talent in the follow-up sample which tends to reduce the magnitude of correlation coefficients proportionately. There are statistical procedures for correcting for this "restriction of range" which may be used appropriately in these situations.

SIGNIFICANT DEVELOPMENTS IN PSYCHOLOGIC SELECTION OF AIRCREW

WORLD WAR I. Aircrew selection had its beginning in World War I when it was realized that courage was not enough and particular qualifications were needed for pilots, even of the relatively simple military aircraft of that day. The earliest selection consisted of physical examinations to insure that "no aviator shall fail in his mission . . . because of discoverable physical defect" (28). Burwell (29) reported that American forces were impressed by the experience of the British Royal Flying Corps in the first year of its participation in the war. Ninety of every 100 British aviators killed during this period "died because of their own individual deficiencies," and of these, "60 were found to have been directly due to physical defects."

Intensive research on methods of aircrew selection in World War I was reported in *Air Service Medical* (28) and the Report of the Psychology Committee of the National Research Council (30) in the United States, and in England in the report *Medical Problems of Flying* (31). Reports by individuals in the United States, England and other countries described tests of mental alertness, simple and complex reaction time, judgment of the speed of moving objects and of the extension of a parabolic curve, reasoning by analogy, choice reactions, equilibrium differential, sway suggestibility and tilt perception. However, very few of them were evaluated adequately and their predictive validity was in doubt. The results for proposed selection tests of adaptability and emotional stability, such as startle tests, free association tests of fear of flying and psychophysiologic tests of tremor, cardiovascular and respiratory responses, which were widely investigated during the same period, were even more equivocal. However, many of the aptitude test approaches of this early period bore fruit in

TABLE 15
The 9 Point Stanine Scale

Stanine	Per Cent of Group Attaining	Per Cent Below
9 (highest)	4	96
8	7	89
7	12	77
6	17	60
5	20	40
4	17	23
3	12	11
2	7	4
1 (lowest)	4	0

later selection research. The need for satisfactory evidence as a basis for acceptance of the utility of selection tests were fully recognized by the psychologists of that period, as evidenced by their reports in the *Medical Research Laboratory Manual* published in 1918 (32).

BETWEEN WORLD WARS I AND II. During the period from the end of World War I through the middle "thirties," some notable progress in aircrew selection research was made in several countries despite considerable reduction of financial support. In the United States this research was centered at the School of Aviation Medicine at Randolph Field, Texas. The review by Razran and Brown in 1941 (33) revealed that this activity continued to follow the two separate directions of ability and adaptability measurement which had begun during World War I.

Research with ability tests apparently produced some successful results, although Flanagan (1) found that validity data on a substantial number of cases was available for only four tests of complex reaction time and psychomotor coordination developed during this period. These were summarized as follows: (1) Between 1926 and 1930, 1274 students tested on the Thorne Reaction Time Test were followed up and a low, but significant, correlation was found between test scores and graduation or elimination for failure to make satisfactory progress in flying training. (2) The other three tests were of the stick and rudder variety. They included, in the United States, the Complex Coordinator and the Automatic Serial Action Apparatus, which were developed by O'-Rourke, Mashburn, Constable and Glenn (34, 35), and a British test by Reid and Flack (36) which was similar to the Complex Coordinator. Follow-up studies of each of these, based on samples of about 1000 cases, showed a correlation (biserial) with graduation or elimination in pilot training around 0.35.

According to Flanagan (1), research by the Royal Air Force, the Royal Canadian Air Force, the United States Navy, the National Research Council for the Civil Aeronautics Administration and the United States Army Air Forces "all agreed in finding coordination tests involving the use of a stick and rudder, lathe-type two-hand coordination tests and pencil-and-paper intelligence tests predictive of success in pilot training." The intelligence tests, similar to Thorndike's earlier "alertness" tests of World War I, were not as stable from sample to sample of trainees, as the other tests. Williams (37) and Whittingham (38) found that "in addition to the Sensory-Motor Apparatus No. 3 and the lathe-type, two-hand tests, a paper-and-pencil test of mechanical comprehension had predictive value in a Royal Air Force study. The Royal Air Force experimented in 1941 with tests to classify men as fighter or bomber pilots, but later abandoned them because of ambiguous results. The Royal Canadian Air Force used the Link Trainer extensively for classifying pilots, observers and aerial gunners, but this device was considered too expensive, time consuming and difficult to standardize, by the Army Air Forces psychologists in view of the promising results of simpler psychomotor devices" (1).

Research on personality measures for pilot selection also continued between the wars with studies of psychogalvanic response, the "ice water immersion test" and other autonomic measures (32). In 1930 Major Raymond F. Longacre (39), at the School of Aviation Medicine at Randolph Field, developed a comprehensive procedure for personality study of prospective aviators which was incorporated into the physical examination for flying. This procedure, based on a "psychiatric type" interview and observation of the candidate by the flight surgeon during the physical examination has continued as part of most flying physical examinations to this day and in the U. S. Air Force is known as the ARMA (Adaptability Rating for Military Aeronautics). Unlike other aspects of the psychologic examination of flyers, no satisfactory evidence of its validity has yet been obtained (17, 29, 32), although there have been several notable contradictory findings (17, 40). In the summer of 1941 the National Research Council was experimenting with a number of personality, interest and biographic inventories for the Civil Aeronautics Administration and the U. S. Navy.

Flanagan summarized the past work on pilot selection research at the beginning of

World War II as follows (1):

| "In summary, it can be said that in the summer of 1941 there was evidence from a number of samples that certain apparatus tests and possibly one or two pencil-and-paper tests had predictive value for success in pilot training. However, the samples for the recently tested populations tended to be small and the results not entirely consistent. Much additional research seemed necessary before a satisfactory procedure for selecting pilots could be based on established relationships" (p. 12).

WORLD WAR II. The most extensive research and development effort on the problems of aircrew selection was that undertaken by the U. S. Army Air Forces Aviation Psychology Program in World War II (1). However, important work in this field was also carried out by the U. S. Navy and the air services of several other combatant nations. The chronology of the actions which created the Psychological Research Agency within the Medical Division of the Army Air Corps and the development and activities of this Agency has been reported in detail elsewhere (1, 6, 8, 29).

The contributions of this program to aircrew selection were substantial. A preliminary selection test was developed, known as the Aviation Cadet Qualification Examination (41) which was officially adopted in January 1942. This test, which contained sections measuring comprehension and judgment, mathematical ability, mathematical comprehension, alertness and leadership qualities, replaced the previous 2 year college or "equivalent" prerequisite for aircrew training and assessed candidates' general potentialities, practical judgment and capacity for absorbing ground school instruction. It was administered by several hundred boards and was used to accept or reject aircrew candidates prior to administration of the classification battery, which gave three separate aptitude scores, for bombardier, navigator and pilot. The specific purpose of this test was to qualify for aviation cadet training those men who were sufficiently alert and intelligent to be capable of learning an aircrew assignment and who could measure up to the intellectual and leadership standards required of officers in the Army. It was designed to measure aptitude rather than specific knowledge obtained through formal education or training.

This test proved highly successful as shown by the following results. With a qualifying score of 90 (out of a possible maximum of 150) 37 per cent of qualified cadets passed pilot training and 58 per cent failed; 18 per cent of qualified cadets passed navigation training and 53 per cent failed. With higher cutting scores, discrimination was better.

The aircrew classification battery, administered subsequently, was used to classify accepted cadets, who had passed the qualifying examination, on the basis of the three specialties. The aptitude composites for this battery have come to be referred to as "stanines." Thus, there were the bombardier stanine, navigator stanine and pilot stanine. Later there was a flight engineer stanine. The final classification battery, which was administered at a few classification centers, consisted of six apparatus tests of coordination and speed of reaction (later reduced to four) and 14 printed paper and pencil tests.

Figure 17 presents a summary of the World War II results for the pilot stanine composite for 185,367 men trained as pilots in wartime classes 43-F through 45-H. The validity coefficient for the pilot stanine with pass-fail in primary training averaged about 0.50 and fluctuated between 0.40 and 0.60 among the various classes. The bars indicate the proportions eliminated for flying deficiency, fear and at own request at each pilot stanine score in primary pilot training. Twenty-four per cent of this total group were eliminated; discrimination is shown by the extremely low rates at the highest stanines and the extremely high rates of elimination at the lowest stanines. The number of men tested at each level reflects both the effects of self preselection in the relative proportions of high and low stanine volunteers represented and also the rejection of low stanine candidates after the classification program was adopted. Most of the men with low stanines in this chart entered primary schools early in 1943. The stanine scores used here were "augmented" by adding points to test scores to reflect previous flying experience (6).

Figures 18 and 19 present similar results for the navigator and bombardier stanines. The data for navigator trainees in figure 18 consist of 15,533 new aviation cadets (pilot eliminees were excluded) from classes 43-12,

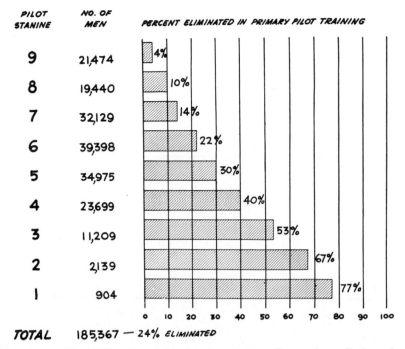

PILOT STANINE	NO. OF MEN	PERCENT ELIMINATED IN PRIMARY PILOT TRAINING
9	21,474	4%
8	19,440	10%
7	32,129	14%
6	39,398	22%
5	34,975	30%
4	23,699	40%
3	11,209	53%
2	2,139	67%
1	904	77%

TOTAL   185,367 — 24% ELIMINATED

FIG. 17. Summary of World War II results for pilot stanine. Proportions eliminated at each pilot stanine for flying deficiency, fear and own request. Flying experience credit is included in stanine score. Data include primary pilot classes 43-F through 45-H. Most of the low stanine cases were admitted in 1943.

-13, -14, -17, -18 and 44-1 through 45-13, with an over-all elimination rate of 14 per cent. The data for bombardiers cover classes 43-8 through 43-18, with an over-all elimination rate of 18 per cent. The average validity of the navigator stanine was about 0.45 and of the bombardier stanine, about 0.20.

Many different tests and procedures were tried out in this research and the test batteries underwent a number of revisions. A comprehensive and reasonably detailed account of the entire program has fortunately been published (1, 6, 8–13, 41, 42). In addition to the basic selection and classification phases described, the research was extended to other special activities, including the selection of low altitude bombardiers, selection of bombardiers for navigator training, selection of radar observers and of flight engineers, and adaptation of the classification battery for use by French and Philippine air services.

The psychologic selection program for United States Naval Aviation Cadets is known as FAR (Flight Aptitude Rating) battery. This had its background in a study

at Pensacola in 1940 (43) which revealed substantial validity for an intelligence test and a psychomotor test against pass-fail in training. The first naval cadet battery consisted of the Wonderlic Personnel Test of Mental Ability, the Bennett Mechanical Comprehension Test and a Biographical Inventory concerned with morale, interests and attitudes (44). The Wonderlic Test was replaced in 1942 by the Aviation Classification Test. The reported validity of the FAR, based on the Mechanical Comprehension Test and the Biographical Inventory, was 0.43 and with the later addition of the Aviation Classification Test, it became 0.50 (3). Channell (45) reported a study in 1941, based on 445 student pilots at Squantum Naval Reserve Air Base which found that the further addition of the Serial Reaction Time Test raised the FAR validity to 0.61. Figure 20 shows representative results for the Mechanical Comprehension Test, Aviation Classification Test and Biographical Inventory on substantial samples, and for the FAR composite of these three tests on 8615 cases. Instead of stanines, these tests

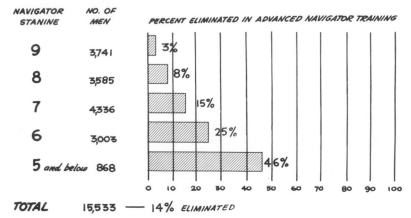

Fig. 18. Summary of World War II results for navigator stanine. Proportions eliminated at each navigator stanine for flying deficiency, fear and own request. Only new aviation cadets, classes 43-12, -13, -14, -17, -18 and 44-1 through 45-13 included.

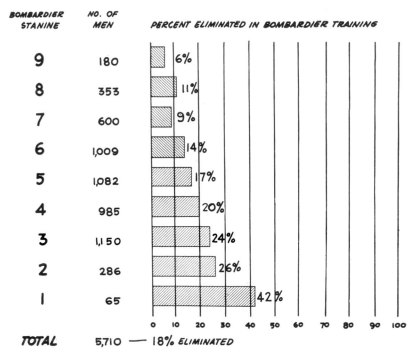

Fig. 19. Summary of World War II results for bombardier stanine. Proportions eliminated at each bombardier stanine for unsatisfactory progress, fear and own request. Only new aviation cadets from classes 43-8 through 43-18 are included.

are scaled by letter grade, from A (highest) to E (lowest).

POST-WORLD WAR II DEVELOPMENTS. The most important developments in aircrew selection following World War II have been in the application of scientific methods and procedures to the selection of airline flight personnel and in research and development on personality and motivational predictors of aircrew success. Research has continued on measures of aptitude and some changes have been made in military selection batteries, but none involving new concepts or additions of fundamental significance.

Airline Selection. In 1948 McFarland, Chapman, Burger, and Graybiel (46) made a

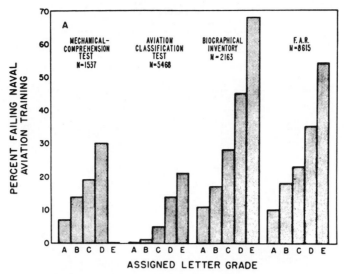

FIG. 20. Summary of results for naval aviation selection tests. Per cent failing naval aviation training at each letter grade. (Based on McFarland (3), fig. 2.1).)

direct follow-up of their Boston Study test battery. This consisted of a battery of psychologic tests administered in 1941 to 191 CAA student pilots with no airline experience (but with an average of 246 hours of flying) and 109 copilots with an average of 895 hours of flying. These tests were given in connection with a government sponsored training program for military transport operations of the airlines.

It was found that if an IQ of 100 on the Otis Test of Mental Ability had been used as a minimum standard, only 4 per cent of the successful pilots and 42 per cent of the eventual failures would have been rejected at the time of selection. According to McFarland, "experience in several airlines has indicated that if a pilot candidate scores below 40 (IQ = 110) on the Otis Test of Mental Ability, he may lack the intelligence required of an airline captain" (3, p. 61). This study also found significantly discriminating predictions for the Bennett-Fry Test of Mechanical Comprehension and two psychomotor tests, Serial Reaction Time and Two-Hand Coordination. Interestingly enough, the predictions over 7 years were equal to or better than for immediate, short term criteria, supporting the practical use of these tests for the selection of airline pilots. As in the case of military experience, prediction by a battery of tests was superior to that of individual tests.

After World War II the American Institute of Research (AIR) undertook studies of the job of the airline pilot under CAA and National Research Council sponsorship (7). On the basis of this research tests were developed to measure the potential of individuals for the job. In July and August 1946 these were tried out on about 100 first officers of one airline (47) and criterion ratings were obtained from Captains and check pilots over a 6 to 12 month period. On the basis of this study, the tests were revised and then offered for commercial use for the selection of pilots and flight engineers for airlines and of pilots and pilot mechanics for companies which operate their own aircraft.

Figure 21 shows the relationship between AIR test stanine score and performance of 568 pilots and flight engineers in the United Airlines Training Course. This airline did not hire personnel with test scores below 4, but the results clearly show the validity of the predictions. The results of this study are impressive because the tests were administered only to experienced, CAA qualified personnel who applied for aircrew jobs with United Airlines and the range of talent in the applicant group was severely restricted in comparison with that of applicants for initial training. Figure 22 is based on a follow-up of 1077 commercial pilots, 2 to 4 years after testing, which made use of CAA medical records. It shows that the proportion of

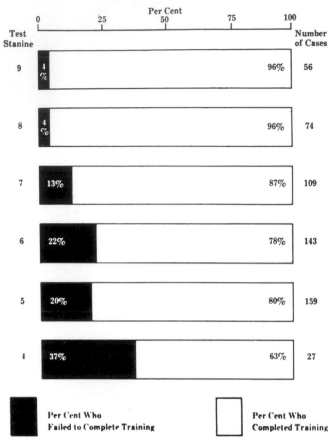

FIG. 21. Relationship of test stanine score to performance of 568 pilots and flight engineers in United Air Lines training courses.

pilots who were still flying increased with AIR pilot stanine. Figure 23 shows results for the same tests on El Al Israel Airlines. In this small sample, all five pilots with high scores (stanines of 7 to 9) were ranked average or above on job performance, whereas only 54 per cent (7 of 13) of the medium stanine group (4 to 6) and 50 per cent (3 of 6) of the low stanine group (1 of 3) achieved such ratings.

The AIR battery consists of 14 tests of three general types: (1) seven job element tests of specific skills and judgments relevant to the operation of aircraft; (2) three background inventories concerned with experiences and accomplishments of the successful pilot; and (3) four personality measures which attempt to evaluate the "poise, interests and attitudes basic to a career in commercial flying" (47). The composite,

over all stanine score is a weighted average of the stanine scores of the separate tests.

The AIR pilot stanine battery consists of the following tests (48), most of which are variants of similar tests in the basic military test batteries:

"*Job Element Tests*

"*Instrument Reading:* Measures speed in reading basic instruments and inferring from them the position of an airplane. Three-dimensional spatial orientation is emphasized.
"*Visualization of Plane Movements:* Measures ability to visualize changes in the movement of an airplane when it is rotated about its vertical, lateral, and longitudinal axes, both singly and in combination.
"*Dial Reading:* Measures accuracy and speed in reading dials typical of those on an aircraft instrument panel.
"*Orientation:* Measures skill in identifying landmarks from aerial photographs.
"*Signal Reaction Time:* Measures speed and

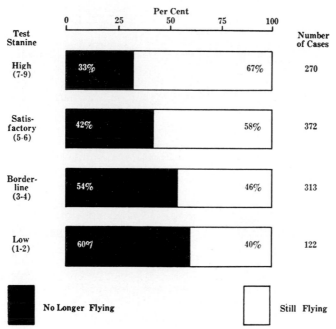

FIG. 22. Relationship of test stanine scores to continuation of 1077 pilots in commercial flying 2 to 4 years later.

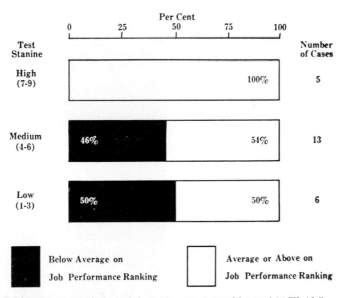

FIG. 23. Relationship of test stanines to job performance rankings of 24 El Al Israel flight personnel.

accuracy of response to complex visual signal patterns.

"Judgment and Comprehension: Measures ability to reason logically in selecting the best solutions to practical problem situations.

"Mechanical Relations: Measures ability to grasp the essentials of the operation of mechanical devices, and reflects the extent to which basic physical and mechanical principles can be applied.

"Background Inventories

"Experience: An evaluation of 20 different kinds of aviation experience, each weighted according to its relation to pilot success.

"Education: An evaluation of general educa-

tional level, as it pertains to a career in flying.
"Personal History: An assessment of varied biographical information related to pilot job requirements.

"Personality and Interest Measures

"Pilot Information: Measures interest in the field of aviation. The amount of information the applicant possesses on such topics as aero-equipment, principles of flight, and navigation affords an objective indication of the extent to which he is genuinely interested in this area.
"General Information: Measures factual knowledge in several areas as an indirect but objective index of interest patterns. This permits evaluation of the similarity of the candidate's interests to the interests characteristic of successful pilots.
"Attitudes: Measures the extent to which the candidate's attitudes are compatible with flying as a career.
"Appearance and Impression: A rating of personal characteristics which can be directly observed. Attributes evaluated include appearance, bearing, courtesy and cooperativeness."

United Air Lines has estimated that it saved $773,604 in previously wasted training costs, plus an additional amount in personnel turnover, since adoption of its comprehensive selection program in 1952. The attrition rate in the Basic First Officer (Convair 340)-Flight Engineer (DC 6-7) Course and Instrument Training was 19.9 per cent in 1951. This was reduced to 8.7 per cent in 1952 and maintained at that level up to the present. As a result of improved selection 114 flyers who would have washed out of this training were rejected. The cost of training to the company was computed as $6786 per trainee. Turnover rate, for First Officers was reduced from an average of 5.7 per cent for 1949, 1950 and 1953 (it was disproportionately high in 1951 and 1952 because of the Korean War) to an average of 1.87 per cent for the years 1954 to 1957. Part of the saving in turnover is reflected in reduced training attrition but it also results in reduced hiring and elimination of processing costs for applicants (at least $388 per applicant).

The United Air Lines selection program includes a company physical examination, psychologic testing, interviews by personnel interviewers and the Flight Manager. All of these employment instruments are reviewed as a whole by the System Board of Review, composed of the Senior Vice President of Flight Operations and his staff, who make the final selection of flight personnel. The psychologic testing includes the AIR Stanine Battery, the Otis Self Administering Test of Mental Ability (higher form), a personal history form and the Humm-Wadsworth Temperament Scale. Despite some reservations on the part of management officials concerning the effectiveness of the Humm-Wadsworth test and the interviewing procedures, company records have shown statistically significant relations between scores on the former and success in training. Research on the effectiveness of the interviews is being conducted.

No changes in selection procedures have been contemplated by this air line in contemplation of the transition to jet aircraft. On the other hand, the importance of its selection program is increased because the complexity of the jet airliners and the newness of many of the systems, flight procedures and the like will require a much more extensive training program, especially in ground school.

Military Selection. The postwar experience of the U. S. Air Force in further validation of the aircrew battery during a period of shifting standards and training organization has been covered thoroughly by Burwell (29). He has also reported the administrative considerations which led in 1955 to the adoption of the Air Force Officer Qualifying Test (AFOQT) in place of the aircrew battery. This new aircrew selection battery, which is revised annually, requires 8 hours to administer and consists of five paper and pencil tests: Officer Aptitude Test, Biographical Information Test, Flying Aptitude Test, Attitude Survey-Information Inventory and Officer Activity Inventory (49). The aptitude items of the first three are very similar in content and format to the written portions of the aircrew battery. The psychomotor apparatus tests, which have shown consistently high validity, were dropped from this battery principally because of the administrative necessity of adapting the test program to use at many locations as the population of AFROTC graduates gradually became the major source for recruiting of new trainees.

The AFOQT is scored on the stanine scale and provides five aptitude composites: officer aptitude, pilot aptitude, observer-technical aptitude, verbal aptitude and quantitative aptitude. It also provides four interest stanines: flying, administrative, technical and quantitative. The pilot and observer-technical aptitude stanines, in conjunction with the officer aptitude stanine have been used with substantial validity for the classification of aircrew candidates; the other aptitude stanines refer to nonaircrew problems. The interest measures for pilot have been analyzed with reference to a criterion of duration of active flying service and in 1957 a Career Retention stanine was validated. It has been claimed (50) that if pilot and observer candidates with career retention stanines below 7 were rejected, dollar savings of 152 million per 1000 careerists would be yielded. That is, for every 1000 career pilots and observers trained, this amount would be realized in savings estimated to be wasted on the training of nonretained personnel.

Table 16 presents a brief summary of the content of the 1953 version of the aircrew battery and of the 1955 version of the AFOQT. The tests are listed by descriptive titles and are checked in the appropriate column if represented in each battery. The tests represented by the same title which appear in both batteries are not necessarily identical. The weights shown indicate how the various tests are combined into separate composites for pilot (P), observer (Obs) and officer aptitude (OA, previously referred to as OQ, officer quality) in the aircrew battery. Weights for the AFOQT are 1 throughout. Sample items are shown in table 16.

In a recent comparative survey of the pilot selection programs of the U. S. Air Force, U. S. Navy, Royal Air Force, Royal Canadian Air Force and French Air Force, Burwell (15) found that, except for the apparatus tests, which have been discontinued by both U. S. air services, there is much agreement in content among military test batteries.

Personality and Motivational Tests in Aircrew Selection. The incorporation of interest

TABLE 16

Composition of the USAF Aircrew Classification Battery (ACB), 1953 Version and of the AFOQT, 1955 Version, Showing Weights for Pilot, Observer and Officer Stanine Composites

Descriptive Title of Test	ACB Weights*			AFOQT Weights*		
	P	Obs	OA	P	Obs	OA
Information—general, aviation	2			1		
Verbal—vocabulary, analogies			3			1
Verbal—reading comprehesion	2	1	2			1
Verbal—spelling						1
Mechanical information	1			1		
Mechanical principles	1			1	1	
Interpretation of data—dials, tables, graphs		2	1		1	1
Perception—spatial orientation (2 parts)		1				
Perception—visualization of maneuvers				1		
Perception—flight orientation				1		
Perception—instrument comprehension	1					
Numerical—computation		1	1		1	1
Numerical—reasoning		2	3		1	1
Reasoning—practical judgement				1		1
Reasoning—coordinate reading				1		
Coordination—rudder control	2					
Coordination—complex coordination	1					
Coordination—rotary pursuit	1					
Coordination—discrimination reaction time		2				
Interests—biographic data	1			1		1

* P = pilot; Obs = observer; and OA = officer aptitude.

and attitude items in the AFOQT and the validation of the Career Retention stanine, discussed above, represents an important research effort to enlarge the aptitude selection battery by the addition of motivational measures. An extensive research program to develop a test battery for adaptability screening of flying personnel has been in progress at the School of Aviation Medicine, USAF, since 1949. A number of personality and motivational tests have been adapted to pilot and observer selection in this research with practically useful incremental validity, after physical and aptitude screening, with reference to both training and post-training criteria (17–19). At the time of this writing, a full scale field test of a proposed test battery was in progress at Lackland Air Force Base on a sample of 10,000 pilot and observer candidates.

ILLUSTRATION OF TEST CONTENT

The brief descriptive notes and illustrations presented in this section explain the rationales of representative technical tests of the types widely used in aircrew selection. The descriptive titles used are keyed to the list in table 16.

Information Tests. Such tests sample technical information that would ordinarily be acquired by persons having the interests appropriate to potential success in aircrew positions: *e.g.*, active sports, navigation, gunnery, aviation and mechanical information.

The maximum number of shells that a hunter may have in his shotgun when hunting game protected by the Federal government is
A. Two
B. Three
C. Four
D. Five
E. Don't know

Acceleration of motorcycle engines is always accomplished by
A. Elevating the throttle control
B. Depressing the throttle control
C. Turning the throttle control inward
D. Turning the throttle control outward
E. Don't know

An "apron" is a
A. Trailing edge of the wing
B. Cover to protect airplane engines outside the hanger
C. Strip of the field where planes are parked
D. Wind protection for a plane which is on the ground
E. Don't know

A tappet in automotive equipment usually is a
A. Valve regulating the oil pressure
B. Breaker point in the distributor
C. Push rod between a cam and a valve stem

For duck hunting, it is generally considered best to use
A. A standard cylinder choke
B. An improved cylinder choke
C. A modified choke
D. A full choke
E. Don't know

"Ground loop" refers to
A. Using two reference points on the ground while making an inside loop
B. An inside loop, in which the plane skims the ground at the bottom of the loop
C. A dangerous 360° turn in taxiing a plane
D. A designated area on a landing field set off for the purpose of ground maneuver practice
E. Don't know

As a light plane is about to make contact with the ground in a three-point landing, it should be
A. Gunned
B. Made to glide
C. Made to climb
D. Stalled
E. Don't know

If an engine that is equipped with a magneto ignition system runs smoothly, then stops firing, the trouble is probably in the
A. Magneto
B. Spark plugs
C. Voltage control
D. Generator

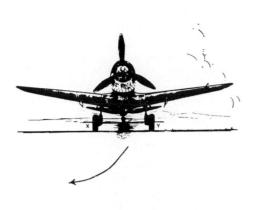

As the plane turns in the direction indicated,

A. wheel X will press harder on the ground.
B. wheel Y will press harder on the ground.
C. wheels X and Y will press equally hard on the ground.

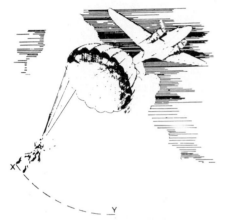

The man will be swinging

A. faster at point X.
B. faster at point Y.
C. equally fast at points X and Y.

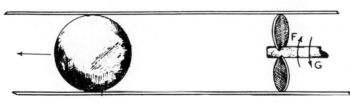

The ping pong ball in the tube will move in the direction indicated,

A. only if the fan turns in direction F.
B. only if the fan turns in direction G.
C. if the fan turns in either direction F or G.

FIG. 24. Mechanical principles. Measures understanding of principles as reflected in responses to practical items as illustrated.

Figures 27, 28 and 29 illustrate three types of perception tests. The two pictures in figure 27 represent the pilot's straight ahead view from the cockpit. The picture at the right was taken after a single maneuver. The examinee must determine which of the following it is: left or right turn, left or right roll, climb up or down. The first picture shows the cockpit view as it appears while flying straight and level toward a mountain range. The second picture shows the view as it appears in a right bank. To move from the

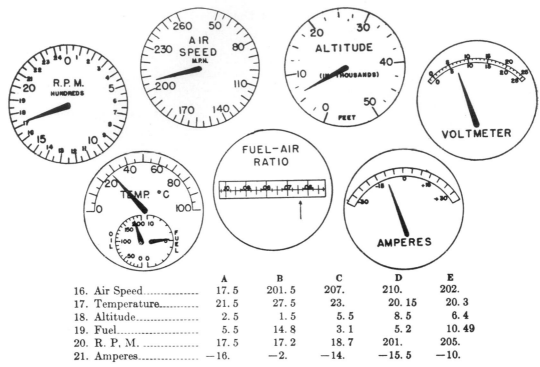

	A	B	C	D	E
16. Air Speed	17. 5	201. 5	207.	210.	202.
17. Temperature	21. 5	27. 5	23.	20. 15	20. 3
18. Altitude	2. 5	1. 5	5. 5	8. 5	6. 4
19. Fuel	5. 5	14. 8	3. 1	5. 2	10. 49
20. R. P. M.	17. 5	17. 2	18. 7	201.	205.
21. Amperes	−16.	−2.	−14.	−15. 5	−10.

FIG. 25. Interpretation of data: dial reading. Measures ability to locate appropriate dial for each question and read the scale position of the pointer quickly and accurately.

first position to the second the pilot had to roll the plane to the right. Speed is a factor in determining score.

The flight orientation test illustrated in figure 28 also presents a cockpit straight ahead view but does not involve the sequential judgment in the previous test. The examinee's task is to identify the attitude of the aircraft which matches the orientation in the picture at the left. Scores depend on number correct under speeded conditions.

The instrumentation test illustrated in figure 29 requires the examinee to visualize the orientation of the aircraft in space on the basis of the instrument data presented. He must choose the aircraft, in this example, which is flying straight and level and due east. Speed and accuracy determines the score.

Reasoning: Practical Judgment.

A man on a very urgent mission during a battle finds he must cross a stream about 40 feet wide. A blizzard has been blowing and the stream has frozen over. However, be-

cause of the snow he does not know how thick the ice is. He sees two planks about 10 feet long near the point where he wises to cross. He also knows where there is a bridge about 2 miles downstream. Under the circumstances he should

A. Walk to the bridge and cross it
B. Run rapidly across on the ice
C. Break a hole in the ice near the edge of the stream to see how deep the stream is
D. Cross with the aid of the planks, pushing one ahead of the other and walking on them
E. Creep slowly across on the ice

A pilot has made a forced landing near a mountain cabin. He finds that the nearest phone is at an isolated ranger's cabin 14 miles across the mountains to the north. It is winter. He sets out on foot for the ranger's cabin at 6 A.M., carrying enough food for only one meal. At 10 A.M., having met no one, he comes to three branches of the trail, all unmarked. It would be best for him to

A. Follow the trail that appears to lead

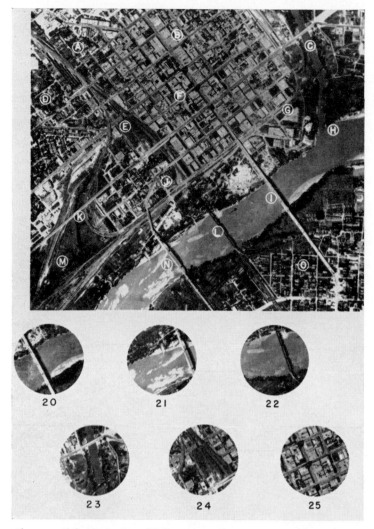

Fig. 26. Perception: spatial orientation. Measures speed and accuracy of location of excerpted "target areas" in aerial maps. This skill depends on the individual's ability to orient himself in space as well as perceptual accuracy.

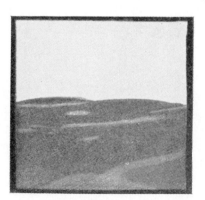 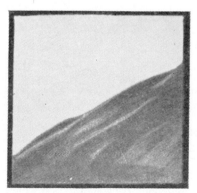

Fig. 27. Perception: visualization of maneuvers. (See text.)

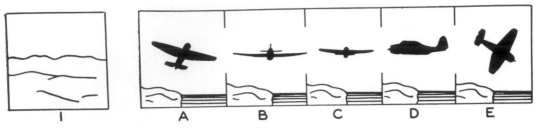

FIG. 28. Perception: flight orientation. (See text.)

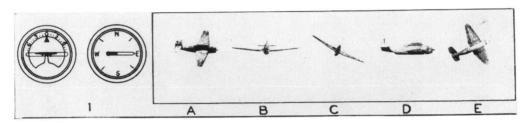

FIG. 29. Perception: instrument comprehension test. (See text.)

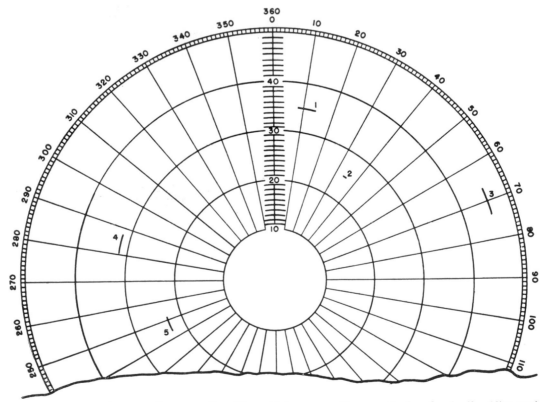

FIG. 30. Reasoning: coordinate reading. The grid below provides a vertical scale of miles (distance) and a circumference scale of degrees (bearing) by means of which the examinee can estimate the direction and distance of each object seen in the "scope" from the center of the circle.

in the right direction until he reaches
the cabin or the end of the trail

B. Turn back immediately toward his
starting point

C. Leave the trail and go due north by
compass

D. Walk until noon along the trail that
appears to lead in the right direction;
then turn back if not sure of his location

E. Stay at the fork in the trail and wait
for someone to come by

Because of motor failure, a fighter pilot is
forced to bail out at night and land in unfamiliar territory near the battle zone. After
he has landed, it is most important for him
to find out the

A. Name and location of the nearest town

B. Strength of the troops holding the
territory

C. Location of the nearest friendly lines

D. Language spoken by the inhabitants

E. Nature of the surrounding terrain

Apparatus Tests. Typical apparatus tests
are shown in figures 31 to 34 inclusive. The

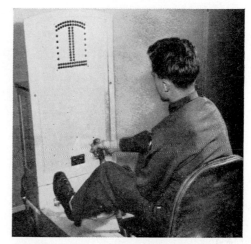

FIG. 32. Complex coordination test

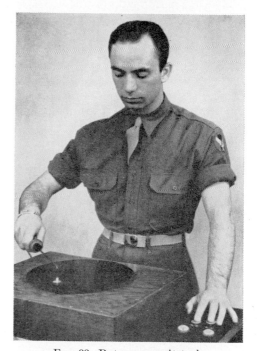

FIG. 33. Rotary pursuit task

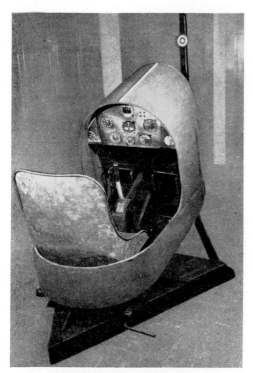

FIG. 31. Rudder control test

rudder control test, shown in figure 31, has
been the single most valid test in the aircrew
battery. Coordination of visual perception
of the alignment of the pointer across the
top of the apparatus with the target light
with adjustments of rudder pedals is required. Score is time on target.

In the complex coordination test, illustrated in figure 32, the examinee must make
three adjustments rapidly and synchro-

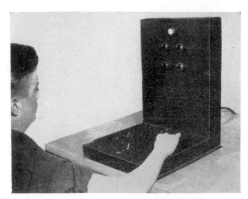

FIG. 34. Discrimination reaction time test

nously to align the response lights in the three parallel banks to a target pattern. The adjustments involve leg movements on the rudder pedals and movement of the joy stick both forward-backward and left-right. Score depends on speed of matching patterns.

The rotary pursuit task (fig. 33) requires the examinee to track a rotating disk on the turntable with a stylus held at arms length. It measures smoothness of arm-hand-shoulder coordination and steadiness as well as visual-motor coordination. The apparatus in the picture also involves divided attention and the examinee must respond to differential signal lights with his left hand while tracking the disk with his right. Score depends on time on target.

In the discrimination reaction time test, shown in figure 34, each of the four toggle switches on the horizontal base of the apparatus is keyed to a different two-light pattern of the four colored lights on the panel. As each pattern is presented the white light comes on and is extinguished when the correct response is made. Reaction time for the correct response is measured.

REFERENCES

(1) FLANAGAN, J. C.: The aviation psychology program in the Army Air Forces. Army Air Forces Aviation Psychology Program Research Reports, No. 1. Washington, D. C., Superintendent of Documents, Government Printing Office, 1948.

(2) FITTS, P. M., AND JONES, R. E.: Analysis of factors contributing to 460 "pilot-error" experiences in operating aircraft controls. Report TSEA-694-12. Wright Field, Dayton, Ohio, Engineering Division, Air Materiel Command, 1947.

(3) McFARLAND, R. A.: Human Factors in Air Transportation, New York, McGraw-Hill Book Co., Inc., 1953.

(4) FLANAGAN, J. C.: Personal communication, 1958.

(5) SELLS, S. B., AND BURWELL, R. R.: The establishment of norms. Symposium on Physical Standards and Selection. Randolph Air Force Base, Texas, School of Aviation Medicine, USAF, 1957.

(6) DuBOIS, P. H.: The classification program. Army Air Forces Aviation Psychology Program Research Reports, No. 2. Washington, D. C., Superintendent of Documents, Government Printing Office, 1947.

(7) GORDON, T.: The airline pilot: a survey of the critical requirements of his job and of pilot evaluation and selection procedures. Report No. 73. Washington, D. C., Division of Research, Civil Aeronautics Administration, 1947.

(8) GUILFORD, J. P.: Printed classification tests. Army Air Forces Aviation Psychology Program Research Reports, No. 5. Washington, D. C., Superintendent of Documents, Government Printing Office, 1947.

(9) MILLER, N. E.: Psychological research on pilot training. Army Air Forces Aviation Psychology Program Research Reports, No. 8, Washington, D. C., Superintendent of Documents, Government Printing Office, 1947.

(10) KEMP, E. H., AND JOHNSON, A. P.: Psychological research on bombardier training. Army Air Forces Aviation Psychology Program Research Reports, No. 9, Washington, D. C., Superintendent of Documents, Government Printing Office, 1947.

(11) CARTER, L. F.: Psychological research on navigator training. Army Air Forces Aviation Psychology Program Research Reports, No. 10, Washington, D. C., Superintendent of Documents, Government Printing Office, 1947.

(12) COOK, S. W.: Psychological research on radar observer training. Army Air Forces Aviation Psychology Program Research Reports, No. 12, Washington, D. C., Superintendent of Documents, Government Printing Office, 1947.

(13) DAILEY, J. T.: Psychological research on flight engineer training. Army Air Forces Aviation Psychology Program Research Reports, No. 13, Washington, D. C., Superintendent of Documents, Government Printing Office, 1947.

(14) VAN LENNEP, D. J., ET AL.: Investigations of the personality of pilots in relation to their operational success. Unpublished. cf. McFarland (3, p. 85).

(15) BURWELL, R. R.: Contemporary pilot selection. A comparison of pilot selection in the air services of the United States, Canada, Great Britian and France. Unpublished

Thesis, School of Aviation Medicine, USAF, Randolph Air Force Base, Texas, 1957.

(16) SELLS, S. B., AND BERRY, C. A.: Human requirements for space travel. Air Univ. Quart. Rev., 1958, in press.

(17) SELLS. S. B.: A research progam on the psychiatric selection of flying personnel. I. Methodological introduction and experimental design. Research Report, Project 21-37-002, No. 1. Randolph Air Force Base, Texas, School of Aviation Medicine, USAF, 1951.

(18) SELLS, S. B.: Development of a personality test battery for psychiatric screening of flying personnel. J. Aviation Med., 26: 35–45, 1955.

(19) SELLS, S. B.: Further developments on adaptability screening of flying personnel. J. Aviation Med., 27: 440–451, 1956.

(20) TRITES, D. K., KUBALA, A. L., AND SELLS, S. B.: Aircraft accidents vs. characteristics of pilots. J. Aviation Med., 26: 486–494, 1955.

(21) THORNDIKE, R. L.: The human factor in accidents with special reference to aircraft accidents. Research Report, Project 21-30-001, No. 1. Randolph Air Force Base, Texas, School of Aviation Medicine, USAF, 1951.

(22) JENKINS, J. G., ET AL.: The combat criterion in naval aviation. National Research Council Committee on Aviation, Psychology, Report No. 6. Washington, D. C., Division of Aviation Medicine, Bureau of Medicine and Surgery, U. S. Navy, 1950.

(23) SELLS, S. B.: Human flight behavior in groups. Aeromedical Review No. 6-58. Randolph Air Force Base, Texas, School of Aviation Medicine, USAF, in press.

(24) NAGAY, J. A.: Revisions of the standard flight-check for the airline transport rating based on airline tryout. Report No. 89. Washington, D. C., Division of Research, Civil Aeronautics Administration, 1950.

(25) TRITES, D. K., AND KUBALA, A. L., JR.: Characteristics of successful pilots. J. Aviation Med., 28: 34–40, 1957.

(26) KUBALA, A. L., JR.: Adaptability screening of flying personnel: preliminary analysis and validation of criteria of adaptability to military flying. Research Report No. 58-121. Randolph Air Force Base, Texas, School of Aviation Medicine, USAF, in press.

(27) THORNDIKE, R. L.: Personnel Selection: Test and Measurement Techniques. New York, John Wiley & Sons, Inc., 1949.

(28) U. S. War Department, Air Service, Division of Military Aeronautics: Air Service Medical. Washington, D. C., Superintendent of Documents, Government Printing Office, 1918.

(29) BURWELL, R. R.: Historical review of aircrew selection—development of psychologic selection of pilots in the United States

Air Force and predecessor organization in the United States Army. Aeromedical Review No. 1-58. Randolph Air Force Base, Texas, School of Aviation Medicine, USAF, 1957.

(30) Report of the Psychology Committee of the National Research Council. Psychol. Rev., 26: 83–149, 1919.

(31) Medical Research Council, London: Medical Problems of Flying. London, His Majesty's Stationery Office, 1920.

(32) U. S. War Department, Air Service, Division of Military Aeronautics: Manual of Medical Research Laboratory. Washington, D. C., Superintendent of Documents, Government Printing Office, 1918.

(33) RAZRAN, G. H. S., AND BROWN, H. C.: Aviation. Chapter 3 in Symposium on Military Psychology. Psychol. Bull., 38: 322–330, 1941.

(34) MASHBURN, N. C.: The complex coordinator as a performance test in the selection of military flying personnel. J. Aviation Med., 5: 145–154, 1934.

(35) MASHBURN, N. C.: Mashburn automatic serial action apparatus for detecting flying aptitude. J. Aviation Med., 5: 155–160, 1934.

(36) REID, G. H., AND BURTON, H. L. Psychomotor responses in relation to flying. Proc. Roy. Soc. Med., 17: Section on War, 43–53, 1923–1924.

(37) WILLIAMS, G. O.: Ph.D. Thesis, London University, 1939.

(38) WHITTINGHAM, H. E.: Medical research and aviation. J. Roy. Nav. M. Serv., 26: 15–24, 1940.

(39) LONGACRE, R. F.: Personality study. J. Aviation Med., 1: 33–50, 1930.

(40) FINESINGER, J. E., ET AL.: An investigation of prediction of success in naval flight training. Report No. 81. Washington, D. C., Division of Research, Civil Aeronautics Administration, 1948.

(41) DAVIS, F. B.: The A.A.F. qualifying examination. Army Air Forces Aviation Psychology Program Research Reports, No. 6. Washington, D. C., Superintendent of Documents, Government Printing Office, 1947.

(42) MELTON, A. W.: Apparatus tests. Army Air Forces Aviation Psychology Program Research Reports, No. 4, Washington, D. C., Superintendent of Documents, Government Printing Office, 1947.

(43) FRANZEN, R., AND McFARLAND, R. A.: Detailed statistical analysis of data obtained in the Pensacola study of naval aviators. Report No. 41. Washington, D. C., Division of Research, Civil Aeronautics Administration, 1944.

(44) FISKE, D. W.: Validation of naval aviation cadet selection tests against training criteria. J. Appl. Psychol., 31: 601–614, 1947.

(45) CHANNELL, R. C.: Psychomotor tests as predictors of success in flight training. Naval

Air Reserve Base, Squantum, Massachusetts, 1942.

(46) McFARLAND, R. A., CHAPMAN, W. P., BURGER, F. D., AND GRAYBIEL, A.: A study of 300 airline pilots in the early stages of their training. Unpublished. *cf*. McFarland (3, p. 85).

(47) A.I.R. Research Notes, No. 13, Pittsburgh, Pennsylvania. American Institute of Research, 1957.

(48) The A.I.R. Stanine Tests for Pilot Selection, Pittsburgh, Pennsylvania, American Institute of Research, 1957.

(49) MILITARY PERSONNEL: Air Force Personnel Evaluation Manual, AFM 35-8. Washington, D. C., Department of the Air Force, 1954.

(50) Personnel Laboratory Brief. Lackland Air Force Base, Texas, Air Force Personnel and Training Research Center, 1957.

8

THE ATMOSPHERE

Harry G. Armstrong, M.D.

The atmosphere at altitude differs in several respects from that at sea level and these differences give rise to many of the problems associated with aviation medicine. It is for this reason that one must have an intimate understanding of the upper atmosphere before being introduced to a discussion of the clinical entities which result from exposure to this environment. The atmosphere may be defined as being the gaseous envelope which surrounds the earth's surface and is composed of a mixture of the gases listed in table 17. As a result of the earth's gravitation, one would expect a marked separation by diffusion of these various gasses because of their differences in weight but this is prevented, up to very high altitudes, by winds and vertical turbulence.

DIVISIONS OF THE ATMOSPHERE

There are a number of agents which act within and upon the atmosphere, such as gravity and solar radiations, which bring about physical and chemical changes at various altitudes. Based on these differences the atmosphere can be divided and subdivided into a number of strata. There are several ways of doing this but the most commonly accepted system begins by dividing the atmosphere into two major segments. The first is called the inner atmosphere which extends from the earth's surface to an altitude of 600 miles and the second is called the outer atmosphere, or exosphere, which extends from the 600 mile level to the outer limit of the atmosphere at about 1200 miles.

The earth's gravitational force acts on the molecules of the atmosphere to pull them down to the surface of the earth. At the same time, however, the atmospheric gas attempts to expand in all directions into every available space including interplanatary space. This tendency of the atmosphere to expand is caused by the kinetic energy of its molecules or, in other words, its temperature. This temperature in turn is principally the result of solar radiation. As a consequence of the interplay of these two forces the atmosphere becomes thinner, or less dense, with altitude. Finally, a point is reached where the molecules are so widely separated that they seldom if ever collide with each other. This point in our atmosphere is at the 600 mile level and is used to mark the border between the inner atmosphere and the outer atmosphere or exosphere. Only as long as collisions between air particles occur can the atmosphere be considered as a continuous material medium and this is, therefore, limited to the inner atmosphere. The exosphere is, on the other hand, not a continuous material medium but a kind of spray or fringe zone, composed of freely moving particles, which very gradually thins out into the vacuum of space where the density of matter is only 10^1 particles per cu. cm.

The inner atmosphere is subdivided into three spheres which are referred to, from below upward, as the troposphere, the stratosphere and the ionosphere, respectively. The outer boundaries of these spheres are re-

*Composition of the Dry Atmosphere in
Volumes Per Cent*

Gas	Volume Per Cent
Nitrogen	78.09
Oxygen	20.95
Argon	0.93
Carbon dioxide	0.03
Neon	1.80×10^{-3}
Krypton	1.00×10^{-4}
Helium	5.24×10^{-4}
Hydrogen	5.00×10^{-5}
Xenon	8.00×10^{-6}

ferred to as the tropopause, stratopause and the ionopause. The subdivisions of the various spheres are called layers.

The subdivision of the two lower spheres is based on thermal considerations and the criterion used is the lapse rate or temperature gradient. The lapse rate is the mean change of temperature in degrees per unit step of altitude and is expressed in ° C. per 300 feet of altitude. The reason for choosing the lapse rate as a criterion for the subdivision of the troposphere and stratosphere is that their most conspicuous physical and meteorologic characteristic is a mixing of air

masses, convection and change of relative humidity. The latter are closely related to the lapse rate of the temperature and, thus, a marked change in the lapse rate determines the boundaries between these spheres and layers.

With this background we are now prepared to describe the various divisions of the atmosphere which we shall do beginning with the troposphere. The troposphere is characterized by decreasing temperature with altitude, vertical convection currents and a variable moisture content. The outer limit of the troposphere, the tropopause, varies with the latitude and the time of year averaging 30,000 feet over the earth's poles and 56,000 feet over the equator as is shown in figure 35.

The lowest layer of the troposphere is the so-called bottom layer, comprising the first 6 feet above the ground. It is set off from the next higher layer because of its peculiar characteristics derived from the kind of soil, vegetation and water.

The next, or ground layer extends from 6 feet up to 1.2 miles. In this layer other influences of the earth's surface are predominant, such as surface friction, causing reduction of wind speed and changes of wind

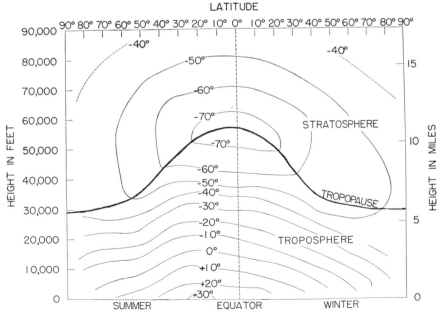

Fig. 35. Variations in the temperature and the height of the tropopause at different latitudes and seasons of the year.

direction. The proximity of the ground is also responsible for a thermal instability or unstable lapse rate caused by warming of the air from the soil which itself has been warmed up by absorption of solar radiation. As a result we observe updrafts and general turbulence. Normally, clouds are not found in this layer but haze and fog may form.

The outer and the main layer of the troposphere is the advection layer, formerly called the cloud layer. It has been so named because horizontal dislocation of air masses prevail over the vertical ones. It is the breeding place of clouds and where the cold and warm fronts move. In brief, the advection layer is the main stage of weather phenomena. This layer has a relatively stable lapse rate of $-1°$ C. per 300 feet of altitude. The advection layer extends from about 1.2 miles above the earth to the variable altitudes shown in figure 35 depending on the latitude and the season. The upper limit of the advection layer is the tropopause which also marks the dividing line between the troposphere and the stratosphere.

The next major division of the atmosphere is the stratosphere. The stratosphere extends from about 8 to 50 miles above the earth's surface and is subdivided into three layers based on thermal differences.

The lowest, or isothermal layer, extending up to about 15 miles above the earth, has a fairly constant temperature of around $-67°$ F. $(-55°$ C.). Being isothermal this layer has little air turbulence and in that regard is an ideal flying zone. Also, these conditions permit a slight gravitational separation of the atmospheric constituents with the volume per cent of oxygen falling to 20.7 at 60,000 feet and to 20.4 at 90,000 feet.

The next, or warm layer of the stratosphere extends from about 15 to 30 miles above the earth's surface. It shows a fairly steady increase in temperature from $-67°$ F. $(-55°$ C.) to 50° F. (10° C.) at a height of 30 miles (see fig. 106, chapter 19). This increase in temperature is probably caused by the effect of the strong absorption of solar ultraviolet light by the layer of ozone which is concentrated at those altitudes and will be discussed later.

The third or outer layer of the stratosphere extends from about 30 to 50 miles above the surface of the earth and is referred to as the upper mixing layer. Here no absorption of ultraviolet takes place, because of the absence of ozone, and the temperature is governed largely by long wave radiation. Consequently, a sharp fall in temperature occurs from 50° F. (10° C.) at 34 miles to about $-100°$ F. $(-72°$ C.) at 50 miles altitude. This temperature change produces a strong turbulence and a thorough remixing of the atmospheric gasses.

The next major division of the atmosphere, the ionosphere, begins at a height of about 30 miles and extends out to a distance of about 600 miles above the earth's surface. The ions in this layer are the result of photochemical and photoelectric reactions between the molecules of the atmosphere and solar ultraviolet radiation. The latter is absorbed in the process with the end product being ions and free electrons. The ionosphere is divided into four layers.

The lowest and most variable of these is the D layer at 30 to 60 miles. It disappears during the night. The E layer, known also as Kennely-Heaviside layer, is normally found between the 50 and 95 mile levels. The F, or Appleton layer, subdivided into the F_1 and F_2 layers extend from the 95 to 150 mile and from the 150 to 250 mile levels, respectively. At night they form a single layer F. The electron density in the E layer is about 10,000 per cubic centimeter at 70 miles altitude at night which increases to about 150,000 per cubic centimeter during the day. In the F layer, at 160 to 190 miles, the values are higher by a factor of 10.

The ionosphere surrounding the earth between 50 and 250 miles acts as a reflector for electromagnetic waves and, thus, is a prerequisite for wireless telegraph and long range radio communication. Inasmuch as the ionizations are caused by solar ultraviolet radiations the ionosphere is under the direct influence of the sun. When we have a normal undisturbed sun we have a normal undisturbed ionosphere and, consequently, normal communications. The sun, however, often shows disturbances in the form of eruptions, flares and sunspots, resulting in a blackout in radio communication. Although the various regions of the ionosphere are called layers they are actually a heavily ionized continuum. In the D, E and F regions

TABLE 18

Atmospheric Strata and Their Altitude Ranges

Atmos-pheres	Spheres	Layers	Approximate Height
			miles
Space			Above 1200
Outer	Exosphere		600 to 1200
Inner	Ionosphere	Atomic	250 to 600+
		F ($F_1 + F_2$)	95 to 250
		E	50 to 95
		D	30 to 60
	Stratosphere	Upper mixing	30 to 50
		Warm	15 to 30
		Isothermal	8* to 15
	Troposphere	Advection	1.2 to 8*
		Ground	6 feet to 1.2 miles
		Bottom	0 to 6 feet

* Average.

the electron density becomes greater or the electron density gradient is greater than in the areas between and it is these regions, with abruptly higher electron density gradients, that act as reflectors of radio waves.

The temperature of the ionosphere rises constantly with height up to about 3600° F. (2000° C.). However, the density of the air in the upper layers of the ionosphere is so reduced that the concept of temperature loses its usual meaning which will be explained later.

The highest layer of the ionosphere, the atomic layer, extends between 250 and 600 miles from the earth's surface. It is assumed that the gases here are more or less dissociated. Oxygen for instance is completely dissociated above the 70 mile level and nitrogen may exist primarily also in the atomic state above the F layer. With this atomic layer we have also reached the outer limit of the inner atmosphere.

The area above 600 miles is the outer atmosphere or the exosphere which extends from 600 to about 1200 miles above the earth and blends gradually with the vacuum of free space. In this marginal region the collisions between molecules become very rare. Those particles with lower kinetic energy move in elliptic trajectories away from the earth and then fall back again as a result of the earth's gravity. Some of the lighter particles with a very high kinetic energy,

mainly hydrogen and helium, attain a speed of 7 or more miles per second and may then escape into space.

Having outlined the various divisions and subdivisions of the atmosphere, with a general description of the characteristics of each, we shall next go into more detail concerning the physical and chemical properties of the atmosphere which are of concern to us in aviation medicine.

WATER VAPOR

Water vapor is not considered as one of the components of the atmosphere and, accordingly, it was omitted from table 17. Actually water vapor is present throughout the troposphere ranging in amount from 1 to 5 per cent. The lower the temperature the less the amount of water vapor required to saturate the air so that by the time the temperature of the stratosphere is reached the water vapor in the air is negligible. It is the condensed or frozen moisture in the air which is responsible for cloud formations of which there are some 21 types.

THE JET STREAM

In the general vicinity of the tropopause high westerly winds are occasionally encountered with velocities up to 200 miles per hour. They are most frequently observed in the circumpolar regions, are fairly narrow in width and tend to shift their position both vertically and horizontally to a limited extent. Along the margins of these jet streams there is strong turbulence but none within the stream itself. These jet streams appear and disappear for no known reason and their cause is also unknown.

TEMPERATURE

In 1924 the U. S. Bureau of Standards developed a "U. S. Standard Atmosphere" based on yearly average figures and assuming gravity to be constant, the absence of moisture, a linear temperature decrease with altitude and a temperature in the stratosphere of −67° F. (−55° C.). This original "Standard Atmosphere" has since been extended and the latest version is shown in table 19. The temperatures at even higher altitudes are shown in figure 106 of Chapter 19.

TABLE 19

Altitude-Pressure-Temperature Relationships Based on the U. S. Standard Atmosphere

Altitude	Pressure†		Temperature	
feet	*mm. of Hg*	*p.s.i.*	*°C.*	*°F.*
0	760	14.70	15.0	59.0
1,000	732.9	14.17	13.0	55.4
2,000	706.6	13.66	11.0	51.9
3,000	681.1	13.17	9.1	48.3
4,000	656.3	12.69	7.1	44.7
5,000	632.3	12.23	5.1	41.2
6,000	609.0	11.78	3.1	37.6
7,000	586.4	11.34	1.1	34.0
8,000	564.4	10.91	-0.8	30.5
9,000	543.2	10.50	-2.8	26.9
10,000	522.6	10.11	-4.8	23.3
11,000	502.6	9.72	-6.8	19.8
12,000	483.3	9.35	-8.8	16.2
13,000	464.5	8.98	-10.8	12.6
14,000	446.4	8.63	-12.7	9.1
15,000	428.8	8.29	-14.7	5.5
16,000	411.8	7.96	-16.7	1.9
17,000	395.3	7.64	-18.7	-1.6
18,000	379.4	7.34	-20.7	-5.2
19,000	364.0	7.04	-22.6	-8.7
20,000	349.1	6.75	-24.6	-12.3
21,000	334.7	6.47	-26.6	-15.9
22,000	320.8	6.20	-28.6	-19.5
23,000	307.4	5.94	-30.6	-23.0
24,000	294.4	5.70	-32.5	-26.6
25,000	281.9	5.45	-34.5	-30.2
26,000	269.8	5.22	-36.5	-33.7
27,000	258.1	4.99	-38.5	-37.3
28,000	246.9	4.77	-40.5	-40.9
29,000	236.0	4.56	-42.5	-44.4
30,000	225.6	4.36	-44.4	-48.0
31,000	215.5	4.17	-46.4	-51.6
32,000	205.8	3.98	-48.4	-55.1
33,000	196.4	3.80	-50.4	-58.7
34,000	187.4	3.62	-52.4	-62.3
35,000	178.7	3.46	-54.3	-65.8
36,000	170.4	3.29	-55.0‡	-67.0‡

Altitude	Pressure	
feet	*mm. of Hg*	*p.s.i.*
37,000	162.4	3.14
38,000	154.9	2.99
39,000	147.6	2.85
40,000	140.7	2.72
41,000	134.2	2.59
42,000	127.9	2.47
43,000	122.0	2.36
44,000	116.3	2.25
45,000	110.8	2.14
46,000	105.7	2.04
47,000	100.7	1.95
48,000	96.05	1.86
49,000	91.57	1.77
50,000	87.30	1.69
51,000	83.22	1.61
52,000	79.34	1.53
53,000	75.64	1.46
54,000	72.12	1.39
55,000	68.76	1.33
56,000	65.55	1.27
57,000	62.49	1.21
58,000	59.58	1.15
59,000	56.80	1.10
60,000	54.15	1.05
61,000	51.63	1.00
62,000	49.22	0.95
63,000	46.92	0.90
64,000	44.73	0.86
65,000	42.65	0.82
		p.s.f.
66,000	40.6	113.2
68,000	36.9	102.9
70,000	33.6	93.52
72,000	30.4	85.01

Altitude	Pressure	
feet	*mm. of Hg*	*p.s.f.*
74,000	27.7	77.26
76,000	25.2	70.22
78,000	22.9	63.8
80,000	20.8	58.01
82,000	18.9	52.72
84,000	17.2	47.91
86,000	15.6	43.55
88,000	14.2	39.59
90,000	12.9	35.95
92,000	11.7	32.7
94,000	10.7	29.71
96,000	9.7	27.02
98,000	8.8	24.55
100,000	8.0	22.31
110,000	5.0	13.92
120,000	3.24	9.026
130,000	2.18	6.071
140,000	1.51	4.213
150,000	1.08	3.003
160,000	0.787	2.190
170,000	0.583	1.624
180,000	0.433	1.206
	μ. of Hg	
190,000	321.6	0.8956
200,000	238.6	0.6645
210,000	174.9	0.4869
220,000	125.9	0.3504
230,000	88.69	0.2470
210,000	61.02	0.1699
250,000	40.9	0.1139
260,000	26.65	0.07422
270,000§	17.34	0.04829
280,000§	11.49	0.03200
290,000§	7.843	0.02184
300,000§	5.493	0.01530

* Sources: 0 to 80,000, Brombacher tables, NACA Report No. 538, 1935; 80,000 to 300,000, NACA Technical Note No. 1200, 1947.

† Conversion factors: 1 mm. of Hg = 0.019339 p.s.i.; 1 p.s.i. = 51.715 mm. of Hg.

‡ Temperature remains constant above this level up to about 22 miles.

§ Day pressure only; gravity constant.

It is important that the reader understand that these high temperatures at extreme altitude refer to the kinetic temperature of the gas molecules which is proportional to the mean square of the particle velocity. From this it must not be assumed that an object in that region would come into thermal equilibrium with the kinetic temperature of the gases present at those altitudes. The reason for this is that the amount of heat transfer from the gas molecules to the object is negligible because of the rarefied nature of the gas. The temperature of the object would be determined almost solely by radiation from the sun and the earth. Inasmuch as various surface materials of such an object differ in the amount of radiation they absorb and reflect this has a marked effect as shown by the following from the calculations of Buettner. At 115 miles altitude the ambient gas particle temperature is 400° C. A polished aluminum body facing the sun, at that altitude and thermally shielded from the rear, would have an equilibrium temperature of 428° C. A similar body, except for a black exterior, would have an equilibrium temperature of 122° C. and one with a white exterior a temperature of −51° C. If the surface of such a body is directed toward the earth and away from the sun the temperature of these various surfaces would range between 295° C. and −29° C. Accordingly, the environmental temperature of an object in space, such as an inhabited missile, can be fairly accurately controlled by the composition and color of the exterior surface of the object.

ATMOSPHERIC PRESSURE

The atmosphere, owing to the pull of the earth's gravitational field, is compressed so that it is densest at the surface of the earth. With increasing altitude the atmospheric pressure falls rapidly at first and then more slowly until it becomes a vacuum at the outer limit of the atmosphere. Air has mass and weight and at sea level exerts a pressure of over 1 ton per square foot, 14.7 pounds per square inch or 760 mm. of Hg under standard conditions. Above sea level the the pressure of the atmosphere progressively decreases as shown in table 19 and in figure 36. It is important to note that equal changes of altitude at various distances from the earth's surface do not result in equal changes in atmospheric pressure. Thus, a change from sea level to 1000 feet altitude results in a change of 27.0 mm. of Hg of pressure while a change of altitude from 15,000 to 16,000 feet results in a pressure change of only 17.0 mm. of Hg. Between 40,000 and 41,000 feet and between 50,000 and 51,000 feet the respective atmospheric pressure changes are only 6.5 and 4.1 mm. of Hg. This must not be confused with the fact that the atmospheric pressure at a constant temperature, decreases exponentially. In other words, the pressure decreases in equal fractions at equal altitude intervals so that at about 18,000 feet the pressure is one-half that at sea level, at twice this height, or at 36,000 feet it is one-fourth, etc. It is also interesting to note that at an altitude of 20 miles, or slightly over 100,000 feet, almost 99 per cent of the total atmospheric mass is below that level and that the remaining 1 per cent occupies all the space from that point to the outer limit of the atmosphere some 1200 miles distant.

DECREASED DENSITY EFFECTS

The decrease of air pressure and density at the outer reaches of the atmosphere results in a loss of the latter's ability to transmit sound, which was first demonstrated by Robert Boyle in the 17th century through the use of a vacuum jar. As soon as the free pathway of the air molecules is in the order of the wave length of sound, transmission of sound ceases. The atmospheric region where this occurs lies between 50 and 120 miles of altitude. In the lower part of this range the higher tones are first affected, and as the altitude increases the lower tones also disappear. On the basis of transmissibility of the air for sound, we can divide the atmosphere into three zones; the acoustic zone from sea level to about 50 miles; the transacoustic zone from 50 to 120 miles and, finally, the anacoustic zone above 100 miles. Here the silence of space begins. In this region of the atmosphere there is also no sound barrier and, consequently, the Mach unit to measure aircraft speed becomes meaningless.

Another result of the decreased density of

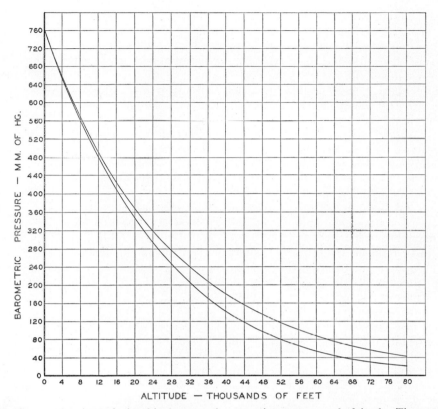

FIG. 36. Curves showing relationship between barometric pressure and altitude. The upper curve assumes a mean temperature of 15° C. whereas the lower curve assumes standard conditions.

the atmosphere is the disappearance of the thermal or heat barrier. In the lower denser regions of atmosphere very fast flying vehicles become extremely hot because of air friction. Above about 120 miles, however, the heat transfer of the rarified air is so small that no heat barrier can be expected at any speed.

At this point it would seem appropriate to define the different aeronautic concepts of altitudes which are as follows:

True altitude is the actual height in feet above sea level. This is the altitude most frequently used by the pilot inasmuch as it is needed in flying over such obstacles as mountains whose altitudes are expressed in feet above sea level.

Tape line altitude is the actual height in feet above the terrain.

Pressure altitude is the height in feet which corresponds to a specific barometric pressure given in the tables of "U. S. Standard Atmosphere."

Density altitude is the height in feet corresponding to a given density ratio in the standard atmosphere. The density altitude is significant to the engineer with regard to airplane performance.

ELECTROMAGNETIC RADIATION

As has already been indicated, radiation from the sun (solar radiation), the stars of our galaxy and other galaxies in the cosmos (cosmic radiation) has a marked influence on the earth's atmosphere. Radiation from these sources is divided into electromagnetic and particle radiation and we shall discuss them in that order. The sun is the principal source of electromagnetic radiation and the basic process involved is nuclear reactions of the fusion type in the sun's interior. The actual radiation which leaves the sun, however, stems from the surface layer called the photosphere. The electromagnetic spectrum of this photospheric radiation ranges from soft x-rays around 6 angstroms to radio waves of more than 10 meters. The spectral energy distribution follows closely that of the radiation of a black body at a temperature of about 6000° K.

This original radiation of the sun, before entering free space, passes through the cooler layers of gas surrounding the sun, the so-called chromosphere. On the way through this chromosphere selective absorption of light by atoms and molecules takes place. This absorption is manifested by a great number of fine dark lines of the spectrum, the so-called Fraunhofer lines.

This absorption spectrum of the chromosphere represents the radiation as it is found in interplanetary space still ranging from soft x-rays to radio waves of more than 10 meters. It is not noticeably altered on the way from the sun through free space to the earth's atmosphere but here a definite change takes place. Generally speaking, when radiation enters the atmosphere it is transmitted unchanged, refracted, reflected, scattered, absorbed, deflected or polarized. Deflection and polarization are of minor importance to us here and will not be discussed.

In the first four cases, namely, transmission, refraction, reflection and scattering, the form of energy remains the same; light remains light and retains the same wave length. In the process of absorption, however, radiation energy is transformed into other forms of energy: chemical energy, heat and electricity and into light of different wave lengths. This transformation of energy takes place in the form of excitation, ionization of atoms or molecules and dissociation of molecules.

In the case of photodissociation molecules are split into smaller molecules and into atoms, essentially by the longer ultraviolet of solar radiation of 2100 to 3000 angstroms. This process takes place in the atmospheric regions above 12 miles throughout the whole atmosphere. In photoionization electrons are knocked off from molecules or atoms which become positively charged and are called ions. This process is produced by absorption of short ultraviolet down to 1000 angstroms and commences in the atmosphere above 40 miles. Radiation that causes ionization is referred to as ionizing radiation. All other radiation is referred to nonionizing radiation.

In the process of excitation electrons are merely lifted from their original orbits to higher orbits. In this way, the molecules or atoms become excited. The electrons return later to lower orbits with the emission of light. Excitation followed by de-excitation with light emission is found in the regions above 50 miles and this light is called airglow. Molecules can also become excited by infrared rays, influencing their vibrations, rotation, etc. When these molecules with higher vibration and rotation frequencies collide with others they attain a higher translatory speed or a higher kinetic energy which means an increase of their temperature.

RADIATION ABSORPTION

The absorption of radiation by the atmosphere will be considered as it occurs from above downward. At the 600 mile level, the spectrum of solar radiation is the same as in free space; namely, the spectrum of soft x-rays to radio waves. Entering the atmosphere, radiation can be absorbed by the gases; oxygen, ozone, water vapor and carbon dioxide; by the fluid raindrops and by the solid bodies; ice crystals, snow, hail and all kinds of dust. The only part of the spectrum that is not absorbed by the gaseous phase of the atmosphere is its visible part. This is, however, absorbed by the liquid aerosols like clouds and by dust aerosols. The nonvisible parts of the spectrum, (i.e., the ultraviolet and the infrared range of solar radiations, both are absorbed by the gases of the atmosphere to a considerable degree.

Beginning with the shortest wave lengths, the rays below 2000 angstroms are absorbed by oxygen and nitrogen in the highest regions of the atmosphere. Dissociations, ionization, excitations and heat production are the result. We also find a strong absorption in the ultraviolet section of the spectrum (2000 to 3000 angstroms). This range of absorption is related to ozone. Ozone is triatomic oxygen (O_3). It is formed by the shorter range of ultraviolet around 2000 angstroms being absorbed by oxygen (O_2). In this process ozone is formed according to the formula $3 O_2 \rightarrow 2 O_3$. There is another photochemical process which destroys ozone. This process is effected through absorption of ultraviolet from 2100 to 2900 angstroms by ozone according to the formula $2 O_3 \rightarrow 3 O_2$. In this way a photochemical equilibrium between formation and destruction of ozone is established. Most of the ozone is formed between 50,000 and 140,000 feet with a maximum concentration of about 8 parts per million by weight at around 75,000 feet. Despite this relatively small amount the existence of ozone in our atmosphere has a far reaching significance for the physics of the atmosphere as well as in a biologic respect.

With regard to physics the process of the destruction of ozone is especially important because in this process heat is liberated in considerable quantities. This heat is held responsible for the increase of the temperature at altitudes above 20 miles. This in turn leads to turbulence of the air and thermodynamic mixing of the atmospheric chemical components, which again counteracts gravitational separation.

The formation and destruction of ozone is of tremendous biologic significance because they almost entirely block the biologically destructive ultraviolet below 3000 angstroms. This ozone umbrella, however, is itself extremely toxic and this would pose a medical problem if the atmosphere at the maximum ozone level around 70,000 to 80,000 feet were to be pressurized to physiologic pressure levels in the cabin of a plane.

Radiation Scattering

A second process that affects solar radiation on its way through the atmosphere is scattering. This process involves essentially the visible part of the spectrum. Light is scattered or dispersed by the air molecules, atoms and fine dust in all directions without changing its wave length. This process produces the so-called skylight. Day skylight is indirect sunlight because the path of light is not directly from the sun to the eye but from the sun to the air particles to the eye. During the night a certain amount of the moonlight and starlight is also scattered.

According to Rayleigh, scattering of light is inversely proportional to the fourth power of the wave length. Accordingly, violet and blue light are scattered the most, followed by green, yellow, orange and red. For this reason during the day the sky appears light blue but before sundown, when the direct sunlight has to travel through many more miles of atmosphere, all of the violet and blue are scattered out and owing to the longer wave lengths of the remaining colors, the sun and the surrounding sky appear yellow and red. However, if we ascend into the upper atmosphere, the atmospheric path of solar light becomes shorter, the air is more rarified and the scattering effect becomes less and less. Thus, the skylight becomes weaker and finally completely disappears; this means that the bright bluish sky gradually turns into the darkness of space with the sun and stars visible at the same time. This condition of a dark sky with a bright sun is reached between 80 to 100 miles altitude. The presence or absence of scattering of light is the main difference between atmospheric optics and space optics. Finally, visible light is also reflected within the atmosphere. To a large degree it is reflected back into space and the reflecting material is mainly the cloud cover.

All of the aforementioned processes—absorption, scattering and reflection—lead to an attenuation of solar radiation as a whole and to an attenuation and extinction of certain sections of the solar spectrum. A considerable amount of the original irradiated solar energy is reflected and scattered back into space, some is absorbed by the constituents of the atmosphere and as a result of all of this—under average atmospheric weather conditions—only a little more than half of it reaches the gound by direct solar radiation and indirect radiation, namely, reflection and scattering.

The solar radiation that reaches the ground is, to a small degree, reflected back into the atmosphere by the earth's surface but the larger part is absorbed by the soil, water and vegetation. This absorbed solar energy is also partly reradiated back into the atmosphere and space.

Particle Radiation

Particle, or corpuscular radiation, consists of the particles which compose the atoms.

The source of corpuscular radiation is the sun as well as the entire cosmos. Those rays coming from the sun are mainly protons and electrons and are responsible for such phenomena as the northern lights, or aurora borealis, and the electromagnetic storms which sometimes disturb radio communications. The cosmic rays, consist of 79 per cent protons, *i.e.*, nuclei of hydrogen, the lightest element, and 20 per cent alpha particles, nuclei of helium, the second lightest element. They also contain nuclei of heavier atoms up to the iron group (about 1 per cent). These cosmic particles have a very high speed which they have probably acquired by accelerations in the electromagnetic fields found between the galaxies or star clusters.

The cosmic rays in their original form are called primary cosmic rays whereas their heavy component is called heavy primaries of cosmic radiation. When these primary cosmic rays strike the atmosphere or collide with any other denser matter, such as metal or the tissue of living organisms, we observe essentially two kinds of effects. The penetrating particles strip off electrons from the molecules lying in their pathway and the atoms that compose the material and in this way produce a track of ions and electrons. Owing to this effect cosmic rays belong to the category of ionizing radiation. The ionization tracks are especially strong in the case of penetration by a heavy cosmic ray particle. Another effect may occur when a cosmic ray particle strikes the nucleus of an atom directly. In such a collision the nucleus is heated to a temperature of billions of degrees in thousandths of a second. This heat causes the nucleus to explode into fragments consisting of protons, neutrons, mesons, electrons, etc., which fly away at very high speed in all directions. A scattering of this type is called an explosion star.

When the primary cosmic rays enter the atmosphere events of the kind just described take place between 60,000 and 120,000 feet. In this zone of absorption they lose their original form and the ionizations and collision products which they create, rain down in showers through the lower layers of the atmosphere. These secondary cosmic rays are less powerful than the primaries but powerful enough to penetrate several hundred feet into water. Accordingly, from sea level up to 60,000 feet, we are exposed only to these secondary cosmic rays. The heavy primaries are seldom found below 70,000 feet (13 miles) altitude but above that level their numbers increase rapidly.

Dr. James A . Van Allen has very recently discovered a doughnut shaped belt of high radiation intensity surrounding the earth opposite both sides of its magnetic equator. This belt starts at about 350 miles from the earth's surface and is thought to extend out for some 7000 or more miles where the intensity drops off sharply. This radiation consists of fast moving protons and electrons which vary in intensity depending upon the activities of the sun. The location and shape of this belt is determined by the effect of the earth's magnetic field on the particles involved.

The major significance of this new finding is that living organisms shot far out into space would have to pass through this lethal zone of radiation. The danger would vary with the time of exposure and the presence or absence of adequate shielding of the passenger compartment. There is an exception to the above based on the fact that the area above the earth's magnetic poles is essentially free of radiation and a space vehicle launched from either of those regions could reach outer space without transversing the Van Allen belt.

Light Phenomena

Radiation also produces light phenomena which can be observed in the sky during the night. They are night airglow, polar auroras or polar lights and zodiacal light. The first two are caused by an intensive photochemical activity in the upper atmosphere whereas the latter is a physical phenomenon outside the atmosphere. The process behind this phenomenon is an excitation of atoms or molecules by radiated energy either of electromagnetic or corpuscular radiation.

It will be recalled that in ionization, electrons are completely knocked off from the orbits of their atom. In the case of excitation, however, they are merely lifted from their normal orbits to outer orbits and are said to be raised to a higher energy. In excited atoms the lifted electron tends to return from its higher stage of energy to its original orbit.

When this happens the energy which pushed it to higher orbits reappears in the form of electromagnetic waves of light. The electron returns to its initial orbit in jumps or "quantum leaps" like a ball tumbling down a stairway and these "jumps" of different amounts are responsible for the emission of light of different wave lengths.

Night airglow and polar auroras are examples, on a gigantic scale, of light emission caused by photoexcitation. The night airglow is a very faint luminance in the upper atmosphere distributed over the whole sky. It is emitted by atomic oxygen, nitrogen and sodium which have been brought into excited states by the ultraviolet of solar radiation. Solar energy absorbed in this way during the day is released during the night.

In contrast to the night airglow which is diffusely distributed all over the sky, auroras are found in the polar regions only. The northern lights are called aurora borealis and the corresponding phenomenon in the southern regions is known as the aurora australis. The fact that auroras are associated with the magnetic poles of the earth supports the theory that they are caused by the bomdardment of air molecules by electrically charged particles, like protons and electrons, ejected from the sun which are then channeled toward the magnetic poles by the earth's magnetic field. These fascinating light phenomena occur at altitudes of 60 to 600 miles. Not only are the air molecules under the auroral bombardment excited but they are also ionized, *i.e.*, they lose outer electrons. These invisible ionized auroras cut through the ionosphere and sometimes produce a complete blackout in radio communication which is of great importance in relation to flights in the polar regions.

Zodiacal light is a faint illumination which appears only in the zodiac, *i.e.*, the zone of the sky within which lie the paths of the sun, moon and planets. It is lenticular in form and best seen after the end of twilight on a very clear evening and before twilight on a clear morning in a moonless sky. It is broadest and brightest near the horizon and thins out to a distance of about 90° from the horizon. This glow along the zodiac is sunlight reflected by micrometeorites which have a strong preference for the ecliptic plane.

METEORS

Meteors in great numbers travel through space with an average velocity of 12 to 36 miles per second. Owing to their tremendous speeds, meteors are usually vaporized when they enter the earth's atmosphere from the intense heat generated by friction. The great majority of meteors are the size of fine dust, a few weigh a gram or more and, over the centuries, there is evidence of some weighing many tons. The two former usually ignite and are vaporized above the 50 mile level and form what is commonly known as shooting stars. The heavier meteors penetrate lower into the atmosphere and the heaviest ones reach the earth's surface before their total mass is completely destroyed. Our principal interest and concern here, of course, is the possibility of meteors striking and destroying a space vehicle in, or beyond, the outer fringes of the atmosphere. Actually, this appears to be unlikely inasmuch as it has been calculated that a meteor large enough to penetrate a three-eighth inch dural metal skin of a space vehicle presenting 1000 square feet of surface area would, in the absence of meteor showers, be encountered on an average of only once in 100 years of space flight.

REFERENCES

(1) STRUGHOLD, H.: Lecture Notes on the Atmosphere. Randolph Air Force Base, Texas, School of Aviation Medicine, USAF 1958.
(2) BUETTNER, K., AND HABER, H.: The aeropause. Science, 115: 656–659, 1952.
(3) HABER, H.: Man in Space. New York, Bobbs-Merrill Co., Inc., 1953.
(4) STRUGHOLD, H., HABER, H., BUETTNER, K., AND HABER, F.: Where does space begin? Functional concept at the boundaries between atmosphere and space. J. Aviation Med., 22: 342–349, 1951.
(5) STRUGHOLD, H.: Space equivalent conditions within the atmosphere. Astronautica Acta, 1: 32, 1955.
(6) STRUGHOLD, H.: The ecosphere of the sun. J. Aviation Med., 26: 323–328, 1955.
(7) WHITE, C. S., AND BENSON, O. O.: Physics and Medicine of the Upper Atmosphere, A Study of the Aeropause. Albuquerque, University of New Mexico Press, 1952.
(8) BUETTNER, K.: Thermal aspects of travel in the aeropause—problems of thermal radiation. In WHITE, C. S., AND BENSON, O. O.: Physics and Medicine of the Upper Atmosphere, A Study of the Aeropause, Albuquerque, University of New Mexico Press, 1952.

9

ALTITUDE SICKNESS

Ulrich C. Luft, M.D.

Altitude sickness may be defined as a state of acute oxygen deficiency (hypoxidosis) resulting from the reduced partial pressure of oxygen (hypoxia) in the inspired air at altitude. Hypoxia was early recognized as the major limiting factor to life at high altitude and remains a subject of paramount importance to aviation medicine.

ETIOLOGY

A continuous supply of oxygen is essential to the life process in each individual cell where energy is liberated by biologic combustion from the energy sources, carbohydrate, protein and fat with formation of carbon dioxide and water. Although the body ordinarily possesses appreciable reserves of these energy sources, it has very limited storage capacity for oxygen itself and is, therefore, extremely susceptible to shortage of this key element. The vital supply line of oxygen from the surrounding atmosphere to the various organs involves the work of muscles, namely in the tidal movements of the respiratory pump and of the heart to provide circulation of the blood conveying oxygen to the periphery. Of equal importance is the process of diffusion which transfers oxygen from the lungs into the blood and from the blood to its destination in the tissues. Diffusion is the passage of molecules from a region of high partial pressure to an area of lower partial pressure. Direction and force of diffusion are governed by the prevailing pressure gradient. What are the factors which determine the partial pressure of oxygen in the atmosphere and in the course of its delivery to the cells?

Partial Pressure of Oxygen

As pointed out in the preceding chapter, the earth's atmosphere consists of a mixture of oxygen, carbon dioxide and nitrogen (including traces of rare gases) in remarkably constant proportion and variable amounts of water vapor. Dalton's law of partial pressures states that when gases or vapors are present in mixture in a given space the pressure exerted by each constituent is the same as if it alone filled the entire space and the total pressure is equal to the sum of partial pressures caused by each gas or vapor present.

$$P_{O_2} + P_{CO_2} + P_{N_2} + P_{H_2O} = B$$

It follows that the partial pressure of each gas will vary with the total pressure in a mixture of constant composition and that the partial pressure of each constituent can be calculated if its volume fraction and the total pressure are known. Thus, in absolutely dry air at sea level the partial pressure of oxygen is

$$P_{O_2} = 760 \times 0.2095 = 159 \text{ mm. Hg.}$$

However, on entering the respiratory passages the inspired air becomes rapidly saturated with water vapor and is simultaneously warmed to approximately body temperature. This has to be taken into account in all considerations of partial pressures for respiratory gases within the body. The water vapor pressure, in contrast to that of dry gases, is not dependent on the total pressure, but is determined entirely by the temperature and the amount of water available for vaporization. If water is present in abundance, as is the case in the respiratory organs, the gas will become fully saturated with water vapor which exerts a constant pressure of 47 mm. of Hg at body temperature (37° C.), regardless of the barometric pressure. Under these circumstances the partial pressures of oxygen, nitrogen and carbon dioxide no longer add up to the barometric pressure (B), but only to the total pressure less the water vapor pressure, or $B - 47$ mm. of Hg. Consequently, the above equation must be modified to obtain the partial pressure of oxygen in air entering the lungs at sea level, as:

$$\text{(Sea level) Tracheal } P_{O_2} = (760 - 47) \times 0.2095 = 149 \text{ mm. of Hg.}$$

It is apparent that with the reduction of barometric pressure at altitude, the water vapor encroaches more and more upon the other gases present so that finally at approximately 63,000 ft. where the barometric pressure is 47 mm. Hg there is theoretically no room for any other gas in the respiratory tract.

TABLE 20

Physiologically Equivalent Altitudes

Altitude	Barometric Pressure	B-47	F_{O_2} Inspired, Dry	Tracheal P_{O_2}
feet	*mm. of Hg*	*mm. of Hg*		*mm. of Hg*
39,000	147	100	1.00	100
10,000	523	476	0.2095	100
Sea level	760	713	0.1400	100

The tracheal oxygen pressure expressed in general form as

$$P_{T_{O_2}} = (B - 47) \times F_{O_2}$$

where F_{O_2} signifies the dry fraction of oxygen in the inhaled gas, is frequently used in aviation medicine to define physiologically equivalent conditions produced at different barometric pressures according to the fraction of oxygen in the inspired gas. For example, the following three conditions are physiologically equivalent with regard to their tracheal oxygen pressures (table 20).

Although the tracheal oxygen pressure can be predicted for any given altitude, the conditions in the alveoli of the lungs where gas exchange takes place involve physiologic events subject to individual variation. On the one hand, oxygen diffuses into the blood stream and carbon dioxide is released into the lungs. This process in itself would rapidly lead to an exhaustion of alveolar oxygen and to an excess of carbon dioxide if it were not closely matched by appropriate pulmonary ventilation controlled by the central nervous system. In fact, the concentration and, therefore, the partial pressures of alveolar gases are found to be remarkably consistent at sea level where the average oxygen pressure is 103 mm. of Hg (range: 96 to 110 mm. of Hg) and that of carbon dioxide 40 mm. of Hg (36 to 44 mm. of Hg). For comparison, data derived from alveolar gas samples taken at various altitudes in a low pressure chamber are presented in table 21 in relation to

TABLE 21

Tracheal Oxygen Pressure, Alveolar Oxygen Pressure and Carbon Dioxide Pressure in the Alveolar Gas When Breathing Air and 100 Per Cent Oxygen at Physiologically Equivalent Altitudes

	Breathing Air					Breathing Oxygen (100 Per Cent)				
Altitude	Barometric pressure	Tracheal P_{O_2}	Alveolar		RER*	Altitude	Barometric pressure	Tracheal P_{O_2}	Alveolar	
			P_{O_2}	P_{CO_2}					P_{O_2}	P_{CO_2}
feet	*mm. of Hg*	*mm. of Hg*	*mm. of Hg*	*mm. of Hg*		*feet*	*mm. of Hg*	*mm. of Hg*	*mm. of Hg*	*mm. of Hg*
Sea level	760	149	103	40	0.85	33,000	196	149	109	40
5,000	632	122	79	38	0.87	36,000	170	123	85	38
10,000	523	100	61	36	0.90	39,000	148	100	64	36
15,000	429	80	46	33	0.95	42,000	128	81	48	33
20,000	349	63	33	30	1.00	45,000	111	64	34	30
22,000	321	57	30	28	1.05	46,000	106	59	30	29

*See Text.

the barometric pressure and the tracheal oxygen pressure. At 20,000 feet, the alveloar oxygen pressure is reduced to less than one-third its sea level value, whereas the barometric pressure is still little less than half an atmosphere. In addition to water vapor with which the tracheal air is already saturated on entering the lungs, carbon dioxide constitutes an appreciable fraction of total alveolar pressure. If the metabolic rate and pulmonary ventilation remained unaltered at altitude, the alveolar pressure of carbon dioxide would remain constant at about 40 mm. of Hg. The observed drop in carbon dioxide pressure is secondary to an increase in ventilation stimulated by hypoxia acting upon chemoreceptors located in the carotid sinus area. In effect, the moderate increase in ventilation which is seldom more than

double the sea level value at rest serves to improve the alveolar oxygen pressure and alleviate hypoxia to a considerable extent. Closely associated with the hyperventilation observed on acute exposure to altitude is an increase in carbon dioxide discharge relative to the oxygen uptake of the blood which is indicated by a rise in the respiratory exchange ratio (RER) toward or above unity (table 21). The respiratory exchange ratio is identical with the respiratory quotient (RQ) only in a "steady state" where respiratory gas exchange is commensurate to the cellular metabolism. This process also tends to raise the oxygen pressure by diluting the nitrogen in the lungs. However, it will be pointed out later that prolonged spontaneous or voluntary hyperventilation at altitude can have serious deleterious effects.

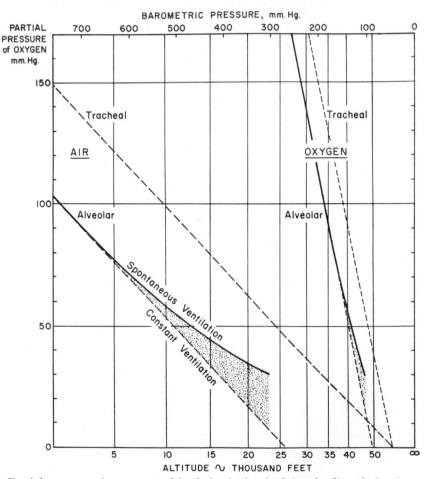

Fig. 37. Partial pressure of oxygen at altitude in the inspired (tracheal) and alveolar gas present when breathing air (left) and oxygen (right). Without increase in ventilation at altitude the alveolar pressure of oxygen would follow the straight line marked "constant ventilation." (Based on data of Boothby *et al.* (2).)

Figure 37 summarizes the respiratory response to altitude on brief exposure up to 22,000 feet with regard to the partial pressure of oxygen in the lungs. The shaded area represents the gain in oxygen pressure acquired by the spontaneous hyperventilation as compared to a hypothetical individual who did not respond to the hypoxic stimulus and did not increase his ventilation at altitude. The latter would encounter a critically low oxygen pressure (30 mm. of Hg) at 15,000 feet, instead of at 22,000 feet as in the average person. Thus, altitude tolerance is to a major extent dependent upon the ventilatory response of an individual to hypoxia.

Oxygen Diffusion and Transport in the Blood

The transfer of oxygen from the gas phase in the lungs into the blood stream coursing through the pulmonary capillaries is accomplished entirely by diffusion and, therefore, is primarily dependent upon the pressure gradient prevailing between the alveolar oxygen and the oxygen tension in the mixed venous blood entering the lungs from the right heart. Only a minute part of the oxygen transferred to the blood is carried in physical solution. Nearly a hundred times more is conveyed in loose chemical binding by the hemoglobin contained in the red cells. The peculiar affinity of hemoglobin for oxygen is best demonstrated by relating oxygen pressure to oxygen saturation in the oxygen dissociation curve of the blood. In figure 38 the alveolar oxygen pressure found at various altitudes, according to table 21, is projected onto the oxygen dissociation curve. At 10,000 feet the oxygen pressure is already 40 mm. of Hg less than at sea level and yet the oxygen saturation is still 90 per cent. On continued ascent to 22,000 feet, however, an

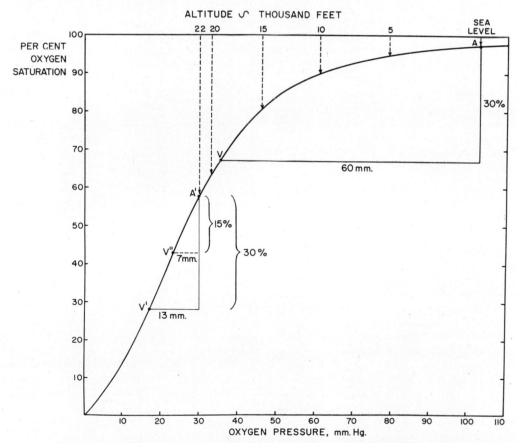

Fig. 38. The oxygen dissociation curve with average arterial oxygen pressures at sea level (*A*) and at 22,000 feet (*A'*). Assuming the same oxygen utilization for both conditions (30 per cent), the arteriovenous pressure difference is much smaller at altitude (*A'-V'*) than at sea level (*A-V*). The contrast is even greater when the oxygen utilization is reduced by increased cardiac output (*A'-V''*) (see text).

additional drop of 30 mm. of Hg leads to a saturation of only 58 per cent in the arterial blood. Thus, the characteristic shape of the oxygen dissociation curve accounts for the relatively mild effects of hypoxia up to 10,000 to 12,000 feet and the serious impairment at higher altitudes.

Another remarkable effect of the steep slope of the oxygen dissociation curve in its middle range is that it minimizes the drop in oxygen pressure associated with the discharge of oxygen to the tissues for metabolism. Ordinarily, the blood is deprived of approximately 6 volumes per cent of oxygen in its passage through the systemic capillaries. This utilization represents 30 per cent of the total oxygen capacity of the blood (normal, 20 volumes per cent). At sea level arterial blood is saturated to 97 per cent and mixed venous blood to 67 per cent. Reference to figure 38 shows that this corresponds to an arteriovenous difference of 60 mm. of Hg oxygen pressure. At 22,000 feet, where the arterial saturation is only 55 per cent, the drop in oxygen pressure for the same utilization would be only 13 mm. of Hg $(A' - V')$. This figure is unrealistic since exposure to high altitude will invariably lead to an increase in cardiac output. According to Fick's principle, the oxygen utilization of the blood is inversely proportional to the cardiac output, provided the oxygen consumption is constant:

$$O_2 \text{ utilization} = \frac{O_2 \text{ consumption}}{\text{cardiac output}}$$

If we assume that the cardiac output was twice as great at 22,000 feet as at sea level under resting conditions, the oxygen utilization would be only 15 per cent and the corresponding difference in oxygen pressure between arterial and mixed venous blood $(A' - V'')$ only 7 mm. of Hg.

What is the relative significance of the various physiologic mechanisms which serve to safeguard the mean oxygen pressure in the systemic capillaries, upon which the individual cells are ultimately dependent? Figure 39 presents the total oxygen pressure gradient between dry atmospheric air and venous blood emerging from the capillaries as a series of cascades for conditions at sea level, 10,000 and 22,000 feet.

The total pressure head can be broken down into four separate steps of which the first is the result of water vapor saturation of the air entering the lungs. The second, between tracheal to alveolar air, is dependent upon respiratory gas exchange and ventilation. The small gradient between alveolar air and arterial blood is caused by physiologic arteriovenous shunts in the pulmonary circuit. The final step between systemic arterial and mixed venous blood is affected by several factors, the most important being the oxygen consumption, the dissociation curve for oxygen and the cardiac output.

At altitude the tracheal-alveolar gradient becomes smaller as a result of the greater pulmonary ventilation. The most striking difference between the examples for sea level and 22,000 feet is seen in the gradient from arterial to mixed venous blood which is only 7 mm. of Hg at altitude as compared to 60 mm. of Hg at sea level for the same oxygen consumption. This phenomenon is attributable to the characteristics of the oxygen dissociation curve, as well as to an increase in capillary blood flow. The mean capillary oxygen pressure indicated in figure 39 represents an average for the entire capillary bed and may vary considerably from one organ to another, depending upon regional conditions of blood flow and oxygen requirement.

Hypocapnia

In the early days of physiologic research in the Alps, it was observed that the carbon dioxide pressure in the alveolar gas and its content in the blood was lower than at sea level. This condition, known as acapnia (from Καπνοσ = smoke), was believed to be a direct effect of low barometric pressure, (1) and was deemed responsible for the symptoms of altitude sickness. Later, it was recognized that acapnia, or better, hypocapnia, is the inevitable consequence of excessive ventilation caused by hypoxia whereby more carbon dioxide is exhausted by the lungs than is being generated by metabolism. The same situation can be readily produced at sea level by voluntary or spontaneous hyperventilation. The acid-base balance of the blood and other body fluids is highly susceptible to alterations in carbon dioxide pressure since the hydrogen ion con-

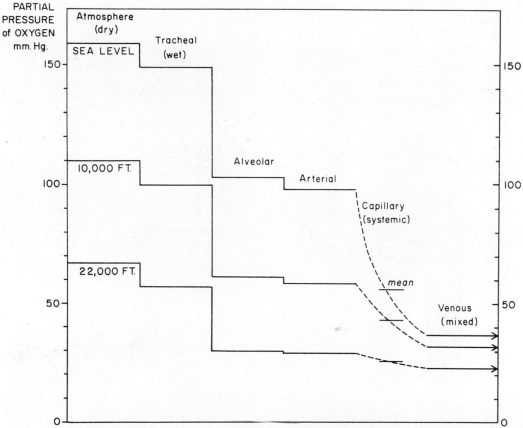

FIG. 39. Cascade of oxygen pressure from dry atmosphere to mixed venous blood at sea level, 10,000 and 22,000 feet. Mean effective oxygen pressure in systemic capillaries is estimated for the resting state.

centration is mainly determined by the proportion of bicarbonate to free carbonic acid present. The effects of hypocapnia can be better understood when related to the manner in which carbon dioxide is transported by the blood. It is indicated in figure 40 that a relatively small fraction is carried as free carbonic acid which varies in linear proportion to carbon dioxide pressure. The total carbon dioxide content, however, which also includes the much larger fraction in form of bicarbonates, follows a parabolic curve. Superimposed on the carbon dioxide absorption curve are straight lines irradiating from the origin which designate points with the same hydrogen ion concentration in terms of pH. When the carbon dioxide pressure falls below the normal value (A), as in hypoxia, the total carbon dioxide also falls, but not at the same rate as the free carbonic acid, so that the blood acquires a higher pH, indicating a state of alkalosis.

In individuals who remain at high altitudes for a period of hours or days, respiratory alkalosis may be partly compensated by elimination of bicarbonate through the kidneys in the process of acclimatization. In acute exposure, a certain degree of hypocapnia is always present and must, therefore, be taken into account as a factor contributing to the manifestations of altitude sickness.

Whereas respiratory activity is governed almost entirely by carbon dioxide at sea level, the stimulus of hypoxia becomes more and more predominant at altitude with a corresponding loss of carbon dioxide stimulation associated with hypocapnia. The net result is a moderately augmented pulmonary ventilation. If the alveolar carbon dioxide pressure is maintained constant by adding appropriate amounts of this gas to the inspired air, hypoxia elicits a much greater respiratory response. Conversely, respiration is markedly depressed in the presence of

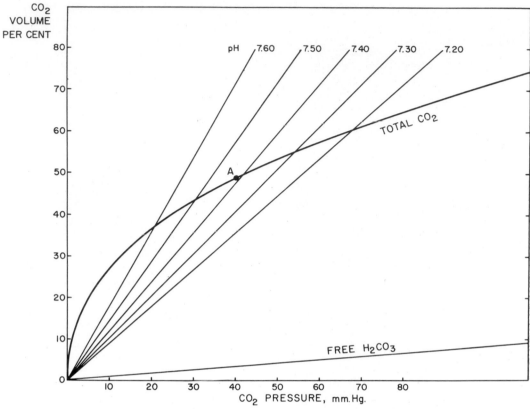

Fig. 40. Carbon dioxide absorption curve for whole blood (after Peters and Van Slyke (3)) with iso-pH lines. *A* is the mean arterial point at sea level.

hypocapnia at altitude when the hypoxic stimulus is suddenly removed by breathing pure oxygen so that a period of apnea may ensue.

Respiratory alkalosis also modifies the transport of oxygen in the blood. If one examines the group of oxygen dissociation curves at different pH values presented in figure 41, it is evident that the curve for high pH is shifted to the left. This means that the blood will be charged to a higher saturation on its passage through the lungs. On the other hand, utilization of oxygen at the tissue level must take place at lower oxygen pressure than usual since the blood will not part with oxygen so readily. This holds true for conditions of alkalosis at sea level where gas exchange takes place on the upper part of the curve. At high altitudes, where oxygen transport is limited to the lower, steeper part of the dissociation curve, alkalosis has little effect on the oxygen pressure in peripheral blood.

Finally, hypoxic hyperventilation leads to a depletion of carbon dioxide in the tissues where it plays an important role in regional vasomotor control, particularly in the central nervous system. Under physiologic conditions, cerebral blood flow is governed by two factors, the systemic blood pressure and the carbon dioxide pressure. Loss of carbon dioxide by hyperventilation at normal oxygen pressures reduces blood flow through the brain and can elicit cerebral symptoms which are indistinguishable from those of hypoxia. Severe hypoxia, on the other hand, is known to cause dilation of the cerebral blood vessels. On ascent to altitude, hypocapnia occurs in the presence of progressive hypoxia so that the vasoconstrictor effects of the former compete against the vasodilating influence of the latter. At altitudes above 20,000 feet where the arterial oxygen pressure falls below 35 mm. of Hg, a moderate over-all increase in cerebral blood flow is observed, indicating that hypoxia has a more

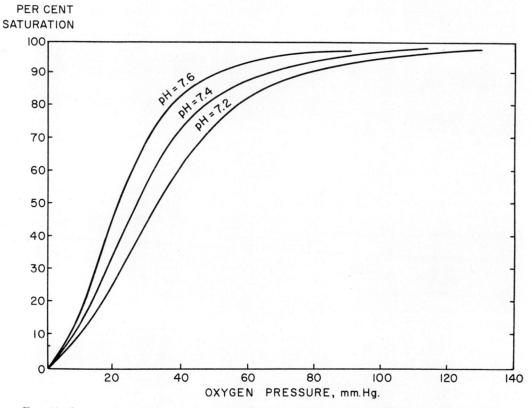

PER CENT
SATURATION

FIG. 41. Oxygen dissociation curve of the blood for different pH conditions (Roughton, (4))

powerful vasodilator effect when the oxygen pressure reaches a critically low level. This contention is supported by observations showing that the blood supply to the brain is much better if normal carbon dioxide pressure is maintained during hypoxia.

The preceding discussion may serve to emphasize the essential difference between the physiologic disturbances caused by hypoxia at altitude, in contrast to asphyxia observed clinically in cases with severe respiratory embarrassment. Insufficiency of oxygen is common to both conditions, but asphyxia is invariably associated with a retention of carbon dioxide leading to hypercapnia whereas altitude sickness is a state of hypocapnic hypoxia. The significance of this differentiation is apparent in the interpretation of symptoms, as well as for prevention and treatment.

SYMPTOMATOLOGY

In the early days of aviation and during the first two decades of its rapid develop-

ment, the effects of altitude were naturally encountered during gradual ascent, without oxygen equipment, in balloons or open cockpit aircraft climbing at a rate of 200 to 1000 feet per minute. With the advent of jet and rocket propulsion systems and the general use of pressurized or sealed cabins, exposure to the altitude environment has become the rare exception rather than the rule. On the other hand, the chances of fatality caused by hypoxia are much greater in emergencies at operational altitudes far beyond the habitable regions of the atmosphere and the manifestations of altitude sickness will differ considerably from the classic pattern encountered in gradual ascent. Nevertheless, the many excellent observations that have been made in the past on the subjective and objective symptoms of altitude sickness in gradual ascent are invaluable since they permit a detailed analysis of progressive functional impairment in the different organ systems and provide, as it were, a slow motion picture of its development.

It is unfortunate that man is not endowed by nature with any specific sensory perception for inadequate oxygen pressure in contrast to his keen sensitivity to many other hazards of the environment, be they mechanical, thermal or chemical. No conscious biologic alarm system exists for hypoxia to compare, for instance, with the acute discomfort caused by an excess of carbon dioxide in the environment. There are, however, certain nonspecific manifestations of which many people become aware, particularly if they have had previous experience. For this reason, practical indoctrination under controlled, simulated conditions of altitude is highly desirable for flying personnel.

Subjective Symptoms

During steady ascent at a rate of about 1000 feet per minute without additional oxygen, the experienced aviator usually becomes aware of a feeling of "air hunger" which is not exactly dyspnea, but a desire to take an occasional deep breath or yawn at 10,000 to 12,000 feet. This is frequently associated with a vague feeling of apprehension and restlessness, sometimes with headache, more often with slight dizziness. On continued ascent beyond 15,000 feet, the elusive feeling of anxiety and alertness gives way to progressive lassitude and indifference in some individuals, in others to increased mobility, hilarity or irritability. Visual and auditory disturbance may be experienced, such as a sensation of darkening of the surroundings and engine noises becoming faint or varying in pitch. One is seldom conscious of increased respiratory effort or of palpitations since these coincide with the progressive failure of sensory perception and critical judgment in approaching unconsciousness. The climax of altitude sickness was described in 1875 by G. Tissandier (5) after his balloon ascent to 25,000 feet, which proved fatal to both of his companions, in words that still ring true today:

"But soon I was keeping absolutely motionless, without suspecting that perhaps I had lost use of my movements. Toward 7,500 m. (24,606 feet) the numbness one experiences is extraordinary. The body and the mind weaken little by little, gradually, unconsciously, without one's knowledge. One does not suffer at all; on the contrary. One experiences inner joy, as if it were an effect of the inundating flood of light. One becomes indifferent; one no longer thinks of the perilous situation; one rises and is happy to rise. Vertigo of lofty regions is not a vain word. But as far as I can judge, this vertigo appears at the last moment. It immediately precedes annihilation, sudden, unexpected, irresistible."

If relief can be promptly provided by immediate descent to below 15,000 feet or inhalation of oxygen, recovery can be remarkably rapid and consciousness returns with a feeling of lightheadedness. Little or no memory exists for events immediately preceding the incident, but tremor and slight muscular incoordination persist for several minutes and are now subjectively recognized.

In the past, a considerable amount of flying was done in unpressurized aircraft between 10,000 and 14,000 feet without additional oxygen. Headaches and lassitude similar to a hangover following such operations were common, but the causal relationship was often not recognized since no discomfort was felt during flight. The sequelae experienced by those who survive extended exposure to altitudes in excess of 23,000 feet, usually caused by interruption of oxygen supply, are much more severe. Delirious and comatose states, paraesthesias and paralysis of various types and duration have been described.

Objective Manifestations

RESPIRATION. One of the early signs of incipient altitude sickness is the mobilization of respiratory excursions with little or no alteration in the number of breaths per minute. The resulting increase in alveolar ventilation is reflected in the alveolar carbon dioxide pressure at altitudes as low as 5000 feet, but is usually not grossly measurable below 10,000 feet. It becomes much more pronounced at greater altitudes, but even in extreme hypoxia the total ventilation per minute is seldom more than double the resting value at sea level. The individual variations in this response to altitude are quite marked. Persons who live permanently at elevations in excess of 5000 feet show a significantly greater increment in pulmonary ventilation when exposed to acute hypoxia than residents at sea level. During physical activity the augmented respiration becomes

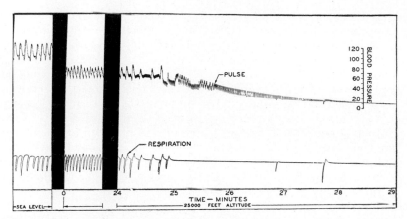

FIG. 42. The accumulative effect of hypoxia produced by exposure to 25,000 feet altitude for 30 minutes (canine).

more noticeable inasmuch as altitude and exertion are synergistic in this respect.

Experimental studies have shown that the hypoxic stimulus is mediated by reflexes from the chemoreceptor organs located in the carotid sinus region and at the arch of the aorta (6). The respiratory response to low oxygen pressure is completely absent when these structures are put out of action. The breathing pattern often becomes irregular at high altitudes and may be of the periodic type which is attributed to the interaction of hypoxia with the normally predominant respiratory control governed by carbon dioxide. In the terminal stages of altitude sickness as observed in animals (fig. 42), rhythmic respiration may cease abruptly although the heart continues to beat for many minutes longer. Respiratory failure during hypoxia is usually an indication of irreversible damage to the respiratory centers in the brain and artificial respiration is mostly in vain. Sudden cessation of breathing can also occur immediately after administering oxygen to a severely hypoxic aviator and cause considerable alarm on the part of the observer. After one or two deep breaths of oxygen, respiration ceases because the hypoxic drive is suddenly removed and the carbon dioxide stimulus is inadequate owing to the preceding hyperventilation. This condition is corrected spontaneously when sufficient carbon dioxide has accumulated by metabolism and regular breathing commences in less than 1 minute. Under these circumstances, artificial respiration would only delay the recommencement of spontaneous breathing.

CIRCULATION. The cardiovascular system responds to altitude first by an increase in heart rate which is perceptible in the resting state at about the same altitude as the initial respiratory changes are observed. If ascent is continued up to the limit of tolerance the pulse rate increases steadily, but not by more than 30 to 40 beats above the value at sea level. Alterations in blood pressure occur above 15,000 feet where the systolic pressure rises with higher pulse pressure. These reactions are associated with an increase in the stroke volume of the heart and of cardiac output (7). The circulatory adaptations encountered in altitude sickness do not originate in the heart since an isolated heart preparation beats slower and weaker when perfused with hypoxic blood (8). Neither does the vasomotor center in the brain respond directly to lack of oxygen, but only to reflexes originating in the chemoreceptors of the carotid sinus and aorta. Numerous investigations concerning cardiovascular adjustments to low oxygen pressure indicate that there is considerable redistribution of blood flow to organs of high oxygen requirement, such as the heart and the brain, with corresponding reduction in other regions.

In the majority of healthy individuals there are no signs of circulatory failure, even in the face of impending unconsciousness at altitude. There are rare exceptions, however, in whom impairment of central nervous functions are preceded and at the same time precipitated by abnormal reactions of the cardiovascular system, with an acute fall in blood pressure and bradycardia. This condition is accompanied by pallor, cold sweat and, occasionally, nausea as in vagovasal syncope, and was called the "fainting type" by Schneider and Lutz in 1920 (9). These authors found that 47 per cent of their subjects, who were young men with no previous experience at altitude, were "fainters." More extensive, recent studies show that, although there may be up to 20 per cent "fainters" on first indoctrination at simulated altitude, only 2 to 3 per cent prove to be reproducible on re-examination. It appears reasonable to assume that most of the men who faint during their first encounter with hypoxia do so for psychologic and emotional reasons, as frequently seen during venesections or mass inoculations. Nevertheless, the few who are of the persistent "fainting type" are

potentially dangerous since they are also more difficult to revive after an hypoxic episode and should not be chosen for flight duties.

The electrocardiogram undergoes characteristic changes revealing inadequate oxygen supply to the heart muscle, depending on the altitude and duration of exposure. An example is given in figure 43 with tracings from Lead II. In addition to the increased heart rate, these reveal a reduction in the amplitude of the T-wave from 0.46 to 0.33 mv. at 16,400 feet after 5 minutes and to 0.23 mv. after 1 minute at 24,600 feet. In the latter there is also a slight depression of the ST segment and the P-wave is higher. All the changes noted disappeared 30 seconds after giving oxygen to the subject and the lower tracing is identical with that taken before ascent with the exception of the reduced frequency typical of the posthypoxic state. In the terminal stages of hypoxia, ob-

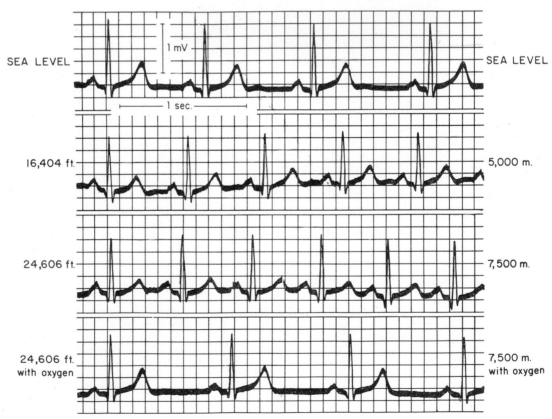

FIG. 43. Electrocardiogram (lead II) in man showing reduced T-wave, increased P-wave and slight depression of ST segment at altitude.

served in experimental animals, the electrocardiogram closely resembles the pattern seen clinically in myocardial infarction.

Prior to the general use of pressure cabins in commercial aircraft, the question as to whether a patient with a history of coronary vascular disease should be advised to travel by air was a serious one for the physician concerned. Even moderate hypoxia at 8000 to 10,000 feet added to a marginal condition of myocardial ischemia might precipitate a critical situation in flight. Currently, jet airliners operate at 35,000 feet or above, but the cabin environment is maintained at pressures equivalent to not more than 6000 feet and additional oxygen is immediately available to each passenger.

THE BLOOD. It has long been known that inhabitants of high mountain regions have, on the average, a greater number of red cells in their blood than people living at sea level. In newcomers to high elevations the red cell count and hemoglobin gradually increase over a period of many days or weeks, depending on the elevation. This process is characteristic of altitude acclimatization and requires a minimum of 24 to 48 hours continuous exposure to altitudes above 10,000 feet to become of measurable significance. There exists no convincing evidence that the number of circulating red cells actually changes during brief exposure to low barometric pressure leading to altitude sickness. It should be realized that the number of red cells counted per cubic millimeter and the hemoglobin concentration determined per unit of blood also reflect fluctuations in the total plasma volume which is subject to fluctuations influenced by the fluid and electrolyte balance.

Armstrong and Heim (10) have demonstrated beyond doubt that exposures as long as 7 hours to 12,000 feet, even when repeated daily over a period of 4 weeks, do not ellicit a hemopoietic response comparable to that found in genuine acclimatization. The same authors (11) reported that other blood constituents such as the white cells, blood nonprotein nitrogen, NaCl and blood sugar were also not altered appreciably during several hours at 12,000 feet.

URINARY SYSTEM. The rate of urine secretion was found to be reduced in dogs breathing low oxygen mixtures to simulate altitudes between 14,000, and 35,000 feet (12). In man this has been confirmed (13) at a simulated altitude of 18,000 feet in the low pressure chamber. The quantity of urine does not appear to be affected at altitudes below 16,000 feet. Urine collected during episodes of hypoxia corresponding to 23,000 feet was sparse, but highly alkaline in its reaction (14) with values reaching pH 8. This finding is explained by the presence of a marked respiratory alkalosis under these circumstances.

GASTROINTESTINAL SYSTEM. According to experimental data from various sources, both gastric mobility and chemistry are affected by altitude sickness. Early studies by Van Liere (15) and his associates indicated that gastric emptying time is delayed at altitudes in excess of 8000 feet in man. Recent observations by Shockett et al. (16) show no certain changes in gastric evacuation even at 15,000 feet. However, at 18,000 feet Mallison (17) found reduced mobility combined with a minimal secretion of free hydrochloric acid on stimulation with 5 per cent alcohol in 8 out of 11 subjects. A normal gastric response was observed when oxygen was breathed at the same altitude. Similarly, the mobility of the intestines is also depressed by hypoxia which leads to a loss of tone, as well as diminished rate and amplitude of peristalsis (18).

In view of morphologic and biochemical investigations performed on animals, there is reason to believe that intermediate metabolism in the liver is seriously impaired during the advanced stages of altitude sickness where rapid mobilization of blood sugar and drainage of glycogen stores takes place. Unfortunately, data on liver function studies in man at altitude are sparse. A significant decline in the utilization of galactose ingested at 18,000 feet was reported by Rittinghaus (13) in healthy male subjects.

METABOLIC RATE AND BODY TEMPERATURE. Numerous investigations on this subject indicate considerable variation in the resting oxygen consumption in man and animals during hypoxia. An interpretation of the contradictory findings is difficult without knowledge of the coincident body temperature which in many cases is lacking. In

1877, Paul Bert (5) made the important observation that exposure to altitude at normal environmental temperature leads to a significant fall in rectal temperature. This phenomenon is more marked in small animals than in those with larger body mass, but it has been well demonstrated in man (19) at altitudes of 16,400 and 23,000 feet. In these experiments the oxygen consumption was considerably below normal during the first 5 minutes of hypoxia, but then showed an increase, finally exceeding the control level. However, the increase in metabolic rate was not sufficient to restore the initial body temperature. A corollary to this is provided by experiments combining hypoxia with a cold environment (20). During hypothermia in hypoxia, the metabolic response was significantly less than to the same degree of cold with adequate oxygen pressure. The implications are that the neural and chemical mechanisms of thermoregulation are impaired by hypoxia causing some variability in metabolic rate depending upon the degree and duration of exposure.

The maximal oxygen consumption attainable in exhaustive physical exertion is markedly reduced at altitude. This is already noticeable well below 10,000 feet.

THE ADRENAL GLANDS. There are rather striking similarities between the physiologic reactions to low oxygen pressure and the effects obtained after the administration of epinephrine. This is evident not only in the behavior of the cardiovascular system, as pointed out by Cannon (21), but also of the gastrointestinal tract and in the hyperglycemia noted under hypoxic conditions. Animal experiments, in which venous blood from the adrenals was sampled directly (22) in the terminal stage of hypoxia, indicate that there is indeed an appreciable discharge of epinephrine with relatively little norepinephrine under these circumstances. There is evidently a reflex mechanism involved, since the secretion of epinephrine in response to hypoxia is diminished or absent when the adrenals are denervated.

In recent years, considerable attention has been given to the hormones of the adrenal cortex in relation to conditions of stress. Giragossintz and Sundstroem (23) reported an extensive study on rats showing that under conditions of very low barometric pressure for extended periods the functional alterations were identical with those observed in corticoadrenal deficiency in adrenalectomized animals. They reasoned that if the cause of abnormal function under hypoxia was due to a lack of the cortical hormone, the administration of this hormone would ameliorate the condition of the animals. This they found to be true. However, in order to sustain the animals under conditions of high altitude they had to supplement much higher doses of cortical hormone than at sea level. It was inferred that animals with intact adrenals exposed to the same altitude required an equal amount of hormone and that the glands were unable to meet this requirement. These observations, which were concerned with the chronic effects of hypoxia, were supplemented later by Armstrong and Heim (10) who exposed rabbits to a simulated altitude of 18,000 feet for 4 hours daily. They first noted an hypertrophy of the entire adrenal glands and, at a later stage, marked degenerative changes in the cortex. The possibility of the fatigue and prostration observed in altitude sickness being the result of adrenal insufficiency cannot be denied. In man, hypoxia equivalent to 18,000 feet sustained for periods up to 45 minutes did not induce a detectable increase in the titer of ACTH in peripheral blood or in the concentration of corticosteroids in the plasma (24). When hypoxia was combined with heat stress and extended over a period of 2 hours, the plasma concentration of corticosteroids was increased in 5 out of 8 subjects.

THE SPECIAL SENSES. The process of dark adaptation of vision is very highly susceptible to oxygen deficiency and significant impairment has been demonstrated at altitudes as low as 6000 to 7000 feet (25), becoming more marked with increasing hypoxia. The normal rate of dark adaptation is completely restored when additional oxygen is breathed and it is wise for pilots to use oxygen equipment or equivalent cabin pressure in flights above 5000 feet at night.

Above 15,000 feet, increasing loss of light perception, particularly in contrast discrimination, becomes evident in quantitative measurements. Similarly, the muscles of accommodation and convergence fatigue more rapidly, whereas stereoscopic vision remains essentially unaltered. The flicker fusion frequency is significantly reduced in moderate hypoxia and has been used to test the efficiency of drugs on performance at altitude (26).

Another very precise criterion of the attenuation of sensory elements at altitude is the loss of perception for sound of high frequency (bone conduction!). With increasing altitudes, the upper frequency limit declines as it does with age. Hearing in the middle and low frequency range, which involves speech intelligibility, monitoring engine noise, etc., is not seriously affected below 18,000 to 20,000 feet. The sense of touch and pain is said to be exaggerated under the initial effects of altitude in gradual ascent to 12,000 to 15,000 feet, but becomes progressively dulled with more severe hypoxia, and individuals have been known to sustain rather serious injuries without being aware of it until returning to lower altitudes when the pain first attracted attention to the lesion.

THE NEUROMUSCULAR SYSTEM. Spinal reflexes play an important part in the integration of voluntary movements. Systematic studies (27) of the knee jerk as a test example of a simple neuromuscular reflex made during ascent to high altitudes have revealed a marked depression in the amplitude of reflex movement beginning as early as 12,000 feet and reaching a minimum at about 16,000 feet. When ascent was continued to 24,000 feet the amplitude progressively increased and became much exaggerated in severe hypoxic states (hyperreflexia).

There is a progressive deterioration of voluntary muscular control at altitudes of about 14,000 feet and above. The first sign to appear is incoordination of the finer muscular movements followed by slowing of movements, tremor and finally paralysis.

Just as in most other symptoms of altitude sickness the time factor is important and several hours of exposure may produce effects which are not present initially. This has been especially noted during experimental studies in the altitude chamber where technicians working at 12,000 to 14,000 feet altitude pressure become slower in movement, awkward and clumsy and develop muscular tremor and incoordination.

A good illustration of the loss of voluntary muscular control in altitude sickness is shown in figure 44. This shows, on the left, a sample of normal handwriting at 2000 feet altitude in flight followed by further writing during a climb at a rate of 1000 feet per minute. At the higher altitudes the subject (H. G. A.) was well aware of the fact that his writing was faulty but in spite of a concentrated effort was unable to improve it. At 25,000 feet altitude collapse was imminent and oxygen was turned on. In the right hand column of figure 44 the oxygen supply was turned off at 30,000 feet altitude during a descent at a rate of 2000 feet per minute. The results are quite apparent although one gets a false impression of the extent of the recovery for during the succeeding hour after the plane had landed the subject was still suffering from marked muscular incoordination and mental confusion. This same phenomenon has been frequently observed by pilots following flights to high altitudes without oxygen in that they are unable to make good landings unless they first descend to a low altitude and spend a considerable time there before attempting to land. The difficulties in these cases consist not only of muscular incoordination but of impaired vision, eye muscle imbalance, diminished depth perception, slowed reaction time and impaired intellectual activity.

CENTRAL NERVOUS SYSTEM. By far the most interesting and the most striking objective symptoms of altitude sickness are those resulting from a change in behavior. These have been studied extensively by McFarland (25) both in flight and in the laboratory and his works should be consulted for a detailed discussion of his results.

Most recent writers agree that there are no significant psychologic changes from hypoxia even during prolonged flights at altitudes below 9000 feet. Above this altitude, however, psychologic changes begin to appear and the degree of change, as in the case of physiologic processes, is in proportion to both the altitude and to the duration of exposure.

In a continuous ascent at a moderate rate of climb psychologic changes are usually not manifested until about 12,000 feet altitude is reached. At this altitude Tanaka found that his average subject's responses were altered. McFarland (25), in a long series of tests, also

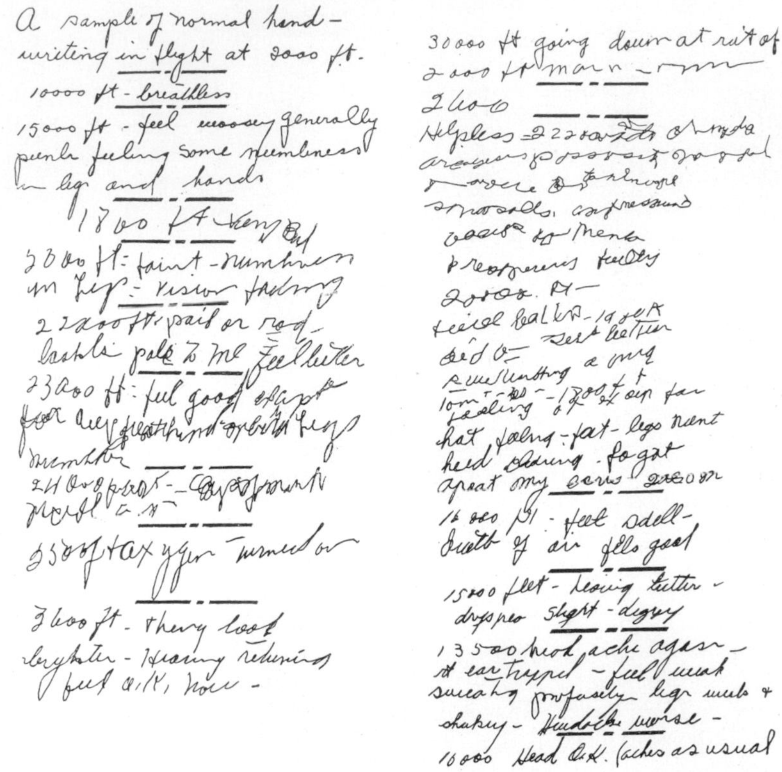

FIG. 44. Handwriting samples obtained during an ascent to 25,000 feet and during descent from 30,000 feet, without oxygen.

found that the initial significant psychologic effects first occurred at this level. These effects consist of a slight decrease in immediate memory and the onset of psychologic complaints. At about 14,000 feet altitude handwriting begins to become impaired and there is a significant degree of mental fatigue as measured by the number of "blocks," as has been described by Bills. At this same altitude there may be a change in moods which are more or less characteristic in each individual and there may be sleepiness, lack of volition and lethargy or there may be a temporary stimulation with euphoria.

At about 18,000 feet the effects become much more pronounced and at this point, in addition to a definite decrease of sensory perception, there is quite marked impairment of neuromuscular control, the field of attention is narrowed and the higher mental processes are affected as indicated by loss of memory, the development of irrational or fixed ideas and the loss of sound judgment and self criticism. This alteration does not take place in a uniform manner but may fluctuate between periods of lethargy and attention peaks so that psychologic tests may show very irregular results.

Between 20,000 feet and the point at which unconsciousness occurs the psychologic effects are quite profound. Simple reaction time tests and simple sensory and motor responses become altered. There is a marked loss of neuromuscular control and there may be twitching, rhythmic movements or even paralysis. Awareness of the lapse of time is lost as well as volitional control except that there is a great persistence in attempting to carry out an assigned task. Explosive emotional outbursts may occur with periods of laughter, anger or pugnaciousness.

Prolonged exposure of several hours to the various altitudes described above is characterized by a marked accentuation of the symptoms and in some instances an alteration in their character. The principal difference is in the increased amount of fatigue, the increased lethargy and lack of volition and the greater number and severity of psychologic complaints. The after effects depend upon the degree and duration of the exposure and vary from a few hours of fatigue and headache to a marked mental confusion and physical prostration which may persist for as long as 48 hours.

The electroencephalogram has been used with success to monitor altitude sickness (28), in particular to define the transition from moderate to severe degrees of cerebral involvement under circumstances where direct observation is difficult or impossible. The normal bioelectric pattern recorded, for instance, from frontoparietal leads (fig. 45) consists of α waves having a potential of 50 to 60 microvolts with a frequency of about 10 c.p.s. and β waves with much smaller amplitude and double the frequency. In progressive hypoxia there is a trend toward slower frequencies and greater amplitudes. Thus, the first disturbances are announced by an activation of the α waves without much change in frequency (fig. 45, second tracing). Later, the frequency is reduced (5 to 6 c.p.s.) and the amplitude increases (fig. 45, third tracing). At a stage where handwriting becomes illegible and perception is dulled, large slow waves of 2 to 3 c.p.s. emerge (fig. 45, lower tracing) and may lead to complete disappearance of electrical activity unless adequate oxygen pressure is restored in the cerebral vessels. When reoxygenation is accomplished promptly the pathologic features disappear in reverse order and normal α waves reappear in 10 to 20 seconds. Slow waves in the electroencephalogram are by no means specific for oxygen deficiency but are seen in different types of cerebral disease. In healthy individuals they occur in hyperventilation and under the effect of drugs such as Metrazol, mescaline and others.

In review of the various subjective and objective manifestations of altitude sickness with regard to their sequence of appearance during gradual ascent and in relation to the altitude at which they generally occur, one can distinguish several phases (27) of progressive physical and mental deterioration:

1. *Indifferent phase* (ground level to 10,000 feet). There is no impairment and the physiologic reserves are essentially intact.

2. *Compensatory phase* (10,000 to 15,000

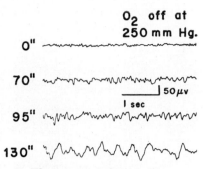

FIG. 45. Electroencephalogram (frontoparietal lead) at ground level and at 27,600 feet (250 mm. of Hg) after removal of oxygen mask. (Courtesy of the *Journal of Applied Physiology*.)

feet). The physiologic adjustments, mainly respiratory and circulatory are adequate to compensate for effects of hypoxia. Additional environmental stress or physical exertion may produce decompensation. There is latent hypoxidosis.

3. *Phase of distress* (15,000 to 20,000 feet). The compensatory mechanisms become inadequate, there is manifest hypoxidosis and the physical and mental reserves are minimal.

4. *Critical phase* (20,000 to 25,000 feet). There is mental and physical incapacitation leading to loss of comprehension and posture with convulsions and cessation of respiration and finally of circulation.

One might call this the classic form of altitude sickness as it was observed and experienced by some of the pioneers in aviation medicine. An important feature of this sequence is the gradual ascent not exceeding 1000 feet per minute. Under these conditions the organism is essentially at an equilibrium with the gaseous environment throughout and physiologic adjustments have ample time to come into play.

The situation is different when an aviator flying at 25,000 feet or above is cut off from his oxygen supply, a frequent cause of hypoxic emergencies during the last war. In this case the rate of onset of altitude sickness is not dependent upon the operational altitude alone, but also upon the rate of pulmonary ventilation, which washes out the oxygen breath by breath, replacing it with atmospheric air. For this reason there is an appreciable delay in the development of critical hypoxia and it is obvious that it can be avoided entirely in voluntary separation

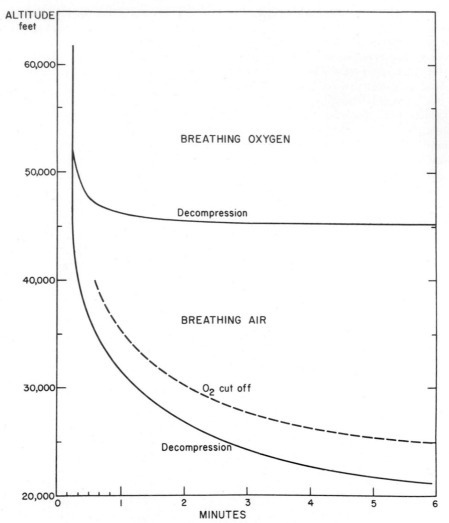

FIG. 46. *Solid curves:* time of useful consciousness at altitude after rapid decompression breathing air (below) and breathing oxygen (above) in pressure cabin. *Interrupted curve:* time of useful consciousness after separation from oxygen supply in unpressurized cabin.

from oxygen as long as one can hold his breath. In figure 46 the interrupted curve indicates the average time of useful consciousness after inadvertent cutoff from oxygen at altitudes between 22,000 and 40,000 feet when using ambient pressure oxygen equipment. Above 30,000 feet altitude sickness sets in acutely leading to the critical phase with little or no premonition or effective physiologic counteraction.

For the present and the future we are more concerned with the form of altitude sickness that results from sudden loss of cabin pressure in vehicles operating at practically unlimited altitudes. In rapid decom-

pression the absolute pressure in the lungs follows that of the cabin atmosphere within fractions of a second, thus instantaneously altering the effective pressure gradient for gas exchange with the blood. As noted in figure 39, the average oxygen pressure in mixed venous blood is 35 to 40 mm. of Hg. Immediately after rapid decompression to 33,000 feet the alveolar oxygen pressure is actually lower than this figure, with the result that oxygen is discharged from the blood instead of being absorbed. Alveolar samples taken under these circumstances show a higher oxygen content in the alveolar gas than in the inspired air (29). When oxygen is breathed during decompression this situation does not arise unless the flight altitude is in excess of 50,000 feet.

The time of useful consciousness after rapid decompression while breathing air is significantly shorter than after interruption of oxygen in an unpressurized cabin, as indicated in figure 46. It is also noted that, at 45,000 feet the time of useful consciousness is at a minimum of 15 seconds which remains constant at higher altitudes. When using oxygen during decompression without additional pressure equipment, the same minimum is reached at 53,000 feet. The sequence of motion picture frames presented in figure 47 with the coincident electroencephalographic tracings below are all taken 14 seconds after rapid decompression (0.2 second) from 32,600 (200 mm. of Hg) to 54,500 feet (70 mm. of Hg). The subject was breathing 100 per cent oxygen throughout. Recompression was accomplished in 2 seconds after exposures varying from 6 to 18 seconds in duration. Complete unconsciousness occurred after 15 to 16 seconds in all exposures of more than 6 seconds to 54,500 feet. The appearance of the subject was the same as that observed in a petit mal seizure in epileptics, with a sudden staring fixation of the eyes and almost complete absence of movements. Subsequently, loss of postural tone and mild convulsive movements were evident after the two longest exposures of 12 and 18 seconds. This phase is associated with severe electroencephalographic changes and temporary, almost complete absence of electrical activity (19th to 20th seconds). Recovery was complete and the electroencephalogram returned to a normal pattern 25 to 30 seconds after recompression to

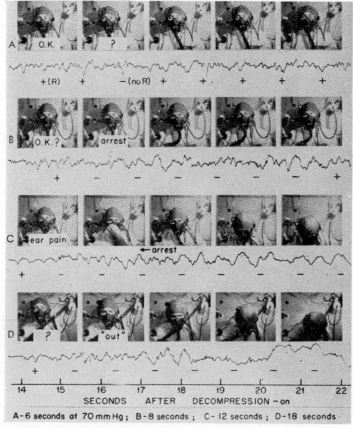

FIG. 47. Posture and electroencephalogram in four tests with decompression from 200 to 70 mm. of Hg in 0.2 second with different durations of exposure to altitude. A, 6 seconds; B, 8 seconds; C, 12 seconds; and D, 18 seconds. Signs + or − indicate presence or absence of signal from subject to mark consciousness. (Courtesy of the *Journal of Applied Physiology*.)

TABLE 22

*Distribution of 100 Subjects According to Their
"Critical Threshold" during Ascent in a Low
Pressure Chamber at 1000 Feet per Minute
with 5 Minutes Stay at Each Step of
1000 Meters (3281 Feet)*

Altitude in Meters	Altitude in Feet	Critical Threshold for:
		per cent
5000	16,404	3
6000	19,685	18
7000	22,966	55
8000	26,247	20
9000	29,528	4

adequate oxygen pressure. The fulminating course of this form of altitude sickness precludes any modification by physiologic adjustments. For the same reason individual differences in the time to unconsciousness are very small.

ALTITUDE TOLERANCE

The ability to withstand low oxygen pressure in the inspired air varies markedly from one individual to another, even if one does not take into account the relatively few cases who tend to react with circulatory collapse at comparatively low altitudes (fainting type). Table 22 gives the results of a survey on 100 healthy service men between 20 and 30 years of age who were tested by gradual ascent in a low pressure chamber. The test was terminated by giving oxygen when the individual had reached his physiologic "ceiling" as determined by failing comprehension and illegibility of a writing test.

Numerous attempts have been made to correlate altitude tolerance with inherent physical characteristics of an individual so that one might predict his performance in hypoxic emergencies on the basis of a medical examination. In general, this has been unsuccessful, although persons in good physical condition, but not necessarily of athletic physique, are, as a rule, above the average in their altitude tolerance. It has also been remarked that men with a high resting pulse pressure and normal diastolic blood pressure are more resistant to hypoxia. Practical experience in altitude tolerance tests has led to the conclusion that inferior adjustments are relatively frequent among younger subjects, particularly in those of less than 25 years of age. However, in a group of men ranging from 25 to 40 years of age there was no significant trend with regard to their performance under hypoxia. Temporary indisposition caused by upper respiratory or gastrointestinal infections, lack of sleep with excess of alcohol and tobacco can seriously reduce a person's physiologic "ceiling". Hypoglycemia, even of a mild degree as found normally in the fasting state, can precipitate the effects of altitude. Obviously, depressant drugs, especially those which are known to act upon the respiratory centers, are deleterious at altitude.

Additional environmental or operational stress when superimposed upon oxygen deficiency can create a critical state at altitudes which are usually tolerable. Extreme heat in the cabin demands circulatory adjustments that are divergent from those which counteract hypoxia, thus reducing the compensatory capacity. High gravitational forces disturb pulmonary and cerebral blood flow, thus adding ischemic insult to hypoxic injury of the brain. Physical exertion increases the demand for oxygen in a system that is already in jeopardy from the lack of it.

With regard to the effects of cold, one might perhaps expect an improvement in altitude tolerance since it is known that, in a state of hypothermia, life can be sustained with much less oxygen owing to the reduced metabolism. However, this applies to the unconscious state of *vita minima* as found in hibernating animals but not to the aviator acutely exposed to cold. Practical experience in operational and simulated bail out tests at high altitudes have proved that cold precipitates altitude sickness.

Considerable effort has been expended on investigations in search of chemical agents or drugs to improve mental and physical performance under marginal conditions of hypoxia. Although valuable basic information was gained thereby, the results have been disappointing from a practical point of view. Much more impressive results have been gained by utilizing the biologic capacity for acclimatization to altitude which is acquired by living at high elevations for several days or weeks. Many inhabitants of high mountain regions in Asia and America live and work all their lives at altitudes above 15,000 feet. Members of high altitude expeditions have lived at 25,000 feet as long as 10 days without additional oxygen (30) in an environment that would be fatal for an unacclimatized individual within a few minutes. Practical tests have demonstrated that even acclimatization at an elevation of 8000 to 10,000 feet for 10 to 14 days is sufficient to raise the physiologic ceiling from 23,000 to 28,000 feet on acute exposure to altitude. This effect is lost within 3 to 4 weeks after return to sea level unless the stimulus is maintained by daily exposure to moderate altitudes for at least 1 hour. This can be accomplished in a low pressure chamber or by breathing low oxygen mixtures.

Differential Diagnosis

There are three other conditions encountered in healthy individuals in flight at high altitudes which should be considered as possible alternatives or complicating factors in establishing a diagnosis. The symptoms are frequently quite similar to those found during or after severe hypoxia.

1. Carbon monoxide intoxication caused by inhalation of exhaust gas from engines or other source of incomplete combustion.

2. Hyperventilation syndrome develops in the course of protracted excess ventilation caused by apprehension and excitement.

3. Neurocirculatory collapse, acute condition of prostration of uncertain etiology, believed to be associated with dysbarism.

These conditions are dealt with in detail in other chapters of this book.

Pathology

There is abundant experimental evidence that severe general disturbance of biologic oxidation from a variety of causes can lead to serious irreversible damage in the cellular structure of the parenchymatous organs with predilection for the liver, the heart and the central nervous system (31). After death caused by acute atmospheric hypoxia, a characteristic pattern in the nature and localization of structural lesions can usually be found. The latter vary in degree and extent with the duration of the lethal hypoxic episode. It appears that the cells around the central veins of the liver lobules are the most highly susceptible to hypoxia. Sharply defined vacuoles containing a hyaline fluid are to be seen in the cell body. Quite similar phenomena occur in the muscle cells of the endocardium, predominantly in the left ventricle along the course of venous capillaries. In the brain the globus pallidus and frequently the corpus subthalamicus show symmetrical lesions. When the lethal hypoxia is of longer duration (hours or days) the vacuolar degeneration is superceded by fatty degeneration of cells or necrosis. If the organism survives, fibrotic areas may be found in the heart and liver. It is difficult to assess precisely how long cerebral cells can be subjected to complete anoxia before irreversible damage occurs and revival is impossible. The occurrence of hypoxia to a degree which produces brain damage in human beings without causing death is rare but that it probably does occur is illustrated by the following case history:

The radio operator of an airplane crew was alone in the rear compartment of an aircraft flying at 25,000 feet when the airplane began a gradual descent. At that time this crew member was known to be conscious and normal. For the next 45 to 60 minutes the aircraft continued its descent, and at the end of the period was at 15,000 feet, at which time an attempt was made to reach the radio operator on the aircraft interphone without success. A second member of the crew went to investigate and found the radio operator lying unconscious on the floor of the plane and disconnected from his oxygen supply. The patient was blue in color and his respirations had ceased. The electrically heated flying suit that he was wearing was also disconnected.

Artificial respiration was started immediately, oxygen was administered and the electrically heated flying suit reconnected. Within a few moments after the artificial respiration was begun the patient gasped and in a few minutes began to breathe fairly regularly. About an hour later the plane landed and the patient was seen by a medical officer. Pulse rate at that time was 160 per minute and the blood pressure 140/82. The patient was still unconscious but very restless and somewhat spastic, the latter occurring intermitently. The respirations were irregular and varied between 25 and 45 per minute. His clothing and skin were drenched with perspiration and his temperature was 105.4° F.

Oxygen inhalations were continued for about 4 hours after the plane landed and the patient's pulse, temperature and respirations gradually returned toward normal during this time. At the end of this 4 hour period there were short intervals of consciousness, whereas at the end of 12 hours the patient was semicomatose and could be aroused to a degree but appeared to be in a vegetated state. He was unable to speak. He vomited several times, once in a projectile manner. At the end of about 24 hours he began to talk for the first time and previous pathologic and neurologic signs mentioned above disappeared. However, he was very restless and difficult to control. When asked what had happened he said that he had been riding a bicycle and had been struck by an automobile. Although apparently in the best of spirits tears would be streaming down his face. At times he became delirious and was obviously hallucinated. He was informed several times that the day was Sunday but in a few minutes told the examiner that it was Tuesday. On the second day after the accident the patient recognized a friend but showed little judgment and could not remember things for more than a minute or two. On the third, fourth and fifth days following the accident the patient continued about the same but showed evidence of having visual hallucinations at times.

During the following 4 weeks improvement continued and at the end of that time the patient appeared to be normal except for spotty memory defects and a tendency to confabulation. A neurologic examination

TABLE 23

Altitudes at Which Hypoxia Death Occurred

Thousands of Feet	Number of Cases
17 to 20	2
20 to 22	4
22 to 24	6
24 to 26	11
26 to 28	23
28 to 30	13
30 to 31.5	11
Not recorded	5
Total	75

which included an electroencephalogram was essentially negative. However, considering the whole picture, especially the length of the coma, the hyperpyrexia, the early neurologic findings and the mania and delirium leads to the conclusion that there had been some diffuse organic brain damage. However, a re-examination of this case some 18 months later failed to disclose any abnormality and he appeared to have recovered completely.

POSTMORTEM FINDINGS

The exact pathology in fatal cases of high altitude hypoxia was not clearly defined until the work of Lewis and Haymaker (32) was published in 1948. Fifty-nine of these cases were collected by Armstrong in the European theater during the course of World War II and the balance of the cases were collected by others in the United States and in various other American overseas theaters of operations. All of the tissues from these various sources were sent to the U. S. Army Institute of Pathology in Washington along with the case histories and the original autopsy reports where they were assembled and carefully studied.

The altitudes at which death occurred were known in 70 cases and were as shown in table 23. It is of special interest that 2 of the fatalities resulted at 17,000 to 20,000 feet. All except 2 of the victims were dead upon the return of the airplanes to their bases. One of those who returned to base alive survived for 40 hours and the other for 21 days. Neither fully regained consciousness and both showed continuous signs and symptoms of cerebral irritation and injury.

The exact duration of the hypoxia was known in only 6 cases. In 2 cases it was 5 to 6 minutes and in 4 cases 3 minutes or less. In 30 cases the duration of hypoxia was not recorded whereas in the remaining 45 cases it was estimated by fellow crew members to be as indicated in table 24.

The principal pathologic changes caused by hypoxia in these cases may be divided into three categories: (1) vascular phenomena characterized by passive congestion, edema and hemorrhages of the internal organs and engorgement of the systemic veins; (2) vacuolar changes, with and without inclusion bodies, in parenchymal cells of various internal organs, especially the heart and liver; and (3) changes in the central nervous system. Engorgement was prominent in virtually all brains affecting capillaries and larger vessels in the parenchyma or leptomeninges or both. Hemorrhages, usually sparse, small and perivascular, were noted in the brains but in the leptomeninges only occasionally. The central nervous system hemorrhages were located most frequently in the cerebral cortex, subcortical white matter and periventricular region including the floor of the fourth ventricle.

Edema, manifested by perivascular sponginess of the parenchyma, was a conspicuous feature being observed in 48 of the 58 brains studied. In some of the brains edema was most prominent in the subcortical white matter, in others subpially and in still others in the tissue subjacent to the subependymal cell plate.

Reactive changes of the central nervous system were frequently observed. In 19 of the 58 brains the resting histiocytes of the arachnoid were diffusely hypertrophied in some regions and in others they had become detached from trabeculae and were free in the arachnoid meshes. Adventitial histiocytes of the cerebral vessels were also occasionally hypertrophied. Perivascular cuffs of inflammatory cells consisting of lymphocytes and a scattering of larger mononuclear cells were observed in 33 of the brains examined. These cuffs were small and sparse and tended to be located in the region of the inferior olivary nucleus and in the internal capsule especially near the striatum. In only 6 cases were collections of lymphocytes observed in the leptomeninges.

Ganglion cells suffered various degenerative changes in about half the cases. Those in the cerebral cortex, including the hippocampus, seemed to bear the brunt of the attack. Swollen ganglion cell bodies and processes were found rather infrequently. On the other hand, shrinkage and hyperchromatosis of cytoplasm and nuclei were often observed. These acute changes, which tended to be spotty, were sometimes visible throughout all laminae of the cortex in a given section but usually predominated in two or three laminae of the midcortex. Other ganglion cell changes included eccentricity of nuclei and nucleoli, disintegration of nu-

TABLE 24

Length of Time without Supplementary Oxygen prior to Death

Time	Number of Cases
minutes	
Less than 3	5
3 to 5	9
6 to 10	13
11 to 20	9
21 to 30	7
31 to 60	0
Over 60	2
Unknown	30
Total	75

clei, vacuolation of cytoplasm and, rarely, tortuosity of apical dendrites. Even more striking abnormalities were present in the pyramidal layer of the hippocampal formation, especially in Sommer's sector. Spotty acute cell changes were also observed in the striatum, thalamus, substantia nigra, globus pallidus, red nucleus, basis pontis, claustrum and amygdala. The cells of the hypothalamus and medulla were largely spared.

REFERENCES

(1) Mosso, A.: Der Mensch auf den Hochalpen. S. Hirzel. Leipzig, 1897.

(2) Boothby, W. M.: Handbook of Respiratory Physiology in Aviation. Randolph Air Force Base, Texas, School of Aviation Medicine, USAF, 1954. p. 44.

(3) Peters, J. P., and Van Slyke, D. D.: Quantitative Clinical Chemistry, Vol. I. London, Bailliere, Tindall and Cox, 1931, p. 897.

(4) Roughton, F. J. W.: Handbook of Respiratory Physiology in Aviation. Randolph Air Force Base, Texas, School of Aviation Medicine, USAF, 1954, p. 57.

(5) Tissandier, G.: In Bert, P.: La Pression Barométrique; Recherches de Physiologie Expérimentale. Paris, Masson et Cie., 1878. (English translation by Hitchcock, M. A., and Hitchcock, F. A.: Barometric Pressure. Columbus, Ohio, College Book Co., 1943, p. 967.)

(6) Heymans, C., and Bouckaert, Y.: Le Sinus Carotidienne. Paris, Masson et Cie., 1933.

(7) Grollman, A.: The Cardiac Output of Man in Health and Disease. Springfield, Illinois, Charles C Thomas, 1932.

(8) Barcroft, J.: The Respiratory Functions of the Blood. Part I. Lessons from High Altitudes. London, Cambridge University Press, 1925.

(9) Schneider, E. C., and Lutz, B. R.: Circula-

tory response to low oxygen tension. In
Air Service Medical, Vol. I. Washington,
D. C., Government Printing Office, 1920,
pp. 86–98.

(10) ARMSTRONG, H. G., AND HEIM, J. W.: Effect
of repeated daily exposures to anoxemia.
J. Aviation Med., 9: 92–96, 1938.

(11) ARMSTRONG, H. G., AND HEIM, J. W.: Factors
influencing altitude tolerance during short
exposures to decreased barometric pressure. J. Aviation Med., 9: 45–56, 1938.

(12) VAN LIERE, E. J., PARKER, H. S., CRISHER,
G. R., AND HALL, J. E.: Effect of anoxemia
on secretion of urine in the dog. Proc. Soc.
Exper. Biol. & Med., 33: 479–180, 1935.

(13) RITTINGHAUS, F. W.: Über Blutzucker und
Zuckerbedarf im Unterdruck. Luftfahrtmed., 9: 95–103, 1943.

(14) LOESCHCKE, H. H., LUFT, U., AND OPITZ, E.:
Die Beteiligung der Niere am Säure-Basen-
haushalt beim Höhenaufenthalt und bei
akuter Hypoxie. Luftfahrtmed., 9: 265–280,
1943.

(15) VAN LIERE, E. J.: Effect of anoxemia on the
alimentary tract. In Anoxia: Its Effect on
the Body. Chicago, University of Chicago
Press, 1942, pp. 159–185.

(16) SHOCKETT, E., JACKSON, M. M., AND DYME,
H. C.: The effect of moderate altitude upon
human gastric emptying time. J. Aviation
Med., 24: 113–122, 1953.

(17) MALLISON, R.: Der Einfluss der Höhe auf die
Magenfunktion. Luftfahrtmed., 4: 156–165,
1940.

(18) WELTZ, G. A., AND v. WERZ, R.: Die Darm-
bewegungen unter Sauerstoffmangel. Luftfahrtmed., 7: 98–117, 1942.

(19) HOUCK, K. TH.: Über Sauerstoffverbrauch
und Wärmehaushalt im Sauerstoffmangel.
Luftfahrtmed., 9: 26–32, 1944

(20) HÜLNHAGEN, O.: Über Störungen der Wär-
meregulation im akuten O$_2$-Mangel bei
Kältebelastung. Luftfahrtmed., 9: 16–25,
1944.

(21) CANNON, W. B.: Endocrinology and Metabolism, Ed. 2. New York, D. Appleton-Cen-
tury Co., Inc., 1929.

(22) HOUSSAY, B. A., AND MOLINELLI, E. A.:
Descarga de adrenalina provocado por la
asfixia. Rev. Soc. argent. biol., 1: 402–425,
1925.

(23) GIRAGOSSINTZ, G., AND SUNDSTROEM, E.:
Cortico-adrenal insufficiency in rats under
reduced pressure. Proc. Soc. Exper. Biol. &
Med., 36: 432–434, 1937.

(24) HALE, H. B., SOYERS, G., SYDNOR, K. L.,
SWEAT, M. L., AND VAN FOSSAN, D. D.:
Blood adrenocorticotropic hormone and
plasma corticosteroids in men exposed to
adverse environmental conditions. J. Clin
Invest., 36: 1642–1646, 1957.

(25) MCFARLAND, R. A.: Human Factors in Air
Transportation. New York, McGraw-Hill
Book Co., Inc., 1953.

(26) ADLER, H. F., BURKHARDT, W. L., IVY, A. C.,
AND ATKINSON, A. J.: Effect of various
drugs on psychomotor performance at
ground level and at simulated altitudes of
18,000 feet in a low pressure chamber. J.
Aviation Med., 21: 221–236, 1950.

(27) STRUGHOLD, H.: Die Höhenwirkung im Lichte
nervenphysiologischer Betrachtung. Luftfahrtmed., 2: 210–222, 1938.

(28) LUFT, U. C., AND NOELL, W. K.: Manifestations of brief instantaneous anoxia in man.
J. Appl. Physiol., 8: 444–454, 1956.

(29) LUFT, U. C.: Handbook of Respiratory Phys-
iology in Aviation. Randolph Air Force
Base, Texas, School of Aviation Medicine,
USAF, 1954, p. 138.

(30) HOUSTON, C. S., AND BATES, R. H.: K2, the
Savage Mountain. New York, McGraw-
Hill Book Co., Inc., 1954.

(31) BÜCHNER, F.: Allgemeine Pathologie. Mün-
chen-Berlin, Urban & Schwartzenberg,
1956, pp. 131–148.

(32) LEWIS, R. B., AND HAYMAKER, W.: High
Altitude Hypoxia. Autopsy Observations
in 75 Fatal Cases and an Analysis of the
Causes of the Hypoxia. Project Report No.
513. Randolph Air Force Base, Texas,
School of Aviation Medicine, USAF, 1948.

10

BREATHING OXYGEN

Charles F. Gell, M.D.

Oxygen was discovered independently by Priestley and by Scheele in 1774. It is a colorless, odorless, tasteless, chemically active gaseous element occurring in the free state in the atmosphere of which it forms about 23 per cent by weight and about 21 per cent by volume at all altitudes at which it has been measured up to 65 miles. Above this altitude oxygen dissociation occurs with the appearance of atomic oxygen. Molecular and atomic atmospheric components decrease in quantity at progressively higher altitudes. Between 600 and 700 miles the effect of the earth's gravity on these atmospheric molecules has been reduced to a degree that the individual kinetic energy of the molecule may be sufficient to allow it to escape into space. This region is called the exosphere and may be considered the extreme limit of the earth's atmosphere.

Oxygen has the molecular formula O_2, the symbol O, an atomic weight of 16.00, a specific gravity referred to air of 1.105 and a liter of the gas weighs 1.429 grams. Oxygen can be reduced to a liquid at $-182.5°$ C. and to a solid at $-223°$ C. The chief commercial source of oxygen is from the liquefaction of air. Of interest to aviation medicine, in view of sealed capsule oxygen recycling requirements, are certain algae which have the ability of releasing oxygen through their metabolism of CO_2, *i.e.*, photosynthesis. Other devices can act as oxygen sources, such as certain electrolytic cells which release oxygen through the action of electrolyte on metallic plates.

Ozone is a triatomic form of oxygen being one and one-half times as dense as oxygen and having the molecular formula of O_3. The theory of ozone formation is that of photochemical action by sunlight. Ozone is highly toxic when inhaled even in minute concentrations. The concentration of ozone in the lower stratum of the atmosphere is not worthy of concern, measuring only two parts to 10^8 parts of atmosphere. There is a moderate increase of concentration with altitude until, at approximately 50,000 feet, a relatively rapid increase occurs up to 60 parts of ozone to 10^8 parts of atmosphere. This concentration persists between 50,000 to 80,000 feet and is known as the ozone layer. Inasmuch as the toxic threshold value is given at 10 parts of ozone to 10^8 parts of atmosphere for 8 hours, the ozone layer is definitely a toxic environment. Ozone has a destructive effect upon rubber and the use of this material is structurally dangerous unless protected from the ambient atmosphere in the ozone layer.

Oxygen is the most vital of the body requirements in higher organisms and the immediate cause of death, except when one is burned alive, is practically always caused by lack of oxygen in the tissues. The body has little internal storage capacity for oxygen but depends upon an almost continuous replacement from the air.

By virtue of the small storage of oxygen in the lungs, a man at rest and under normal conditions can hold his breath for 1 to $1\frac{1}{4}$ minutes. If the oxygen in the lungs and blood is washed out by breathing any inert gas such as nitrogen, sudden and complete loss of consciousness will occur in about 50 seconds.

There are many conditions which may bring about a decreased oxygen supply to the body tissues but we are concerned here only with that which results from a decrease of partial pressure of oxygen in the inspired air during aircraft flights at high altitudes. The mechanism by which oxygen want is created in the body by aircraft ascents and the effects of such oxygen want has already been discussed in detail in chapter 9. In the present chapter we will concern ourselves with the various methods and means of preventing altitude sickness in aviation through the use of oxygen added to the inspired air.

Oxygen Utilization in the Body

A comprehensive review of the physiology of normal respiration at sea level can give us a better understanding of the need for supplemental oxygen at altitude. As the normal person breathes at sea level, he inhales approximately 500 cc. of air with each inspiration. This inhaled volume of gas consists of 79.03 per cent nitrogen, 20.93 per cent oxygen, 0.04 per cent carbon dioxide and traces of rarer gases. Inasmuch as the total atmospheric pressure is 760 mm. of Hg, it is a simple matter to calculate the partial pressure of oxygen as 159 mm. of Hg. Hence, as the normal volume of air at sea level is inspired, the initial pressure of oxygen as it enters the breathing orifices is the equivalent of 159 mm. of Hg. As the air traverses the bronchial tree to the alveolar spaces, however, three things happen to reduce its oxygen partial pressure. It becomes mixed with residual gas that has a reduced oxygen partial pressure, it becomes saturated with water vapor and it is diluted by carbon dioxide. The total effects of these diluents on the oxygen content of the inspired air is to reduce its partial pressure to 100 mm. of Hg by the time it reaches the alveoli.

Inasmuch as the transfer of oxygen molecules across the pulmonary capillary membrane is a simple gradient effect, we have then only 100 mm. of Hg oxygen pressure as the driving mechanism. As venous blood returns from the tissues, we find that its oxygen content, as a result of tissue oxygen utilization, has been reduced to 40 mm. of Hg, or less. This blood from the right heart enters the pulmonary capillaries where, through the mechanism of gradient transfer from the high oxygen partial pressure in the alveoli to the low oxygen tension in the pulmonary capillaries, the oxygen tension of the whole blood is replenished to a pressure almost as high as that in the alveoli. Both the red blood cells and the fluid element of whole blood can carry oxygen.

The blood fluid carries only a small amount of oxygen in simple solution. Oxygen in solution in the plasma of the arterial blood never exceeds 0.3 per cent by volume. A far greater amount of oxygen is carried by the hemoglobin in the red cells. This oxygen is combined chemically as oxyhemoglobin which, when fully saturated, can carry 20.9 per cent oxygen by volume in arterial blood. The total potential oxygenation of whole arterial blood is 21.2 per cent by volume, or 21.2 cc. of oxygen per 100 cc. of blood. The association of hemoglobin with oxygen never reaches 100 per cent. The normal saturation of oxygen in the blood cells is approximately 97.5 per cent in arterial blood.

The metabolic requirement of the body tissues demands a continuous reoxygenation of tissue cells by the arterial blood. Tissue cell oxygen pressure ranges from 0 to 60 mm. of Hg, depending upon the rate of metabolism and the distance of specific tissue cells from the capillaries. Here, too, the transfer of oxygen from capillaries to cell is a simple gradient effect. As arterial blood with a high oxygen content is exposed to cells with a greatly reduced oxygen tension, the oxygen dissociates from the hemoglobin and diffuses into the tissue cells. Arterial blood in the capillaries will be depleted to approximately 40 mm. of Hg oxygen pressure depending upon the tissue requirement. The tissue requirement for oxygen will be dictated by the activity of these tissues. The carbon dioxide tension, pH and temperature of the tissues will also influence oxygen dissociation from hemoglobin, but these are the results of tissue activity.

Of importance to the understanding of oxygen requirement at altitude is the graph (fig. 48) known as the oxygen dissociation curve. This graph demonstrates that the

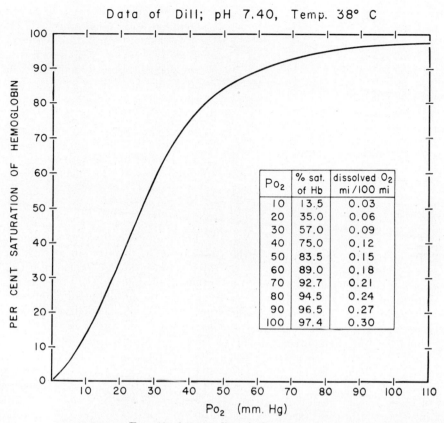

Data of Dill; pH 7.40, Temp. 38° C

Po₂	% sat. of Hb	dissolved O₂ ml/100 ml
10	13.5	0.03
20	35.0	0.06
30	57.0	0.09
40	75.0	0.12
50	83.5	0.15
60	89.0	0.18
70	92.7	0.21
80	94.5	0.24
90	96.5	0.27
100	97.4	0.30

FIG. 48. Oxygen dissociation curve

uptake of oxygen by hemoglobin is not a linear relationship. Examination of the curve shows that hemoglobin is 13 per cent saturated at 10 mm. of Hg oxygen pressure, 35 per cent at 20 mm. of Hg, 75 per cent saturated at 40 mm. of Hg, 88 per cent saturated at 60 mm. of Hg, 94 per cent saturated at 80 mm. of Hg, and 97.5 per cent saturated at 100 mm. of Hg. This oxygen dissociation curve illustrates why, to certain limited altitudes, the arterial oxygen tension will sustain life which would not be possible if hemoglobin were saturated linearly by the associated alveolar oxygen tension. Other factors of importance in the application of oxygen at altitude is the indication that increasing the alveolar oxygen pressure above 100 mm. of Hg will result in only a small increase in oxygen-hemoglobin combination and, secondly, it demonstrates that hemoglobin will give up oxygen rapidly when the oxygen tension is less than 60 mm. of Hg.

Preoxygenation, or the breathing of 100 per cent oxygen at sea level, is a procedure that was utilized prior to high level flights in airplanes without pressurized cockpits or in the absence of pressurized suits. This procedure, sometimes called denitrogenation, is not as commonplace as in the past because of the advanced design of present-day aircraft. The physiology involved in the procedure, however, is worthy of review.

The effect on the composition of lung gases is of the first order of discussion. As 100 per cent oxygen is breathed, the nitrogen in the lungs is not replaced by its normal 79 per cent component. Hence, it is rapidly diluted and washed out from the alveoli. Alveolar nitrogen is almost completely removed in less than 2 minutes. There follows a resultant diffusion of nitrogen from the tissues and blood to the low nitrogen pressure area in the lungs with an ultimate reduction of nitrogen stores in the body. It is estimated that 50 per cent of nitrogen can be eliminated from the body in 1 hour of breathing 100 per cent oxygen at sea level. Nitrogen elimination is not rapid because it

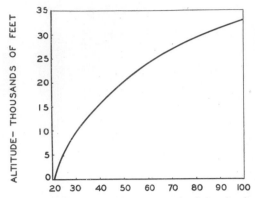

Fig. 49. Per cent oxygen required in the inspired air at various altitudes to maintain a normal alveolar oxygen tension.

lacks any special transport mechanism in the blood.

The effect of preoxygenation on the carbon dioxide content of the tissues and alveoli is not as spectacular. This is the result of the fact that the carbon dioxide is a product of tissue metabolism and the source of higher pressure lies within the tissues and blood rather than in the alveoli. Hence, the use of 100 per cent oxygen will not cause unusual removal of alveolar carbon dioxide. It may possibly interfere with the normal carbon dioxide transport from the tissues, however, by immobilizing oxyhemoglobin and, consequently, reducing the amount of reduced hemoglobin available for carbon dioxide transport.

The blood picture in the breathing of 100 per cent oxygen alters in the following manner. The hemoglobin becomes completely saturated instead of the usual 97.5 per cent. A greater amount of oxygen goes into simple solution in the blood plasma. The sum total of additional oxygen in the hemoglobin and plasma amounts to 11 per cent of normal. Under these conditions the oxygen tension in the venous blood is found to be 60 mm. of Hg instead of the usual 40 mm. of Hg.

The effect of 100 per cent oxygen on respiration is one of slight depression followed by a moderate stimulation of the breathing cycle. The depression is considered to be caused by the effect of high oxygen tension on the chemoreceptor activity in the aortic and carotid bodies. The subsequent stimulation may be caused in part by the

irritant action of 100 per cent oxygen in the bronchioles and alveoli and/or a dilation of the pulmonary capillaries. Other systemic changes in preoxygenation are a consistently reduced pulse rate, a marked reduction in cardiac output and a moderate constriction of the peripheral vessels. The effect of preoxygenation on tissue cells seems to be innocuous. There is no evidence that increased blood oxygen tension causes a variation in the utilization of oxygen by the tissues or causes an abberation in the enzymatic action involved.

OXYGEN REQUIREMENTS AT HIGH ALTITUDE

The amount of oxygen which must be added to the inspired air at high altitude to maintain sea level conditions in the lungs is influenced by many factors. The altitude, of course, is of primary consideration but the per cent oxygen needed is not directly proportional to the pressure change because of the presence of a constant water vapor and CO_2 tension in the lungs. As a consequence, the percentage of oxygen in the inspired air must be increased more rapidly than the pressure decreases with ascent and when this relationship is presented graphically we get the curve shown in figure 49.

Having determined the amount of oxygen required at various altitudes it is next necessary to determine the amount of activity which may be indulged in. It has been shown by various authors that the amount of air breathed and oxygen consumed by an individual varies with his activity as shown in table 25. As can be seen from this table the consumption of oxygen while walking 5 miles per hour increases about 10 times and the air breathed about eight times over that

TABLE 25

Oxygen Consumed and Volume of Air Breathed
(Cubic Feet per Hour)

Activity	O₂ Consumption	Air Breathed
Rest (in bed)	0.5	16.25
Rest (standing)	0.69	22.05
Walking (2 m.p.h.)	1.65	39.4
Walking (3 m.p.h.)	2.26	52.6
Walking (4 m.p.h.)	3.38	79.0
Walking (5 m.p.h.)	5.40	129.0

required at rest. As a consequence the amount of oxygen which must be added to the inspired air in flight must be varied according to the ventilation rate in order to keep the oxygen percentage constant.

A further and very important consideration is the fact that each method of administration varies tremendously in its efficiency and, in most cases, the amount of oxygen supplied to the individual is no criterion of the amount available to him for respiration. In practice the only satisfactory means of determining the amount of oxygen required for any particular piece of equipment is to determine experimentally the flow necessary to give a sea level value to the partial pressure of the oxygen in the lungs or in the blood.

Oxygen Utilization in Flight

All high altitude military airplanes are provided with oxygen equipment and military personnel are required to utilize oxygen at all times while participating in flight above 10,000 feet. One of the first indications of incipient oxygen lack occurs at night where a measurable reduction in night vision usually occurs at altitudes as low as 5000 feet. The decision establishing the mandatory altitude at which military personnel must use oxygen equipment is based on the factor of dispensing with the annoyance of the use of oxygen equipment until an altitude is reached where hypoxia may create an equal or greater handicap. The physiologic changes caused by the development of minor hypoxia from sea level to 10,000 feet are of a moderate nature. In most cases the airmen are unaware of them. They consist of a slight increase of pulmonary ventilation resulting from an increase in the rate and depth of breathing. There is a slight to moderate increase of blood pressure and pulse rate. In military aircraft capable of flight above 35,000 feet, the cockpits are usually pressurized. Pressurization varies from 12,000 to 18,000 feet. In aircraft capable of flight above 35,000 feet, positive pressure breathing equipment is used. In military aircraft capable of flight above 55,000 feet, full or partial pressure suits with their ancillary oxygen equipment are required. Individuals are encouraged to use oxygen at lower altitudes than those prescribed whenever it is deemed necessary by reason of low altitude tolerance, undue physical activity in flight or other circumstance which cannot be covered by general regulation.

In commercial aviation, oxygen equipment is installed in accordance with civil aeronautics regulation. In commercial carriers with unpressurized cabins, a separate oxygen system is maintained for the crew and passengers, respectively. The passenger oxygen equipment requirement consists of a 10 per cent passenger availability at 8000 to 14,000 feet to 100 per cent equipment availability for passengers above 15,000 feet for the duration of the flight. Pressurized cabin commercial carriers are covered by additional civil air regulations. At present, the average commercial carrier flies at a maximum altitude of 20,000 feet with an internal pressurization of 8000 feet. Under these circumstances civil aeronautics regulation requires that crew members be provided with oxygen equipment for the duration of the flight above 10,000 feet. Ten per cent of the passengers will be provided with oxygen equipment with 30 minutes capacity if the altitude does not exceed 25,000 feet.

Jet transports flying at altitudes of 40,000 feet will have an internal pressurization of 8500 feet. In view of the possibility of failure of plane pressurization of jet aircraft which for economical operation must invariably fly above 25,000 feet altitude, the existing civil aeronautics regulation stipulates oxygen equipment for all passengers. In addition, the pilot will wear an oxygen mask at all times above 25,000 feet. Automatic presentation systems are installed in this type of commercial carrier. With this system the pilot can make the masks available to passengers in case of emergency by simply pressing a button. The passenger then holds a rubber cup over his nose and mouth until subsequent descent to safe levels has been accomplished.

The physiologic effects of loss of pressurization of jet transports will not be caused by explosive decompression, but to the effect of acute oxygen deprivation. The onset of hypoxia will depend upon the type of equipment failure and the altitude of the plane. In the case of compressor malfunction the internal pressurization will drop slowly and corrective measures will be less urgent. In the case of loss of pressurization owing to rupture of the cabin, rapid decompression may occur with an urgent requirement for supplemental oxygen by all on board.

Pressurized aircraft flying above 40,000 feet may be in danger of cabin contamination by ozone. A cabin pressurized to 10,000 feet at a 40,000 foot ambient altitude would be below the toxic threshold standard of 10 parts ozone to 10^8 parts of atmosphere, but at 48,000 feet, it would be 10 times the standard toxic threshold. This would be reduced somewhat if the cabin air is fortified with oxygen. The indications are, however, that in pressurized cabin flight where pressurization is accomplished by compressing ambient air, the occupants of the plane must use oxygen for the prevention of the deleterious effect of ozone if the flight is conducted above 45,000 feet.

With respect to the use of oxygen on commercial carriers for persons who may require it at altitudes below 8000 feet because of constitutional disturbances, the air lines are faced with a difficult problem. Obviously it is impractical to attempt a physical examination of every prospective air traveler and there are many among them with healthy appearing exteriors who may be internally debilitated. Persons with cardiac disease associated with decompensation are definite risks whereas well compensated cardiacs usually can tolerate the moderate reduction in atmospheric pressure in pressurized aircraft. Postcoronary disease, angina pectoris and arterial hypertensive states should be evaluated according to the gravity of the condition. This is true of blood diseases, principally the anemias. Asthma and emphysema, and diseases of the respiratory system, also fall into this category. Persons with artificial pneumothorax should not fly because of the increase in gas volume occurring even at pressure cabin altitudes. Fatalities in pneumothorax patients resulting from exposure to moderate altitudes have occurred. The commercial aviation carrier apparently must take the risk of persons in the foregoing category being sensible enough to consult their physicians before exposing themselves to flight.

OXYGEN EQUIPMENT

The continuous development and refinement of oxygen equipment over the past 20 years has resulted in fairly standardized configurations. Aircraft oxygen systems consist of the following basic components: (1) an oxygen reservoir consisting of a container for liquid, gaseous or chemically produced oxygen; (2) a metering device to control pressure and flow of oxygen. This device may fortify ambient air intake with sufficient oxygen to preserve life in accordance with the percentage requirement at altitude; (3) a mask covering the aviator's respiratory orifices and continuous with the oxygen system; and (4) the necessary tubing and connections to integrate the system.

Oxygen may be carried as a peroxide, a liquid or a gas. Peroxides and superperoxides are in a state of imminent practicability as an oxygen source and the method of its use will be briefly described. Liquid and gaseous oxygen are in common use and will be discussed in some detail.

Peroxides

If the peroxides of the alkali earths, such as calcium or barium, or the peroxides of the alkali metals, such as sodium or potassium, are added to water they will react to form free oxygen and a hydroxide. This fact has fascinated many scientists who have visualized the possibility of devising a simple effective piece of oxygen equipment which would be light, compact and almost automatic in its operation. To this end, in the past, attempts have been made to construct a closed system which would operate as follows:

The peroxide is carried in granular form in a canister into which the wearer breathes. The moisture of the breath liberates oxygen from the peroxide and at the same time a hydroxide is formed. As the breath passes through the hydroxide the carbon dioxide of the exhaled air is absorbed and the air is then reinspired having had its oxygen replaced and carbon dioxide removed. This process is then repeated and presumably could continue until all of the oxygen in the peroxide is exhausted. In practice this actually does occur although such a system presents many difficulties.

The addition of water to most peroxides not only evolves oxygen but a tremendous amount of heat. The presence of a caustic alkali in a breathing circuit is dangerous as is also any nitrogen which may inadvertently get into the system and, by displacing oxygen, lead to asphyxia. The amount of oxygen evolved from any peroxide is difficult to control and in freezing temperatures the moisture will congeal and, thus, interrupt the generation of oxygen completely. Despite these difficulties the use of chemical sources of oxygen for potential extended flight above the atmosphere is being presently actively investigated.

Liquid Oxygen

Liquid oxygen is bluish colored and has a boiling point of $-182.5°$ C. It is produced commercially by the liquefaction of ordinary air after which the nitrogen is distilled off. In order to maintain liquid oxygen in its liquid state it must be kept at a temperature below its boiling point of $-182.5°$ C. This is accomplished in field servicing of aircraft by storing it in a liquid oxygen cart (fig. 50) which is essentially a double-walled insulated tank with a means for charging liquid oxygen converters. For laboratory use the liquid oxygen is usually stored in a vacuum flask which is encased in a protective metal housing to prevent it from being broken in handling or shipping. The top of the storage containers are never provided with anything but a vented, loose fitting cap for as the oxygen evaporates, it expands to 860 times its liquid volume and, if confined, would develop tremendous pressures and blow the container to pieces. The field servicing carts for liquid oxygen are fitted with pressure release valves for the same reason.

Liquid oxygen cannot be stored for extended periods of time because of evaporation loss which amounts to a minimum of 2.5 pounds every 24 hours. The design of small liquid oxygen production plants for field use makes this problem unimportant today, whereas, it was a serious problem in the past. Liquid oxygen containers can be secured now in any desired capacity.

For use in aircraft (1), liquid oxygen is

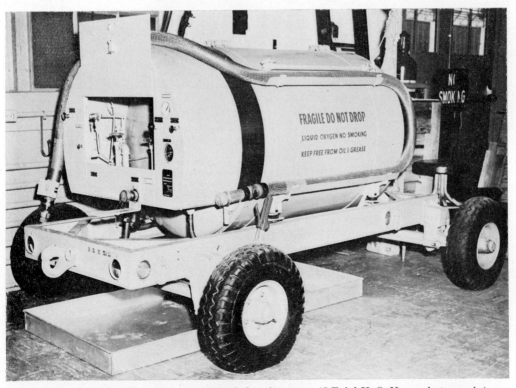

FIG. 50. Field liquid oxygen storage and charging cart. (Official U. S. Navy photograph.)

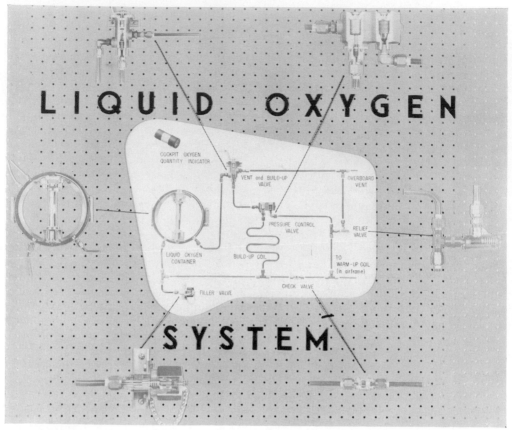

FIG. 51. Schematic cross section of a 5 liter liquid oxygen system for aviation use. (Official U. S. Navy photograph.)

placed in a special liquid oxygen converter shown diagrammatically in figure 51. The liquid oxygen container of the converter system is from 1 to 15 liters capacity and is vacuum insulated to keep heat transfer to a minimum. A capacitance probe is centrally located in the container which senses the liquid quantity. The system has a spring loaded filler valve, a buildup coil which acts as a heat exchanger, pressure closing and pressure opening valve, manual vent and buildup valve, spring loaded, pop type valve and check valve.

The container is filled by forcing liquid oxygen under pressure into the container through the filler valve. It is full when liquid issues from the vent and buildup valve. At this point the cockpit oxygen quantity indicator will show full. With proper valve settings, the liquid oxygen flows from the container into the buildup heat exchanger where it absorbs heat and changes into the gaseous

state which, in turn, causes pressure buildup. These warm gases circulate through various valves back to the gaseous phase of the container enabling more liquid to flow to the heat exchanger. This circulation and pressure buildup continues until the predetermined pressure setting is reached. At this point the pressure closing valve closes, stopping further pressure buildup.

After the converter has attained operating pressure, the unit is ready to deliver gaseous oxygen as required by the crew. As the flow of gaseous oxygen causes the pressure to drop in the system the pressure closing valve opens and pressure buildup again occurs. By this action the system pressure is maintained while the converter is delivering gaseous oxygen. The valving system will compensate for excessive pressure buildup and exert pressure relief if necessary.

As compared to gaseous oxygen, liquid oxygen has a marked advantage in aviation in two respects. For a given quantity of gas the liquid requires much less space and is very much lighter. The matter of weight, of course, is entirely a difference in the weights of the containers required in the two cases and in practice favors the liquid by a ratio of approximately four to one. In other words, the equipment required to supply a given quantity of gaseous oxygen will weigh at least four times as much as the equipment required to supply the same quantity of oxygen carried in the liquid state. This advantage of low weight and small space for liquid oxygen is rapidly bringing about its extensive use in aircraft. The difficulties of manufacturing, shipping and storing have been eliminated to a great degree by the development of field liquid oxygen generators and the perfection of servicing equipment. Practically all new military combatant craft are now fitted for liquid oxygen. Extended flight, long range aircraft still use the gaseous oxygen system to a large extent.

Gaseous Oxygen

Gaseous oxygen is always carried in aircraft in cylinders. These cylinders are specially designed of light weight metal alloys for aviation use. The standard compressed gas shipping cylinder is made of a much heavier steel. Two types of aviation oxygen cylinders are in common use. The cylinder designed for 1800 pounds per square inch pressure is standard in Naval aircraft. It is a wire wound, metal alloy container. The standard oxygen cylinder in use in the Air Force is a low pressure type stressed for a pressure of 450 pounds per square inch. Although considerably lighter, it naturally displaces a greater volume for an equivalent amount of oxygen as compared to the high pressure type of cylinder. The increased bulk is a handicap in the low pressure cylinders, but they are utilized in Air Force aircraft in the assumption that they are safer insofar as potential shattering is concerned. All cylinders are fitted with a needle valve and an attachment for a regulator.

There are several very important things to be kept in mind with reference to the filling of oxygen cylinders. The cylinders when empty should be stored in a cool, dry place away from open flames. No substances other than a mixture of litharge (red lead oxide)

and glycerine should be used for sealing the threads of the valve assembly, or regulator outlet, or any other part of the oxygen equipment for oil or grease used in any of these places may cause fire or explosion when in contact with oxygen.

In preparing an oxygen cylinder to be filled the valve should be removed and all dust, dirt, moisture and metal scales removed from inside the cylinder by blowing it out with compressed air.

Aviation oxygen should be at least 99 per cent pure, completely free of noxious substances, odorless and tasteless. It should not contain more than 0.02 mg. of water per liter at 760 mm. of Hg and 20° C. to eliminate the possibility of stoppage from freezing if water should collect in the system.

With an oxygen source mounted in the airplane it is then necessary to have some means of getting the oxygen to the pilot in the required amounts. This may be accomplished by means of various types of regulators connected to suitable outlets and masks. The standard types will be discussed.

Oxygen System Regulators and Masks

As previously stated, gaseous oxygen in a cylinder is at an initial pressure of 400 to 1800 pounds per square inch and liquid oxygen converters deliver at 70 pounds per square inch. Inasmuch as these pressures constantly fall as oxygen is consumed, it is necessary to place a regulator in the line to control the oxygen pressure and flow. The ideal oxygen system should: (1) deliver automatically to the user the required amount of oxygen at all altitudes; (2) indicate the amount of oxygen supply still remaining in the reservoir; (3) give some positive evidence that oxygen is flowing at the proper rate; (4) be simple and sturdy in construction and, at the same time, be compact and light in weight; and (5) be foolproof and reliable.

Oxygen regulators are designed to function at the service ceiling of the aircraft in which they are installed. They are, consequently, of increasing complexity as the altitude requirement is increased. Oxygen regulators can be grouped in the following categories: (1) continuous flow regulators; (2) demand and diluter-demand regulators; (3) positive pressure and positive pressure diluter-de-

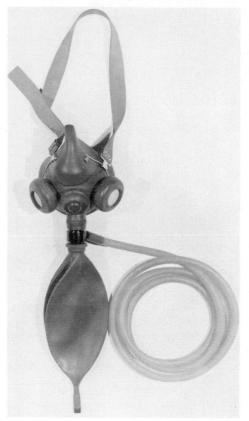

FIG. 52. BLB Oxygen Mask. (Official U. S. Navy photograph.)

mand regulators; and (4) miniaturized 100 per cent demand regulators.

The continuous flow regulator is used to supply oxygen to passengers in transport type of aircraft. In this system a high pressure gaseous oxygen source is used, hence, a pressure reducer is inserted between the cylinder and the regulator inlet. This type of system utilizes the BLB mask (fig. 52). This mask was developed by Boothby, Lovelace and Bulbulian (2) in 1938.

When the mask is in use the oxygen is delivered through a tube to the lower end of the reservoir bag, then up through the connecting and regulating device and into the nose piece from where it is inhaled by the wearer. The exhaled gases pass down through the tubes and part pass out through any ports in the rotary sleeve that may be open. The remaining portion of the exhaled gases pass on downward into the reservoir where it mixes with the incoming oxygen. When the bag becomes distended with the mixture of expired air and oxygen, the slight back pressure then produced permits the excess exhaled air to escape through the expiratory valve. The expired air thus escaping will be from the latter part of the expiration and will contain the most carbon dioxide and least oxygen. Conversely, that part of the expired air which passes into the bag first and contains the least carbon dioxide and most oxygen is available for rebreathing, thus helping to increase the efficiency of the apparatus. On the next inhalation, the mixed oxygen and expired gases, further admixed with atmospheric air entering through the portholes, are again drawn in. This type of equipment, beside its use in aviation, is also used widely in clinical medicine for the administration of oxygen.

The demand regulator is named in accordance with the principle in which it functions. In this system there is an intermittent flow of oxygen controlled by the user's breathing. This is accomplished by the use of a demand valve and an air tight oxygen mask. With such an arrangement, inspiration causes a negative pressure to develop in the system which trips the demand valve and allows oxygen to flow into the mask for whatever length of time and in whatever amount is required depending on the length and depth of inspiration. The amount of negative pressure required to activate the demand valve is only a few millimeters of water and, thus, does not noticeably interfere with respiration. As soon as the inspiration ceases and the negative pressure in the system falls the demand valve closes and shuts off the flow of oxygen. During expiration the exhaled air is discharged from the mask through a flapper valve which prevents the entrance of air into the mask during inspiration.

In addition to the system employing the demand regulator there is also a diluter-demand system which contains an automatic mixing device in the regulator which gives the correct proportion of air and oxygen required at various altitudes. This mixing is controlled by a valve which admits only air and no oxygen to the mask up to about 10,000 feet after which oxygen is also admitted. As ascent continues the per cent of oxygen is increased automatically and that of the air accordingly decreased until, at between 25,000 and 30,000 feet, the valve closes off the air intake completely and pure oxygen only is fed into the mask.

The diluter-demand oxygen system is very efficient being entirely automatic in its operation and normally requires no attention from the wearer. One of its greatest advantages is that it not only feeds oxygen in the correct proportion at the various altitudes but also the amount of oxygen is automatically regulated in accordance with the varying needs of the body under conditions of rest or of any degree of physical activity.

This system requires an absolutely air tight mask which will not allow air to leak into the system under conditions of small negative pressures. Such leaks are especially dangerous at the higher altitudes inasmuch as they cause a dilution of the oxygen being breathed. The standard military A14 mask fulfills this requirement (fig. 53).

Diluter-demand regulators are equipped with an emergency manually operated control which allows the automix or diluter to be turned off so that 100 per cent oxygen can be obtained at any altitude. Although the use of 100 per cent oxygen at moderate altitudes is wasteful and tends to rather quickly deplete the supply, it should be used in certain emergencies. These include the revival of individuals suffering from hypoxia; to compensate for a leak in the oxygen mask or defective operation of a regulator; the presence of toxic fumes or chemical agents inside the airplane; and for denitrogenation during ascent or for treating shock cases during evacuation.

For very high altitude flying another type of oxygen equipment is available known as the pressure-breathing type. With this equipment the oxygen in the mask is at a pressure above the ambient barometric pressure which results in an increased alveolar oxygen tension and increased oxygenation of the arterial blood. The amount of added oxygen pressure must be carefully controlled and ordinarily should not exceed 30 cm. of water (15 mm. of Hg) inasmuch as higher pressure may cause an individual to collapse.

Pressure-breathing equipment is practical only at altitudes of 40,000 feet and above where the other systems fail to provide adequate oxygen to the tissues and only then at the expense of a certain amount of dis-

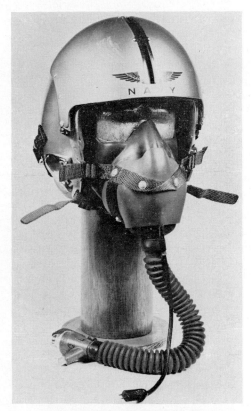

Fig. 53. Standard A14 oxygen mask, for use with demand or diluter-demand regulator systems. (Official U. S. Navy photograph.)

comfort and possible danger. Inasmuch as the oxygen in the mask in pressure-breathing is under positive pressure a special mask with an inner face seal is required. The military A13A positive pressure mask gives a good seal if properly fitted (fig. 54). Fatigue results from the effort required to exhale against the positive pressure. The increased intrathoracic pressure is transmitted to the great vessels of the chest causing a rise in arterial pressure, a damming back of the venous blood to the heart, a reduced cardiac output and an elevated peripheral venous pressure. Pressure breathing may induce hyperventilation with a resultant lowered CO_2 and unconsciousness from acapnia. To minimize these difficulties a positive pressure of not more than 15 mm. of Hg should be used and then for only as short a time as possible.

The amount of gain in altitude through the use of pressure breathing as compared to 100 per cent oxygen from the conventional

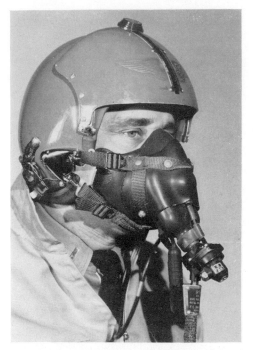

Fig. 54. A13A positive pressure mask for aviation oxygen systems with mask mounted positive pressure regulator. (Official U. S. Navy photograph.)

oxygen system varies with altitude and the amount of positive pressure used as shown in table 26.

If higher pressures are necessary a counterpressure vest covering the entire chest can be used. This vest has an inelastic covering with a pneumatic lining and exerts a pressure on the external chest wall equal to the positive pressure in the lungs. A more complete counterpressure support is accomplished by the use of the partial pressure suit at pressure breathing altitudes. This suit provides counterpressure to the entire body with the exception of the hands and feet. Venous pooling in the extremities with loss of plasma into the tissues is avoided as well as providing counterpressure to the thorax and abdomen.

The physiologically ideal equipment for use at altitudes where pressure breathing is required is the full pressure suit (fig. 55). This suit has a pneumatic lining covering the entire body from neck to feet with an inelastic outer covering. The head is covered with a plastic helmet atmospherically con-

tinuous with the suit with the exception of the face which has a separate compartment for breathing oxygen. In effect the pneumatic lining is automatically inflated above 35,000 feet to a pressure which compensates for the decrease in ambient pressure. The compensation keeps the body at a 35,000-foot pressure equivalent regardless of the ambient pressure caused by altitude. The oxygen pressure in the face compartment is likewise maintained. Thus, normal breathing is maintained at any altitude eliminating the necessity for pressure breathing.

A new miniature positive pressure, 100 per cent oxygen, demand type of regulator has recently been designed for either mask mounting or chest wear (fig. 54). This regulator operates from a liquid oxygen 70 p.s.i. source or a reduced high pressure gaseous system. This regulator in addition to being small and light has an additional advantage. Being mounted on the man instead of the airframe, it is so arranged that it automatically connects to his bail-out oxygen system in case of ejection from the aircraft. In case of submersion, this system will also provide the aviator with bail-out oxygen underwater.

TABLE 26

The Relationship between Flight Altitudes and Equivalent Oxygen Altitudes with Various Settings of the Pressure Breathing Equipment when the Added Pressure is Expressed in mm. of Hg.

Flight Altitude	Equivalent Oxygen Altitude					
	40,000	41,000	42,000	43,000	44,000	45,000
40,000	0					
41,000	6.6	0				
42,000	12.8	6.2	0			
43,000	18.8	12.2	6.0	0		
44,000	24.5	17.9	11.7	5.7	0	
45,000	29.8	23.2	17.0	11.0	5.3	0
46,000		28.5	22.3	16.3	10.6	5.3
47,000			27.2	21.2	15.5	10.2
48,000			31.9	25.9	20.2	14.9
49,000				30.4	24.7	19.4
50,000					28.9	23.6
51,000					33.0	27.7
52,000						31.6

OXYGEN POISONING

The term oxygen poisoning is an unfortunate one insofar as its relationship to the use of oxygen in aviation is concerned. The knowledge that there is such a syndrome and in the absence of complete information has caused some aviators to conclude that the use of 100 per cent oxygen at altitude may bring about some debilitating effect. It should be remembered that oxygen poisoning is a function of both the excess of oxygen partial pressure in the inspired air and the duration of exposure.

The possibility of toxic effects of high oxygen pressure decreases as the altitude increases. At 18,000 feet the aviator breathing 100 per cent oxygen will actually be breathing this oxygen at a pressure of one-half of 1 atmosphere. At 33,000 feet he will be breathing oxygen at 20 per cent of 1 atmosphere even though he is excluding all ambient air and breathing 100 per cent oxygen. Inasmuch as, as stated before, the duration of exposure as well as the oxygen partial pressure are the controlling factors in oxygen poisoning, we have had little to worry about to date in aviation because of the short exposures. This may not be true in future space flight, however, where it might be necessary to continuously expose men to a high oxygen partial pressure in a sealed cabin environment for long periods of time.

Paul Bert in 1878 was the first to demonstrate that high partial pressure of oxygen had a toxic effect on the body and may cause death. Since that time many others have studied this problem and, even now, the etiology and pathology of oxygen poisoning is not completely understood. The symptoms attendant on continuous inhalation of 100 per cent oxygen at 1 atmosphere are primarily related to the respiratory system. The symptoms elicited by continuous inhalations of oxygen at pressures greater than 1 atmosphere are generally related to the nervous system. Where oxygen pressures above 3.5 atmospheres are breathed, death in experimental animals may occur in 2 or more hours. In these cases, the physically dissolved oxygen in the blood is sufficient to supply the tissues without dissociation of oxyhemoglobin. As a result, the transport of carbon

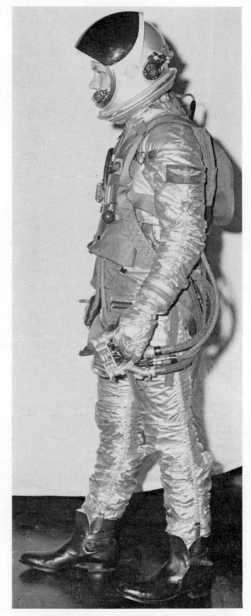

FIG. 55. Military aviator's full pressure high altitude suit. (Official U. S. Navy photograph.)

dioxide from the tissues is interfered with and it rapidly accumulates to the extent that it produces convulsions and death.

In breathing pure oxygen at sea level, the process is somewhat different. Comroe and Dripps (3) exposed 34 young men to 100 per cent oxygen at sea level pressure for 24 hours. Other investigators exposed themselves or others to similar concentrations. In all cases respiratory symptoms were elicited. Predominantly these were substernal pain, reduction in vital capacity, indications of pulmonary congestion and atelectasis.

It is apparent that at some level above the normal oxygen partial pressure of 1 atmosphere, oxygen toxicity symptoms ap-.pear. This was determined first by Armstrong (4) to be approximately 70 per cent of oxygen at 1 atmosphere of pressure or 100 per cent of oxygen at 12,500 feet altitude, both of which are equivalent to an oxygen partial pressure of 530 mm. of Hg. Gell *et al.* (5), however, recently exposed 6 men to 418 mm. of Hg oxygen pressure for 7 days continuously. All of the subjects experienced substernal tightness early during the exposure. There was a decrease in vital capacity of 2 subjects and a roentgenographic indication of atelectasis in 1 subject. The indications were that in 7 days' exposure to 418 mm. of Hg oxygen partial pressure, the toxic effects of high oxygen concentration were beginning to appear. From this data, it appears that an oxygen partial pressure in excess of 55 per cent of 1 atmosphere exceeds the permissible limit for 7 days' exposure.

Unrelated to oxygen poisoning, but certainly annoying to aviators breathing pure oxygen, is its dehydrating effect on the respiratory system. The drying out of the mucosa of the mouth and throat is a frequent complaint of flying personnel following prolonged breathing of 100 per cent of oxygen.

PREVENTION AND TREATMENT OF ALTITUDE SICKNESS

The syndrome known as altitude sickness ranges from the incipient discomfort provoked by flying without using oxygen equipment at altitudes where low grade hypoxia occurs, to the acute fulminating attack resulting from failure of oxygen equipment at critical altitudes. Obviously, if the rule for the use of oxygen equipment at all times above 10,000 feet is carried out or if a pressurized cabin is in use, altitude sickness will not occur. If oxygen equipment is defective or pressurization cannot be maintained, the most effective prophylaxis is descent to altitudes below 10,000 feet. Extended flight without oxygen at altitudes between 10,000 and 15,000 feet may result in symptoms of headache, sleepiness and fatigue. At higher

altitudes there may also be abnormal behavior, nausea, vomiting and, in extreme cases, mental confusion and prostration. For the milder symptoms of headache and fatigue a good night's sleep is usually sufficient for recovery. In more severe cases, a 24 hour rest may be necessary.

In the event of respiratory failure artificial respiration should be initiated immediately and the patient given 100 per cent oxygen. This treatment should be continued as long as there is any evidence of life. The practice of utilizing a mixture of CO_2 and oxygen is definitely contraindicated. The reason for this is that upon cessation of respiration, CO_2 accumulates in the tissues to the extent that there may be a partial or complete paralysis of the respiratory center resulting from the CO_2 poisoning. Accordingly, the use of CO_2 mixtures under these circumstances only aggravates the existing CO_2 poisoning and consequent respiratory paralysis.

Time of Useful Consciousness

The time of useful consciousness is a term expressing the length of time between an individual's suddenly being totally deprived of his oxygen supply at various altitudes and the onset of physical or mental deterioration and, also, the onset of unconsciousness. For our purpose in this discussion, we will use the term time of useful consciousness to indicate the interval between the loss of oxygen supply and the first evidence of disability as manifested by a deterioration in the individual's handwriting. The term time to unconsciousness will be used to describe the time interval between the loss of an individual's oxygen supply and the time he becomes unconscious. The former is of the greatest practical importance to the aircraft crew inasmuch as it represents the time during which they can re-establish their oxygen supply, descend to lower altitudes or otherwise correct the difficulty if possible. The latter is of primary importance to passengers who have no function to perform in operating the airplane but whose lives would be endangered should unconsciousness occur.

The length of time between the loss of one's oxygen supply and the loss of useful consciousness and the time to unconscious-

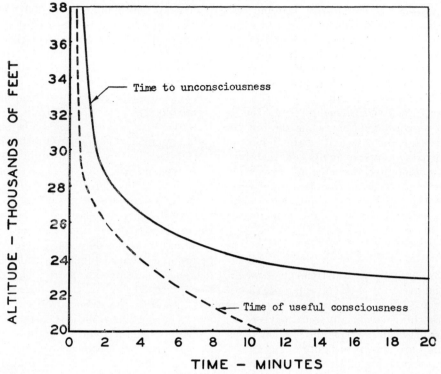

FIG. 56. The time of useful consciousness and the time to unconsciousness at various altitudes caused by a sudden loss of oxygen supply.

ness is determined primarily by the altitude. It is also influenced to some extent by the inherent tolerance of the individual and is markedly influenced by the amount of his physical activity. Thus, it has been shown that exercise sufficient to double the pulmonary ventilation reduces the time of consciousness at 30,000 feet to approximately 50 per cent of the resting value and that tripling the pulmonary ventilation reduces the time of consciousness to approximately one-third that of the resting state. In healthy young adults at rest the average times of useful consciousness and the time to unconsciousness at various altitudes are as shown in figure 56. It will be noted that at the higher altitudes the difference between the time of useful consciousness and the time to unconsciousness is minimal but increases quite rapidly at the lower altitudes. At the higher altitudes the time of useful consciousness is very short being, on the average, some 30 seconds or less at 40,000 feet, 45 to 60 seconds at 35,000 feet, 70 to 90 seconds at 30,000 feet and 2 to 3 minutes or longer at 25,000 feet.

It is to be emphasized that in the paragraphs above we have been discussing time intervals in relation to a sudden loss of oxygen supply at high altitude. An explosive decompression in a pressurized cabin airplane will greatly decrease these intervals in the altitude range of 25,000 to 65,000 feet.

The reason for the very rapid onset of unconsciousness when the oxygen supply is cut off at high altitude is that, in this situation, the oxygen reverses its direction of flow and passes from the blood back into the lungs and thence out to the atmosphere until equilibrium is established with the oxygen of the atmosphere. In the event of a foreseen oxygen failure, this loss of oxygen from the blood and lungs can be delayed for a minute or 2 by the following procedure. While still breathing pure oxygen, overventilation is practiced for about half a minute and then, just before the oxygen supply is cut off, a deep breath is taken and held as long as possible. This accomplishes two things. The overventilation washes carbon dioxide out of the system and allows the breath to be held about twice the normal length of time by temporarily delaying the stimulation of the respiratory center by an excessive accumulation of carbon dioxide in the blood. The holding of the breath maintains a high partial pressure of oxygen in the lungs and in the blood and does not allow this oxygen to escape back to the atmosphere. When this procedure is utilized it must be remembered that while the breath is being held the oxygen in the lungs is being consumed by the body and that hypoxia is developing. As a consequence the use of oxygen should always be resumed by the time the breath can be no longer held or otherwise collapse will quickly follow.

THE LIMITS OF HIGH FLYING WITH OXYGEN

In 1939, Armstrong and Heim (6) studied the partial pressure of the alveolar gases and the oxygen saturation of the arterial blood while breathing essentially pure oxygen at altitudes between 24,000 and 40,000 feet. The results are shown in figure 57.

Accurate analyses of the inspired oxygen showed that it contained about 1 to 2 per cent of nitrogen while the alveolar air showed a nitrogen partial pressure of 5 mm. of Hg. The alveolar carbon dioxide, as was expected, stayed constant at about 36 mm. of Hg at all altitudes.

Beginning at 24,000 feet, the alveolar oxygen amounted to 195 mm. of Hg and decreased steadily with ascent and reached its average normal sea level value of 105 mm.

of Hg at approximately 33,000 feet which corresponds closely to the calculated value at that altitude. At 40,000 feet the alveolar partial pressure of oxygen in the lungs amounted to only 55 mm. of Hg or about half that at 33,000 feet.

The sea level oxygen saturation of the arterial blood for the group studied averaged 96.9 per cent at sea level while breathing ordinary air and is indicated in figure 57 by the dotted line across the top of the graph. The oxygen saturation of the arterial blood varied according to the altitude, being slightly above normal from 24,000 to 27,500 feet and then below normal. At 40,000 feet the arterial oxygen saturation was 88 per cent and from the shape of the curve it may be assumed that at higher altitudes it would decrease at an increasing rate. This dissociation curve at high altitude has a close resemblance to the dissociation curve at sea level when ordinary air is breathed.

From the data given in figure 57 it would appear that the oxygen saturation of the blood begins to fall below normal at about 27,500 feet and when it is considered that this result was obtained under ideal laboratory conditions it may be assumed that this would not ordinarily be improved in actual practice. This point does not necessarily mark the limit of high flying with oxygen, however. Inasmuch as it is permissible to ascend to 10,000 or 12,000 feet above sea level without oxygen, where the oxygen saturation of the arterial blood is decreased

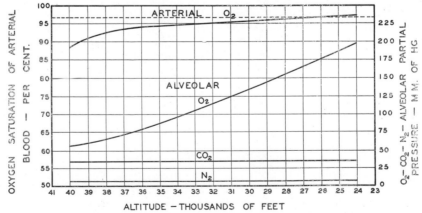

FIG. 57. The average oxygen, carbon dioxide and nitrogen partial pressures in the alveolar air and the oxygen saturation of arterial blood while breathing essentially pure oxygen at various high altitudes.

to about 88 per cent, it would seem equally reasonable to allow one to ascend to 40,000 feet while breathing pure oxygen where the average arterial oxygen saturation is likewise about 88 per cent. It is interesting to note in this connection that with normal respiration at 40,000 feet while breathing pure oxygen, the calculated partial pressure of oxygen in the lungs would amount to only 55 mm. of Hg. Actually, as shown in the graph, the average oxygen partial pressure in the lungs did amount to 55 mm. of Hg. A further point of interest not shown by the graph is the fact that certain individuals did not respond with an increased ventilation and consequently showed an oxygen saturation of the arterial blood of only 83 per cent which is about equivalent to that found at 15,000 feet while breathing normal air.

The absolute limit of high flying using oxygen is not known but on September 28, 1934, Commendatore Donati of Italy, attained an altitude of 47,358 feet in an unsealed cockpit airplane. If Donati had been breathing normally at that altitude, he would have had only 12 mm. of Hg oxygen partial pressure in his lungs (atmospheric pressure (99) − water vapor pressure and carbon dioxide pressure in the lungs (87) = 12). This would have resulted in an arterial oxygen saturation of only about 7 per cent which would have produced almost immediate death. As a consequence he must have had a respiratory center which was very sensitive to oxygen want and which caused him to greatly overventilate with a consequent marked increase of alveolar oxygen and decrease of alveolar carbon dioxide.

Reports indicate that Donati, upon landing, suffered a nervous and physical reaction which left him practically unconscious and it was necessary to lift him from the cockpit of the airplane. At that time his pulse was 105 and remained at about 100 for some time. After 24 hours, during most of which time Donati slept, he was reported to be again in a normal physical condition.

Experiments with animals breathing pure oxygen at these high altitudes show (4) that they experience hypoxia at 35,000 feet and above 40,000 feet die after variable periods of time depending on the altitude. Thus,

rabbits exposed to 43,000, 45,000, 47,000 and 50,000 feet altitude died in 120, 32, 7 and 3 minutes, respectively, from oxygen want.

From the practical standpoint, taking into consideration not only our ability to create normal concentrations of oxygen in the lungs, but also the limitations of present oxygen equipment, the frailties of human nature and the consequences of a loss of oxygen supply at high altitude, flights requiring the use of oxygen are definitely more hazardous than those below that level, other things being equal. The greater the altitude the greater this hazard becomes. In the region of 25,000 feet and above any serious defect in the oxygen system or its improper use will quickly lead to disaster.

The Posthypoxic Paradox Effect

The posthypoxic paradox effect is defined as an abrupt fitlike incident which occurs in rare cases immediately after a marked oxygen deficiency is suddenly relieved by the breathing of an ample supply of oxygen. The term "paradox effect" refers to the fact that in the normal course of events the relief of the hypoxia should improve the condition of the individual rather than impair it. The symptoms of a posthypoxic paradox effect may last from 15 seconds to several minutes and may be varied in character.

In the 4 cases described by Noell (7), 1 displayed a syndrome similar to a narcolyptic episode with a marked decrease of muscle tonus. The second case exhibited a hypertonia of the skeletal muscles manifested by signs similar to those of Parkinson's syndrome. The third case showed hyperkinesis and signs of apraxia whereas the fourth suddenly became unconscious as in an epileptic attack. Upon repeated tests each of these individuals always reacted with the same set of symptoms as before and nothing could be found to explain their reactions.

It was found that hyperventilation just before oxygen was administered aggravated the symptoms whereas a gradually increasing oxygen supply diminished or abolished the attacks. Three to 5 per cent carbon dioxide inhalations had no effect. Investigations of known narcoleptic and epileptic patients gave no positive response.

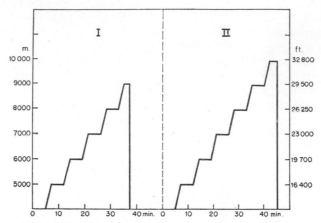

FIG. 58. The physiologic ceiling during gradual ascent in the decompression chamber in 8 subjects (mean values) before (*I*) and after (*II*) return from a Himalayan expedition. (After Luft.)

ALTITUDE ACCLIMATIZATION

It has long been known that individuals who stay for several days or weeks in the mountains develop a tolerance to high altitude to the extent that ascent to 28,000 feet without oxygen has been accomplished and several days have been spent at 23,000 feet.

This whole question has been thoroughly studied by Luft (8). He found that 8 mountaineers who spent 3 months above 14,000 feet, 6 weeks above 20,000 feet and 7 days at 23,000 feet had developed an increased altitude ceiling as shown in figure 58. Other studies in Germany showed that the time required to reach complete acclimatization at various altitudes is as shown in table 27. The factors which were determined to be the most accurate measure of complete acclimatization were the increase in hemoglobin in the blood to a degree which assures the same oxygen capacity of the blood as at sea level and a heart rate which is equal to or less than that at sea level both at rest and with exercise.

In order to use acclimatization on a practical basis further studies were carried out in the Alps at about 10,000 feet altitude. It was found that a fair degree of acclimatization could be acquired in 10 days but that full acclimatization required 3 to 4 weeks. Upon descent to sea level the altitude tolerances began to be lost immediately and had completely disappeared within 3 to 4 weeks. The next step was to devise a method of maintaining this tolerance at sea level and after various trials it was found that this could be accomplished by subjecting the individual concerned to 16,400 feet conditions in an altitude chamber each day, 6 days a week. Under this program the acclimatization was sustained for a test period of 40 days whereas the controls returned to normal. The ceiling of those acclimatized was increased from 23,000 feet without oxygen and 44,300 feet with oxygen to 26,250 feet without oxygen and 47,600 feet with oxygen, a difference of 3250 and 3300 feet respectively.

The above described method of increasing an individual's ceiling obviously has a very limited practical use because of the effort involved to produce a rather limited gain. It was studied in Germany during World War II as a means of increasing their fighter pilots' oxygen ceiling with the introduction of jet and rocket aircraft inasmuch as they did not have pressure breathing oxygen equipment. It is entirely possible that other special situations may arise where this method would be useful.

TABLE 27

Time Required for Complete Acclimatization

Altitude		Time
meters	*feet*	*weeks*
6000	19,700	11 to 12
5000	16,400	9 to 10
4000	13,100	5 to 6
3000	9,800	3 to 4

REFERENCES

(1) MANCINELLI, D.: Liquid Oxygen Instructions. U. S. Navy Manual, 1958.

(2) BOOTHBY, W. M., AND LOVELACE, W. R.: Oxygen in aviation. The necessity for the use of oxygen and a practical apparatus for its administration to both pilots and passengers. J. Aviation Med., 9: 172–195, 1938.

(3) COMROE, J. H., JR., AND DRIPPS, R. D.: Oxygen toxicity. J. A. M. A., 128: 710–717, 1945.

(4) ARMSTRONG, H. G.: The toxicity of oxygen at decreased barometric pressures. Mil. Surgeon, 83: 148–151, 1938.

(5) GELL, C. F., MICHEL, E. L., & LANGEVIN, R. W.: Unpublished data.

(6) ARMSTRONG, H. G., AND HEIM, J. W.: Unpublished data.

(7) NOELL, W.: German Aviation Medicine, World War II, Vol. I. Washington, D. C., Government Printing Office, 1950.

(8) LUFT, U.: German Aviation Medicine, World War II, Vol. I. Washington, D. C., Government Printing Office, 1950.

11

AEROTITIS MEDIA AND AEROSINUSITIS

Harry G. Armstrong, M.D.

In one of the earliest balloon flights ever made, on December 17, 1783, to be exact, the balloonist reported severe pains in his ears. This is of interest principally because it constitutes the first known record of a deleterious effect on the body as a result of flight. In a general way the cause of these ear pains during descent in aircraft have been known since they were first reported but little attention has been paid to them until recent years. During the period of World War I the interest of aviation otologists was concentrated on the vestibular portion of the ear while the middle ear was almost completely ignored. It was finally recognized, however, that pilots who had difficulty ventilating their middle ears were greatly handicapped in their flying and regulations were adopted requiring candidates for flying training to have patent Eustachian tubes. This resulted in a marked improvement in the situation but by no means completely solved it for even with perfectly normal tubes some pilots have difficulty ventilating their middle ears during rapid change of altitude.

With the establishment of commercial passenger air transportation this effect of flight on the middle ear developed with respect to the traveling public. It was obviously impractical to examine the middle ears and Eustachian tubes of prospective airline passengers and as a consequence many were subjected to a considerable amount of discomfort or pain.

In view of the magnitude and importance of the middle ear problem in both military and commercial aviation it is interesting to note that no formal study of this question was attempted until the work of Armstrong and Heim appeared in 1937 (1). As was pointed out by these authors the deleterious effects of flight on the middle ear depends partly on the peculiar structure and functioning of the Eustachian tube and partly on the presence or absence of pathology in this aural appendage. Inasmuch as an intimate and detailed knowledge of the anatomy and physiology of the Eustachian tube is not generally well known a brief review of the more important points in this connection will be presented at this time.

Anatomy and Physiology

ANATOMY. The Eustachian tube is a slitlike, potential tube extending from the middle ear to the nasopharynx. It is formed of bone, cartilage and fibrous tissue.

The bony portion begins at the upper part of the anterior wall of the tympanic cavity and, gradually narrowing, passes downward, forward and mediad for about 12 mm., ending at the angle of the junction of the squamous and petrous portions of the temporal bone.

The cartilaginous portion of the tube extends from the bony portion to the nasopharynx. This section is about 24 mm. in length and is formed of a triangular plate of

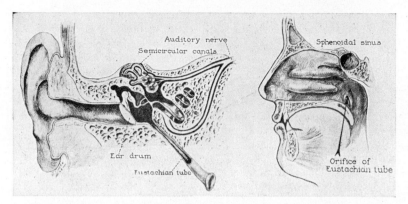

FIG. 59. Schematic representation of the ear and Eustachian tube

elastic fibrocartilage with its apex attached to the bony portion and its base placed directly under the mucous membrane of the nasopharynx where it forms a prominence, the torus tubarius. The upper edge of the cartilage is bent laterally and takes the form of a hook on cross section, open below and laterally. These walls of the canal are completed by fibrous tissue.

The lumen of the Eustachian tube is narrowest at the junction of the bony and cartilaginous portions, the isthmus, and expanding rapidly in both directions reaches its largest diameter at the pharyngeal orifice. At rest the lumen of the cartilaginous portion of the tube is a vertical slit with its walls opposed.

The mucous membrane of the Eustachian tube is a direct extension of that of the nasopharynx and continues backward to line the middle ear completely. The mucous membrane of the bony portion of the tube is thin but in the cartilaginous portion it is thick and very vascular, contains numerous mucous glands and is composed of ciliated columnar cells. Near the mouth of the Eustachian tube is a variable amount of adenoid tissue known as Gerlach's, or the tubal tonsil. The pharyngeal ostium of the Eustachian tube is located high up on the lateral wall of the nasopharynx. This opening is triangular, bounded behind by the torus tubarius and in front by the nasal cavity.

The muscles that are attached to the Eustachian tube and their actions are as follows:

1. *Levator Veli Palatini.* Origin: inferior aspect of the pyramidis ossis temporalis and from the lateral end of the medial lamina of the Eustachian tube. Insertion: downward,

medially and forward parallel to the inferior margin of the medial lamina of the Eustachian tube uniting in the soft palate with the corresponding muscle of the opposite side. Action: elevates the soft palate, narrows the Eustachian ostium and dilates the isthmus.

2. *Tensor Veli Palatini.* Origin: scaphoid fossa of the sphenoid bone, lateral and membranous lamina of the Eustachian tube and angular spine of the sphenoid bone. Insertion: the fibers run downward and forward around the sulcus of the pterygoid hamulus and radiating mediad into the soft palate it attaches to the hard palate and to the corresponding muscle of the opposite side. Action: tenses the soft palate and opens the Eustachian tube.

3. *Salpingopharyngeus.* Origin: inferior part of the ostium of the Eustachian tube. Insertion: blends with the posterior fasciculus of the pharyngopalatinus muscle. Action: raises the upper and lateral parts of the pharynx, opens the ostium of the Eustachian tube.

NORMAL PHYSIOLOGY. The Eustachian tube drains the middle ear and ventilates it. The motion of the cilia and the flutter valvelike action of the tubes favors the motion of material from the ear to the nasopharynx and opposes motion in the opposite direction. The tube, while normally closed, is opened by contraction of its dilator muscles and at such times any air pressure differential existing between the middle ear and the atmosphere is equalized. This may occur during swallowing, yawning and other similar physiologic acts.

SPECIAL PHYSIOLOGY. Aircraft flights involve changes in altitude and this in turn involves changes in atmospheric pressure.

The rates and degrees of atmospheric pressure changes during flight depend on the rates and degrees of ascent or descent and these factors become important when it is remembered that the ear is an air filled closed cavity with pressure equalization possible only when the Eustachian tube is opened.

During ascent it has been found that the effects on the middle ear vary considerably in different individuals and also in the same individual but on the average the following may be noted. At somewhere between 110 and 180 feet altitude (3 to 5 mm. of Hg) there is a slight sensation of fullness in the middle ears and examination will show the tympanic membranes to be slightly bulging. This bulging and the sensation of fullness increase with the decrease of atmospheric pressure until at an average of 500 feet altitude (15 mm. of Hg) there is a sudden annoying "click" in the middle ear as the tympanic membrane snaps back to its normal position. When this occurs it indicates that the Eustachian tube has been forced open by the excess pressure in the tympanic cavity and that the excess pressure in the ear has been relieved by a sudden rush of air from the ear to the nasopharynx.

As ascent continues this cycle is repeated except that all succeeding "clicks" occur at an average interval of only 11.4 mm. of Hg pressure change. This indicates that it requires about 15 mm. of Hg excess pressure in the middle ear at sea level conditions to force the Eustachian tube open and that it remains open until the pressure is reduced to about 3.6 mm. of Hg, when it again closes, leaving 3.6 mm. of Hg excess pressure in the ear. It might be assumed that, inasmuch as the pressure altitude curve is not a straight line, the Eustachian tube would open at equal intervals of pressure but at increasing intervals of altitude during ascent. Actually the reverse has been found to be true for the tubes open at approximately 425 foot intervals (except the first), at both sea level and at 35,000 feet which in terms of pressure difference is equal to 11.4 mm. of Hg in the former but only 3.5 mm. of Hg in the latter. The probable explanation of this phenomenon is that the rarified air of the higher altitudes passes outward through the Eustachian tubes more readily than the denser air of the lower altitudes.

During descent, that is when the atmospheric pressure is being increased, a totally different effect is obtained. Here the Eustachian tube, because of its flutter valvelike action, remains closed regardless of the pressure differential created in the middle ear.

For both ascent and descent the above description applies only to instances in which no attempt is made to ventilate the middle ear by voluntary acts. In individuals with normal patent Eustachian tubes either positive or negative pressure differentials in the tympanic cavity can usually be equalized by voluntary effort except that after a negative pressure of 80 to 90 mm. of Hg or more has developed it is then impossible for the Eustachian muscles to overcome the pressure which holds the fibrocartilaginous portion of the tube tightly collapsed.

AEROTITIS MEDIA

As a result of their studies on the effect of flight on the middle ear Armstrong and Heim (1) concluded that they were justified in describing the resulting condition as a new clinical entity to which they applied the term aerotitis media.

Definition

Aerotitis media is an acute or chronic traumatic inflammation of the middle ear caused by a pressure difference between the air in the tympanic cavity and that of the surrounding atmosphere. It is characterized by various combinations of the following signs and symptoms: marked discomfort or pain in the affected ear, inflammation and invagination or bulging of the tympanic membrane, effusion and hemorrhage in the middle ear, a temporary partial loss of hearing and, on rare occasions, a rupture of the drum membrane.

Etiology

Aerotitis media is caused by inadequate ventilation of the middle ear during ascent or descent in flight. This results in a positive or negative pressure differential developing in the tympanic cavity with a consequent trauma to the tissues involved. Aerotitis media caused by ascent is exceedingly rare. In the few cases observed, there was a stenosis of the Eustachian tube but the cause of this stenosis was not apparent.

During descent, aerotitis media is caused by inadequate ventilation of the tympanic

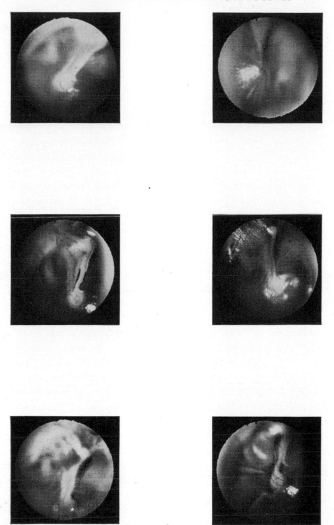

Fig. 60. Photographs of ear drums demonstrating varying degrees of aerotitis media. Upper left, retraction of the handle of the malleus; upper right, mild degree of aerotitis media with mild engorgement along the handle of the malleus; middle left, moderately severe aerotitis media with tympanic retraction, engorgement of the drum and discrete hemorrhage along both sides of the malleus; middle right, moderately severe aerotitis media showing hemorrhage along the anterior surface of the malleus, discrete hemorrhage in Schrapnel's membrane and fluid in the middle ear; lower left, aerotitis media of 4 days duration showing severe retraction, coalescing hemorrhage along the anterior aspect of the handle of the malleus and desquamation of the external layer of the tympanic membrane; and lower right, acute severe aerotitis media demonstrating serosanguineous fluid and bubbles in the middle ear. The outline of the fluid bubbles may be seen shining through the drum membrane. The spokelike lines radiating from the umbo represent the margins of the bubbles. (Courtesy of Col. Paul Campbell.)

cavity resulting either from a failure or an inability to voluntarily open the Eustachian tube. Failure to keep the middle ear ventilated during descent in aircraft may be owing to the inability to learn how to do so, to ignorance of the necessity to do so, to carelessness, to being asleep or it may occur in individuals under the influence of sedatives or who are in coma. The first three of these most frequently occur among inexperienced aircrew members and passengers, the fourth in sleeping passengers and the fifth in patients on ambulance airplanes.

Some of the more frequent causes of Eustachian stenosis, and, thus, the inability to open the Eustachian tubes, are acute and chronic infections of the upper respiratory tract, nasal obstructions, sinusitis, tonsillitis, tumors and growths of the nose and naso-pharynx, paralysis of the soft palate or superior pharyngeal muscles, enlargement of the pharyngeal or tubal tonsil and inflammatory conditions of the Eustachian tube. Another possible cause of Eustachian stenosis is the presence of excessive subepithelial lymphoid tissue within the lumen of the tube which has occasionally been observed from histologic studies of such tissues.

In addition to the above, the effect of malposition of the mandible in relation to stenosis of the Eustachian tube has been reported on by Costen (2) and applied to aviation by Willhelmy (3). The former believed that in individuals with edentulous mouths, ill fitting dental plates, marked overbite, malocclusion, worn or lack of molar teeth or a shortening of the vertical position of the lower jaw that a compression stenosis of the Eustachian tube is likely to occur from a relaxation of the surrounding soft tissues. The latter advocated the repositioning of the mandible in the case of pilots who have difficulty in ventilating their middle ears during ascent and descent and has indicated that deafness in pilots might be corrected by this same procedure. For the most recent opinion on this question see chapter 24.

A form of aerotitis media which is not caused by altitude pressure changes *per se* is caused by the presence of essentially pure oxygen in the tympanic cavity. When oxygen is breathed during descent from altitude it is this gas which enters the middle ear to relieve the negative pressure. After ground level is reached, this oxygen is gradually absorbed by the surrounding tissues, a negative pressure develops in the tympanic cavity and the patient suffers discomfort or pain beginning some 2 to 6 hours after descent. This form of aerotitis media usually occurs only in jet fighter pilots who descend very rapidly and breathe pure oxygen throughout their descent.

Chronic aerotitis media is probably caused by a partial stenosis of the Eustachian tube of such a degree that while the middle ear may be ventilated voluntarily, the tube tends to close before the pressure differential is completely equalized. The result is a repeated slight trauma of the tympanic membrane extending over a period of years.

A fact not generally realized is that, except in experienced aircrew members, a high percentage of the cases of aerotitis media are not owing to pathology in or about the Eustachian tube but to a failure to ventilate the middle ear through carelessness or an inability to master the technique of opening the Eustachian tube. As an example of this, Stewart, Warwick and Bateman (4) reported that 10.1 per cent of airmen trainees on their first altitude chamber run developed aerotitis media during descent from 25,000 and 35,000 feet altitude at a rate of descent of 2500 feet per minute. All of these men were initially free of Eustachian tube pathology and had been thoroughly instructed in how to protect their middle ears just prior to the test.

Another factor which needs to be stressed is that upper respiratory infections and other pathology in or about the Eustachian tubes does not usually produce a stenosis of these tubes, as is generally believed, but only in a relatively small per cent of such cases. For example, Stewart *et al.*, cited above, tested a large number of airmen with acute upper respiratory infections and found that 83.5 per cent of them had no difficulty during descent as compared to 89.9 per cent in their normal controls. Thus, there was a difference of only 6.4 per cent in these two groups. In this series, a small number of the affected trainees were excused from the chamber run but the authors point out that, even had all these cases been included and failed, the percentage of all those with upper respiratory disease who had extreme difficulty during descent would only have been 4.6 per cent as compared to 3.0 per cent in the normal controls. Other authors have reported similar results including those studying deep sea diving trainees (5) where the pressure change was equivalent to diving in an aircraft at a rate of approximately 18,000 feet per minute.

Symptomatology

AEROTITIS MEDIA, ACUTE. *Subjective Symptoms.* During ascent positive pressures of from 3 to 5 mm. of Hg in the middle ear are perceptible in consciousness to most individuals as a feeling of fullness in the middle ear. At about 10 to 15 mm. of Hg pressure the feeling of fullness is distinct and somewhat annoying and affects the hearing by making sounds seem distant and of a lessened intensity. In normal cases about 15 mm. of positive pressure is sufficient to force air out through the Eustachian tube which relieves the pressure in the tympanic cavity and consequently the accompanying symptoms. This relief is initiated by an annoying "click," which is both felt and heard as the tympanic membrane snaps back to its normal position. In stenosis of the tube the pressure required to force it open varies with the degree of stenosis.

This series of events is physiologic and not pathologic in nature and does not produce aerotitis media. However, if there is a stenosis of the Eustachian tube of a nature, and to a degree, that a positive pressure of 50 to 100 mm. of Hg or more develops in the tympanic cavity then the manifestations and symptoms of this disease will be observed.

If the stenosis is complete, pain develops in the ear at between 3000 and 5000 feet altitude and becomes progressively worse with continued ascent. If the stenosis is partial the degree of difficulty depends upon the rate of ascent and the degree of stenosis. Those having marked difficulty are usually forced to give up flying whereas those with minimal symptoms may continue in aviation and it is possible that these are the individuals who develop chronic aerotitis media.

During descent if the middle ear is not ventilated the following train of subjective symptoms may be observed. As the negative pressure develops in the middle ear there is first discomfort followed by pain. The pain is usually first noted when the pressure differential in the tympanic cavity amounts to approximately 100 mm. of Hg and resembles that experienced in acute otitis media. As the descent continues the pain becomes progressively more severe and tends to radiate to the temporal region, the cheek and the parotid gland. At about 200 mm. of Hg pressure difference the tympanic membrane may rupture but this is a very rare event (4) and it usually only occurs in individuals with previous drum membrane pathology.

With negative pressure during descent voluntarily opening the Eustachian tube will prevent the development of acute symptoms. It is to be remembered, however, that it is impossible to overcome a negative pressure in excess of about 80 or 90 mm. by muscular action and immediate relief is obtained only by a return to a higher altitude. In cases in which the pressure has already produced

trauma opening the Eustachian tube will not relieve all the symptoms of that trauma and they will persist until recovery has taken place. Moderate trauma is followed by a sense of soreness in the ear and there may be an occasional sharp stabbing pain caused by movement of the inflamed tympanic membrane. Patients notice a change in the quality of sounds and especially the sound of their own voices which they liken to "talking into a rain barrel." Other sounds appear to be more distant than normal and patients usually complain of a temporary partial loss of hearing.

Objective Symptoms. Aerotitis media developing during ascent will show a bulging of the tympanic membrane with a decrease or loss of the light reflex. As long as there is an excess pressure in the middle ear the drum membrane tends to appear ischemic but as soon as the pressure is relieved it becomes inflammed to a degree depending on the extent of the trauma sustained.

The signs of aerotitis media caused by descent also vary with the amount of trauma sustained. The sequence of events and the signs which may be observed are as follows. The tympanic membrane is, of course, retracted a variable amount initially but by the time the patient is examined this may have been more or less restored to its normal position if the patient has been able to ventilate the ear in the meantime.

In mild cases there is an injection of the blood vessels running over Shrapnell's membrane and the handle of the malleus. At the next stage there is an erythemia of the upper and posterior portion of the drum. With increased trauma the whole surface of the tympanic membrane and the adjacent portions of the external auditory canal become red and inflammed, the drum develops a translucent appearance and small droplets of fluid may be seen on its medial surface. Beyond this stage gross fluid and air bubbles collect in the tympanic cavity and there may be hemorrhage in the substance of the tympanic membrane and in the middle ear. These hemorrhages are usually completely masked, initially, by the erythemia of the tympanic membrane. However after 24 or more hours, when the erythemia has subsided somewhat, these hemorrhages can usually be seen as a dark area adjacent to the handle of the malleus or as a small dark mass behind the drum.

An audiogram of patients with acute aerotitis media will usually show a conduction type hearing loss amounting to 15 to 30 decibels. This loss may be fairly uniform for the various frequencies or may affect principally the lower or the higher frequencies in individual cases. The amount of hearing loss, if any, is determined by the amount of negative pressure in the middle ear, and, thus, the immobility of the tympanic membrane, and also by the presence or absence of fluid in the tympanic cavity.

Traumatic ruptures of the tympanic membrane are usually linear, quite extensive and may involve any portion of it. The margins of fresh ruptures are red and the whole drum is highly inflamed. There is usually a small amount of blood in the external auditory canal. If the labyrinthic wall is visible through the freshly ruptured drum membrane, it is seen to be red, congested and swollen.

AEROTITIS MEDIA, CHRONIC. *Subjective Symptoms.* In these cases there is a "full and stuffy" feeling in the ears and difficulty in "clearing" them. Head noises may be present but rarely pain. The condition is worse after flights or during acute infections of the upper respiratory tract.

Objective Symptoms. The ear drums are retracted, the drum membrane dull, lusterless and slightly thickened and the light reflex is diminished or absent. Whether or not hearing acuity is diminished in this condition is not known at the present time. Of importance in this connection is the fact that deep sea divers and workers in compressed air who are exposed to atmospheric pressure changes but not to noise, are sometimes found to suffer from deafness. Vail (6) has reviewed the literature on this latter subject and states in part as follows:

"The ear may be affected in two ways by the direct action of compressed air. (1) There may be a more or less mild form of trauma when the damage is confined to the middle ear. (2) There may be trauma when, besides damage to the middle ear, injury is done to the internal ear.

"Alexander thought that the inner ear symptoms appearing in caisson workers were caused by hyperemia and small hemorrhages in the internal ear, and that the symptoms might appear acutely after the injury or could at times have a chronic progressive course.

"Boot was of the opinion that tubal tympanic catarrh caused exaggerated symptoms in those working in an atmosphere of compressed air; that when the patient showed symptoms referable only to the vestibular apparatus, recovery was complete, and that the most characteristic result when the ears were injured was a loss of a considerable portion of the upper range of hearing with a marked lessening of bone conduction. In some cases the organ of Corti seemed to have been suddenly destroyed."

The findings of the authors cited by Vail would seem to indicate that changes of atmospheric pressure are capable of producing injury to both the middle ear and cochlear portion of the inner ear. If this is true then we might expect the same thing to occur in aviators especially during long descents in which they fail, or are unable, to ventilate their middle ears.

In other words it is possible that the loss of hearing in a pilot may not be the result of noise but to mechanical trauma of the middle and inner ear induced by atmospheric pressure changes. A possible example of such an occurrence is illustrated by the audiogram shown in figure 61. This audiogram was obtained by the author from a pilot whose left ear drum had been ruptured several years previously during a rapid descent. The drum healed without incidence but all useful hearing was lost indicating that serious damage to the inner ear had also occurred. The bone conduction loss for all frequencies in this case was not measurable inasmuch as they were beyond the range of the audiometer used.

Diagnosis

The diagnosis of aerotitis media is simple if the history is known. The different signs and symptoms of this condition closely resemble the various stages of infectious otitis media or external otitis and as previously stated, have frequently been mistaken for them. Likewise, chronic aerotitis media may be easily mistaken for a chronic infectious middle ear process unless a history of exposure to repeated changes in altitude is obtained. Table 28 will assist in the differential diagnosis.

Another possible source of confusion is that individuals suffering from an upper respiratory disease will sometimes show a hyperaemia of the tympanic membrane and this same thing will occasionally be observed in an individual after he has employed the Valsalva technique. It has also been observed

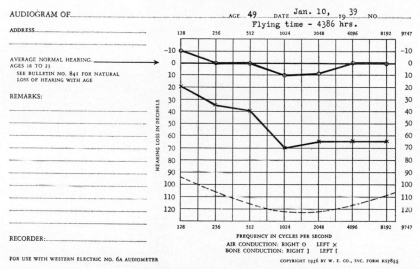

FIG. 61. Audiogram of a pilot whose left ear drum had been ruptured several years previously during a dive.

TABLE 28

Differential Diagnosis of Aerotitis Media, Otitis Media and External Otitis

	Aerotitis Media	Otitis Media	External Otitis
1	Due to barometric pressure changes	Inflammatory	Inflammatory
2	Retraction of drum	Bulging of drum	View of drum may be obstructed
3	Drum land mark accentuated	Drum landmark obliterated	—
4	Rupture of vessels	Diffuse erythema	—
5	No thickening of drum	Thickening of drum	May be thickening of drum if visible
6	Usually no fever	Fever usually present	May be fever
7	White blood cell count normal	White blood cell count elevated	White blood cell count elevated
8	Sero sanguinous fluid in middle ear	Serous or seropurulent fluid in middle ear	No fluid in middle ear
9	Hearing normal or slightly reduced	Deafness profound	Hearing normal if canal not obstructed
10	No pain on pressure over tragus and movement of auricle	No pain on pressure over tragus and movement of auricle	Pain on pressure over tragus and movement of auricle
11	No swelling of canal	Slight if any swelling of canal	Swelling of canal

(4) that about 50 per cent of all individuals who descend from high altitude, without difficulty and without subjective symptoms, will likewise show a hyperaemia of the drum upon examination. In all three of these situations, the hyperaemia is generally confined to an injection of the vessels along the handle of the malleus or to the upper two quadrants of the drum. From a purely technical viewpoint, both the Valsalva induced cases and those without symptoms following descent are, by definition, aerotitis media. However, in actual practice most authorities arbitrarily make such a diagnosis only in the presence of both signs and symptoms.

In addition to establishing the primary

diagnosis of aerotitis media it is essential for purposes of proper treatment to determine which of the following contributary causes was involved: (1) inadvertent failure to ventilate the middle ear during descent; (2) an inflammation of the Eustachian tube or of the adjacent tissues; (3) a mechanical obstruction of the Eustachian tube orifice; or (4) an obstruction of the lumen of the Eustachian tube caused by the presence of excess lymphoid tissue. This latter is quite rare and can only be assumed to exist when there are repeated attacks of aerotitis media for which there is no other reasonable explanation.

Complications

Although pilots usually avoid flying during periods when they have an acute infection of the upper respiratory tract, nevertheless, a considerable amount of such flying has been done. It might be expected in these cases that during descent the intermittent blasts of air from the pharynx to the tympanic cavity would carry with it septic material to the mechanically irritated tympanum and set up an acute infectious process. That this does not usually occur in evidenced by the fact that an infection of the middle ear following an attack of aerotitis media is an extremely rare event. The probable explanation for this is that the function of the Eustachian tube is to drain the middle ear, as well as to ventilate it, and that the motion of the cilia in the tube favors the movement of material from the ear to the nasopharynx and opposes motion in the opposite direction.

Treatment

PROPHYLAXIS. All candidates for flying training should be carefully tested as to the patency of their Eustachian tubes. Those that have a partial or complete stenosis of these tubes should be rejected until the condition corrects itself or is corrected by appropriate treatment.

The most useful prophylactic measure for all those who fly is proper instructions. This requires an explanation of how the Eustachian tube functions followed by instructions as to how to ventilate the tympanum, when to ventilate it and how frequently this is necessary. The simplest maneuver to actuate the Eustachian tube is to swallow. Unfortunately this is not effective in many individuals,

especially in the presence of an upper respiratory infection. A more effective method is difficult to describe but may be learned by practicing the suppression of a simulated yawn. In this maneuver the lips are kept closed, the jaws are moderately separated and the throat ballooned outward. A roaring in the ears will indicate when the effort is successful. An even more effective method is the Valsalva maneuver and its effectiveness is enhanced by relaxing the jaw and throat muscles, opening the bite slightly and moving the lower jaw back and forth latterly.

The two latter maneuvers can be sustained over a period of several seconds and, thus, are very useful in high speed dives. However, a sustained Valsalva with its prolonged pulmonary inflation and stimulation of the stretch reflex may produce a cardiac arrhythmia in individuals with hypersensitive carotid sinuses. Lamb discusses this reflex in chapter 22 and he is of the opinion that any prolonged pulmonary inflation is potentially dangerous and should be avoided, especially during flight.

It has repeatedly been observed that experienced aircrew members have, on the average, much less aerotitis media than students or inexperienced crews indicating the value of practice. This strongly suggests that student flyers are not being properly or adequately trained in regard to ear ventilation and much unnecessary suffering and loss of time is the result.

Those suffering from a permanent stenosis of the Eustachian tubes should be enjoined from flying except under controlled conditions of gradual changes of altitude through a maximum range not to exceed 3000 feet. Those with an acute infection of the upper respiratory tract who have an urgent need to fly should be prepared by gargling a hot physiologic solution of sodium chloride or by having a detergent spray directed well back into the nasopharynx followed by the instillation or inhalation of atropine, ephedrine or benzedrine compounds. A fairly good index of whether or not these individuals will experience difficulty is to have them attempt a Valsalva maneuver. If such an attempt is unsuccessful they are fairly certain to develop aerotitis media. However, if they can readily perform the Valsalva maneuver the probability of their having difficulty is only slightly greater than would be experienced in the absence of the respiratory infection.

The introduction of pressure cabin aircraft was a great advance in the prevention of aerotitis media but in spite of this the incidence of this disease among military fighter pilots has shown a sharp increase in recent years. Studies by Dickson and King (7) have shown that in aircrews trained on jet fighters the incidence of aerotitis media is three times greater than in aircrews on piston engined aircraft and that for aircrew under training in jet fighters the incidence is six and a half times that of comparable trainees using piston type aircraft. Their explanation for this is the increased diving rate for jet aircraft which they cited as being in the range of 8000 to 16,000 feet per minute. To explain the failure of pressure cabins to prevent aerotitis media in jet fighter operations, these authors considered the hypothetical case of an aircraft at 40,000 feet with a cabin pressure equivalent to that at 30,000 feet which descends at a rate of 20,000 feet per minute. When this aircraft reaches an altitude of 10,000 feet the pilot has passed through a pressure change equivalent to 20,000 feet of descent in $1\frac{1}{2}$ minutes. This is equal to a descent rate of 13,000 feet per minute which exceeds the diving capability of any existing piston engined aircraft by a factor of two.

When an individual develops a negative pressure in his middle ear to the degree that he is unable to force his Eustachian tubes open by the usual means relief can be obtained by ascending to a higher altitude. This also permits him to regain voluntary control of his middle ear ventilation after which descent may be resumed.

Aerotitis media from an oxygen filled tympanic cavity can usually be prevented by switching off the oxygen as early as practical during descent so that the middle ear is filled with air instead of oxygen by the time ground level is reached. This may not be fully effective in jet fighters because of the extremely limited time element involved. In spite of this, great care should be taken that pilots are not encouraged to turn off their oxygen prematurely for reasons which are quite obvious.

Pilots who land with oxygen filled tympanic cavities usually have no difficulty unless they go to sleep shortly thereafter. The reason for this is that during sleep the middle ear is not regularly ventilated and the oxygen is absorbed instead of being gradually replaced by air entering the Eustachian tube as would otherwise occur. Such attacks can be prevented by having the airman perform about six reverse Valsalvas before retiring. This maneuver is accomplished by taking a mouthful of water, holding the nostrils closed with the fingers and swallowing. This creates a negative pressure in the pharynx and secondarily in the middle ear drawing off some of the trapped oxygen. This oxygen is then replaced by air as the negative pressure in the ear is subsequently relieved.

In airline operations with unpressurized cabins, descent should be as gradual as is practical and passengers should be told how and when to ventilate their middle ears. Gum chewing, eating and drinking increases the swallowing rate from a normal of once every 60 to 75 seconds to an interval of from 1 to 30 seconds and accordingly are useful means of preventing aerotitis media. This applies especially to children who cannot understand or carry out instructions. Infants pose a difficult problem but may be helped by having them nurse during descent. Sleeping passengers should be awakened inasmuch as the swallowing rate of sleepers is slowed or absent and they are thus much more susceptible than those who are awake.

In airline operations with pressure cabins, the cabin pressure should be kept as near that at ground level as is practical. Where it is necessary to operate the cabin at, for example, 8000 feet equivalent pressure, this pressure should be increased as gradually as possible during descent.

These airline procedures for both pressurized and unpressurized cabins apply also to all other types of flying and the magnitude of the middle ear problem will depend on the degree to which these procedures can be, and are, carried out.

Active Treatment

Acute aerotitis media is usually self limited and in most cases the treatment is essentially palliative and should be conservative. Marked discomfort or pain should be relieved by appropriate medication. If the tympanic membrane has been ruptured it should be treated expectantly. Sterile cotton placed loosely in the external auditory meatus will add to the patient's comfort during cold weather.

If there is a negative pressure in the tympanic cavity, an attempt should be made to relieve it by shrinking the nasal mucosa and the Eustachian orifice. After allowing time for the medication to be fully effective ask the patient to perform a Valsalva maneuver and if this fails, politzerize. This should produce favorable results in all but a very small percentage of cases. Inasmuch as the patient's ear remains sore and even a small pressure differential produces marked discomfort, the patient's subjective symptoms should not be the criteria in deciding that the above described treatments have failed.

If examination of the tympanic membrane, at this point, shows it to be still markedly retracted, the next step is to gently catheterize the Eustachian tube and inflate. This should not be attempted except in the more severe cases and only by those who are properly trained to accomplish this procedure. Myringotomy or paracentesis have been advocated from time to time (8, 9) but most authorities strongly oppose their routine use. The reason is that both of these procedures may implant an infection in a perfect culture medium which otherwise would remain sterile. Cases in which myringotomy or paracentesis may be justified are those that fail to respond to all other treatment and have a negative pressure and fluid in the tympanic cavity after conservative therapy. A myringotomy or paracentesis should be performed in the posteroinferior quadrant of the tympanic membrane after meticulous cleansing

TABLE 29

Frequency of Operations Performed in Cases of Aerotitis Media*

Operation	Frequency
Submucous resection of nasal septum	34
Intranasal antrostomy	7
Caldwell-Luc antrostomy	2
Intranasal frontal sinus drainage	1
Clearance of ethmoids	1
Removal of nasal polyps	1
Tonsillectomy	1
Myringotomy	4
Total number of operations	51

* From Dickson and King.

of the external auditory canal. When no fluid is present a sucking noise will be heard when air rushes into the middle ear. When fluid is present the procedure should be followed by politzerization which will force the fluid from the tympanic cavity and hasten recovery.

The follow-up treatment of these cases consists of the application of dry heat to the external ear for 15 minutes every hour, rest, removal from flying and the concurrent treatment of any existing upper respiratory or local infection. The application of heat to the ear offers considerable relief to the patient and may facilitate serum displacement within the middle ear through hyperemia. Flying personnel should remain grounded not only until the middle ear has essentially returned to normal but also until any contributing cause has been eliminated.

The type and relative frequency of surgical procedures that may be required is suggested by 51 operations reported by Dickson and King (7) which is shown in table 29. In their series, 80 per cent of the patients were returned to full flying duties, 5 per cent to limited flying and the remaining 15 per cent were permanently grounded.

In cases where excess lymphoid tissue in the Eustachian tube or over its pharyngeal opening is the etiologic factor in aerotitis media both radium and Roentgen treatments have been utilized to destroy or cause a recession of this tissue. During World War II radium treatments, in accordance with the technique developed by Crowe (10), were given an extensive trial with results that are difficult to evaluate. Later Shilling and his group (11) concluded from their experience that, where indicated, radium treatments produced good results in 90 per cent of cases. More recently Roentgen therapy has been reported as being successful in 32 per cent of cases treated (7) all of whom would otherwise have been permanently grounded. The technique employed has been described by Dickson and McGibbon (12) who devised this treatment. Briefly stated the treatment consists of dosage to the affected tube of 1180 to 1640 r spread over 14 to 21 days followed by 3 weeks sick leave and finally a decompression test to evaluate the results.

Cases of chronic aerotitis media seldom present themselves for treatment and are usually found during routine examinations of the ears of airmen with several years of flying experience. If questioned, they will usually admit to a continual feeling of fullness or "stuffiness" in their ears but seem to accept this without complaint. Low grade chronic infections in, or adjacent to, the Eustachian tube or moderate amounts of excess lymphoid tissue within the tube are the most likely causes of this condition although any of the other factors which produce acute aerotitis media may be responsible. Where such causes are found they should be corrected.

AEROSINUSITIS

As is generally known, the nasal accessory sinuses are mucous membrane lined, air filled cavities in the bony skull which open separately into the nose by means of patient orifices. If these orifices are normal, air will pass into and out of the sinuses without any difficulty during ascent or descent. However, if these orifices are obstructed, pain will result because of the pressure or partial vacuum in the sinuses (13).

The incidence of aerosinusitis is quite rare and usually only one sinus is affected. The frequency of distribution of aerosinusitis among the various sinus cavities (7) is indicated in table 30. An attack may occur either during an ascent or descent but the latter is the more frequent. The severity of an attack will depend on the range and speed of ascent or descent and also whether the ostium of the sinus involved is partially or completely stenosed. The stenosis of the affected ostium may be caused by the presence of fluid, mucus, pus, redundant tissue, polyps, anatomical deformities, inflammations or tumors in or about the ostium making the sinus a closed cavity.

The subjective symptoms of aerosinusitis usually consist of severe pain in the affected sinus during flight which tends to increase as the change of altitude continues. Reversing the direction of altitude change usually brings relief, at least temporarily. If a frontal sinus is involved, the pain extends over the forehead above the bridge of the nose whereas the pain from the maxillary sinuses is localized in the cheek bones on either side of the nose. In the latter instance, the pain is sometimes referred to the teeth of the upper jaw and may be mistaken for aerodontalgia. A sucking

TABLE 30

Frequency of Distribution of Aerosinusitis Among Sinus Cavities

Sinus Involved	Frequency
Frontal	70
Antrum	19
Frontal and antrum	10
Ethmoid	1
Total	100

* From Dickson and King.

noise high up in the nose is described by some patients and a few of them will exhibit lacrimation.

Upon examination, local tenderness will be found over the affected sinus in most cases and frequently a purulent or mucopurulent discharge will be seen about the sinus opening. Further examination may reveal a mechanical obstruction caused by the presence of tumors, polyps, redundant tissue or anatomical deformities. Roentgenography may give evidence of a sinus lesion such as a thickened lining or polyps but does not clearly differentiate between the contributing factors of pre-existing disease from the results of aerosinusitis.

The best prophylactic measure to prevent aerosinusitis is a very careful initial examination of candidates for flying training with the elimination of those who are susceptible. Among trained flyers those with acute upper

TABLE 31

Frequency of Operations Performed in Patients with Aerosinusitis*

Operation	Frequency
Submucous resection of nasal septum	26
Intranasal antrostomy	25
Caldwell-Luc antrostomy	3
Intranasal frontal sinus drainage	2
Clearance of ethmoids	5
Removal of nasal polyps	5
Middle turbinectomy	3
Middle turbinal infracture	1
Tonsillectomy	2
Adenoidectomy	1
Total number of operations	73

* From Dickson and King.

respiratory or sinus infections should be grounded until recovery has taken place.

The immediate treatment of aerosinusitis is a return to the altitude where the pain first became perceptible. The flight should then be terminated with the return to ground level at as slow a rate as possible. The therapy of these cases should first be directed to relieving the pain and the pressure differential in the affected sinus as quickly as possible by the simplest possible means. Vasoconstrictors locally applied in the form of inhalators, sprays or drops and hot or cold packs (whichever gives the most relief) should constitute the initial treatment. Should this prove to be ineffective and severe pain persists the middle meatus should be anesthetized and the anterior half of the middle turbinate infracted. At this point, if no relief has been obtained and a maxillary sinus in involved, it may be entered with a cannula passed through the ostium or by puncture with a small needle through the inferior meatus.

It will be found in many of these cases that they are suffering from a concurrent upper respiratory infection, an allergic rhinitis or an infected sinus. If so these should also be given immediate appropriate treatment. In all cases search should be made for mechanical obstructions of the ostium and if found should be dealt with after the acute symptoms have subsided. This may involve surgery of the types shown in table 31, from Dickson and King (7) which also indicates the relative frequency of the operations performed in their series. In a follow-up of these cases it was reported that 77 per cent were successfully returned to full flying duties, 18 per cent to limited flying and 5 per cent were permanently grounded.

Tissue specimens in cases of recurrent aerosinusitis exhibit the changes found in subacute infectious sinusitis namely; edema, congestion, mucous and submucous hemorrhages, infiltration with polymorphonuclear leucocytes, lymphocytes, plasma cells and some fibroblastic hyperplasia.

REFERENCES

(1) ARMSTRONG, H. G., AND HEIM, J. W.: The effect of flight on the middle ear. J.A.M.A., 109: 417–421, 1937.

(2) COSTEN, J. B.: A syndrome of ear and sinus symptoms dependent upon disturbed function of the temporomandibular joint. Ann. Otol. Rhin. & Laryng., 43: 1–15, 1934.

(3) WILLHELMY, G. E.: Ear symptoms incidental to sudden altitude changes and the factor of overclosure of the mandible: preliminary report. U. S. Nav. M. Bull., 34: 533–541, 1936.

(4) STEWART, C. B., WARWICK, O. N., AND BATEMAN, G. L.: Acute otitic barotrauma resulting from low pressure chamber tests. J. Aviation Med., 16: 385–408, 1945.

(5) SHILLING, C. W., HAINES, H. L., HARRIS, J. D., AND KELLY, W. J.: Aerotitis media. J. Aviation Med., 18: 48–55, 1947.

(6) VAIL, H. H.: Traumatic conditions of the ear in workers in an atmosphere of compressed air. Arch. Otolaryng., 10: 113–126, 1929.

(7) DICKSON, E. D. D., AND KING, P. F.: Results of treatment of otitic and sinus barotrauma. J. Aviation Med., 27: 92–99, 1956.

(8) CANFIELD, N., AND BATEMAN, G. H.: Myringo-puncture for reduced intratympanic pressure, J. Aviation Med., 15: 340–346, 1944.

(9) TRAWBRIDGE, B.: A new treatment of acute aero-otitis media. Arch. Otolaryng., 50: 255–263, 1949.

(10) CROWE, S. J.: Irradiation of the nasopharynx. Tr. Am. Acad. Ophth., 51: 29–35, 1946.

(11) SHILLING, C. W., HAINES, H. L., HARRIS, J. D., AND KELLY, W. J.: Prevention and treatment of aerotitis media. U. S. Nav. M. Bull., 46: 1529–1558, 1946.

(12) DICKSON, E. D. D., AND McGIBBON, J. E. G.: The treatment of recurrent otitic barotrauma by irradiation (with special reference to lymphoid tissue in the submucosa of the Eustachian tube). J. Laryng. & Otol., 63: 647, 1949.

(13) CAMPBELL, P. A.: Aerosinusitis—a resume. Ann. Otol Rhin. & Laryng., 54: 1–15, 1945.

12

DECOMPRESSION SICKNESS

Hans G. Clamann, M.D.

Decompression sickness in general has been defined as a unique syndrome resulting from a pressure reduction in a surrounding atmosphere of any magnitude, providing a living body has been—at least partially—equilibrated to the higher atmospheric pressure prior to decompression. When humans, such as divers, have been exposed to pressures higher than the normal or sea level pressure of 14.7 p.s.i. (760 mm. of Hg) and then are decompressed to lower pressures the resulting symptoms are called caisson disease or compressed air illness. Flying personnel who are decompressed from sea level pressure to subatmospheric pressures by ascent in an airplane or in a high altitude chamber may exhibit altitude decompression sickness or simply decompression sickness.

Armstrong (1) was the first to demonstrate the presence of gas bubbles in the blood stream, following ascent to high altitude, and to this he applied the term aeroembolism. Subsequently (1952), this same author recommended the use of the term decompression sickness be applied to the total symptom complex resulting from a reduction of the barometric pressure exclusive of hypoxia and the expansion of the gases contained in the hollow air filled cavities of the body. In the meantime, Adler (2) had suggested the use of the term dysbarism which he divided into two types as follows: disturbances in the body resulting from an excess of gas pressure within the body fluids, tissues or cavities over the ambient gas pressure he named hypobarism whereas for those disturbances in the body resulting from an excess of the ambient gas pressure over that within the body fluids, tissue or cavities he applied the term hyperbarism.

From the above discussion it is evident that the terms decompression sickness and dysbarism are essentially synonymous and they are both in common use. In this chapter the term decompression sickness will be employed in conformity with its use throughout the other portions of this book.

HISTORICAL REVIEW

In 1670, Robert Boyle (3) reported seeing a bubble within the eye of a viper exposed to a high vacuum and Hoppe (1857) (4), asserted that if animals were rapidly exposed to a vacuum of 50 mm. of Hg pressure, absolute or less, that gas bubbles were formed in their blood just as might occur on sudden decompression from pressure greater than 2 atmospheres. A French engineer, Triger, about 1850 built and used the first caisson for tunnel work. The term "compressed air illness" (caisson disease) was first used by Pol and Watelle in 1854. References to the above papers and many other early workers are cited in the books by Paul Bert (5) and Hill (6). Paul Bert, who performed a large number of decompression experiments, denied that nitrogen bubbles were ever formed at less than 1 atmosphere pressure. Hill and Greenwood (7) were unable to find bubbles in mice, guinea pigs or kittens at decreased atmospheric pressure but in one rabbit decompressed in 3 minutes to 50 mm. of Hg

175

absolute pressure they found the heart and large vessels filled with what was assumed to be air.

Pol and Watelle seem to be the first to have recognized that exposure to high pressure was not dangerous but the subsequent decompression was. The danger was proportional to the degree and period of compression and especially to the rapidity of the decompression. They recommended slow decompression and, when symptoms occurred, recompression as treatment. Heller, Mager and Von Schroetter, quoted by Hill (6), described many cases of caisson disease and the complex symptoms, for instance, the painful itch produced by air bubbles in the fat of subcutaneous tissue.

Jongbloed seems to be the first (Thesis to the University of Utrecht in Holland) who reported the effects of simulated altitude other than hypoxia in a low pressure chamber. This thesis was presented at the International Air Congress in 1930 (8). The report gave descriptions of pain ("bends") in the wrists, knees and hip joints and attention was called to some of the similarities and differences between compressed air illness and decompression sickness. Barcroft *et al.*, quoted by Fulton (9), on experiments carried out in the low pressure chambers, in

TABLE 32

Solubility of Oxygen, Nitrogen and Helium in Water, Expressed in cc. of Gas in 1 cc. of Solvent, as the Function of Temperature at Atmospheric Pressure

Gas	Temperature in °C				
	0	10	20	30	40
Oxygen	0.0489	0.038	0.031	0.0261	0.0231
Nitrogen	0.0235	0.0186	0.0155	0.0134	0.0113
Helium	0.0094	0.0089	0.0086	0.0083	0.0081

TABLE 33

Solubility of Various Gases in Water and Olive Oil Expressed as cc. of Gas Dissolved in 1 cc. of Solvent at 38° C. at Atmospheric Pressure

Liquid	Helium	Nitrogen	Oxygen	Argon	Carbon Dioxide
Water	0.0087	0.0127	0.023	0.0262	0.592
Olive oil	0.0148	0.0667	0.112	0.1359	—

1931, described "sore legs" at 30,000 feet and acute pain in both knees at 36,000 feet. In this country, Armstrong (10) in 1934 described "bends" experienced in a decompression chamber. All these studies formed the foundation for subsequent research in aviation medicine and physiology.

ETIOLOGY

Theories of Etiology

The various theories of the etiology of decompression sickness have a common basis. This basis rests mainly on two physical laws. *Henry's Law* states that the concentration of gas molecules dissolved in a liquid (solvent) is proportional to the pressure of the gas to which the liquid is exposed or proportional to the partial pressure of the gas components in case of a gas mixture, like air. The gas concentration is also influenced by the kind of solvent and by the temperature. Table 32 shows values of solubility for three gases and demonstrates that the solubility of a gas decreases with increasing temperature. Table 33 denotes that fat (olive oil) dissolves more gas than water. The solubility ratio of oil and water, however, differs considerably for various gases: 1.7 for helium versus 5.32 for argon. The *Law of Diffusion* states that gas molecules exhibit a random movement at high velocity, the latter increasing with increasing temperature. When the concentration of gas molecules is greater at some point than at another the average number of molecules moving from the higher toward the lower concentration is greater than *vice versa*. Increase of the area of exchange also facilitates diffusion. All these conditions being equal, diffusion is characterized for a certain gas by its "coefficient of diffusion," denoting the speed of exchange between different concentrations of a gas, different gases or both in any system containing such gases. Obviously, the coefficient of diffusion depends on the kinetic energy determined by temperature and mass of the molecules in question.

Expressed as an equation, it is

$$M = KA \frac{(c_1 - c_2)t}{h}$$

where M is the amount of substance which

diffuses through the cross section A in the time t, if the concentration on one side of the layer (thickness h) is c_1 and at the other side c_2. The diffusion coefficient K equals

$$K = vRT$$

where v is the speed of the molecules, R Boltzmann's molecular gas constant and T the absolute temperature. The dimension of K is the area per time; in metric units; for instance, square centimeters per second. Expressed in these units, for a system of gas to gas, K lies between 0.1 and 1 for the various gases in question at normal pressure and temperature. For the gas exchange between a gas and a 1 to 3 per cent agar solution, K is less than 1/100,000 of this value. This explains why a sufficiently fast gas exchange between a gas phase and a colloidal system (agar, tissue) is only possible either in very thin layers or very large areas or both (*i.e.*, in the lung). Solubility of a gas in water exerts an influence insofar as, at the same pressure, the gas with the higher solubility has the higher concentration compared to a gas of lesser solubility (see table 32). More details on the growth of a bubble by diffusion can be found in Fulton's book (11). Under conditions as they exist in the living body, however, bubble formation will rarely occur under a steady state but will be influenced by many factors such as movement of the tissues, circulation of fluids, rapid changes of gas pressure, etc.

The Bubble Theory

During return of a man from the depth to the surface of the water, ascent in aircraft or any other situation in which the atmospheric pressure is decreased, the partial pressure of the body nitrogen is above that of the nitrogen in the lungs. As a consequence the nitrogen dissolved in the blood begins to be given off in the lungs, the nitrogen in the tissues begins to enter the blood stream and by this dual process the excess of nitrogen will be eliminated. It is obvious if one ascends slowly enough to high altitude the nitrogen will be eliminated completely by diffusion. It will be shown in the paragraph "Nitrogen Elimination" that indeed such a time-concentration relationship has been determined successfully for the safety of deep sea divers.

It has been pointed out before that bubbles were observed in early experiments on decompression. A great amount of evidence has been accumulated, as will be shown later, in favor of bubbles being the primary cause of symptoms of decompression sickness such as bends, shakes, etc. However, the situation is not so simple that a certain pressure differential or a certain pressure-time rate necessarily produces bubbles. A very thorough study, both theoretic and experimental, on bubble formation on animals has been worked out by Harvey and his collaborators (12). Although for details the reader is referred to the original paper or to the chapters written by the same author (11), a short summary will be presented here, modified from Adler's presentation (2). Harvey states that the tendency of a gas to come out of a solution is determined by

$$\Delta P = t - P$$

in which ΔP is the differential pressure or tendency for a gas to leave the liquid phase, t equals the total tension of gas in the medium and P equals the absolute pressure (*i.e.*, the total pressure of the gas (or gases) in the liquid phase plus the hydrostatic pressure). The hydrostatic pressure is understood as any mechanical pressure acting upon the liquid except gaseous pressure. Thus, the hydrostatic pressure for an artery would be the arterial blood pressure.

EXAMPLES. *Arterial ΔP at Sea Level.* In the above equation, t for nitrogen would have a value of 79 per cent of 760 mm. of Hg, or 600 mm. of Hg for water or blood outside an artery. The absolute pressure P in the artery at sea level, assuming an arterial blood pressure of 125 mm. of Hg, would be 600 + 125 = 725. The equation would read ΔP = 600 − (600 + 125), therefore ΔP = −125 mm. of Hg.

Great Vein ΔP at Sea Level. Assuming the same partial pressure for nitrogen of 600 mm. of Hg and the blood pressure of a great vein in the chest to be zero mm. of Hg, ΔP = 600 − (600 + 0), therefore ΔP = 0 mm. of Hg. It can be seen from the above equations, ΔP in the artery is negative at sea level. This means there is no tendency of the nitrogen to come out of the solution to form bubbles. The blood pressure of 125 mm. of Hg may be thought of as a hydrostatic pressure helping to keep the nitrogen in solution even at a decreasing atmospheric pressure. Only if the differential pressure becomes more and more positive will there be an increasing tendency for a gas to leave a liquid and to form bubbles. Thus, at high altitude, bubble formation should occur first in capillaries and veins rather than in arteries.

But a positive pressure differential is only a prerequisite for bubble formation. To form bubbles *de novo*, ΔP has to be of the order 100 to 1000 atmospheres. In active animals, where movements occur and tensions are developed in tissues from the pull of muscles, it is conceivable that a ΔP of considerable magnitude (by mechanical pull or negative pressure) might develop. Inasmuch as pressure is the quotient force/area, a relatively small force acting upon an extremely small area may easily produce enormous positive (*i.e.*, sewing needle, stinger of a mosquito) as well as negative pressures, depending on the direction of force.

In small resting animals, the author believes, bubbles rarely form under greatly decreased atmospheric pressure. Bubbles in resting animals are believed to come from minute invisible spheres of gas (nuclei), whose origin is at present obscure. Such gas nuclei may be formed in minute cracks of hydrophobic material on the outside of cells. By growth caused by diffusion the nuclei appear as bubbles in blood, lymph or intercellular fluids and their final use depends on the gas available. Considerable consideration is spent on the hypothesis of formation of nuclei, dependent on surface tension, contact angles between bubble and hydrophilic and hydrophobic surfaces, etc. Pressure pulses, sound waves and turbulence may be important in bubble formation. Also changes in blood flow and, thus, gas exchange as affected by vasoconstriction and vasodilation in local areas may exert their particular effects on the tendency of a tissue to form bubbles.

Other Theories of Decompression Sickness

In his report, Adler (2) mentions three theories which try to explain the pain: (1) paroxysmal muscle contraction initiating agglutination and consequently emboli in small blood vessels, (2) angiospasm of arterioles with reduced blood flow producing hypoxia in muscles and the contractions of hypoxic muscles causing pain and (3) bends were ascribed to a shift in electrolytes in the body so that water was shifted to the intercellular fluid. This in effect produced a syndrome similar to surgical shock similar to the mechanism producing "miner's cramps" where mineral ions are lost and water shifts into the tissues. Unfortunately, the report of Adler (2) based upon results obtained on large numbers of aviation cadets has never been published and the references cited as CAM reports cannot easily be obtained.

Effect of Bubbles

It is mostly assumed that the displacement of tissue by a bubble and, therefore, its volume is responsible for the pathologic effects. Inasmuch as the relative increase of a gas volume in a container with a "frictionless piston" is the same, when decompressed from 5 atmospheres to 1 or from 1 to $\frac{1}{5}$ atmosphere the expected effect should be the same. This is not fully true; experience shows that decompression is more dangerous for the diver than for the aviator for a given pressure ratio. First, it should be considered that bubbles in living beings are often surrounded by elastic tissues opposing free expansion. Prevented from expanding a bubble of 5 atmospheres decompressed to 1 atmosphere will exert five times the force compared to a bubble the same size but decompressed from 1 to $\frac{1}{5}$ atmosphere, corresponding to the pressure ratio of $4:\frac{4}{5} = 5$. Second, according to Henry's Law, the amount of gas dissolved in a liquid increases with increasing absolute pressure. Thus, a larger amount of gas is available on decompression from absolute higher pressures and more bubbles can be formed. As Behnke (13) indicates, central nervous symptoms, such as from the spinal cord, are rare in ascents to altitude and there is a rapid amelioration of symptoms when descent is affected. In caisson workers pathologic changes in the spinal cord and brain are common.

Although, for the reasons cited, decompression is, in general, far more dangerous for the deep sea diver than for the aviator, the mechanism of gas bubble formation is, in principle, the same: bubbles may be formed either by very high negative pressure (locally restricted to very small areas) or from nuclei at hydrophobic surfaces. Once produced, bubbles may grow by diffusion of any gases into the bubbles supported by a "hydrostatic" pressure differential gradient toward (or into) the bubbles or *vice versa*. This was demonstrated in a model (12) which consisted of a glass tube in vertical position closed at the lower end. This tube was filled with water and saturated in layers alternately with air and carbon dioxide. When small bubbles of air moved from an air stratum upward, they increased in size moving through a carbon dioxide layer and decreased just as rapidly passing through a layer of water saturated with air.

Thus, bubbles formed in the body may not be expected to consist of 79 per cent nitrogen or amounts of carbon dioxide and oxygen corresponding to their partial pressures in the tissues. Although governed by Henry's Law and the Law of Diffusion, the complicated interrelationship between so many other factors make it impossible to predict accurately the composition of a gas mixture in a bubble, especially in the state of muscular activity and increased blood circulation. From this it is obvious that the composition of bubbles may change very easily. Besides various amounts of nitrogen, oxygen and carbon dioxide, bubbles will always contain water vapor corresponding to its saturation pressure at the existing temperature.

In physics, "boiling" denotes a situation where the pressure over a liquid is maintained equal to the vapor pressure of this liquid for a given temperature. Under such conditions, heat supplied to a liquid will not raise its temperature any farther but only convert liquid to vapor. Thus, at a temperature of 100° C. the vapor pressure of water becomes equal to the normal atmospheric pressure. The water will "boil," *i.e.*, produce vapor under bubble formation, at a rate corresponding to the amount of heat supplied although the temperature remains constant at 100° C.

This daily experience lets us forget that water will "boil" at a much lower temperature than 100° C. provided the pressure over the water equals the lower water vapor pressure at such temperature. Thus, the water vapor pressure is 47 mm. of Hg at body temperature of 37° C. When a living body is subjected to such a low ambient pressure corresponding to an altitude of approximately 63,000 feet, theoretically all body fluids should start boiling. Actually, the presence of electrolytes and the fact that the body fluids do not form an open surface but are enclosed in compartments under elastic forces (cell walls, blood vessels), shift the boiling point to still lower pressures. Experimentally such boiling effects have been demonstrated on animals. For man this effect has but minor importance, inasmuch as altitudes of such magnitude without a pressure suit means fatal hypoxia (see chapter 13).

In fatty tissues with their higher solubility of nitrogen (see table 33), bubbles should contain a relatively large percentage of nitrogen. Inasmuch as fatty tissues are often supplied by capillaries, generation of bubbles could here be expected first. Armstrong (14) showed in goats that the composition of the bubbles in venous blood (fig. 62) did not show as much nitrogen as theoretically assumed. In blood from the jugular vein he found the bubbles had 6.7 per cent oxygen, 28.3 per cent carbon dioxide and 65.0 per cent nitrogen. In the right ventricle of the heart the analysis revealed 11.4 per cent oxygen, 28.3 per cent carbon dioxide and 60.3 per cent nitrogen.

SYMPTOMATOLOGY IN BENDS AND CHOKES

Bends

Bends are a clinical manifestation of decompression sickness consisting of pain referred to the joints, bones or muscles.

LOCATION OF THE PAIN OF BENDS. The location of the pain is most often described as deep in the joints, bones or muscles of the extremities. Very rarely pain in regions such as the sternum, ribs, vertebrae and cranium has been reported. But even in an extremity the pain is diffuse and poorly localized. Only when localized in the fingers, wrist or a periosteal insertion of a tendon (patella, deltoid) is the localization more definite. As to the anatomical distribution, 54 per cent are recorded as joint pains, 26 per cent as

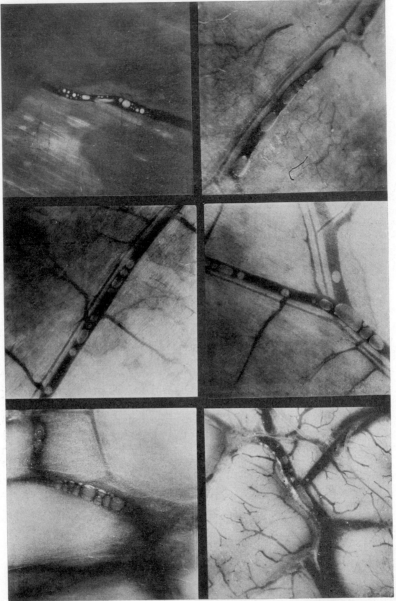

FIG. 62. Nitrogen bubbles in the veins of experimental animals produced by ascent to high altitude.

chiefly muscle pain and 20 per cent as being felt deep in the bone. The greatest number are located in the knees and the shoulders. The incidence of incapacitating bends seems greater in the knees than in the shoulders. The occurrence of bends is equally distributed to both sides of the body. However, some investigators found a slight predominance on the right side. The quality of the pains is described as deep, boring, aching or dull.

Concerning the pain mechanism, the first assumption according to the bubble theory would be production of pain by mechanical distortion of the tissue. But large collections of gas have been detected by x-rays with little or no pain recorded (15) whereas, on the other hand, x-rays did not reveal such collection of gas in cases of definite bends symptoms at altitude during flight (16). Thus, other mechanisms than the simple distortion of tissues and direct stimulation of pain receptors have been theorized, such as pressure on blood vessels and ischemia or pressure by initiating reflex vasoconstriction which produces ischemia.

SKIN MANIFESTATION. Pruritus and thermal sensations of hot and cold have been noted without any objective signs. These are probably caused by the formation of gas bubbles immediately under the skin and in the pores and sweat glands. Another very interesting and frequently noted symptom is a type of formication which does not stay localized but feels like a small compact colony of ants moving over the surface of the body. Emphysema has been observed subcutaneously in various parts of the body and collections of gas have been observed in the fascial planes between muscle layers.

FACTORS INFLUENCING BENDS. Factors influencing bends may be subdivided into two groups: physical factors and physiologic factors. Because of variation in experimental design and technique the data of various investigators cannot always be compared directly. But the following conclusions, as drawn by Adler (2), Fulton (11), and others, may be offered.

Physical Factors. 1. Rate of Ascent. It would be logical to assume that a rapid rate of ascent to altitude or rapid decompression increases the incidence of bends and other symptoms which is true in caisson or diving operation. But data on decompression sickness do not show a distinct relationship between rate of ascent and incidence of symptoms, though Armstrong (10) reported the appearance of bubbles in animals at lower altitudes when faster rates of ascent were used. Evelyn (17) and Gray (18) used rates of ascent varying from 500 to 4000 feet per minute without significant effect on the incidence of serious symptoms. The strongest support for the rate of ascent being relatively unimportant can be seen in the effects of rapid decompression. Hitchcock, quoted by Fulton (9), explosively decompressed humans from 20,000 to 40,000 feet. Although there was an increased incidence of bends and chokes from 55 to 65 per cent as compared with other ascents, the differences were not thought to be significant. Explosive decompression from 10,000 to 38,000 feet showed a significant increase from 62 per cent to 88 per cent, decompression from

27,500 to 45,000 feet, using pressure breathing, resulted in only 55.2 per cent incidence as compared to 40.6 per cent for the controls.

2. Altitude Attained. Altitude of the flight is an important factor. Bends very rarely occur below 20,000 feet. Above this altitude they occur with increasing frequency. Again, the reports of Adler (2) and Gray (19) are quoted because they were collected from unusually large numbers of aviation cadets and, therefore, are correspondingly valuable. The effect of altitude on bends is expressed in the percentage of cadets forced to descend because of the severity of symptoms classified with four grades. The subjects were sitting quietly in the altitude chamber during routine indoctrinations. Rate of ascent was between 1000 and 5000 feet per minute. Oxygen was probably administered in all cases above 10,000 feet. It can be seen that no severe cases (grade 3 and 4) of bends occur before 30,000 feet. From 35,000 feet, the number of severe cases is greater than the number of light cases; above 38,000 feet at exposure times longer than 1 hour, this relationship is reversed only to change again at exposure to 40,000 feet without pressure breathing (see table 34).

3. Duration of Exposure. The longer the exposure, the greater the number of individuals affected. However, the number of incidents per unit of time reaches a peak and then diminishes. In other words, the

TABLE 34

Incidence of Bends at Various Altitudes: No Exercise

Altitudes	Duration of Flight	Number of Tests	Bends Symptoms; Grades		
			1 and 2	3 and 4	Total
feet	*hours*		*per cent*	*per cent*	*per cent*
26,000	0.33	65	1.5	0	1.5
28,000	0.33	80	1.3	0	1.3
30,000	0.33	92	4.3	0	4.3
33,000	2.0	100	18.0	13	5.
35,000	2.0	3744	15.3	18.7	33.
35,000	3.0	584	5.6	7.5	13.1
38,000	1.0	7664	11.3	16.1	27.4
38,000	2.0	239	16.3	15.0	31.3
38,000	3.0	4228	13.5	4.9	18.4
40,000	1.0	105	21.9	31.1	53.0
47,500*	1.0	50	22.0	22.0	44

* Intermittent pressure breathing.

TABLE 35

*Incidence of Bends at Various Altitudes:
With Exercise*

Altitude	Duration of flight	Number of Tests	Bends Symptoms; Grades		
			1 and 2	3 and 4	Total
feet	*hours*		*per cent*	*per cent*	*per cent*
17,000 to 20,000	0.25	387	3.3	0.6	3.9
23,000	1.0	117	6.8	0.9	7.7
23,000	2.0	195	12.8	0	12.8
25,000	2.0	128	10.2	1.6	11.8
26,000	0.33	71	16.9	1.4	18.3
27,000	2.0	93	7.5	1.1	8.6
28,000	0.33	65	12.3	12.3	24.6
30,000	0.33	122	18.0	11.5	29.5
35,000	1.0	1000	17.2	7.2	24.4
38,000	1.5	167	27.6	34.7	62.3

chance of any individual who is not affected developing bends decreases with increasing exposure time.

4. Temperature. No correlation between the frequency of bends and temperature could be found between 70° and 94° F. However, at a temperature of −10° F the incidence of severe symptoms was about twice as high compared to the number at 70° F. although the number of milder symptoms was only slightly increased. These observations seem to indicate the importance of the circulation in the etiology of bends. Increased activity of muscles—shivering—as a factor is not mentioned.

5. Time of the Day. Thompson *et al.* (20) have reported that of 2076 men in low pressure chamber flights to 35,000 feet between 0900 and 1200 in the morning, 41 per cent exhibited decompression sickness, while of 1558 men at the same altitude between 1300 to 1600 in the afternoon only 29 per cent were affected. Other investigators obtained similar results. This may be owing to the fact that metabolism in general is lower during the morning.

Physiologic Factors. 1. Exercise. Exercise while at altitude is one of the most important factors influencing susceptibility to bends and chokes. Deep knee bends, push-ups and other performance of exercise at altitude lower the threshold for the outbreak of symptoms several thousand feet, increase the total number of incidents and shift the ratio of light to severe bends for equality from 38,000 to 28,000 feet (see table 35). Gray (19) showed that by increasing the frequency of the exercise the threshold may be decreased still farther. Gray also mentions that Haldane, in 1908, predicted that bends would occur at an altitude of 23,000 feet on the basis of his study of compressed air illness. The physical and chemical mechanisms whereby muscular activity intensifies the incidence and severity of decompression sickness has been and still is controversial. Production of lactic acid and carbon dioxide increasing with increasing physical work will favor local high tension of carbon dioxide and bubble formation but likewise initiate an increase in blood circulation and cause high local mechanical tensions. The net result of these opposing factors is further modified by the type, intensity and duration of the exercise employed.

2. Age and Obesity. It is well known that in caisson workers and divers the susceptibility of an individual to decompression sickness increases with increasing age. According to Gray, this seems to be true also for the aviator as demonstrated by the number of descents enforced by the severity of the symptoms (see table 36).

It seems not too surprising that age should be a factor inasmuch as with increasing age there is an increase in body weight, often obesity and alteration in circulation. The correlation between obesity and age and susceptibility to decompression sickness may alter predictions regarding the behavior of weight or age groups but not of individuals.

Other Factors. Many other factors, such as physical fitness, hypoxia, diet and fluid intake, repeated exposure, previous injuries

TABLE 36

Relationship between Age and Susceptibility to Decompression Sickness by the Percentage of Descents in Altitude Chamber Flights

Age	Number of Cadets	Descents
		per cent
18 to 19	595	4.2
20 to 21	1806	6.4
22 to 23	1478	9.7
24 to 25	796	11.2
26 to 27	680	13.5

and others have been investigated but did not yield definite results.

Chokes

Chokes may be defined as manifestations of decompression sickness characterized by several interrelated symptoms (2): substernal distress (sense of constriction or tightness in the chest, accompanied by a burning, gnawing, sometimes lancinating pain. Cough while at altitude is usually nonproductive. The substernal distress and cough are aggravated by attempts to take a deep breath.

Difficulty in breathing while at altitude is accompanied by a sense of suffocation and apprehension. Chokes occur at the same altitude as bends but only in a ratio of 1 case in 5 to 8 cases of bends. The evidence available at present suggests that chokes is the result of the circulation of miliary gas emboli in the pulmonary circulation. As in the case of bends, severe chokes may lead to secondary reactions such as pallor, sweating, nausea, vomiting, faintness and unconsciousness. These reactions are closely related to the next group of factors.

Circulatory and Neurologic Symptoms

In about 10 per cent of severe bends and 25 per cent of chokes syncope occurs, accompanied by bradycardia and hypertension probably produced by reflex stimulation. In some cases the syncopic reaction is not remedied by descent and syncope may even occur after the descent secondary to decompression sickness. In cases following chokes, where lung damage may be present, there may be pulmonary edema and pericardial effusion leading to local plasma loss. When the syncopic reaction persists for a prolonged period there is danger of its transformation into a secondary shock with hemoconcentration in its most dangerous form associated with neurologic symptoms. The secondary shock may develop into so-called neurocirculatory collapse.

Neurologic symptoms develop at altitudes where bends and chokes occur. A variety of such symptoms has been noticed. Most common are visual disturbances, such as blurring of vision, diplopia, "blindness" and visual field defects in the form of scotomata, concentric contraction and related phenomena.

Hemiplegia and monoplegia are less common and are mostly, as are other neurologic symptoms, of transitory character if they occur at altitude. Symptoms with delayed onset usually last longer and may take several weeks to disappear.

Case Reports

Fortunately, not too many severe cases and only a few fatal cases of decompression sickness have been reported. In all instances, for details the reader is referred to the original literature.

Most of these cases occurred in high altitude chamber tests. Some cases are described by Fulton (11). Two fatal cases were published by Masland (21); 5 more fatal cases were reported by Haymaker (22). The latter cases occurred at simulated altitudes between 30,000 and 38,000 feet. The ages of 4 of the men ranged from 22 to 26 years; the fifth was 38 years old. In all these cases symptoms developed during the progress of the flight. Bends and/or chokes occurred in only 2 of the 5 cases and symptoms of visual damage followed shortly thereafter in both. In 1 case, neither bends, chokes nor neurologic symptoms were observed and without detected preliminaries, shock developed. Two of the patients were obese and the other three robust. Of particular interest was the presence of fat emboli in the lungs in 4 of the cases and in the brain of the fifth. Fat emboli, so far as the author knows have not been reported in caisson or diver's sickness.

As to the source of the fat emboli the author assumes they may have come from the bone marrow and brought into circulation by nitrogen bubbles, which expanded, ruptured the walls of the venous channels and disrupted and tore the fat. Aeroembolism, which led secondarily to fatal shock, was regarded as the determining factor in the outcome.

A case of a severe neurocirculatory collapse who recovered was reported by Halbouty and Heisler (23). This report is very informative as to therapy. The turning point toward improvement and eventual recovery was marked by tracheotomy, by which much thick, tenacious and clear mucoid material was removed by suction from the trachea thus removing a serious obstacle to respiration.

A case of decompression sickness in an airplane at a cabin altitude of only 24,400 feet was reported by Schneck (24). This case, who also fully recovered, may emphasize that this disease never follows a rigid scheme.

Nitrogen Desaturation

In those instances where it is deemed necessary to ascend to those high altitudes at which decompression sickness is likely to occur the danger of this condition developing can be lessened by several different means. The most obvious of these is to maintain a rate of ascent slow enough such that the saturation of nitrogen in any tissue of the body will never reach double its normal value at any prevailing altitude pressure. This was the first procedure adopted in deep sea diving to avoid compressed air illness but the slowness of the ascent required made this procedure impractical.

In 1907 in England, Haldane and others began a thorough investigation of compressed air illness with special reference to decompression rates. They found that the approved method of slow even ascent was impractical, owing to the changes of tide and weather, and began to search for a more rapid procedure. Reconsidering the whole physiologic problem involved Haldane and his co-workers reasoned as follows.

Inasmuch as there was complete immunity from symptoms caused by bubbles, however long the exposure and however rapid the decompression as long as the excess of atmospheric pressure did not exceed about 1 atmosphere, bubbles of nitrogen would not be liberated within the body unless the supersaturation corresponded to more than a decompression from a total pressure of 2 atmospheres. The volume of nitrogen which would be liberated would be the same when the total pressure was halved, whether the pressure was high or low. Thus, it was postulated that it would be just as safe to diminish the pressure rapidly from 4 atmospheres to 2, or 6 atmospheres to 3, as from 2 atmospheres to 1. Thus, a system of stage decompression would be possible and would enable a diver to get rid of his excess nitrogen through his lungs far more rapidly than if he came up at an even rate.

In 1908 the above theory was tested experimentally by Boycott, Damant and Haldane, first on animals and then on human subjects, and was proved to be valid. Having established his theory Haldane (25) then proceeded to work out decompression tables based on both the depth of the exposure and the duration of exposure. In this respect compressed air illness differs from decompression sickness for in the former, unless the exposure is over a period of several hours, the saturation of the body is incomplete whereas in the latter the body is always completely saturated at the beginning of the ascent. As a consequence we need only consider Haldane's decompression tables based on complete tissue saturation.

For complete saturation of the tissues with nitrogen Boycott, Damant and Haldane estimated that for a man weighing 154 pounds the body would take up about 1 liter of nitrogen for each atmosphere of excess pressure—about 70 per cent more nitrogen than an equal weight of blood would take up. Hence, the amount of nitrogen in the body would be about 26 times as great as that held in the blood alone. From this it was calculated that the body would desaturate according to the logarithmic curve shown in figure 63. However, this rate of desaturation cannot be applied to the body as a whole for the rate will vary widely in different tissues of the body and for any tissue the form but not the position of the curve on the scale of figure 63 is correct.

For a completely saturated diver under a pressure of an excess of $6\frac{1}{2}$ atmospheres ($7\frac{1}{2}$ absolute), which requires an exposure of 5 or more hours under $35\frac{1}{2}$ fathoms (213 feet) of water, Haldane (25) calculated the difference in time required for safe decompression by the stage method and by the uniform method. The results are shown in figure 64 and illustrate clearly that the former can be accomplished in 5 hours whereas the latter requires 10 hours.

By converting figure 64 to a comparable decompression in aviation where an ascent to 46,886 feet is contemplated we would obtain the curves shown in figure 65. In this latter, sea level corresponds to the $35\frac{1}{2}$ fathoms of water and 46,886 feet altitude corresponds to sea level in figure 64. Thus,

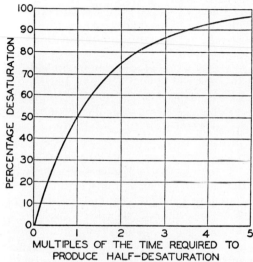

FIG. 63. Curve showing the progress of nitrogen desaturation of the body after any given decrease of pressure. (Modified from Haldane.)

if one wished to ascend to 46,886 feet without encountering nitrogen bubble formation it would be necessary to use either a uniform ascent of only 78 feet per minute or a stage ascent of 156 feet per minute both of which are too slow for practical purposes in aviation.

Two other methods of rapidly desaturating the body of nitrogen which could be utilized in aviation have already been worked out for diving operations. Zuntz (1897) suggested that the breathing oxygen would hasten the elimination of nitrogen from the body as did von Schroetter (1907) and Boinet (1907) also. More recently Behnke (26) and his associates studied the use of oxygen in the prevention of compressed air illness and highly recommended its use. In deep sea diving the use of high partial pressures of oxygen is dangerous, however, because of its

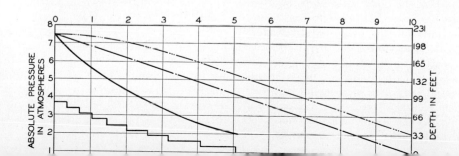

toxic effect but inasmuch as this does not apply at pressures of less than 1 atmosphere this method of nitrogen desaturation offered great possibilities in aviation.

The rate at which nitrogen is eliminated from the body at sea level when pure oxygen is breathed has been worked out in detail by Behnke (26) whose results have been reproduced here in figure 66. The curves in this figure represent the elimination of gaseous body nitrogen during a 4 hour period of oxygen inhalation by a young man weighing 132 pounds. Inasmuch as the nitrogen solvents of the body are water and fat which comprise about 70 and 15 per cent of the body weight, respectively, the broken lines in figure 66 were drawn to represent the elimination of nitrogen from these constituents and the solid line the total nitrogen elimination.

One other possible method of eliminating nitrogen from the body is through the use of a mixture of oxygen (21 per cent) and helium (79 per cent) as was suggested by Sayers, Yant and Hilderbrand (1925). This has found great favor in diving as it replaces the body nitrogen without the use of dangerous high partial pressures of oxygen. However, inasmuch as this latter is not a problem at pressures of less than 1 atmosphere this method appears to offer no advantage over pure oxygen inhalation for use in aviation. Even assuming a slight advantage for the oxygen-helium mixture the use of this mixture would involve the necessity of procuring extra equipment and supplies in addition to that already available for oxygen.

In actual practice in military flying the breathing of oxygen from the ground up or from 10,000 feet at the usual rate of climb is in itself a denitrogenation process which explains why we see fewer attacks in actual flying than during chamber runs where the rate of ascent is usually quite high. For very high flights it is best to have the crew members breathe pure oxygen for a period just prior to ascent. Usually $\frac{1}{2}$ to 1 hour is adequate for denitrogenation and if exercise is indulged in concurrently with the oxygen breathing the elimination of nitrogen from the body is more rapid and, correspondingly, more protection against attacks is afforded.

Using the Lilly-Anderson nitrogen meter, Boothby et al. (27) were able to separate quantitatively the gaseous pulmonary nitrogen from the gaseous tissue nitrogen by the characteristic forms of the curves obtained for total accumulated nitrogen when plotted on logarithmic coordinates. These studies were continued (28, 29). The data obtained are valuable in indicating quantitative methods for the prevention of bends.

A more recent study by Marbarger *et al.* (30) on 33 normal subjects in a low pressure chamber confirmed that prebreathing of 100 per cent oxygen for 2 hours at ground level materially decreased the incidence of bends during a 2 hour stay without exercise at 38,000 feet simulated altitude.

REFERENCES

(1) ARMSTRONG, H. G.: Principles and Practice of Aviation Medicine. Baltimore, The Williams & Wilkins Co., 1939.

(2) ADLER, H. F.: Unnumbered report. Randolph Air Force Base, Texas, School of Aviation Medicine, USAF, 1948.

(3) BOYLE, R.: New pneumatical experiments about respiration, Philosophical Tr., **5:** 2011–2058, 1670.

(4) HOPPE, F.: Ueber den Einfluss, Welchen der Wechsel des Luftdrucks auf das Blut Ausuebt. Arch Anat. Phys. u. Wissensch. Med., **24:** 63–73, 1857.

(5) BERT, P.: La Pression Barometrique: Recherches de Physiologie Experimentale. Paris, G. Masson et Cie, 1878. (English translation by Hitchcock, M. A., and Hitchcock, F. A.: Barometric Pressure, Columbus, Ohio, College Book Co., 1943.)

(6) HILL, L.: Caisson Disease. New York, Longmans, Green & Co., Inc., 1912.

(7) HILL, L., AND GREENWOOD, M.: On the formation of bubbles in the vessels of animals submitted to a partial vacuum. J. Physiol., **39:** xxiii, 1910.

(8) JONGBLOED, J.: The composition of the alveolar air in man at altitudes up to 14,000 meters; partly without oxygen supply. The mechanical effect of very low atmospheric pressure. *In* International Congress of Aerial Navigation, 5th, 1930, The Hague, Vol. 2. p. 1418. La Haye, M. Nijhoff, 1931.

(9) FULTON, J. F.: Aviation Medicine in Its Preventive Aspects. London, Oxford University Press, 1948.

(10) ARMSTRONG, H. G.: The Development of Caisson Disease at High Altitude. Engineering Section Memorandum Report Q-54-59. Wright Field, Ohio, 1938.

(11) FULTON, J. F.: Decompression Sickness, Caisson Sickness, Diver's and Flier's Bends and Related Syndromes. Philadelphia, W. B. Saunders Co., 1957.

(12) HARVEY, E. N., *ET AL.*: Bubble formation in animals. J. Cell. & Comp. Physiol., **24:** 1–290, 1944.

(13) BEHNKE, A. R.: A Review of Physiologic and Clinical Data Pertaining to Decompression Sickness. Naval Medical Reserve Institute, Project X-443, Report No. 4, Bethesda, Md., 1947.

(14) ARMSTRONG, H. G.: Analysis of Gas Emboli. Engineering Section Memorandum Report EPX-17-54-653-3. Wright Field, Ohio, 1939.

(15) THOMAS, S. F., AND WILLIAMS, O. L.: High altitude joint pains (bends); their roentgenographic aspect. Radiology, **44:** 259–261, 1945.

(16) BURKHARDT, W. L., *ET AL.*: A roentgenographic study of "bends" and "chokes" at altitude. J. Aviation Med., **17:** 462–467, 1946.

(17) EVELYN, K. A.: The Effect of Simulated High Altitudes on Human Subjects. Reports No. 1 through 3. London, Ontario, Canada, London Association for, War Research, University of Western Ontario, and the Royal Canadian Air Force. Report to National Research Council, April, July and September, 1941.

(18) GRAY, J. S.: Certain Advantages of a Simulated Flight at 38,000 Feet for High Altitude Classification. Project No. 14, Report No. 1. Randolph Field, Texas, School of Aviation Medicine, USAAF, 1942.

(19) GRAY, J. S.: Present Status of the Problem of Decompression Sickness. Project No. 450, Report No. 1. Randolph Air Force Base, Texas, School of Aviation Medicine, USAF.

(20) THOMPSON, J. W., *ET AL.*: Relationship of Certain Factors to the Incidence of Decompression Sickness, Appendix II. Report to National Research Council, Canada, Report No. F.P.M.S., No. D-3, 1944.

(21) MASLAND, R. L.: Injury of the central nervous system resulting from decompression to simulated high altitudes. Arch. Neurol. & Psychiat., **59:** 445–456, 1948.

(22) HAYMAKER, W., AND DAVISON, C.: Fatalities resulting from exposure to simulated high altitudes in decompression chambers; clinicopathologic study of 5 cases. J. Neuropath. & Exper. Neurol., **9:** 29–59, 1950.

(23) HALBOUTY, M. R., AND HEISLER, J. H.: Severe neurocirculatory collapse at simulated altitude. U. S. Armed Forces M. J., **6:** 1363–1370, 1955.

(24) SCHNECK, S. A.: Decompression sickness at medium altitude. U. S. Armed Forces M. J., **8:** 1366–1370, 1957.

(25) HALDANE, J. S., AND PRIESTLEY, J. G.: Respiration, Ed. 2. New Haven, Yale University Press, 1935.

(26) BEHNKE, A. R.: The application of measurements of nitrogen elimination to the problem of decompressing divers. U. S. Nav. Bull., **35:** 219–240, 1937.

(27) BOOTHBY, W. M., LUNDIN, G., AND HELMHOLZ, H. F., JR.: A gaseous nitrogen elimination test to determine pulmonary efficiency. Proc. Soc. Exper. Biol. & Med., **67:** 558–561 1948.

(28) BOOTHBY, W. M., LUFT, U. C., AND BENSON, O. O., JR.: Gaseous Nitrogen Elimination. Project No. 21-53-003, Report No. 1, Ran-

dolph Air Force Base, Texas, School of
Aviation Medicine, USAF, 1951.

(29) BOOTHBY, W. M., LUFT, U. C., AND BENSON,
O. O., JR: Gaseous nitrogen elimination. J.
Aviation Med., 23: 141–158, 1952.

(30) MARBARGER, J. P., KADETZ, W., PALTAVOKAS,
J., VARIAKOJIS, D., HANSEN, J., AND
DICKINSON, J.: Gaseous Nitrogen Elimination at Ground Level and Simulated Altitude and the Occurrence of Decompression
Sickness. Chicago, Aeromedical and Physical Environment Laboratory, University
of Illinois. Randolph Air Force Base, Texas,
Air University, School of Aviation Medicine, USAF, 1956.

13

MEDICAL ASPECTS OF PRESSURIZED EQUIPMENT

Richard W. Bancroft, Ph.D.

Many of the most serious medical problems associated with flights at high altitudes are directly related to the reduced barometric pressure and particularly to the reduced partial pressure of oxygen in the ambient air. In both commercial and military aviation the development of aircraft capable of operating at increasingly high altitudes far beyond man's limited tolerance to hypoxia and low barometric pressure has made it necessary to provide increasingly complex protective equipment and environmental control systems within the aircraft cabins to insure safe and practical conditions for the crews and passengers.

Both the aeromedical specialist and the aeronautical engineer have long recognized that the most satisfactory method for providing this necessary protection against the hostile conditions encountered at altitude is to pressurize the crew and passenger compartments of high flying aircraft and to maintain, as well as possible, a normal pressure environment within the aircraft cabin regardless of the actual flight altitude (1). By properly controlling the pressure environment of the flyer, based on well defined physiologic requirements and limitations, the major hazards encountered at high altitudes can be either virtually eliminated or dealt with effectively. Moreover, only by this means is it possible for manned vehicles to penetrate above the earth's atmosphere into the vacuum of space.

THE PRESSURE CABIN

In general, during high altitude flights, cabin pressurization can be accomplished by two methods. The conventional and least complex method is to compress and force the outside air continuously into the duly stressed cabin by means of appropriate compressors and to control the desired cabin pressure and ventilation with properly balanced outlet valves. This method is dependent on the ambient air for its source of compressible gas and is applicable for all aircraft designed for flights within the greater portion of the atmosphere. This type of cabin is simply referred to as a "pressure cabin" and the aircraft as a "pressurized aircraft." For manned vehicles capable of sustained flight in the upper limits of the earth's atmosphere and in outer space, the necessary cabin pressure and cabin environment must be created and maintained by self-contained systems that are completely independent of the outside physical conditions (2). Such a cabin, because it must be hermetically sealed and can tolerate only the barest minimum of leakage, differs considerably from the conventional pressure cabin and is better known as a "sealed cabin." Because the design requirements and the biologic considerations for the sealed cabin become increasingly complex in relation to the number of occupants and the duration of flight, this special type of cabin is described in detail in chapter 31. The following discussion will be mainly concerned with the general principles, physiologic requirements and limitations on which cabin pressurization is based.

Advantages of the Pressure Cabin

As implied in the foregoing introduction, the primary purpose of the pressure cabin is to prevent the occurrence of hypoxia and decompression sickness caused by the reduced barometric pressure encountered at high altitudes. The occupants of a well pressurized cabin are also able to enjoy a variety of additional advantages and benefits that are not possible in unpressurized aircraft. With the cabins of high flying aircraft maintained at a pressure altitude equivalent to 10,000 feet or lower, the use of oxygen equipment is no longer necessary (except in certain emergency situations) and the occurrence of decompression sickness in its various manifestations, such as bends, chokes and neurocirculatory collapse, can be completely avoided. The expansion of trapped gas in the gastrointestinal tract, causing abdominal distention, pain and occasionally incapacitating symptoms, is no longer a problem. The temperature, humidity and ventilation of the cabin can be controlled within any desired comfort range despite the sub-zero conditions of the thin ambient air.

During descents from high altitudes the pressurized cabin affords considerable protection against the occurrence of pain and possible complications in the middle ear and nasal sinuses caused by too great and too rapid an increase in the barometric pressure. Pressure changes within the cabin can be kept to a minimum and can be controlled so as to change only slowly. Of great practical importance also is the freedom of movement offered to the occupants of the pressure cabin, in many instances unencumbered by oxygen masks and other specialized high altitude equipment. Not only in multiplace military aircraft but particularly in commercial aviation this freedom to move around in a comfortable environment contributes immeasurably to the success of operational missions with a minimum of fatigue and makes possible passenger flights at extremely high altitudes where the jet airliners and high performance military aircraft operate most efficiently.

Although, from an aeromedical viewpoint, the ideal pressurized cabin environment should be maintained as close to sea level conditions as possible to obtain the maximum benefit and protection during high altitude flights, several engineering and technical factors place certain limitations on the degree to which an aircraft cabin can be pressurized. The increased structural weight of the cabin, the additional equipment and extra power requirements for pressurization significantly limit the performance and payload capacity of the aircraft and add to the maintenance and upkeep. Most important, the high internal pressures that must be sustained within a fully pressurized cabin enhance the problems of excessive leakage and increase the possibility of structural failure and the grave danger of a sudden or explosive decompression, with all of the disastrous consequences that can be involved in such an episode. For these reasons, the extent to which a cabin can be safely and economically pressurized must be carefully considered in terms of both the physiologic requirements and the design limitations imposed by the type of aircraft and the nature of the mission. Fortunately, the normal human is physiologically able to tolerate without difficulty a limited decrease in both the barometric pressure and the partial pressure of oxygen so that considerable latitude is permissible for the design and control of pressurized cabins that will still remain within an acceptable pressure range that is compatible with safety and comfort.

Physiologic Requirements for Pressure Cabins

The main considerations for the design and control of pressurized cabins, as well as for other types of high altitude protective equipment, are based primarily on the hypoxic thresholds and critical altitude limits for the normal unacclimatized man and particularly on the concept of physiologically "equivalent altitudes" with regard to the partial pressure of oxygen in the lungs and arterial blood (3). For a further discussion of equivalent altitudes see chapter 9.

These key equivalent altitudes are listed in table 37 and are characterized by various altitude situations in which the alveolar oxygen tensions are essentially identical. For the unacclimatized man to function normally

TABLE 37

*Equivalent Alveolar Oxygen Altitudes**

Equivalent Altitudes	Barometric Pressure	Breathing	Alveolar Oxygen	Arterial Oxygen
feet	*mm. of Hg*		*mm. of Hg*	*per cent saturation*
Sea Level	760	Air	100	97
34,000	187	Oxygen	100	97
10,000	522	Air	60	89
39,000	147	Oxygen	60	89
50,000	87	Air or oxygen	0	—
Space	0	Air or oxygen	0	—

* Assuming normal carbon dioxide tensions and no hyperventilation.

at altitudes above 10,000 feet, it is necessary to enrich the inspired air with oxygen, the higher the altitude the higher the required percentage of oxygen, until at an altitude of 34,000 feet pure oxygen must be breathed to insure an adequate oxygenation of the blood and tissues equivalent to sea level conditions. At a pressure altitude of 39,000 feet, when breathing pure oxygen, the partial pressure of oxygen in the lungs and arterial blood is approximately the same as at 10,000 feet breathing air. Above 39,000 feet, because of the continuing decrease in the barometric pressure and also because of the characteristic shape of the oxygen dissociation curve for hemoglobin, even when breathing oxygen, hypoxia becomes progressively and strikingly severe. And above 50,000 feet, as a result of the increasingly keen competition between the respiratory gases and water vapor for the limited pressure and available volume that must be shared within the lungs, without hyperventilation this hypoxic situation verges into true anoxia and becomes physiologically equivalent to the anoxic conditions of outer space. Finally, at about 55,000 feet, essentially no oxygen can pass from the oxygen mask or inspired air into the lungs, filled as they are with carbon dioxide and water vapor, regardless of how vigorously one breathes or hyperventilates.

With these equivalent altitudes in mind, the physiologic limits and certain threshold altitudes for various types of pressurized protective equipment are graphically shown in figure 67. With an altitude equivalent to 10,000 feet when breathing air considered as

the critical threshold for hypoxia, flights up to approximately 40,000 feet without pressurization are feasible by using conventional oxygen equipment. Above 40,000 feet, however, pressurization of some type becomes absolutely essential. Because of the limited gain in altitude tolerance provided by simple pressure breathing equipment and the severe physiologic disturbances induced by this unbalanced method for pressurizing the lungs, normal operations and prolonged survival at altitudes much in excess of 40,000 feet can be accomplished in a practical manner only by the pressurized or sealed cabin and, in emergencies, by a pressure suit.

Although the unavoidable hypoxia above

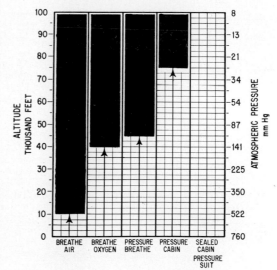

FIG. 67. Physiologic limitations at various altitudes with and without various pressurized protective equipment. (Modified from Luft (4).)

40,000 feet is the most critical factor for minimum pressurization requirements, the threshold altitudes at which other forms of decompression sickness can occur must also be carefully considered when fixing safe physiologic limits for cabin pressurization during operational flights at high altitudes. Without adequate denitrogenation prior to flight, manifestations of decompression sickness become increasingly critical at altitudes above 25,000 feet, the severity of the symptoms being dependent not only on the altitude but also on the duration of the exposure and the amount of muscular activity. Although the occurrence of severe bends below 23,000 feet is unlikely and the incidence below 30,000 feet is low, incapacitating symptoms severe enough to terminate the flight can occasionally occur within this altitude range. Also, abdominal distention and trapped gas pains, though fortunately not serious in most individuals, can be extremely uncomfortable and occasionally incapacitating at altitudes in the order of 25,000 feet or higher.

These most critical threshold altitudes are listed in table 38, which briefly summarizes the major physiologic limitations on which the control of cabin pressurization is based.

Pressure Cabin Control and Pressure Schedules

In the light of these various altitude thresholds and physiologic limits for both hypoxia and decompression sickness, it is apparent that several options are possible for the manner in which the cabin pressure can be most advantageously controlled and maintained. For commercial airliners and military transport planes in which the use of oxygen equipment is impractical and undesirable, it is essential that the cabins be maintained at a pressure altitude equivalent to no higher than 10,000 feet, although to increase passenger comfort and to minimize fatigue and ear difficulties an environmental pressure equivalent to 8000 feet or lower is preferable. To accomplish this the aircraft cabins must be safely stressed to withstand the high pressure differentials that develop between the inside of the cabin and the low outside atmospheric pressure during high altitude flights.

When pressurized cabins are considered in terms of the absolute barometric pressures, both within and outside the cabin and the difference between these two pressures or the "pressure differential" across the cabin walls, the altitude capability of an aircraft for safe and practical flight can be estimated.

TABLE 38

Threshold Altitudes and Physiologic Limitations

Altitude	Barometric Pressure		Physiologic Limitations
feet	*mm. of Hg*	*p.s.i.*	
8,000	564	10.91	Maximum for prolonged flights without undue fatigue from mild hypoxia
10,000	522	10.11	Maximum without supplemental oxygen
23,000	307	5.94	Threshold for occasional symptoms of decompression sickness
25,000	282	5.54	Threshold for occasional severe manifestations of decompression sickness
30,000	225	4.36	Critical threshold for high incidence of decompression sickness
40,000	141	2.72	Maximum, breathing pure oxygen, without additional pressure (pressure breathing, pressure suit or pressure cabin)
45,000	110	2.14	Maximum for reasonably prolonged emergency pressure breathing without pressure suit
50,000	87	1.69	Maximum for brief emergency pressure breathing with immediate descent; pressure suit required for adequate emergency protection

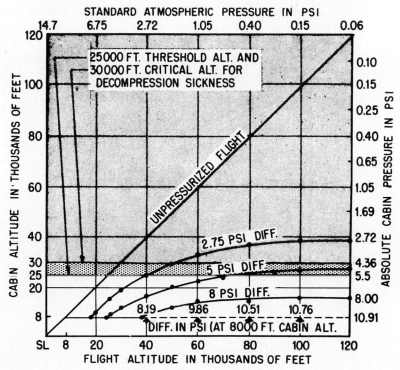

FIG. 68. Various possible cabin pressure schedules with regard to the pressure differential and physiologic limits. (From Konecci and Shannon (5).)

In figure 68 several possibilities are shown for cabin pressurization schedules in relation to various pressure differentials and the critical threshold altitudes.

The cabins of jet airliners and comparable military aircraft are usually designed to support maximum pressure differentials of between 8 and 8.5 pounds per square inch (p.s.i.) or more than half an atmosphere (1 atmosphere being equal to 14.7 p.s.i. or 760 mm. of Hg). Thus, as shown in figure 68, with the cabin environment maintained at a pressure altitude equivalent to 8000 feet (10.91 p.s.i. absolute), operational flights without the use of oxygen equipment are possible at altitudes up to the order of 40,000 feet (2.72 p.s.i.) with a differential pressure across the cabin walls of 8.19 p.s.i. For aircraft to maintain a cabin pressure equivalent to 8000 feet during flights above 40,000 feet, the pressure differential becomes increasingly stressful, developing to more than 10.5 p.s.i. at a flight altitude of 80,000 feet (fig. 68, bottom dotted line). On the other hand, by controlling the cabin pres-

sure so as to maintain a pressure differential that does not exceed 8 p.s.i., the absolute cabin pressure gradually decreases to a pressure altitude equivalent to nearly 15,000 feet during flights at 80,000 feet. In this case supplemental oxygen would have to be used by the crew and passengers when the cabin altitude exceeded 10,000 feet.

For high performance military aircraft, where maximum speed and altitude capability are important, the possibility of cabin decompression either accidentally or in combat situations must be carefully considered. Excessively high cabin pressures and pressure differentials can be reduced substantially during high altitude flights without danger of hypoxia or decompression sickness by using appropriate oxygen equipment and maintaining the cabin at a pressure altitude where the incidence of decompression sickness is not significant. This can be accomplished by limiting the pressure differential to 5 p.s.i. This, as noted in figure 68, permits flights to any altitude, including space flights, without exceeding the critical threshold altitude for decompression sickness of 30,000 feet within the cabin. During flights to 70,000 or 80,000 feet with a 5 p.s.i. differential the cabin altitude remains below 25,000 feet. The same altitude capability is possible, from the standpoint of hypoxia, with a minimum pressure differential of 2.75 p.s.i. providing pure oxygen is breathed during flights above 50,000 feet. Under these marginal conditions, however, the cabin pressure no longer protects against decompression sickness and for flights of long duration the incidence of this syndrome can be expected to be high unless adequate denitrogenation is accomplished before exposure to such low cabin pressures.

In the case of a "sealed cabin" during flights above the atmosphere it is possible to avoid the continuous use of individual oxygen equipment by increasing the percentage of oxygen in the environmental gas with which the cabin is pressurized. It is important to point out, however, that in such a cabin with an absolute pressure of less than 5 p.s.i., and particularly with a minimum pressure of 2.75 p.s.i., it is necessary to pressurize the cabin with essentially pure oxygen to avoid hypoxia. Such a situation may create a grave fire hazard within the cabin even though the pressure of the undiluted oxygen is practically the same as the partial pressure of oxygen in air at sea level. Combustion characteristics depend not only on the oxygen pressure itself but more importantly on the ratio of oxygen to nitrogen, and by reducing the quenching qualities of the inert nitrogen, oxygen partial pressure remaining constant, combustion or even spontaneous combustion is greatly facilitated (6).

Physical Considerations and Limitations for Cabin Control

Although it is clear that the pressurized cabin, to fulfill its proper function, must conform to certain physiologic requirements and must maintain an adequate cabin environment at all operational altitudes, pressurized cabins and conventional pressurization systems have inherent structural and physical characteristics that place definite limitations on their maximum operational capability.

The presure differential ($\Delta P = P$ cabin − P altitude), which represents the internal pressure that must be sustained within the pressurized cabin, is limited by structural considerations and the necessity to avoid the possibility of structural failure and a rapid decompression. From this standpoint, the high internal forces that must be supported by the cabin walls, windows, canopies, hatches, etc., can be appreciated when it is considered that a pressure differential of 8 p.s.i. is equal to an internal pressure of 1152 pounds, or well over half a ton per square foot (8 × 144 square inches). In relation to the total surface area of a cabin, the over-all total pressure is indeed impressive.

On the other hand, the mechanical ability of the compressor system to pressurize, ventilate and air condition a cabin properly at extreme altitudes also has definite limitations that directly influence the pressure differential, the cabin environment and the operational flight altitude. The operating capacity of a compressor system can best be considered in terms of the compression ratio or simply the pressure ratio (P cabin to P altitude), which expresses the extent to which the rarified outside air at high altitudes must be compressed within the cabin to maintain either a constant cabin pressure or a constant pressure differential.

For a constant cabin pressure during ascent to high altitudes, both the pressure ratio and the pressure differential become functions of the altitude, increasing with the decreasing ambient barometric pressure. To illustrate this relationship, the pressure ratio and the pressure differential with reference to various cabin and atmospheric pressures are plotted in figure 69. Both the pressure ratio and the pressure differential for any given cabin pressure and altitude can be found at the intersect of the cabin and flight altitudes. It can be seen in figure 69 that at flight altitudes above 70,000 feet, with a cabin pressure maintained at 10,000 feet, the pressure ratio becomes increasingly high and approaches infinity at altitudes above 100,000 feet as the outside barometric pressure approaches zero. Even with the cabin reduced to a minimum acceptable pressure, equivalent to 40,000 feet, the compression of the ambient air becomes increasingly

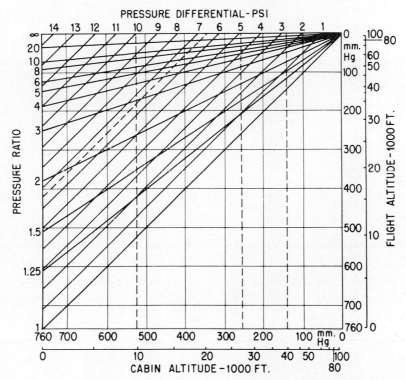

Fig. 69. The pressure ratio and pressure differential for any given cabin altitude and flight altitude. (From Luft (4).)

difficult at these extreme altitudes. According to Mayo (7), the power requirements for adequate pressurization and cabin ventilation become exorbitant at altitudes above 70,000 feet, increasing 10-fold above 100,000 feet, where all available fuel and power are important for flight itself. Furthermore, as pointed out by Mayo (7), because of the extreme pressure ratios at these altitudes the temperature of the compressed air within the cabin becomes excessively high. Figure 70 shows the temperatures of the compressed air at the compressor exit for various flight altitudes and pressure ratios when a cabin is maintained at an absolute pressure of 10 p.s.i. (equivalent to a cabin altitude of approximately 10,000 feet). Under such conditions it can be noted that at a flight altitude of 75,000 feet the temperature is in the order of 600° F. with a pressure ratio of 20. At altitudes above 100,000 feet the compression temperature is measured in 1000's of degrees. The problem of adequate air conditioning in such situations is not only formidable but can be compounded still further by the additional generation of heat caused by air friction and high stagnation temperatures on the surface of hypersonic aircraft flying within the upper layers of the atmosphere. For these reasons, pressurization during flights above approximately 70,000 to 80,000 feet by compression of the outside air becomes increasingly prohibitive and for sustained flights beyond these altitudes it becomes necessary to resort to sealed cabins with their completely independent pressurization and environmental control systems.

Rapid (Explosive) Decompression

Although the development of the pressurized cabin has virtually eliminated many of the problems associated with high altitude flights, the possibility of a structural failure resulting in a rapid, accidental loss of cabin pressure has introduced a new potential hazard for the flyer. Even the remote possibility of such an occurrence must be carefully considered in order to evaluate the physiologic consequences and the marginal limits of safety and to develop adequate protective

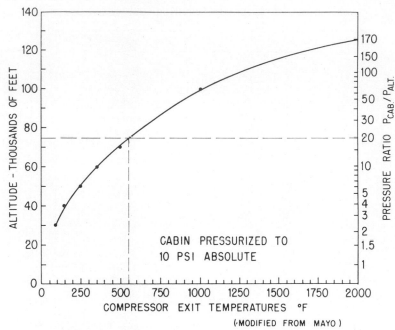

(·MODIFIED FROM MAYO)

FIG. 70. Compressor exit temperatures in a cabin when atmospheric air is compressed to 10 p.s.i. absolute at various altitudes and pressure ratios with a compressor efficiency of 80 per cent. (Modified from Mayo (7).)

equipment and emergency procedures. With pressurized aircraft flying routinely at altitudes above 40,000 feet and with manned vehicles ascending into the vacuum of space, the possible physiologic consequences resulting from a rapid decompression are becoming increasingly formidable.

In the event a perforation should suddenly occur in a pressurized cabin caused, for instance, by the structural failure of a window or canopy or by enemy action, the air in the cabin would immediately rush out through the opening and the cabin pressure would rapidly decrease and equalize with the ambient atmospheric pressure. The occupants of the cabin at the same time would be subjected to this sudden decompression which, depending on the size of the opening, might reach violent and explosivelike proportions. For this reason, extremely rapid decompressions occurring within less than 1 second are commonly called "explosive decompressions." It should be noted, however, that the rush of air through an opening in a pressurized cabin, for thermodynamic reasons, can not exceed the speed of sound regardless of the size of the opening and that one of the physical characteristics for an

explosion in one sense of the word is that the air blast is supersonic. Because of this, a clear distinction between a "rapid" and an "explosive" decompression is uncertain and in the following discussion all such decompressions will simply be referred to as rapid decompressions.

In general, the severity of a rapid decompression on the occupants of a pressurized cabin is dependent on the rate of decompression and the pressure range through which the decompression occurs. The basic physical factors that govern the decompression rate and directly influence the possible physiologic effects are:

VOLUME OF THE PRESSURIZED CABIN. A large cabin will decompress slower than a small cabin, other factors remaining the same.

SIZE OF THE OPENING IN THE CABIN. A cabin with a large perforation will decompress faster than with a small perforation. The relationship between the volume of the cabin and the cross-sectional area of the perforation or orifice determines one of the main factors for the rate and total time of decompression.

PRESSURE RATIO. The time of decompression is also dependent on the pressure ratio (P cabin to P ambient). The larger the pressure ratio the longer the decompression time. This relationship is discussed more thoroughly at the end of the section on rapid decompression.

PRESSURE DIFFERENTIAL. The pressure difference between the cabin pressure and the ambient atmospheric pressure directly influences the severity of a rapid decompression but not the time of decompression. A large pressure differential will result in a more severe decompression than a small pressure differential.

FLIGHT ALTITUDE. The altitude at which a rapid decompression occurs directly influences the seriousness of the physiologic consequences following the decompression, particularly the effects of acute hypoxia. Also, with a given pressure differential, the higher the flight altitude the longer the decompression time. This apparent paradox is owing to the fact that the higher the altitude (with any given pressure differential) the larger the pressure ratio.

Any rapid decompression that unexpectedly occurs in a pressurized aircraft during flight, even though it may be well tolerated by the occupants of the cabin, can often cause a certain amount of excitement and confusion which in turn can lead to more serious consequences that otherwise could have been avoided. The dynamic nature of such an event as a rapid decompression, usually accompanied by a loud noise, a rapid drop in temperature and the sudden appearance of dense fog in the cabin, can give the impression that a real explosion or fire has suddenly occurred and, particularly to the uninitiated, can be extremely disconcerting. For this reason, all Air Force flying personnel undergo a rapid decompression as a routine part of their physiologic training in high altitude indoctrination chambers. In this way they can become familiar with the subjective sensations of such an experience and can learn to adjust and use their oxygen equipment quickly and properly after the decompression.

In evaluating the physiologic effects of a rapid decompression it is first of all important to distinguish between (1) the primary mechanical effects on the body that occur *during* the decompression itself, that is, the possibility of being physically blown through the opening or otherwise severely injured or the possibility of sustaining internal trauma by the sudden expansion of gas in the body cavities such as the lungs, and (2) the secondary physiologic consequences that can occur *after* the decompression, as a result of the acute exposure to low barometric pressures, particularly the hypoxic effects and at altitudes above 63,000 feet the overwhelming combination of anoxia and the formation of water vapor bubbles in the blood and other body fluids.

Accidental Decompressions during Flight

The number of rapid decompressions that have occurred during actual flight have fortunately been relatively few compared to the number of pressurized aircraft that are in the air at any given time. The fact that they do occasionally occur, however, presents a potential danger that can not be underestimated.

From past experience the most serious consequences resulting from the rapid, accidental decompression of pressurized aircraft have been the few unfortunate incidents in which an occasional passenger or crew member located in the direct vicinity of the opening has been physically blown out of the cabin with the blast of escaping air or has been severely injured by striking or being struck by other objects in the cabin. The rush of air through communicating tunnels or narrow passage ways is often sufficient to propel an object or person within these areas with projectilelike velocities. For military personnel, proper indoctrination and training in the in-flight use of restraint harness and seat belts can largely eliminate this hazard but in passenger aircraft it is still a potential danger.

In practically all accidental decompressions that have so far occurred during actual flight the pilots and air crews have managed to land their aircraft safely. The most striking exceptions to this have been the two jet Comet aircraft disasters (8) that occurred in 1954 and which serve to emphasize the violent destructive forces that are generated by a massive structural failure of a pressurized cabin. Reconstruction of these two accidents indicates that at approximately 30,000 feet with a pressure differential of 7.5 p.s.i. the cabin structure suddenly split, creating, at least for one of the Comets, an estimated opening in the fuselage of about 160 square feet with a decompression time that was probably somewhat longer than the theoretically calculated time of 0.059 second. Passengers with seat belts unfastened were apparently hurled violently upward and forward against the cabin structures and as the aircraft broke apart were ejected and fell into the sea. Skull fractures and similar damage to the thorax and back, together with extremely severe internal thoracic and abdominal injuries, were the most predominant findings. After careful evaluation of all the factors involved (8) it has been concluded that the violent ejection and the subsequent water impact at terminal velocities were sufficient to account for all the external and internal injuries. Although considered unlikely, the possibility of pulmonary damage caused by the expansion of gas in the lungs can not be excluded with certainty.

In the relatively few accidental decompressions involving military aircraft (5), particularly with regard to high performance jets, the primary cause has been the sudden loss or structural failure of the bubble canopies. Here again, the most serious injuries and difficulties resulting from these decompressions were caused by shattered fragments of plexiglass or other objects and the bitter cold and windblast following the decompressions. Oxygen masks and helmets were occasionally lost during or immediately after the decompressions because the chin straps were not fastened. Swirling dust in the eyes was one of the most common complaints. The altitudes at which these decompressions took place ranged between 10,000 feet to above 40,000 feet with about 30 per cent above 30,000 feet. The pressure differentials through which the decompressions occurred ranged up to 7.45 p.s.i. with the majority at 3 p.s.i. or less. The only incident in which momentary difficulty in breathing was reported was a decompression through 5 p.s.i. with the theoretically fast decompression time of 0.006 second, although the actual time for aerodynamic reasons was probably much slower than this. Several of the decompressions, however, were apparently faster than 0.1 second without injury to the pilots.

Experimental Rapid Decompressions to Simulated Altitudes

The human body is essentially a liquid system and the tissues and body fluids are not in themselves directly affected by rapid changes in the environmental pressure, providing the drop in pressure is not below the vapor tension of the body fluids (47 mm. of Hg). In figure 71 it can be noted that there is virtually no direct physical effect on the arterial blood pressure of a dog when subjected to a moderately fast decompression with open airways from about 10,000 feet (500 mm. of Hg) to 47,000 feet (100 mm. of Hg) within approximately 1.3 seconds. On

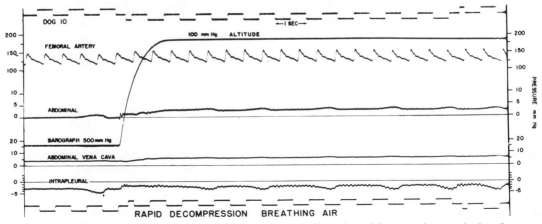

Fig. 71. Arterial, intrathoracic and abdominal pressures in a dog with open airways during decompression from 10,000 to 47,000 feet.

the other hand, during a rapid decompression, gases within the body cavities will immediately tend to expand in accordance with the gas laws and if the escape of this gas from the body is impeded or blocked, excessively high internal pressures can develop depending on the volume of the contained gas and the elastic properties of the surrounding tissues and organs. The sudden impact of such internal gas pressures, if severe enough, can be instantly transmitted through the adjacent body tissue and in this way a rapid decompression can indirectly affect the body fluids and blood pressure. Because of the relatively large amounts of gas contained in the gastrointestinal tract and particularly in the lungs, these two organs are the most susceptible to possible traumatic injury during a rapid decompression. The air in the middle ears, owing to the anatomical structure of the eustachean tubes, tends to escape readily even during the most severe decompressions and rarely, if ever, has caused difficulty, at least in human decompressions. This is also true for the escape of air from the sinus cavities providing the sinus passages are reasonably clear. Only on descent from high altitudes or during recompression do the middle ears and sinuses tend to cause trouble.

HUMAN TOLERANCE TO RAPID DECOMPRESSION. Because of the serious physiologic implications involved in an over distended and over pressurized thorax and abdomen during rapid decompressions, particularly at fast rates and to high altitudes, a considerable number of both human and animal studies have been carried out in order to at least approximate the safe marginal limits. Virtually all of these studies indicate that the healthy human can tolerate relatively severe decompressions without apparent difficulty, providing the pulmonary airways are open. The rigorous series of rapid decompressions conducted by Sweeney (9) have shown that it is possible for man to withstand decompressions from 8000 to 35,000 feet (7.5 p.s.i. differential) in the reported time of 0.09 second and from 10,200 to 35,000 feet (6.55 p.s.i. differential) in 0.075 second without ill effects. As in all rapid decompressions with open airways, there was the sensation of a deep inspiration and inflation of

the chest and abdomen, with a rapid rush of air out of the nose and mouth sufficient to cause fluttering of the lips and cheeks. These and even faster decompressions through smaller pressure changes, 27,000 to 45,000 feet (2.75 p.s.i. differential), were probably approaching the limits of human tolerance and risk. Twinges of pain in the upper regions of the abdomen were reported by Sweeney during the decompressions to 45,000 feet, possibly caused by the sudden internal pressure impact on the diaphragm or the excessive stretching of the diaphragmatic attachments.

THE LUNG DURING RAPID DECOMPRESSION WITH OPEN AIRWAYS. Because of the delicate nature of the pulmonary tissue and the intricate system of airways for ventilation, the lungs are potentially the most vulnerable part of the body during a rapid decompression. Their ability to withstand and quickly compensate for a sudden change in the environmental pressure is probably the limiting factor in the rate and range of decompression that can be tolerated by man. Although no serious injuries have occurred so far in human decompressions with open airways, it has been shown by a wide variety of animal studies that extremely fast decompressions through large pressure changes can invariably cause structural damage to the pulmonary tissue, with coincident injury to other organs during the most severe decompressions (10–12).

The pulmonary trauma and lesions most commonly seen in animals when sacrificed immediately after such rapid decompressions have been described as hemorrhagic, emphysematous and atelectatic areas in various lobes of the lungs with hemorrhages of a lesser degree found in the heart and brain. Rarely, however, were these lesions associated with any detectable disability of the animals. Other animals that were repeatedly decompressed and then several months later sacrificed and examined were completely negative at autopsy (10). Even though it appears that these injuries, at least in animals, are usually transitory in nature if given enough time for recovery, the fact that such structural damage can be produced in the lungs by rapid decompressions, even with open airways, indicates that the mechanical forces generated within the thorax can be of considerable magnitude.

Intrathoracic pressures of more than 200 mm. of Hg have been recorded in dogs when decompressed from 3300 feet to 19,600 feet (6.18 p.s.i.) in 0.015 second (13). Simultaneously recorded pressures in the superior vena cava were over 150 mm. of Hg, followed by high frequency, high amplitude pressure oscillations in both the thorax and blood vessels. In other studies (14) during decompressions from 10,000 feet to 72,000 feet (9.52 p.s.i. differential) in 0.15 second, average intrathoracic pressure of over 95 mm. of Hg were measured, with a coincident pressure wave in the carotid artery of 40 mm. of Hg.

Several mechanisms may possibly play a role in producing the structural damage seen in the lungs of animals as the result of high intrathoracic pressures during extremely fast decompressions. It has been suggested that a sudden over distention of the lungs with stretching and tearing of the alveolar structures and capillaries, as in decompressions with closed airways, may be an important factor. During extremely rapid decompressions, however, the inertial resistance of the thoracic tissue mass to sudden distention may instead result in a severe impact by a pressure wave against the momentarily rigid thoracic cage somewhat similar to that described in blast effects. The pulmonary contusions and bruises caused by decompressions faster than the resonant frequency response of the lungs and thorax may be the result of this effect inasmuch as the distention of the thorax would not be able to follow adequately the sudden build-up of pressure within the lungs. With a resonant frequency of 6 c.p.s. reported for the human chest-lung system, severe decompressions that were considerably faster than 0.16 second might produce damage by such a pressure impact. It has also been suggested (13) that some of the injuries may be caused by high frequency pressure oscillations that are set in motion and transmitted through the thoracic tissue and vascular system. Oscillating pressures such as these may also help to explain the vascular damage that has occasionally been been found in the heart, brain and inner and middle ears after extremely severe animal decompressions. Vail (14) has pointed

out that an unequal ventilation of the lungs with a disproportionate volume of air suddenly escaping from various groups of alveolae during a rapid decompression may possibly create unequal pressures and volumes within the lung tissue itself sufficient to cause rupture or collapse of adjacent alveolar structures and capillaries.

The magnitude and duration of the transient pressure that can develop within the lungs and chest during a rapid decompression with open airways is basically dependent on several factors. The most important considerations that must be taken into account are (1) the rate of decompression of the cabin, (2) the rate of decompression of the lungs, (3) the change in cabin pressure during decompression, (4) the volume of air in the lungs and (5) the rate at which the lungs and thorax can expand during the decompression. Both the escape of air through the trachea and the expansion of the lungs and thorax during a decompression will tend to reduce the intrapulmonic pressure considerably.

The decompression rate of the lungs, however, is definitely limited by the flow resistance offered by the pulmonary airways. Thus, any decompression that is faster than the inherent decompression rate of the lungs will result in a transient positive pressure difference between the inside of the lungs and the surrounding cabin environment, which itself will be in a state of change during the decompression. The faster the decompression rate of the cabin, the greater will be this transient pressure difference.

One possible way to consider this rather complex process of decompression is to visualize the occupant of a pressurized cabin as somewhat similar to a small container or bottle (lungs with open airways) placed within a larger container (the cabin). This concept is schematically illustrated in figure 72, where the small bottle, representing the lungs and airways, is assumed to have a smaller opening in relation to its volume than the large bottle representing the cabin. With such a system it is possible to trace simultaneously the pressure changes within the two bottles and to measure the important pressure differentials that temporarily occur during a decompression. *Curve I* indicates the pressure drop in the large bottle, with an initial "cabin" pressure of 600 mm. of Hg, when it is suddenly opened to an ambient pressure of 400 mm. of Hg. The small bottle also begins to decompress immediately as shown by *Curve II*, but because of its physical characteristics and also because it is in "series" with the large bottle and the ambient atmosphere, its rate of pressure change lags behind that of the large bottle. Thus, *Curve III* is the pressure difference between *Curves I* and *II* and represents the transient "transthoracic" pressure across the wall of the small bottle. This pressure difference rapidly builds up to a peak and then declines more gradually as the "lungs" decompress completely. It can be noted that when the large bottle has equalized with the ambient pressure, the smaller bottle is still in the process of decompression. The initial peak phase of *Curve III* is directly influenced by the decompression characteristics of both the large and small bottles, but the latter part of the curve, beyond the point where the large bottle is at its final pressure, reflects only the decompression characteristics of the small bottle as it decompresses independently to the static ambient pressure.

Measurements such as these have been obtained for the decompression characteristics of the human chest with open airways when the thorax was voluntarily held in a fixed position by muscular tension during rapid decompressions (15). These decompressions were carried out through various selected pressure differentials that ranged from 3 p.s.i. (150 mm. of Hg) to 9.7 p.s.i. (500 mm. of Hg) with decompression times for the cabin of approximately 0.06 to 0.25 second depending on the pressure ratios. From the data obtained and by calculations based on the General Theory of Rapid Decompression of Haber and Clamann (16) it was possible to show that the resistance to air flow through the respiratory passages appears to be considerably greater during rapid decompression (7 cm. of H_2O per liter per second) than during normal quiet breathing (1.8 cm. of H_2O per liter per second). Rapid decompressions may create a situation in the thorax similar to that produced by a cough or forced exhalation. Pulmonary function studies by others have shown that

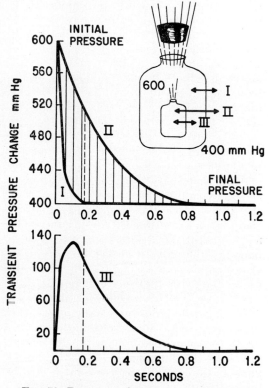

FIG. 72. Decompression of two containers, one within the other, analogous to the cabin and thorax. Decompression *Curves I* and *II* indicate the absolute pressure change in the cabin and thorax, respectively. *Curve III* is the transient pressure difference across the chest wall (15).

the flow resistance during a forced exhalation may increase as much as 20-fold. This is attributed to excessively high intrathoracic pressures which tend to collapse and narrow the bronchial and tracheal airways within the thorax. Partial collapse of the trachea has been observed during the act of coughing. Intrathoracic pressures equivalent to those produced by a cough were measured during the more severe decompressions. A peak chest pressure of 73 mm. of Hg was recorded during a decompression from 4000 feet to 39,000 feet (9.7 p.s.i. differential) in approximately 0.25 second.

The decompression characteristics of the chest when held in a fixed position with open airways was found to be equivalent to the decompression rate of a cabin with a ratio V/A (volume to effective orifice) of 200 M^3/M^2 or 655 feet³/feet². Consequently, a cabin with these characteristics during a decompression will cause no significant increase in the chest pressure regardless of the pressure change in the cabin. These conditions coincide closely with the limits for absolute safety suggested by Violette (13), although as both human and animal studies have shown there is still a considerable margin of safety for much faster decompressions with open airways, the rates of which must be finally limited by consideration of the pressure change in the cabin and the pressure ratio (see also fig. 80 and its accompanying text).

The dynamic influence of water vapor on the intrathoracic pressure during rapid decompressions even to altitudes below 50,000 feet is indicated by comparison of peak chest pressures that were recorded during a series of decompressions to increasingly high altitudes, but with the same differential pressure. As shown by the data in table 39 for five pairs of decompressions, the peak intrathoracic pressures were consistently greater, for the same pressure change in the cabin, whenever the decompressions were to lower final pressures. This effect is most probably caused by the excessive generation of water vapor within the lungs together with the efflux of carbon dioxide and other evolved

gases from the tissue fluids and pulmonary blood, the influence of which becomes increasingly significant at higher altitudes. In some respects this is consistent with the concept of "relative gas expansion" (RGE) as postulated by Sweeney (9) and Lovelace and Gagge (3) for gases saturated with water vapor within the body cavities during rapid decompression. By taking into account the water vapor pressure at body temperature (47 mm. of Hg), the RGE theory is an estimate of the relative change in volume of body gases when the initial cabin pressure (P_c) is reduced to a final ambient pressure (P_a) by the relationship:

$$RGE = \frac{P_c - 47 \text{ mm. of Hg}}{P_a - 47 \text{ mm. of Hg}} \quad \text{(equation 1)}$$

The RGE, however, as determined by this relationship is essentially a comparison of two static conditions and it has been found to be inconsistent and not entirely correct for evaluating or quantitatively defining the dynamic process of a rapid decompression. This becomes particularly complex when the elastic thorax and abdomen may have become distended and an undetermined quantity of gas has escaped during the decompression. As a more exact estimate of gas expansion (E) within the relatively elastic body cavities, based on thermodynamic considerations, Violette (13) has proposed a modified form

$$E = \left(\frac{P_c}{P_a}\right)^{0.9} \quad \text{(equation 2)}$$

which tends to agree more closely with both theory and experimental findings.

RAPID DECOMPRESSION WHILE WEARING OXYGEN MASKS. Inasmuch as the increased intrapulmonic pressure that develops during a rapid decompression is directly influenced by both the abundant production of water vapor at high altitudes and by an increased airway resistance for the escape of air from the lungs at high airflow velocities, any additional restrictions to the pulmonary airways may momentarily tend to increase the intrapulmonic pressure still further. Such a condition can occur when the pressure-demand oxygen mask (type A-13) has been tightly secured on the face prior to decompression. The balanced exhalation valve in this type

TABLE 39

Comparison of Peak Intrathoracic Pressures in Man during Five Pairs of Rapid Decompressions, Each Pair with the Same Pressure Differential, but with Different Initial (P_c) and Final (P_a) Pressures, in mm. of Hg, with Decompression Times in Seconds

$P_c - P_a$	P_c	P_a	t	P_{chest}
150	700	550	0.065	4
	400	250	0.105	10
252	700	448	0.100	17
	400	149	0.170	31
305	700	395	0.130	22
	400	96	0.260	50
405	700	295	0.170	40
	600	196	0.210	59
452	700	248	0.200	30
	600	147	0.255	52

* Data from Luft and Bancroft (15).

of pressure-breathing mask, because of the nature of its construction, becomes temporarily blocked during a rapid change in the ambient pressure and if other pathways for the escape of air from the lungs are not available dangerously high intrapulmonic pressures may develop. On the other hand, because of the overwhelming onset of hypoxia following a decompression to high altitudes, it is important under certain flight conditions that the oxygen mask be worn securely in place at all times in the event such a decompression should occur.

Consequently, this type of pressure-breathing equipment was physiologically evaluated during 35 rapid decompressions from a simulated cabin altitude of 20,000 to 25,000 feet to a simulated flight altitude of 47,000 to 52,000 feet in 0.3 to 0.5 second (17). In this study, the intrapulmonic pressure, as indicated by the recorded mask pressures, reached an average peak of 62 mm. of Hg during the initial phase of the decompressions and then adequate pressure relief invariably occurred by a large leakage of air around the edges of the mask. In all of these decompressions no subjective or objective indications of pulmonary damage were noted. At 50,000 feet after the decompressions all subjects continued pressure breathing for 5 minutes without undue embarrassment.

It is interesting to note that while wearing the same type of equipment, a similar decompression from 30,000 feet (225 mm. of Hg) to 61,500 feet (50 mm. of Hg) was also sustained without ill effects, recompression to 30,000 feet occurring within 10 seconds. A peak intrathoracic pressure of 74 mm. of Hg was recorded during this decompression which, according to the RGE theory (equation 1) involved a relative gas expansion of 60 times the initial gas volume in the lungs. On the other hand, a calculated gas expansion (E) by the method proposed by Violette (equation 2) is approximately 3.9 times the initial lung volume and may possibly indicate a more reasonable value for evaluating the actual conditions at extremely high altitudes.

RAPID DECOMPRESSION WITH CLOSED AIRWAYS. As animal experiments have shown, as well as a few rare human incidents, the most disastrous and even fatal consequences can result if the respiratory airways are completely closed (breath-holding, swallowing, closed glottis) during even relatively slow decompressions of 1 second or longer. When the escape of the intrapulmonic air is thus blocked during the entire course of a decompression, excessively high pressures can develop within the grossly over distended lungs leading to actual rupture of the pulmonary tissue and capillaries with subsequent pneumothorax and mediastinal emphysema. It has been determined by animal experiments that when the lungs and thorax are over expanded by relatively static intrapulmonic pressures of more than 80 mm. of Hg air bubbles are actually forced into the pulmonary circulation as well as into the pleural spaces and can result in a generalized aeroembolism throughout the vital organs of the body (18, 19). Indications of a temporary cerebral insult by this mechanism have been described by Benzinger (20) for a rapid decompression from 10,000 to 39,000 feet with voluntary breath-holding at the moment of decompression. Fatal accidents similar to this have been reported in submarine escape training when the breath was inadvertently held during this type of underwater emergence, one from a depth of only 15 feet (19).

During the routine indoctrination of literally thousands of flying personnel in the process of rapid decompression, one such fatality has occurred that can be directly attributed to a full inspiration with breath-holding at the moment of decompression. This particularly dangerous situation has been carefully analyzed by Luft (4) in an approach toward predicting the marginal conditions for decompression with closed airways and for defining the essential variables and their approximate magnitudes. In accordance with Boyle's Law, it is possible to estimate, at least theoretically, the magnitude of the intrapulmonic pressure after any decompression with closed airways if it is assumed that the respiratory muscles are completely relaxed such as at the end of a normal exhalation. The volume of trapped air in the lungs and the initial and final cabin pressures are the main factors that must be considered. If these factors are known, the intrapulmonic pressure that will come to bear across the chest wall after a sudden reduction in the surrounding cabin pressure can be estimated by the following pressure-volume relationships within the closed, elastic lung, with due regard for the water vapor pressure at body temperature:

$$\frac{P_L - 47}{P_c - 47} = \frac{V_1}{V_2} \qquad \text{(equation 3)}$$

in which P_L equals total (absolute) intrapulmonic pressure after decompression, mm. of Hg; P_c equals barometric (absolute) pressure in cabin before decompression, mm. Hg; V_1 equals lung volume before decompression; V_2 equals lung volume after decompression; and 47 equals vapor tension of body fluids, mm. of Hg. Inasmuch as the expanded lung volume after decompression (V_2) cannot exceed the full lung capacity, the absolute intrapulmonic pressure resulting from a change of lung volume from V_1 to the maximum lung capacity (V_{max}) can, with rearrangement of equation 3, be expressed as

$$P_L = \frac{V_1}{V_{max}} (P_c - 47) + 47. \qquad \text{(equation 4)}$$

The important pressure difference (ΔP_L) between the inside of the lung and the ambient barometric pressure (P_a) after decompression is thus:

$$\Delta P_L = \frac{V_1}{V_{max}} (P_c - 47) + 47 - P_a. \qquad \text{(equation 5)}$$

Theoretically, a slightly more exact estimate of this intrapulmonic pressure difference can be made by taking into account the fact that the lungs and thorax, although distensible, do not behave as a frictionless piston. A positive intrapulmonic pressure is required to hold the relaxed thorax and closed lungs in an expanded position, the greater the thoracic expansion the higher the required intrapulmonic pressure, until, with a positive pressure within the closed lungs of about 20 to 25 mm. of Hg, the lungs and relaxed thorax are expanded to their full vital capacity. The intrapulmonic pressure under these conditions is called the "relaxation pressure" (P_R). If at the instant before decompression with closed airways the relaxed thorax is in an expanded position, such as at the end of a normal inspiration, the intrapulmonic pressure will be somewhat higher than the surrounding cabin pressure. Inasmuch as it is the actual intrapulmonic pressure changes rather than the cabin pressures that are of critical interest under these conditions, a more exact form of equation 5 can be written if this relaxation pressure (P_R) is also taken into consideration. The following equation incorporating P_R is modified somewhat from the original equation of Luft (4).

$$\Delta P_L = \frac{V_1}{V_{max}} (P_c + P_R - 47) + 47 - P_a$$

$$\text{(equation 6)}$$

In figure 73, this equation has been graphically evaluated for decompressions with closed airways from 8000 feet to various altitudes. The resulting intrapulmonic pressures are plotted as a function of the initial lung volumes which are shown on the ordinate as fractions of the total lung capacity. The conventional subdivisions for the various lung volumes are shown for reference on the left side of the figure, with the region for normal tidal volumes as one of the main points of interest. For instance, with the airways closed at the end of a normal exhalation (where the initial lung volume is about one-half the total lung capacity) a decompression to an altitude of 30,000 feet would result in a dangerously high intrapulmonic pressure of approximately 80 mm. of Hg. On the other hand, such a decompression with a smaller initial lung volume of about one-third the total lung capacity would produce essentially no increase in the intrapulmonic pressure inasmuch as the change in the ambient pressure would tend to be completely compensated by expansion of the lungs toward their full capacity with only a relatively slight relaxation pressure maintaining this expanded position. The worst situation under such conditions would be a decompression after a full inspiration with closed airways, for example to 30,000 feet, resulting in a theoretic intrapulmonic pressure in this case of approximately 360 mm. of Hg. A decompression to 20,000 feet would be correspond-

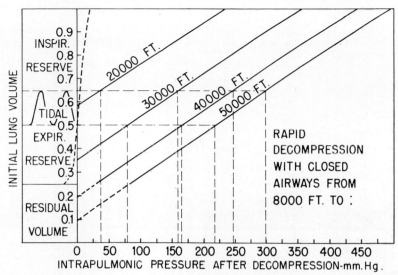

Fig. 73. Intrapulmonic pressures, calculated from equation 6 as a function of the initial lung volume, after decompression with closed airways from 8000 feet to various altitudes between 20,000 and 50,000 feet. (Modified from Luft (4).)

ingly less severe and to 50,000 feet considerably more severe. Intrapulmonic pressures produced after decompressions, either at the moment of a normal exhalation or a normal inhalation in the tidal volume range are shown in figure 73 by the corresponding dashed lines for the several altitudes. The conventional relaxation pressure curve is also shown as the small dashed sigmoid curve on the lung volume scale in the upper left hand side of the figure, from which the value for P_R in equation 6 can be estimated depending on the initial lung volume.

Although such an evaluation as illustrated in figure 73 and equation 6 is admittedly theoretic, it nevertheless can be helpful for at least approximating the essential factors and estimating possible limits of safety.

ABDOMINAL EFFECTS DURING RAPID DECOMPRESSION. Contrary to theoretic expectations, abdominal distress caused by sudden decompression is usually no more severe than that resulting from slower decompressions to the same altitude. On occasion, when the expanding gas in the gastrointestinal tract is excessive or can not be satisfactorily relieved, severe discomfort and pain can result which may lead to more general neurocirculatory reactions and collapse. Abnormally high gastric pressures in the expanded stomach tend to displace the

diaphragm in an upward position and embarrass the respiration.

The gastrointestinal tract of experimental animals (dogs) when decompressed from 10,000 to 50,000 feet at rates as fast as 0.012 second invariably showed no gross pathology (10). Only by subjecting the animals to extreme decompressions, to pressures less than the vapor tension of body fluids, have gastrointestinal lesions been demonstrated, usually of a hemorrhagic nature (11). It has been difficult to produce an actual rupture of the gastrointestinal tract, even with the most severe decompressions.

Vail (14) has recorded the intra-abdominal pressure changes in dogs that were decompressed from 10,000 feet (520 mm. of Hg) to 72,000 feet (30 mm. of Hg) within 0.15 second. The average increase in the abdominal pressure during such severe decompressions was approximately 59 mm. of Hg with an almost immediate decrease after the decompressions to about half this value as gas was expelled from the gastrointestinal tract. Similar results have been reported by Gelfan and Werner (12) in the macaque monkey.

Intra-abdominal pressures (gastric and abdominal vena caval pressures) measured in anesthetized dogs during and after mod-

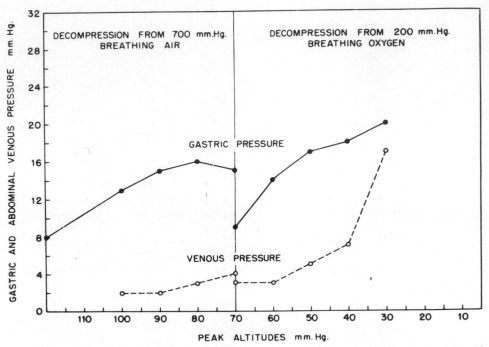

FIG. 74. Average gastric and abdominal venous pressures *during* decompressions to increasingly higher altitudes between 43,000 feet (120 mm. of Hg) and 72,000 feet (30 mm. of Hg).

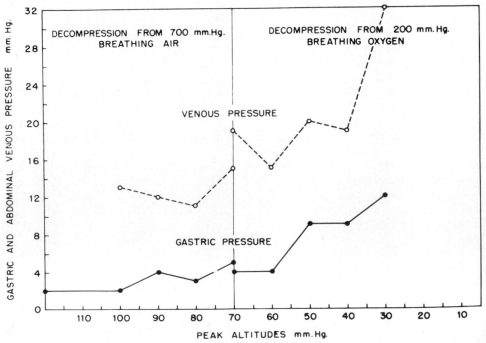

FIG. 75. Average gastric and abdominal venous pressures 1 minute *after* decompression at increasingly higher altitudes.

erately fast decompressions of about 1 second to various peak altitudes are shown in figures 74 and 75. Here again, as expected, the greatest increase in gastric pressures occurred during the most severe decompressions (fig. 74) followed by a decrease within a few seconds at the peak altitudes (fig. 75). On the other hand, the abdominal venous pressure remained relatively unaffected during these rapid decompressions providing the peak altitudes were below 62,000 feet, *i.e.*, to final pressures that were greater than 50 mm. of Hg. Within a minute after the decompressions, however, as the gastric pressures tended to decrease, the venous pressures increased significantly owing to the severe hypoxia and gradual cardiovascular failure, coinciding with the decreasing arterial blood pressure. These abdominal pressure changes can be seen in relation to the arterial pressure and heart rate in figure 76. With decompressions to extremely high altitudes, to less than 50 mm. of Hg, the combined effects of water vapor formation within the low pressure side of the cardiovascular

system and body cavities and the essentially complete anoxia, as shown in figure 77, is reflected in both the gastric and venous pressures coincident with the profound decrease in the arterial blood pressure and heart rate.

CARDIOVASCULAR EFFECTS DURING RAPID DECOMPRESSION. As demonstrated in figure 72, decompressions with open airways in the order of 1 second duration or slower, when there is no appreciable increase in the intrathoracic pressure, produce in themselves no noticeable effect on the heart and circulation. During considerably faster decompressions, however, the rapid build-up of pressure within the lungs and distention of the thorax will cause, first, a positive pressure wave to be transmitted through the heart and great blood vessels, followed almost immediately by a decrease in the arterial blood pressure, often with a pronounced bradycardia. There is evidence that this cardiovascular response immediately following severe decompressions is, at least in part, mediated through cardiopulmonary reflexes that are predominantly vagal in

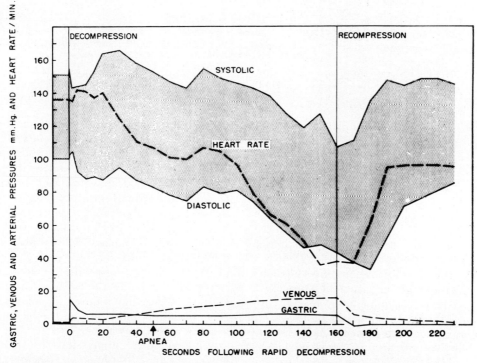

FIG. 76. Effect of rapid decompression with open airways from ground level (700 mm. of Hg) to 55,000 feet (70 mm. of Hg) on the cardiovascular system and gastric pressures in the anesthetized dog. Average effect of eight decompressions (7 dogs).

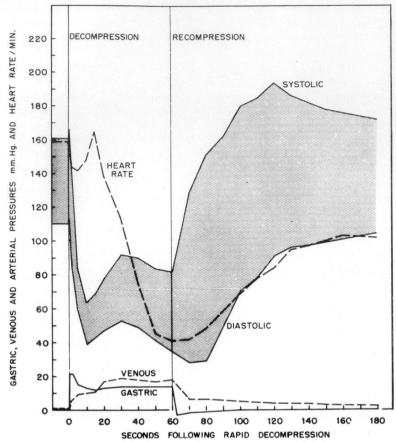

Fig. 77. Effect of rapid decompression with open airways, breathing oxygen, from 32,500 feet (200 mm. of Hg) to altitudes above 66,000 feet (40 to 30 mm. of Hg) on the cardiovascular system and abdominal pressure. Average of 6 decompressions on 4 dogs.

origin (12, 21). The stimulation of stretch receptors within the lungs probably elicits this reflex action and it has been shown that bilateral vagotomy tends to abolish it, whereas denervation of the carotid sinus has very little or no effect.

When the airways are restricted, such as by a tightly fitted oxygen mask, the excessive increase in the intrapulmonic pressure during rapid decompression can greatly intensify this cardiovascular effect, particularly if the high intrathoracic pressure is prolonged by the immediate onset of pressure breathing. As shown in figure 78, the temporary decrease in both the heart rate and blood pressure of an anesthetized dog, fitted with automatic pressure breathing equipment, following a relatively slow decompression of about 1 second to 50,000 feet, can be quite pronounced. Even though the animal was probably somewhat depressed by the anesthetic, cardiovascular recovery appeared to be adequate after several seconds, despite the high breathing pressure and slow respiratory efforts recommenced after about 65 seconds just prior to recompression. In this situation, not only do the cardiopulmonary reflexes play a role during decompression but also the effect of pressure breathing itself after decompression tends to reduce the cardiac output and to initiate vascular reflexes for maintaining the circulation and restoring the blood pressure.

When rapid decompressions are sustained with open airways, the conditions are much more favorable and the severity of the cardiovascular response is dependent on

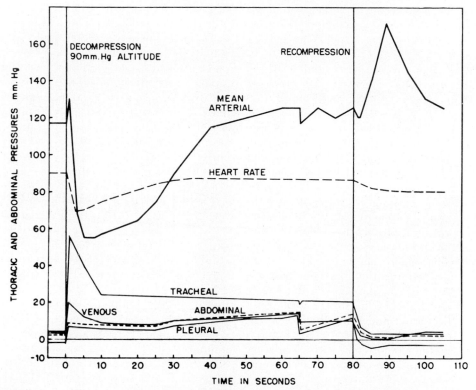

FIG. 78. The cardiovascular response in the anesthetized dog to the combined effects of rapid decompression and pressure breathing. Decompression from 32,500 feet (200 mm. of Hg) to 49,500 feet (90 mm. of Hg).

both the rate and range of decompression, with the final altitude and the influence of hypoxia and water vapor also being of particular importance as can be seen by a comparison of the arterial pressures and the heart rates in figures 77 and 78.

DECOMPRESSIONS TO PRESSURES LESS THAN THE VAPOR PRESSURE OF BODY FLUIDS. With the possible exception of a rapid decompression with closed airways, the most severe conditions are encountered when the unprotected body is suddenly exposed to an altitude where the environmental pressure is less than the vapor pressure of water at body temperature (47 mm. of Hg, 63,000 feet). Unless adequate pressurized garments are immediately activated or recompression to a lower altitude is initiated promptly, serious cardiopulmonary and neurologic damage can be expected, with possibly fatal results if the exposure is prolonged for much more than 1 minute. At these extremely high altitudes above 63,000 feet, not only

are the body tissues immediately subjected to virtually complete anoxia, but at the same time the body fluids and moist surfaces that anatomically are at the same pressure as the ambient environment will begin to vaporize spontaneously and actually boil in the true physical sense of the word.

The fact that biologic fluids can be made to boil at body temperature by lowering the ambient pressure below the vapor tension of the liquids has been known for nearly 300 years when Robert Boyle published his original observations in 1670. One of the first careful studies of such a phenomenon, however, as an aeromedical problem was carried out and reported by Armstrong in 1938 (22). The actual boiling effect was observed in the circulation of rabbits through special glass canulas, placed in the blood vessels, when the animals were decompressed to altitudes above 63,000 feet (47 mm. of Hg). Since then a considerable number of measurements have been made on animals that were exposed to these extremely high altitudes for varying periods of time.

Within the lungs, thorax and gastrointestinal tract upon exposure to pressures less than 47 mm. of Hg, the vaporization of water can proceed at a vigorous rate, completely filling these body cavities and building up sufficient pressure for the rapidly evaporated water vapor to rush out through the mouth and trachea together with other evolved body gases. Respiration usually ceases within a few seconds after the decompression as the abnormally high water vapor pressure within the pleural space, termed "vapothorax," causes at least a partial collapse of the lungs (14). At the same time, vaporization of the blood will commence with a massive formation of water vapor bubbles, first in the great veins within the thorax and the right heart. The cardiac output virtually ceases as a result of this vascular vapor lock, with circulatory arrest, a precipitous drop in the arterial blood pressure and an abnormal increase in the venous pressure (fig. 78).

Edelmann and Hitchcock (23) rapidly decompressed several groups of rats and dogs to a simulated barometric pressure of 30 mm. of Hg (72,000 feet) in 0.03 second and carefully observed the gross appearance and behavior of these animals while at this extreme altitude. The marked distention of the abdomen immediately upon decompression was the first of the most typical signs observed. Not only was respiration embarrassed by the upward deflection of the diaphragm but the action of the heart and the circulation was also probably affected by this abnormal condition. For the first few seconds a deep, rapid respiration was noted and then within 6 to 10 seconds the animals collapsed, followed by mild convulsions. A few gasping respiratory efforts were observed following the convulsive episodes but by the end of 30 seconds respiration stopped completely, the eyes became glazed and the animals appeared to be dead. Upon recompression to ground level, the hearts were still beating and all animals survived providing they were recompressed within 1 minute. Exposure times of 2 minutes re-

sulted in the death of 4 out of 10 dogs and 2 of these survivors later succumbed after a subsequent 4 minute exposure. Respiration usually began spontaneously within 30 seconds after return to ground level for the animals exposed to 72,000 feet for 1 minute, and by the end of 20 to 30 minutes the animals seemed to be essentially normal. During the exposure period at 30 mm. of Hg, lacrimation, salivation and urination occurred and these fluids were observed to bubble. In some cases there was projectile vomiting and defecation.

Further striking evidence of water vapor formation was noted within 30 to 40 seconds at 72,000 feet by a swelling under the skin of the animals which in some cases crept into adjacent areas and in others spread by a series of sudden explosivelike extensions. Upon recompression this swelling of the skin suddenly deflated at a barometric pressure of about 58 mm. of Hg.

The principal pathology found in the animals that died or were sacrificed after exposure to 30 mm. of Hg consisted mainly of edema, hemorrhage and atelectasis in the lungs.

Even though the vaporization of tissue fluids at body temperature when subjected to extremely low barometric pressures is a true "boiling" effect, Ward (24) has suggested that the term "ebullism" be used to describe this unique medical syndrome with all the signs and symptoms that occur as a result of this boiling phenomenon at very high altitudes.

HYPOXIA AFTER RAPID DECOMPRESSION (see also chapter 9). Although the possibility of pulmonary damage during rapid decompression is a potential hazard that cannot be underestimated, past experience with human decompressions has fortunately shown that the possibility is remote providing the airways are unobstructed and also that the incidents of decompressions with closed airways have been extremely rare.

On the other hand, the very real danger of overwhelming hypoxia following a sudden decompression to high altitudes is inevitable unless adequate emergency oxygen equipment is provided and used correctly. A rapid decrease in the cabin pressure is followed within a fraction of a second by the same pressure decrease in the lungs as the expanding respiratory gases escape through the trachea. Consequently the partial pressure of oxygen in both the surrounding air and the alveolae decrease simultaneously with the decompression of the cabin and the lungs. When breathing air, decompressions to 33,000 feet reduces the oxygen partial pressure in the lungs to about 35 mm. of Hg, a value that is approximately that for oxygen in the mixed venous blood (25). As a result, oxygen uptake by the pulmonary blood ceases immediately and within a matter of seconds the onset of hypoxia is rapid and severe. With decompressions to altitudes above 33,000 feet, when breathing air, the alveolar oxygen tension is correspondingly reduced still further so that an actual reversal of the oxygen diffusion gradient across the alveolar membranes is established and oxygen now passes back into the lungs from the venous blood. As a result, immediately following rapid decompressions to these high altitudes, the arterial blood leaving the heart is virtually desaturated, with fulminating hypoxia in the brain and other organs and tissues an inevitable consequence.

Luft *et al.* (25) have shown that immediately following rapid decompressions to altitudes above 40,000 feet there is considerably more oxygen in the lungs than in the ambient air as both oxygen and carbon dioxide pour out of the pulmonary blood. When breathing oxygen prior to decompression this same situation occurs with decompressions to altitudes above 48,000 feet, followed by a similar rapid onset of hypoxia.

Because the rush of air from the lungs during a rapid decompression is much greater than a normal respiratory movement, the incapacitating hypoxia following such a decompression occurs much quicker than by simply removing the oxygen mask while at altitude and washing out the oxygen in the lungs with several breaths of the ambient air. The time of consciousness that remains after rapid decompressions to various altitudes when breathing either air or oxygen and after mask removal at altitude is shown in figure 46 of chapter 9. It can be seen that the time of consciousness when breathing air prior to decompression is considerably shorter than after mask removal at the same altitudes between 25,000 and 40,000 feet and then both tend to reach a minimum time of 12 to 15 seconds at about 45,000 feet. Also, the air and oxygen time curves converge at about 52,000 feet. This brief time of consciousness after sudden exposure to altitudes above 52,000 feet is essentially the same regardless of whether air or pure oxygen is breathed during the decompression. At these altitudes the lungs are completely filled with evolved carbon dioxide and water vapor leaving no room for inspired oxygen or air. With subsequent recompression, however, to lower altitudes, it should be emphasized that the chances for survival are much better and recovery will occur much sooner and at a higher altitude if oxygen is being breathed continuously.

Further studies have also shown that following rapid decompressions to altitudes above 52,000 feet, even when breathing pure oxygen, loss of consciousness is unavoidable if the exposure time before recompression exceeds 5 to 6 seconds (26). With an exposure time above 52,000 feet of more than 6 seconds, unconsciousness inevitably occurs after an interval of about 15 seconds even though recompression to a normally safe altitude has already been accomplished.

DECOMPRESSION SICKNESS FOLLOWING RAPID DECOMPRESSION. The incidence of decompression sickness following rapid decompressions to bends producing altitudes has been found to be only slightly greater than after slow decompressions to the same altitudes (27). Contrary to some early expectations, there is no such thing as "explosive decompression sickness," with no sudden formation of nitrogen bubbles in the tissues and body fluids, providing the decompressions are to altitudes below the critical 63,000 feet where water vapor bubbles begin to be a serious factor.

Determination of Decompression Times for Pressurized Cabins

A general theory of rapid decompression has been developed by Haber and Clamann (16) which, because it takes into account several significant factors associated with a rapid decompression, permits a more accurate analysis of decompression times than is possible by other, more simplified methods. The following brief summary describes the essential considerations and relationships with which the time of decompression for any pressurized cabin can be readily calculated. For a complete mathematic analysis of the theory of rapid decompression the reader is referred to the original report (16).

The time of decompression depends essentially on two factors. One factor is the relationship between the volume of the cabin and the cross-sectional area of the orifice or opening in the cabin. This factor takes into account the geometric constants of the cabin and determines whether a decompression will be relatively fast or slow. A large cabin with a small opening will decompress much slower than a small cabin with a large opening. Haber and Clamann define this relationship as the *time-constant* of the cabin (t_c) and express it in the general form:

$$t_c = \frac{V}{A \cdot C} \qquad \text{(equation 7)}$$

in which V is the volume of the cabin, A is the area of the effective orifice and C is the speed of sound. By introducing the speed of sound as a characteristic of air flow, the influence of density can be eliminated and only the pressure relationships need then be considered. For most calculations a speed of sound of about 1100 feet per second can be used. It is interesting to note that one of the main considerations in the theory of decompression is that the flow of air through an opening in a pressurized cabin can not exceed the speed of sound and that at least the last portion of a decompression occurs at less than the speed of sound.

The "effective" orifice is always smaller than the actual geometric orifice because a variety of factors tend to reduce the flow of air through an opening such as friction, turbulent air flow and shape of the orifice. In aircraft cabins where the sudden loss of a window or canopy may create a fairly clean opening, the effective orifice is about 90 to 95 per cent of the geometric orifice. Thus, the "orifice coefficient" is about 0.9 to 0.95. In altitude chambers where rapid

decompressions are carried out through decompression valves and curved ducts, the effective orifice may be as small as 25 per cent of the actual orifice area.

The second factor on which the time of decompression depends is a pressure dependent factor (P_1) and can be expressed as a function of the pressure ratio:

$$P_1 = f\left(\frac{P_c}{P_a}\right) \qquad \text{(equation 8)}$$

in which P_c is the cabin pressure before decompression and P_a is the cabin pressure after decompression or the pressure of the ambient air. For the total time of decompression, the values for P_1 for any given pressure ratio up to 100 can be obtained from the top curve in figure 79.

Haber and Clamann have shown that the total time of decompression (t_E) is equal to the product of the time-constant (t_c) and the pressure factor P_1.

$$t_E = t_c \cdot P_1 \qquad \text{(equation 9)}$$

Thus, the total time of decompression can be determined if the volume of the cabin, the effective orifice area and the initial and final cabin pressures are known.

For example, assume a rapid decompression in a passenger aircraft under the following conditions:

Flight altitude equals 40,000 feet (2.72 p.s.i.).

Cabin altitude equals 8000 feet (10.91 p.s.i.).

Effective cabin volume equals 9000 cubic feet.

Decompression orifice (window) equals 2 square feet.

Orifice coefficient equals 0.95.

Effective orifice equals 0.95 $\times$ 2 equals 1.9 square feet.

Also assume that the aircraft does not descend during the decompression and the influence of the cabin pressurization system on the rate of decompression is not considered.

The time-constant (t_c)

$$= \frac{9000 \text{ cubic feet}}{1.9 \text{ square feet} \times 1100 \text{ feet per second}}$$

$$= 4.306 \text{ seconds}$$

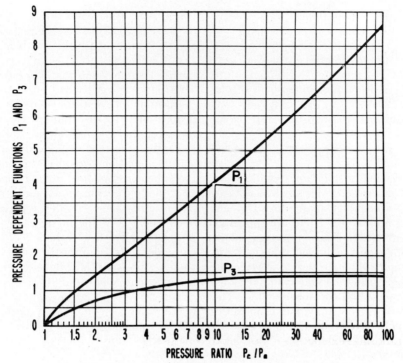

FIG. 79. Pressure function (P_1) for the total time of decompression and pressure function (P_3) for a "constant rate time" of decompression as derived from the pressure ratio (P_c/P_a).

Note that the time-constant, when factored out, is in units of time (seconds).

The pressure dependent factor (P_1) is obtained from the top curve in figure 79 by first computing the pressure ratio.

$$\frac{P_c}{P_a} = \frac{10.91 \text{ p.s.i.}}{2.72 \text{ p.s.i}} = 4.01$$

Note that this ratio is without units so that any units of pressure can be used such as mm. of Hg. Also, P_1 is a ratio (t_E/t_c) and consequently is a unitless factor.

From Figure 79, $P_1 = 2.55$. The total time of decompression $t_E = t_c \times P_1 = 4.306$ sec. $\times 2.55 = 10.98$ seconds.

In the case of an aircraft with a small cabin volume, such as a jet fighter, and assuming the following conditions:

Flight altitude equals 50,000 feet (1.69 p.s.i.).

Cabin altitude equals 25,000 feet (5.45 p.s.i.).

Effective cabin volume equals 60 cubic feet.

Effective orifice (canopy) equals 18 square feet.

The time-constant, t_c equals 0.003 seconds.

The pressure ratio equals 3.22.

From figure 79, $P_1 = 2.20$. The total time of decompression = $0.003 \times 2.2 = 0.0066$ second.

Under certain conditions such as flights in the upper limits of the atmosphere and space flights, the total time of decompression tends to become extremely long because, under these conditions, the pressure ratio becomes very large and consequently P_1 also tends to become large. The drop in cabin pressure, however, may very quickly become physiologically significant even though the last few molecules of air in the cabin may take a long time to find their way out through the opening. For this reason, the lower curve in figure 79 can be used to obtain a pressure factor, P_3, with which a decompression time can be computed if it is assumed that the initial rate of decompression remains constant throughout the course of the decompression.

For example, a rapid decompression occurs in a manned vehicle flying at 200,000 feet.

Cabin pressure equals 200 mm. of Hg.

Ambient pressure equals 0.2 mm. of Hg.

Pressure ratio equals 1000.

Cabin volume equals 100 cubic feet.

Effective orifice equals 1 square foot.

Time-constant, t_c equals 0.091 second.

Calculated P_1, for total time equals 13.9.

Total time of decompression equals 0.091×13.9 equals 12.65 second.

From figure 79, for constant rate time, $P_3 = 1.4$.

Constant rate time $= 0.091 \times 1.4 = 0.127$ second.

The time constants for any combination of cabin volumes and orifice areas have been plotted logarithmically in figure 80 in accordance with equation 7 and are shown as parallel diagonals. In addition an equivalent time constant for the human lungs is also shown in figure 80 in order to relate and compare the decompression characteristics of a cabin to that of the human lung. The characteristics of the human lung and airways are such that when decompressed at the end of a normal exhalation with a rigid

thorax, the time constant is approximately 0.55 second (15). This is equivalent to the time constant of a cabin with a volume of about 200 cubic meters and an effective orifice of 1 square meter or 655 cubic feet per square foot as mentioned previously.

Inasmuch as the time constant is directly proportional to the volume (equation 7), a lung volume that is different from that at the end of a normal exhalation, such as after a full inhalation, would accordingly change the time constant for the lungs. In figure 80, as a guide for approximating either safe or potentially dangerous decompressions with open airways, if the intercept of cabin volume and orifice lies to the left of the human equivalent no significantly dangerous transthoracic pressures will develop regardless of the pressure change in the cabin. On the other hand, for intercepts falling to the right of the human equivalent, decompressions will always be associated with a transient increase in transthoracic pressure, which wil

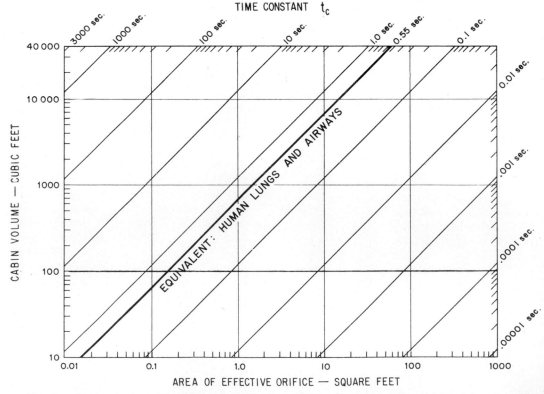

Fig. 80. Chart relating cabin volume and effective orifice to the time constant of decompression. The time constant for human lungs as shown corresponds to that of a cabin of 655 cubic feet with an effective opening of 1 square foot. (Modified from Luft and Bancroft (15).)

be increasingly severe with decreasing time constants for the cabin. Animal experiments have indicated that decompressions with cabin time constants of less than 0.01 second invariably result in intrapulmonic trauma, the severity of which is also dependent on the pressure change in the cabin, (the pressure differential).

The fact that the pressure ratio rather than the pressure differential is one of the main factors that influences the time of decompression is demonstrated in figure 81, which shows the pressure tracings obtained during two series of rapid decompressions with a system similar to that described in figure 72. The top series of decompressions was carried out with the same pressure differential of 200 mm. of Hg, but with different initial cabin pressure, thus, different pressure ratios. Note the longer duration of decompression with lower initial cabin pressures or larger pressure ratios, but essentially the same amplitude for the transient bottle pressures. In the bottom series of decompressions in figure 81, the pressure ratio remains

constant, but the pressure differentials are different. Note the identical decompression times, but decreasing amplitude for the transient bottle pressures with smaller pressure differentials.

THE PRESSURE SUIT

As discussed in the foregoing sections on pressure cabins and rapid decompression, the overwhelming onset of hypoxia within a matter of seconds, following an accidental loss of cabin pressure at altitudes above 40,000 feet, is unavoidable unless adequate pressurized oxygen equipment is available and used immediately. Between 40,000 and 45,000 feet the positive pressures delivered to the lungs from the standard pressure-breathing oxygen mask and regulator can be tolerated reasonably well for a limited period of time by otherwise unprotected individuals. At 45,000 feet, however, a positive mask pressure of 30 mm. of Hg is necessary to provide an alveolar oxygen tension equivalent to 40,000 feet when breathing pure oxygen. Mask pressures less than this will

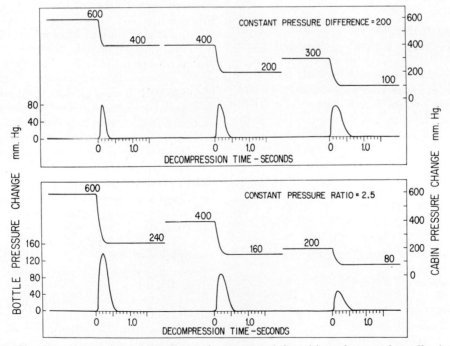

FIG. 81. Simultaneous tracings of the changes in pressure of the cabin and across the walls of an open bottle during two series of rapid decompressions, similar to the arrangement shown in figure 72. Top series, constant pressure differential, but different pressure ratios. Bottom series, constant pressure ratio, but different pressure differentials. Note decompression times and amplitudes of transient bottle pressures.

result in a certain amount of hypoxia. The use of this relatively simple pressure-breathing equipment becomes increasingly limited at altitudes above 45,000 feet because of both the excessive mask leakage with the higher breathing pressures that are required and the profound effect of such high intrapulmonic pressures on the unsupported thorax and cardiovascular system.

For this reason, during emergenices at altitudes above 45,000 feet, and particularly above 50,000 feet, adequate protection can only be accomplished by the use of fully pressurized helmets and proper garments for effective counterpressure over the surface of the body.

Table 40 lists the suit and helmet pressures that are necessary for maintaining the body at a pressure environment equivalent to 40,000 feet (141 mm. of Hg) when exposed to extremely high altitudes. Using pure oxygen for pressurization, life can be sustained even in the vacuum of outer space with a minimum pressure of 141 mm. of Hg without undue hypoxia.

The Full Pressure Suit

Theoretically, the full pressure suit, creating essentially a "micropressurized cabin" around the flyer is the most ideal type of protective garment for high altitude emergencies and approaches most nearly the basic requirements for a true "space suit." Only recently, however, have most of the major technical difficulties in the design and development of such a garment been overcome. Of prime importance has been the problem

TABLE 40
Minimum Helmet and Suit Pressures Required during Exposure at Extreme Altitudes

Flight Altitude	Ambient Barometric Pressure	Necessary Suit and Helmet Pressure
feet	*mm. of Hg*	*mm. of Hg*
40,000	141	0
45,000	111	30
50,000	87	54
60,000	54	87
80,000	21	120
100,000	8	133
150,000	1	140
Outer Space	0	141

of providing adequate internal ventilation to dissipate excessive perspiration and body heat within the gas-tight suit, even when worn uninflated.

In addition to this basic need for maintaining a reasonably comfortable thermal environment within the full pressure suit, the technical difficulty in preventing the suit, when inflated, from becoming unduly rigid and virtually immobilizing the wearer, has also been one of the primary drawbacks in the development of this type of suit as an operational item. A considerable amount of technical ingenuity has been required to design a full pressure suit and helmet that will remain flexible when pressurized to the necessary 2 to 5 p.s.i. (100 to 250 mm. of Hg), depending on the altitude, and which will permit a reasonable amount of mobility and dexterity on the part of the flyer for either continuing the mission or otherwise coping with an emergency situation.

The Partial Pressure Suit

Because of these technical problems associated with the development of the ideal full pressure suit, it has been necessary in the meantime to use an alternative, although less desirable approach toward providing reasonable protection for the flyer in the event of cabin decompression at altitudes above 50,000 feet. This has resulted in the development of the standard *partial pressure suit* and helmet which permits the flyer to tolerate, even for an extended period of time, the high breathing pressures that are necessary at extreme altitudes.

By substituting a helmet with an adequate neck seal for the simple oxygen mask, the entire head can be evenly pressurized without congestion or discomfort in the eyes and ears and without leakage. Over distention of the lungs and thorax by the necessarily high breathing pressures in the helmet is also prevented by a pneumatic bladder system covering the chest and abdomen under the close fitting fabric of the suit. Thus, with the thorax and trunk firmly supported, breathing pressures of about 3 p.s.i. (155 mm. of Hg) can be comfortably tolerated, which otherwise would result in an immediate and fatal over distention and rupture of the lungs. Experimental studies by Henry (18) for establishing the limits for pulmonary pressurization have shown that the lungs within the unprotected thorax will rupture at 70 to 80 mm. of Hg, while firm counter-pressure applied to the chest permits intra-pulmonic pressures of over 170 mm. of Hg without harm. High breathing pressures such as this with pure oxygen are more than adequate for maintaining the intrapulmonic pressure at an equivalent altitude of 40,000 feet, even when exposed to altitudes above 100,000 feet.

HIGH BREATHING PRESSURES AND LOSS OF BLOOD VOLUME. Not only is it necessary to protect the chest and trunk when breathing against high helmet pressures but the remaining parts of the body including the arms, legs and hands must also be enclosed within gloves and the close fitting fabric of the suit for the most effective use of this type of protective garment. With the head, chest and trunk adequately protected from congestion and over distention, but with the rest of the body unprotected, a breathing pressure of 50 mm. of Hg can be tolerated for only a few minutes by the average individual before generalized symptoms of faintness, cold sweat and possibly nausea occur. A breathing pressure such as this is only sufficient to reduce a 50,000 foot altitude to the equivalent of 40,000 feet. With higher breathing pressures under these conditions, for example, 100 mm. of Hg at 65,000 feet, collapse can occur within 2 minutes.

It has been shown by Henry (18) as well as other investigators that this limited tolerance to high pressure breathing when only the chest and trunk are protected, is caused by the shunting of a considerable quantity of blood into the distended veins and capillary beds of the legs and arms sufficient to reduce the effective blood volume almost immediately by as much as 500 ml. If the pressure breathing is continued, an additional quantity of blood can be gradually lost from the effective circulation by the accumulation of fluid within the tissue spaces in the unprotected parts of the body. The pooled blood in the extremities together with this fluid loss to the tissues can amount to as much as 1 liter, which, for a great many persons, is more than sufficient to induce a vaso-vagal reaction and syncope. Often a blood donation of 500 ml. can cause a fainting episode.

For these reasons, the partial pressure suit is designed to cover the arms and legs as well as the trunk even though some mobility of the extremities is sacrificed by doing so In addition to the chest bladders, the suit is constructed with pneumatic tubes or *capstans* which run down the sides and along the legs and arms in such a manner that when the helmet and lungs are pressurized, these capstan tubes are also inflated and tend to draw the suit material tightly over the surface of the body. The higher the helmet pressure, the tighter becomes the suit so that the pressure within the body is more or less perfectly counterbalanced by the mechanical pressure of the suit.

In the event of decompression when flying above 43,000 feet, the partial pressure suit is automatically activated by an ananeroid controlled regulator which is so designed that an altitude equivalent to at least 40,000 feet is maintained in the pressurized suit. Because of this, the partial pressure suit is not adequate for preventing the possible onset of the "bends" if descent to a lower altitude is not commenced soon after decompression. Only with a full pressure suit is it possible to provide sufficient pressure to maintain a suit environment that is equivalent to an altitude below 30,000 feet and below the critical threshold for decompression sickness.

REFERENCES

(1) ARMSTRONG, H. G.: The medical problems of sealed high-altitude aircraft compartments. J. Aviation Med., 7: 2–8, 1936.

(2) CLAMANN, H. G.: Continuous recording of oxygen, carbon dioxide and other gases in sealed cabins. J. Aviation Med., 23: 330–333, 1952.

(3) LOVELACE, W. R., AND GAGGE, A. P.: Aero medical aspects of cabin pressurization for military and commercial aircraft. J. Aeronautical Sc., 13: 143–150, 1946.

(4) LUFT, U. C.: Physiological aspects of pressure cabins and rapid decompression. In BOOTHBY, W. M. (Editor): Handbook of Respiratory Physiology. Randolph Air Force Base, Texas, School of Aviation Medicine, USAF, 1954, Chapter 8.

(5) KONECCI, E. B., AND SHANNON, R. H.: Accidental and Intentional Decompressions in USAF Aircraft. M-30-56, Aero Medical Safety Division, Directorate of Flight Safety Research, Office of the Inspector General, Norton, AFB, Calif., 1956.

(6) SIMONS, D. G., AND ARCHIBALD, E. R.: Selec-

tion of a sealed cabin atmosphere. J. Aviation Med., 29: 350–357, 1958.

(7) MAYO, A. M.: Basic environmental problems
relating to man and the aeropause. In
WHITE, C. S., AND BENSON, O. O., JR.
(Editors): Physics and Medicine of the
Upper Atmosphere. Albuquerque, Univer-
sity of New Mexico Press, 1952, Chapter I.

(8) ARMSTRONG, J. A., FRYER, D. I., STEWART,
W. K., AND WHITTINGHAM, H. E.: Interpretation of injuries in the Comet aircraft
disasters. Lancet, 268: 1135–1144, 1955.

(9) SWEENEY, H. M. Explosive decompression.
Air Surgeon's Bull. 1: 1–4, 1944.

(10) EDELMANN, A., WHITEHORN, W. V., LEIN,
A., AND HITCHCOCK, F. A.: Pathological
lesions produced by explosive decompression. J. Aviation Med., 17: 596–601, 1946.

(11) COLE, C. R., CHAMBERLAIN, D. M., BURCH,
B. H., KEMPH, J. P., AND HITCHCOCK, F.
A.: Pathological effects of explosive decompression to 30 mm. Hg. J. Appl. Physiol., 6: 96–104, 1953.

(12) GELFAN, S., AND WERNER, A. Y.: Cardiovascular responses following explosive decompression of Macaque monkeys to extreme
altitudes. J. Appl. Physiol., 4: 280–310,
1951.

(13) VIOLETTE, F.: Les effets physiologiques de
decompression explosive et leur mecan-
isme. Med. Aeronaut., 9: 223, 1954.

(14) VAIL, E. G.: Forces produced in the thorax
by explosive decompression. J. Aviation
Med., 23: 577–583, 1952.

(15) LUFT, U. C., AND BANCROFT, R. W., Transthoracic pressures in man during rapid
decompression. J. Aviation Med., 27: 208–
220, 1956.

(16) HABER, F., AND CLAMANN, H. G.: A General
Theory of Rapid Decompressions. Project
Number 21-1201-0008, Report No. 3. Ran-
dolph Air Force Base, Texas, School of
Aviation Medicine, USAF, 1953.

(17) LUFT, U. C., BANCROFT, R. W., AND Carter,
E. T.: Rapid Decompression with Pressure-
Demand Oxygen Equipment. Project Num-

ber 21-1201-0008, Report No. 2. Randolph
Air Force Base, Texas, School of Aviation
Medicine, USAF, 1953.

(18) HENRY, J. P. Problems of escape during
flight above 50,000 feet. In WHITE, C. S.,
AND BENSON, O. O., JR., (Editors): Phys-
ics and Medicine of the Upper Atmosphere.
Albuquerque, University of New Mexico
Press, 1952.

(19) POLAK, B., AND ADAMS, H.: Traumatic air
embolism in submarine escape training.
U. S. Nav. M. Bull., 30: 165–177, 1932.

(20) BENZINGER, T.: Explosive decompression.
In Chapter IV-M, German Aviation Medicine, World War II, Vol. I. Washington,
D. C., U. S. Government Printing Office,
1950.

(21) WHITEHORN, W. V., LEIN, A., AND EDEL-
MANN, A.: The general tolerance and cardiovascular responses of animals to explosive decompression. Am. J. Physiol., 147:
289–298, 1946.

(22) ARMSTRONG, H. G.: The Effects of Decreased
Barometric Pressures on Living Organisms.
Engineering Memorandum Report, Wright
Field, Ohio, March 25, 1938.

(23) EDELMANN, A., AND HITCHCOCK, F. A.: Observation on dogs exposed to an ambient
pressure of 30 mm. Hg. J. Appl. Physiol.,
4: 807–812, 1952.

(24) WARD, J. E.: The true nature of the boiling
of body fluids in space. J. Aviation Med.,
27: 429–439, 1956.

(25) LUFT, U. C., CLAMANN, H. G., AND ADLER,
H. F.: Alveolar gases in rapid decompressions to high altitudes. J. Appl. Physiol.,
2: 37–48, 1949.

(26) LUFT, U. C., CLAMANN, H. G., AND OPITZ,
E.: The latency of hypoxia on exposure to
altitude above 50,000 feet. J. Aviation
Med., 22: 117–122, 136 (1951).

(27) HITCHCOCK, F. A., WHITEHORN, W. V., AND
EDELMANN, A.: Tolerance of normal men
to explosive decompression. J. Appl. Physiol., 1: 418–429, 1948.

14

AIR SICKNESS

Harry G. Armstrong, M.D.

Motion sickness is probably as old as the human race and it has been referred to in medical literature since the time of Hippocrates and Galen. Although all forms of motion sickness are basically the same it has been the custom in recent years to break it down into types, depending on the cause, and we speak of sea sickness, car sickness, train sickness, swing sickness, air sickness, etc.

In view of the great amount of suffering and disability from sea sickness among sailors and passengers traveling by water during the past centuries it is interesting to find that very little serious attention was given to this malady until 1931. In that year Sjöberg (1) published the results of his classic studies on motion sickness which constitute the outstanding work available on the basic factors involved in that condition.

In aviation, air sickness was largely ignored until Armstrong (2) carried out a series of studies, prepared the first clinical description of the disease and published his findings in 1939. Shortly after this it was realized that air sickness was having an adverse effect on the World War II effort and a number of additional investigations were initiated. From these studies it was learned that 10 to 11 per cent of all flying students became air sick during their first 10 flights (3, 4) and that 1 to 2 per cent of them were eliminated from flying training for that reason. Other aircrew members in training had even greater difficulty and the air sickness

rate among them ran as high as 50 per cent in some cases. It was also found that fully trained combat crews, other than pilots, sometimes became air sick which affected their combat efficiency. An even more serious situation was found to exist among air-borne troops. Under very unfavorable conditions as high as 70 per cent of these individuals became air sick and upon landing were more or less temporarily disabled at a time when their services were most urgently needed.

Attempts to solve the air sickness problem, during and subsequent to World War II, were directed primarily to discovering a drug to be used as a prophylactic measure or as a treatment and secondarily to clarifying the physical, physiologic or psychologic mechanisms through which the disease was made manifest. The net result of the early studies of drugs was that hyoseine (Scopolamine) in 0.65 mg. doses was the most effective compound available. This remedy left much to be desired, however, inasmuch as it was not completely effective and in some cases had undesirable side effects. No further progress was made until 1949 when Gay and Carliner (5) reported spectacular results with Dramamine in the prevention and treatment of sea sickness. This resulted in a new series of investigations of this and other antihistaminic drugs as to their effectiveness in air sickness. Studies on Dramamine were disappointing in the sense that Strickland et al. (6) found that hyoseine was 10 to 12 per cent more effective than Dramamine in preventing experi-

219

mentally produced air sickness in flight and that Dramamine was no more effective than a placebo in preventing swing sickness. In addition, Strickland's group found that Dramamine, in the 100 mg. doses utilized, produced undesirable side effects in 8.7 per cent of all subjects tested.

At about this same time Chinn *et al.* began their monumental work on antihistaminic and related drugs as well as others, especially among the vitamin group, that had been reported as being effective in air sickness. This study group was soon expanded to include all three of the military services and was known as the Army, Navy, Air Force motion sickness team.

After several years of effort well over 50 compounds had been evaluated and 14 were finally selected as showing the most promise. These 14 were then further evaluated during a carefully controlled test on 7000 subjects and the results published in 1956 (7). Three of the 14 compounds were found to be highly effective and superior to the other drugs tested. These drugs were meclizine (Bonamine), cyclizine (Marezine) and promethazine (Phenergan). Among these three the effectiveness was essentially identical and the only side effect noted was sedation with promethazine.

The studies undertaken, during and since World War II, to clarify the basic mechanism by which motion sickness is produced were without success and this remains one of nature's well guarded secrets. These efforts were not completely fruitless, however, for a number of facts about motion sickness were discovered which had previously been unknown. Most of these had to do with the physical factors which increased or decreased the incidence of motion sickness and the role that psychologic factors play in producing this condition. Before the beginning of these wartime studies three factors of major importance had already been established. The idea that motion sickesss is the result of vestibular stimulation originated well over 100 years ago when it was noted that deaf-mutes or other individuals whose labyrinths had been destroyed by disease were completely immune to this malady. Sjöberg (1) provided the final proof by destroying the labyrinths of motion susceptible dogs and showing that they were then no longer susceptible. Sjöberg also found that animals encased in plaster casts, to reduce the kinesthetic impulses from motion to a minimum, resulted in a decreased incidence of motion sickness. The third major factor was Armstrong's (2) observation that visual disorientation increased the susceptibility to air sickness and conversely that visual orientation in space tended to decrease this susceptibility.

Up until World War II there was a number of authors who had expressed the view that motion sickness was produced principally or entirely by psychogenic stimulae. Further investigations failed to find evidence to support this idea and most authorities now agree with the findings of Wendt (8) that although psychic factors are operative to some degree, the physical and physiologic factors outweigh them in importance. For example, the idea that fear produced or increased the incidence of air sickness was shown to be erroneous by the observation that there was no increase in air sickness among aircrews when they entered combat. Similarly other personality traits and disagreeable environmental conditions which had previously been credited with having a marked psychic influence were shown to be of no great significance and this whole matter was finally placed in its proper perspective.

A number of advances were also made regarding the physical and physiologic factors which influenced motion sickness. Posture was found to play an important role as evidenced by the fact that in a controlled experiment the incidence of swing sickness was 5 per cent with the subjects in the supine position whereas in the seated position the rate was 27.5 per cent (9). It was also determined that keeping the head fixed by means of a headrest and a restraining device also markedly reduced the incidence of both swing (10) and air sickness. In actual flight tests Johnson and Magne (11) found this procedure to be from 60 to 83 per cent effective in susceptable Canadian paratroop trainees. Another study revealed that two-thirds of the sea sickness of troops in landing barges could be prevented by having the men stand erect instead of assuming a crouching position.

That age and sex have an influence is

indicated by airline medical reports that women are more susceptible to air sickness than adult males, and the findings of Chinn (7) that among adult males the sea sickness rate varies inversely with age as follows: at age 30 and above vomiting occurred in 9.7 per cent; at ages 25 to 29 in 16.1 per cent; at ages 20 to 24 in 22.3 per cent; and at ages 17 to 19 in 25.1 per cent of the subjects.

Further evidence of the influence of vision on motion sickness was provided by a number of experiments including the use of a "witch house." This is an amusement park device in which the subject sits in a chair in the middle of a room. While the subject, the chair and the floor remain stationary the remainder of the room revolves on its horizontal axis producing the optical illusion that it is the subject that is rotating. This produced violent illness with nausea, vomiting and the other cardinal symptoms of motion sickness. In other words, it demonstrated the fact that motion sickness can be produced in the absence of motion. Other evidence that vision has an important influence on air sickness was supplied by Green's (12) observations of bomber crew trainees. He reported that 80 per cent of the attacks of air sickness in these crews of 10 men occurred in the 3 men who occupied the navigator's compartment. These men could not see out of the aircraft and, thus, were unable to orient themselves in space by visual means. Green further noted that to suppress an impending air sickness attack these men would usually go to the pilot's compartment or to the nose of the airplane where they could see the horizon or objects on the ground and, thus, orient themselves visually. Green's observations have been confirmed by Manning and Stewart's (9) swing tests of subjects who could see and those who could not. The former had a sickness rate of only 27.5 per cent as compared to 64 per cent in the latter.

All of these observations on visual influences tended to confirm Armstrong's (2) earlier observations that trained pilots practically never get air sick while flying an airplane but may become ill when riding as a passenger as a result of the fact that in the former instance the pilot must constantly keep himself oriented visually whereas in the latter situation he usually does not. Thus, there is not only evidence that a lack of vision and visual orientation increases susceptibility to motion sickness but also that constant and exact visual orientation in space is a powerful suppressor of motion sickness.

Up to this point we have been discussing air sickness and motion sickness in general as a military problem but this is not to be construed to mean that a similar problem does not exist in civil aviation. The difficulty here is that there are practically no published studies of this question in the literature and the extent of the problem that exists is largely a matter of speculation. If we assume that the air sickness rate among civil flying trainees of all types is the same as military student pilots we can then arrive at a rough approximation of the magnitude of the problem and the probable consequences. On this basis we could expect that among the 80,000 civilian trainees in 1955, some 10 per cent or 8000 of them became air sick one or more times during their first 10 flights and that 1 to 2 per cent or 800 to 1600 of them either failed or withdrew from training for this reason.

A civil problem of even greater magnitude, of course, is the incidence of air sickness among the more than 50 million aircraft passengers carried annually in this country alone. Here also there is a lack of carefully controlled experimental data and in this instance any attempts to draw conclusions from military experiences with air-borne troops would no doubt be quite misleading because of the difference in the types of flying involved in the two situations. Nonetheless, motion sickness has been, and probably will remain, a formidable problem to a number of air passengers just as it has been and will continue to be a problem to the great hordes who travel in ships, trains or cars or ride in elevators and amusement devices.

With the above information as a background we can now describe air sickness as a clinical entity.

Definition

Air sickness may be defined as a clinical condition, produced primarily by aircraft accelerations in flight, which is manifested by pallor, sweating, vertigo, nausea, vomiting and prostration.

ETIOLOGY

That air sickness is produced by aircraft accelerations is indicated by two well established facts. The first is that the incidence of air sickness and its severity is closely related to the duration and severity of the accelerations experienced. The second is that persons without functioning labyrinths never become air sick. In current operations the highest incidence of air sickness is produced by angular or rotary accelerations of the type produced by acrobatics. Other accelerations involved are intermittent irregular accelerations in a vertical direction incident to flying through turbulent air, a periodic lateral acceleration from sitting in the nose or tail section of a plane that is "hunting" or yawning and a corkscrew type of acceleration from flying a pattern of that configuration. Making a turn while flying fairly close to the ground is a relatively frequent cause of air sickness and it is not unusual for an individual to be free of symptoms during a long journey by air until the approach for a landing is made. There is experimental evidence that accelerations of different frequencies, wave patterns and magnitude influence the incidence of motion sickness but this finding is of limited significance in flying because of the extreme irregularity of the motion in aircraft.

In considering the mechanism through which motion produces air sickness there is no question that the vestibular apparatus is of primary importance (1) inasmuch as there is no illness if this organ is not functioning. The question as to which sense organ in the nonauditory labyrinth is involved is a matter of dispute among those who maintain it is the christa, those who favor the otolith organs and a group that feel both are necessary. The general consensus of opinion is that the utricular maculae are the receptors chiefly stimulated by linear accelerations, that the sense organs of the canals respond to angular accelerations and that it is the macula which is primarily involved. The nervous pathway from the labyrinth to the central nervous system has not been fully traced nor has the interplay of nerve impulses from the labyrinth and the other sensory organs, which produce air sickness, been satisfactorily explained even on a theoretic basis.

In addition to the vestibular apparatus the ocular system and the muscle and joint kinesthetic sense have an influence on the incidence and severity of air sickness. Continuous exact visual orientation in space is a powerful suppressant of air sickness while lack of such orientation tends to induce or aggravate motion sickness. As mentioned previously visual illusions of rotation in the absence of motion can produce the motion sickness syndrome. In flight the three situations where visual impressions are most apt to cause difficulty are when the individual cannot see outside the airplane, when the individual allows the nearby landscape or clouds to "swim" past his vision instead of fixing his eyes on a point of reference and when the individual suffers sensory confusion. This latter usually occurs when an aircraft changes its attitude without the person concerned sensing it visually or otherwise. If an individual looks out the window and finds, for example, that he is not in straight and level flight as he had assumed but perhaps tilted to the left in a steep turn he may immediately develop motion sickness.

The kinesthetic sense, the viscera and the sense of touch have all been investigated as to their role in motion sickness but only the first of these seems to be involved (1) and it only to a limited degree. The effect of posture on the incidence of air sickness is not believed to be related to any of these kinesthetic factors but to result from variations in the position of the head and especially the amount of head movement.

It is probable that no one with a normal vestibular apparatus is completely immune to air sickness. However, there are marked differences in the degree of susceptibility among individuals. Individuals who are susceptible to one type of motion sickness are generally susceptible to all other types of motion sickness. Most individuals develop an increased tolerance to motion with experience but not all. Thus, among military flying trainees (4), where about 10 per cent of them suffered from air sickness during the first 10 flights, only 1 or 2 per cent had difficulty subsequently. Most of the latter had to be eliminated from flying training because of their inability to adapt and illustrate the fact that certain individuals are unable to develop a tolerance to motion.

Several surveys of air sick personnel have been made to determine the individual's opinion as to the factors which produced his illness, and only 10 to 38 per cent of them (8) gave rough air as the cause. Accordingly, in 64 to 90 per cent of the cases other factors were cited which included such things as hypoxia, lack of fresh air, a warm environment, indigestion, general indisposition, being hungry, alcoholic or food indiscretions, food odors, grief, fear and a host of others. This no doubt explains why there has previously been so much confusion concerning the etiology of motion sickness not only among patients but also among the medical profession who apparently accepted the patients' statements at their face value. This in turn leads to another interesting facet concerning motion sickness which should be mentioned. That is that motion sick patients are inclined to be the subject of ridicule rather than sympathy probably on the basis of it being a disease which is more embarrassing than serious and that it is considered a sign of weakness or an inability to "take it." In addition, vomiting is not socially acceptable and for these reasons the patient is usually ashamed to admit he is getting sick, generally makes every effort to conceal it and finally makes every possible excuse to explain it on socially acceptable grounds.

In view of the above the practitioner must not permit himself to be misled by a patient's statements. He should accept the fact that motion sickness is caused by motion and that other factors have very little influence on the onset or course of the disease. If this attitude is adopted the physician can better prepare a susceptible individual for a journey by air or treat an actual attack of the disease.

SYMPTOMATOLOGY

SUBJECTIVE SYMPTOMS. If the onset of an attack of air sickness is gradual the first symptom is usually a slight nausea and a generalized feeling of ill-being. If the disease progresses, this is followed by increased nausea and the patient usually begins to feel hot and notices that he is beginning to perspire. At the next stage the patient feels acutely ill, loses his volition and may develop vertigo and mental depression. The final stage is vomiting and there may be prostration. Vomiting may occur only once and bring relief but this latter is usually only temporary and vomiting will then recur one or more times. Generally the illness persists, in varying degree, during the remainder of the flight and complete recovery does not take place until several minutes or hours after landing.

In many cases the disease does not develop gradually but will have an explosive onset with vomiting developing in a matter of seconds or minutes without any preliminary warning. This type of attack generally occurs in a situation where visual disorientation is a contributing factor. Vomiting is generally, but not necessarily, an index of the severity of a patient's subjective symptoms. Certain individuals will feel deathly ill without vomiting although they usually have severe nausea and the other manifestations of the disease. It should also be kept in mind that most of the mild or moderate cases of air sickness do not vomit and that this latter is not necessary to establish a diagnosis of the illness.

OBJECTIVE SYMPTOMS. The objective symptoms of air sickness consist initially of facial pallor and sweating especially about the face. Retching or vomiting may be observed in the later stages and at this time the patient will appear listless and acutely ill. The blood pressure and pulse may rise or fall with a majority of individuals showing a moderate fall before vomiting and a moderate rise subsequent to vomiting. The oral temperature tends to fall at all stages of the disease (13). The diagnosis of air sickness is simple if the history is known but might temporarily be confused with other diseases manifested by nausea and vomiting such as food poisoning.

There are no complications in the normal healthy person, but patients suffering from any condition or disease that would be aggravated by vomiting should not be exposed to the possibility of developing air sickness. Patients who have their jaws wired together to splint a fracture should not fly unless the wires are replaced by rubber bands to remove the danger of vomitus being aspirated into the lungs.

TREATMENT

PROPHYLAXIS. Much can be accomplished to prevent air sickness through the control of the airplane. Banks and turns should be as gentle and of as small a degree as is practical. The aircraft should not be allowed to yaw or to porpoise, turbulent air should be avoided if possible and efforts should be made to fly around or over storms.

Pilot trainee applicants who give a history of repeated attacks of motion sickness should be disqualified on the initial physical examination and those who continue to get air sick after the first 10 training flights should also be eliminated. Trainees should not normally be eliminated for air sickness prior to the 10th flight inasmuch as about 80 to 90 per cent of them become adapted during this period and have no further difficulty. Thus, flying experience is an effective prophylactic measure which applies to passengers as well as trainees. Among passengers, air-borne troops and patients an attack of air sickness can usually be prevented by having the individual assume the supine position or by suppressing head motion by means of a headrest and proper instructions to keep the head in a fixed position. Crew members and passengers both should be able to see out of the airplane and instructed not to allow the landscape or nearby clouds to "swim" past their vision but to fix their eyes on definite objects and to keep visually orientated in space at all times. The use of encouragement and suggestion may be helpful as well as indoctrination and training to develop habituation and, if this is successful during the initial flights, it will avoid adverse conditioning and expectation of future sickness on subsequent exposures.

The best prophylactic measure of course is antimotion sickness remedies taken about 1 hour before flight time. As previously stated the most effective of these now available are meclizene (Bonamine) in 50 mg. doses, cyclizine (Marezine) in 50 mg. doses or Promethazine (Phenergan) in 25 mg. doses. Meclizine is a long acting drug and one dose is adequate for a full day's journey, whereas the other two should be given three times a day for prolonged trips. Promethazine has a mild sedative effect and, if this is considered undesirable, one of the two other drugs mentioned should be prescribed.

ACTIVE TREATMENT. Drug treatment of active air sickness may be difficult or impossible owing to the patient's inability to retain the medication in his stomach long enough for it to be effective. However, attempts at this should be made and if it fails the patient should be placed in the supine position or have his head immobilized against a headrest. The drugs of choice are those mentioned above under prophylaxis. Air sickness is self limited and will cure itself without treatment soon after a flight. However, it is a most disagreeable experience to the patient and every reasonable effort should be made to prevent an attack from occurring.

REFERENCES

(1) SJÖBERG, A. A.: Experimentelle Studien über den Auslosungmechanismus der Seekrankeit. Acta oto-laryng., 14: 1–136, 1931.

(2) ARMSTRONG, H. G.: Principles and Practice of Aviation Medicine, Ed. 1. Baltimore, The Williams & Wilkins Co., 1939.

(3) RUBIN, H. J.: Airsickness in a primary Air Force training detachment. J. Aviation Med., 13: 272–276, 1942.

(4) HEMINGWAY, A., AND GREEN, E. L.: Airsickness during early flying training. J. Aviation Med., 16: 409–416, 1945.

(5) GAY, L. N., AND CARLINER, P. E.: Prevention and treatment of motion sickness. I. Seasickness. Science, 109: 359, 1949.

(6) STRICKLAND, B. A., HAHN, G. G., AND ADLER, H.: Studies on airsickness. J. Aviation Med., 21: 90–97, 1950.

(7) CHINN, H. I., et al.: Evaluation of drugs for protection against motion sickness aboard transport ships; Report of study by Army Navy, Air Force motion sickness team. J. A. M. A., 160: 755–760, 1956.

(8) WENDT, G. R.: Of what importance are psychological factors in motion sickness? J. Aviation Med., 19: 24–33, 1948.

(9) MANNING, G. W., AND STEWART, W. G.: The Effect of position on the incidence of swing sickness. Association Commission on Aviation Medical Research, National Research Council, Canada, Report No. C2426, 1942.

(10) JOHNSON, W. H., STUBBS, R. A. KELK, C. F., AND FRANKS, W. R.: Stimulus required to produce motion sickness. I. Preliminary report dealing with importance of head movements. J. Aviation Med., 22: 365–374, 1951.

(11) JOHNSON, W. H., AND MAYNE, J. W.: Stimulus required to produce motion sickness. J. Aviation Med., 24: 400–411, 1953.

(12) GREEN, D. M.: Airsickness in bomber crews. J. Aviation Med., 14: 366–372, 1943.

(13) HEMINGWAY, A.: Cardiovascular changes in motion sickness. J. Aviation Med., 16: 417–421, 1945.

15

VERTIGO AND RELATED STATES

Harry G. Armstrong, M.D.

Vertigo, in its broadest sense, is defined not only as a sensation as if the external world were revolving about the subject or as if he himself were revolving in space but also as being a state of mental bewilderment or confusion (1). This chapter will deal with vertigo in flying, as defined above, and also with a number of related states based on a lack of or the ignoring of sensory impressions. These various states are extremely dangerous for they involve not only such things as the development of illusions and the loss of aerial equilibration and orientation but a loss of effective control of the aircraft as well. In order that these aerial difficulties may be better understood we shall first very briefly consider how man maintains his equilibrium and orients himself on the ground.

It is generally acknowledged that man on the ground maintains his equilibration and orients himself in relation to his environment by means of sensory impressions from his eyes, vestibular apparatus, deep sensibility (muscle, joint and tendon sense), viscera and skin. Terrestrial man is acted upon continuously, to a uniform degree and in a constant direction by gravity. He normally accelerates, decelerates and rotates slowly. He seldom revolves more than 90 degrees about any of the principal axes of his body and then only at a low rate. He is in continuous physical contact with the earth's surface (or structure fixed thereon)

and is always in such close contact with some point of reference that the slightest deviation of position may be visually detected.

In aircraft centrifugal force may modify the normal action of the pull of gravity and for all practical purposes may be said to increase its effect, decrease it, neutralize it or even reverse its direction. Motion is also altered not only in rate but also in extent and direction and accelerations and decelerations are markedly increased. Rotations may consist of an irregular series of rapidly alternating excursions through small degrees of arc, as in the rough air, or they may consist of very rapid wide excursions through 360 or more degrees about any one of the three principal axes of the body as may occur in acrobatics. Of paramount importance in aerial equilibration and orientation is the fact that here man does not have physical contact with the earth but only with the airplane which operates independent of both the force and direction of gravity as far as the occupant's sensory impressions are concerned. Even aerial vision is modified by the remoteness of fixed points of reference such that only relatively great deviations of position and distance can be recognized when flying at high altitude. The greater the distance between an aircraft and the ground the slower the former appears to move and the less accurate the pilot's spatial orientation. For example, a pilot at high altitude cannot fly a course exactly parallel to the earth's surface without the aid of his aircraft instruments. These numerous new and novel situations inherent in flying pose a fairly difficult problem to the student aviator initially but with experience he usually learns to deal with them without too much effort. However, there comes a time in the pilot's training or experience when he must fly without the aid of his normal vision, such as at night or in clouds, at which time he becomes especially susceptible to the development of false or misinterpreted sensory impressions.

How or why these various illusions develop will next be considered beginning with a description of the problem of blind flying, as it has been dealt with over the years, and this will be followed in turn by a discussion of other related phenomena.

BLIND OR INSTRUMENT FLYING

Blind flying may be defined as that flying accomplished in which visible reference to the earth for the purpose of recognition of position is impossible by reason of fog, clouds, dust, darkness or any other natural or artificial phenomenon. Instrument flying is that flying which is accomplished by means of reference to instruments in the airplane.

Serious efforts to study and solve the blind flying problem did not get underway until after World War I. However, during that war there were a number of studies carried out at the Air Service Medical Research Laboratory (2) concerning the function of the vestibular apparatus in an attempt to prove that highly sensitive labyrinthine reactions were an aid in learning to fly and to enable a pilot to keep oriented in space. In these studies five different groups of subjects were tested, namely; normals, deaf-mutes lacking vestibular perception, deaf-mutes possessing vestibular perception below normal, tabetics with impaired deep sensibility and whirling (ballet) dancers. These studies showed that:

1. Tactile and deep sensibility (muscle joint and tendon sense; splanchnic and visceral sense) each participate in the composite of general motion perception in flying but are not capable individually or as a group of correctly interpreting changes of position and, hence, of providing orientation in the air.

2. Normal persons suffer an illusion of reversal of motion during decelerations of vertical or rotary motion whereas deaf-mutes with below normal or absent vestibular perception usually do not.

3. Normal persons are more accurate than deaf-mutes in detecting tilts, banks and turns in flight when blindfolded.

4. Normal pilots, when coming out of a spin, suffer an illusion of reversal of motion and, as a consequence, frequently fall into a second spin with usually fatal results.

5. Professional ballet dancers with normal vestibular reactions when whirling suffer dizziness and nausea unless they jerk their heads around rapidly and keep their eyes fixed on a definite point of reference at all times except for the instant the head is turning.

These findings not only proved that the vestibular apparatus, in the absence of vision, is incapable of maintaining aerial equilibrium and orientation but also that in spins it produces an illusion of reversal of motion and loss of aircraft control. At about this same time Horn (3) provided additional evidence that a highly sensitive vestibular apparatus is not desirable when he reported that 10 per cent of all pilots he saw in France during World War I complained of having been nauseated, of having vomited or of having suffered from dizziness while flying.

As stated previously none of these studies at the Air Service Medical Laboratory were conducted in relation to blind flying but a few years later the results obtained were to prove invaluable in that connection as we shall now see.

Shortly after the end of World War I officers of the U. S. Army Air Corps began experimenting with various types of instruments to serve as a mechanical substitute for a terrestrial point of visual reference. The two types of instruments which seemed to show the most promise was the bank-and-turn indicator and the artificial horizon. Although, theoretically, either of these instruments should have been found successful experience showed that in actual practice the pilot using them soon became confused and disoriented. This occurred even when either the bank-and-turn indicator or the artificial horizon was used, not because the instruments did not function properly, but because pilots were convinced that their sensations of motion were correct and that the instruments were faulty.

In an attempt to discover the reasons for the discrepancies between the theory and practice of instrument flight several very interesting experiments were carried out principally by Ocker and Crane of the United States Army Air Corps. It was found, for example, that a blindfolded man who attempted to walk or guide a vehicle in a straight line invariably traveled in a curved path, either to the right or left, which finally took the form of a spiral which became smaller and smaller in radius. It was also noted that once the direction of turn was established that it was never reversed and that the greater the rate of turn the greater the tendency for this rate to increase further which explains the spiral nature of the path in each case.

Believing that the flight of birds might furnish a valuable clue to the problem of blind flying several varieties were subjected to many interesting experiments. To everyone's surprise it was discovered that birds, including homing pigeons, cannot "fly blind" and that when they encountered fog or clouds or were blindfolded and released from an airplane that they simply set their wings for a glide and landed at once.

By 1926, in spite of all the work that had been done by aeronautical engineers, the problem seemed no nearer solution than it had in the beginning and finally the aid of medical science was solicited. In that year Major David A. Myers, a flight surgeon of the Army Medical Corps, began a study of the physiologic factors involved in instrument flying and shortly thereafter demonstrated the fundamental principles which have made possible blind flying as we know it today. The results of Myers' (4) work was not published until 1936 and no clearer understanding of the physiologic principles involved in instrument flying can be obtained than by consulting his original article. The following is a general summary of his reasoning and deductions.

Equilibration in the air requires that each of the three principal senses concerned, *i.e.*, sight, muscle sense and vestibular sense, function correctly and that their sensory stimuli be interpreted correctly in consciousness. Although these three senses are normally coordinated each of them can be brought into separate action and send its message to the brain. In equilibration sight is a reliable sense, muscle sense is variable acting whereas the vestibular sense is sensitive and powerful acting but very unreliable.

If the body is rotated in any dimension of space certain definite and fixed messages will be sent to the brain by the vestibular sense acting in coordination with sight and muscle sense. Provided this body motion is not too violent or long continued the brain will receive reliable information from this trinity of senses and will maintain equilibrium and one will know accurately at all times what position the body occupies with relation to the earth's surface and what direction, if any, it is moving. If, during this rotation the body is stopped or retarded one will have a momentary sensation of giddiness but will immediately, by the use of sight, adjust the position of the body to a point of reference on the earth and maintain equilibrium.

Whenever the human body is rotated and there is no visual point of reference messages will be sent to the brain but each and every one of these messages will be false. This is exactly what happens in blind flying where all visual reference to the earth is absent and only muscle sense and vestibular sense remain. Consequently, in flying blind without visual reference to gravity the pilot will be unable to sense the position of his ship with relation to the earth's surface, unable to sense the speed and direction of motion and will eventually go into circular motion, experience vertigo and crash.

Merely restoring sight to the equilibrium sense, however, is not enough. There must be something within the pilot's range of vision to act as a point of reference and tell him what position his airplane is in with reference to the earth. Furthermore, while the hand on the bank and turn indicator will show the direction of rotation the false impressions will still exist and vertigo result unless the pilot is taught to ignore his sensations and believe the instruments.

This last observation of Myers was, and still remains, of fundamental importance for no matter how easily the student flyer learns to read his instruments and to interpret them, the ignoring or suppression of his sensations is always an extremely difficult task which requires long and repeated practice not only as a student but throughout the individual's whole flying career.

Thus far we have been speaking of the difficulties during blind flight and we shall now consider the added difficulties that may occur during a sudden and unexpected shift from visual to instrument flying. When a pilot has to suddenly transition from visual to instrument flight he may become disoriented and the aircraft go out of control before the transition is complete. The time interval involved is about 45 seconds and a great deal can happen during that interval. This is especially so inasmuch as a sudden transition is usually based on the fact that the pilot is in difficulty and may already have become disoriented. Man inherently prefers to see where he is going and pilots are no exception to the rule. There is, therefore, a tendency for them to fly contact until the last possible moment or to attempt to split their attention between visual and instrument rules. This is especially so during night flying, in hazy conditions and when flying through scud clouds just above or below an overcast. Other situations in which a sudden switch may have to be made is when shifting from wing formation to solo flight or when flying just above or below an overcast and solid clouds are unexpectedly encountered. Finally, a pilot flying contact at dawn or dusk toward the lighter half of the hemisphere may have no difficulty. However, if he makes a 180 degree turn toward the darker half of the hemisphere he may then find the horizon and the landscape totally obscured and must quickly revert to instruments.

From what has been said concerning these early studies of blind flying the reader has no doubt gained the impression that disorientation in the air invariably leads to a set pattern of events consisting of a spin, a recovery from the spin, the development of vertigo and a second spin leading to a crash. Actually there are at least eight other well defined patterns of events during banks and turns during blind flight which lead to disorientation, the causes and results of which are outlined in the paragraphs below.

FALSE SENSATIONS FROM BANKS AND TURNS IN BLIND FLIGHT

1. UNPERCEIVED MOTION. The vestibular apparatus and other functioning equilibratory senses are fairly insensitive to gradual changes of directions or to small amounts of acceleration or deceleration so that in blind flight there may be motions of the airplane which are not recognized. For example, blindfolded individuals can be tilted from 4 to 10.6 degrees downward and from 7 to 24.0 degrees upward (2) before they can detect any change.

With reference to the amount of rotation necessary to stimulate the vestibular apparatus, Ter Braak (5) found that in the rabbit an angular acceleration of 0.25 degree per second per second was sufficient to elicit deviation of the eyes. Tumarkin (6) from his experiments in the human, found the threshold of acceleration to be about 0.2 degree per second per second, Buys gives a value of 1 to 2 and Mach found that an acceleration of 2 to 3 degrees per second per second acting from 14 to 16 seconds gave a threshold stimulus. Mulder and Buys found that a uniform acceleration of 2 degrees per second per second gives the impression of uniform rotation. The threshold for vertical accelerations has been found to be between 4 and 12 cm. per second per second whereas for the horizontal it lies between 2 and 20 cm. per second per second.

Within the above limitations the aircraft can climb, dive, turn or roll without there being any sensation of change from straight and level flight and the pilot may become disoriented accordingly.

2. SENSATION OF CLIMBING WHILE TURNING. In a horizontal turn the banking of the airplane is not usually sensed but there is an awareness of the body being pressed more firmly into the seat as a result of the centrifugal force. As a consequence, the sensation is that of a zoom upward, it is interpreted as such and the natural reaction is to push forward on the stick.

3. SENSATION OF DIVING DURING RECOVERY FROM A TURN. During recovery from a turn the pressure of the body on the seat is decreased which results in a sensation similar to that when the airplane is nosed over from level flight into a dive. As a conse-

quence return to level flight creates the false sensation of diving, causing a tendency to pull back on the control column resulting in a steep climb and possible stall.

4. ESTIMATING THE DEGREE OF BANK. Because the amount and rate of bank of an airplane, in going into a turn, is below the threshold of the organs of equilibrium the degree of bank attained during blind flying is usually underestimated. This causes the the pilot to bank too steeply in going into a turn and to overcorrect in a return to level flight which results in a bank in the opposite direction.

5. UNPERCEIVED BANKS. Under ordinary circumstances, if one tilts the body sideways, this can be easily sensed inasmuch as the pull of gravity on the body makes us aware of this tilt. In an aircraft turn such a sensation of tilting does not exist because the body is acted upon not only by gravity but by centrifugal force as well and the resultant of these two forces acts in a line perpendicular, not to the earth, but to the transverse axis of the airplane which creates a sensation of sitting erect.

6. SENSATION OF OPPOSITE TILT IN A SKID. If an airplane skids during a turn the centrifugal force on the body no longer acts perpendicular to the transverse axis of the airplane and there is a sensation that the airplane is banked in the opposite direction from its true position.

7. ILLUSION OF TURNING. If, during instrument flight, the aircraft gradually turns away from its proper heading and this is eventually corrected by a sharp movement of the rudder this may be followed by an illusion of the aircraft being in a continuing turn.

8. SENSATION OF DIVING BEYOND THE VERTICAL. If in a very sharp turn or in a spin, the head is suddenly turned downward, as might occur from looking at an object on the floor of the cockpit, the vestibular apparatus of the inner ear is acted upon by two distinct rotary motions at the same time with the result that there is a sensation of falling forward. Thus, the airplane feels as though it had suddenly nosed downward beyond the vertical and the natural response of the pilot is to pull back on the control column which, in a spin, only aggravates the situation.

This type of motion, *i.e.*, when an active movement of the head is made in a plane at right angles to a plane of passive rotation, is known as a Coriolis (7) acceleration. This may take place, for example, during a spin if the pilot should mean-while move his head up or down. If the head is moved (turned) downward during a left hand spin the resultant sensation is of rotation to the left and downward and the falling reaction is to the right and downward. When present the Coriolis reaction usually produces marked vertigo and is especially dangerous in aviation for that reason.

9. SENSATION OF REVERSAL OF ROTATION. This has been discussed previously.

THE LEANS

There is still another type of labyrinthine reaction owing to accelerations in aviation during instrument flying which was first described by Armstrong (8) in 1939. Among airplane pilots this condition is commonly referred to as "the leans." If, while the pilot is not watching his blind flying instruments, the airplane, because of rough air, should suddenly roll several degrees to the left and then recover very slowly it is evident that the labyrinth will record the tilt of the body to the left but not its recovery to the vertical position. As a result the pilot has the distinct feeling that he and the airplane are tilted to the left.

Even looking at the blind flying instruments, which show the airplane to be back on an even keel, sometimes fails to destroy the illusion and the pilot still feels that he is flying along left wing down and that he is correspondingly leaning to the left instead of sitting straight up. In order to overcome this feeling, which is very disconcerting and uncomfortable, the pilot leans over in his seat to his right to what he feels to be the vertical. This of course actually causes him to lean to the right. This maneuver satisfies the pilot with reference to his own position in space and inasmuch as he realizes that the instruments are correct he flies the airplane properly according to their indications but still has the sensation that the airplane is flying left wing down (fig. 82).

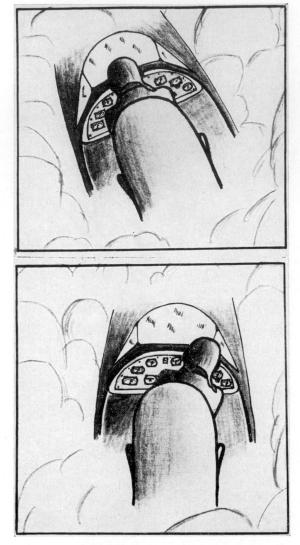

Fig. 82. The leans. The upper sketch shows the position the pilot "feels" he and the airplane are in. The lower sketch shows the actual position of the airplane and the position which the pilot assumes in his seat.

The same type of reaction may sometimes occur during pitching of the airplane. When this happens the pilot gets the impression that the airplane is either climbing or descending although the instruments show the airplane to be in level flight.

A second method by which either of the above described phenomena could occur is the reverse of that already explained. In such a case the airplane would roll or pitch very slowly through several degrees of rotation and then return suddenly to level flight. In this event the direction of "lean" would also be reversed inasmuch as a roll to the left would cause the pilot to lean to the left in order to sit in what he feels to be the vertical position.

All of the above conditions, that is whether left or right, forward or back, or whether caused by the airplane movement having its first component fast or slow, are all the result of the same physiologic manifestation. This consists in the creation of false vestibular sensations through which the labyrinths lose their correct "zero" setting for the vertical and come to rest in a new position either to the left, right, forward or back of the true "zero." Recovery may occur gradually through the action of vision which is given a correct impression of the direction of gravity by the blind flying instruments or the condition may persist until the ground is actually sighted. On the other hand, the condition may disappear suddenly because of a motion of the airplane which is the exact opposite to that which induced the condition initially.

THE OCULOGYRAL ILLUSION

In 1946 Graybiel and Hupp (9) described a form of apparent motion which may be observed following stimulation of the semicircular canals. To this phenomenon they applied the term the oculogyral illusion. In the daylight and if visual cues are plentiful relatively strong stimulation of the cresta ampullaris is necessary before visual illusory effects are observed, but in darkness a weak stimulation of the labyrinth will cause strong illusions of apparent motion which may persist after all other sensations of the rotation have disappeared. In darkness this apparent motion has a threshold of about 0.2 to 0.3 degree of rotary accelerations per second per second.

If a person in the dark fixes his eyes on a lighted target (which turns with the subject) and he is given a sufficiently strong stimulus consisting of being rotated for 20 revolutions at a rate of 25 r.p.m. several illusory effects may follow in succession as follows.

If the subject is rotated to the left the target appears to move to the left with the onset of rotation and may appear to be displaced to a maximum of 30 degrees of arc. An illusion of rapid motion lasts for about 7 to 8 seconds followed by slowing and finally the target appears to come to rest after an elapsed time of about 30 seconds. In some cases this first illusion is followed by a second one consisting of an apparent slight, slow movement of the target to the right.

If now the rotation is suddenly stopped the target then appears to move rapidly to the right in a series of jerks and may appear to be displaced to the right as much as 60 degrees of arc. The apparent movement of the target gradually slows and finally disappears within 30 seconds. This may be

followed, in a few seconds by an apparent small movement of the target to the left and this in turn may be followed by still another movement of the target after a short latent period. This latter is of short duration and the apparent movement is slow and indefinite.

Graybiel and Hupp explain the oculogyral illusion largely on the basis of nystagus with the apparent motion of the target being caused by the tracking of the image over the retina. They also point out that night flying involving angular accelerations of considerable magnitude, while exceptional, could produce this illusion in a pilot with possible serious consequences.

THE OCULOGRAVIC ILLUSION

In 1820 Purkinje noted that on a merry-go-round one involuntarily leans to the center in order to bring the long axis of the body into line with the perceived vertical. Mach also noted this effect of acceleration and that one senses the direction of the resultant vector force and tends to regard it as the vertical.

In 1946 an investigation of a series of night takeoff accidents in the R.A.F. led Collar (10) to the belief, which was verified by flight tests, that the forward acceleration of an aircraft on takeoff causes a false sensation of a nose-high attitude of the plane. This can cause the pilot to lower the nose and dive into the ground during which time he experiences a sensation of steady climb. This type of illusion is most likely to develop on a clear but very dark night where the takeoff is in the direction of an unlighted area, the horizon is not visible and the pilot fails to follow his artificial horizon but attempts to watch the ground.

The reverse of the above may also occur, especially during high decelerations, such as following the opening of dive brakes during descent. This may result in an illusion of a nose-down attitude the correction of which could lead to a stall and subsequent spin.

In 1952 Graybiel (11) made a detailed laboratory study of these manifestations and termed them oculogravic illusions based on the fact that they arise as a result of stimulation of the otolith organs. Different positions of the subject on the centrifuge produced different patterns of the illusion. His original works should be consulted for details. For our purpose here we will mention only one of his experiments which gave an effect similar to the actual takeoff effect described above. In this experiment the subject faced the center of rotation of the centrifuge and was accelerated in 3 seconds at a rate such that the resultant vector force on the subject's body was at a 45 degree angle with the vertical. This resulted in the subject having a sensation of his body, the seat and other supporting structures being smoothly but firmly tilted backward while the lighted target on which his eyes were fixed appeared to rise. These apparent movements were rapid at first, then slow and finally there was no apparent movement. On stopping the centrifuge these apparent movements were reversed and the subject sensed his true position and that of the target light correctly.

The Oculoagravic Illusion

In 1958 Gerathewohl and Stallings (12) investigated the oculogravic illusion employing accelerations of less than the force of gravity up to the point of weightlessness. The studies were carried out with the subject in the rear seat of a two place, fighter type airplane which was flown on a smooth parabola course creating a short period of weightlessness during the parabola and up to 3 plus g during the pullout from the dive. During these maneuvers the observer induced a strong visual after-image and recorded its apparent motion.

It was found that an increase of g forces produced a downward movement and weightlessness an apparent upward movement of the visual after-image and the latter was termed the oculoagravic illusion. In this illusion there was a direct relationship between the direction of the accelerative force and target displacement and also between the magnitude of the acceleration and of the illusory displacement. The visual after-image appeared to rise into the upper part of the apparent visual field when weightlessness was reached and maintained that position during most of the weightless period and then returned to its normal position when a normal 1 g condition was resumed.

The authors attribute the oculoagravic illusion to an otolith response and noted that the direction of apparent movement of the image was the opposite of that expected from the previous work of Graybiel and others on the oculogravic illusion. Further work on this question is needed to clarify these conflicting results.

The Autokinetic Illusion

In 1945 Graybiel and Clark (13) reported on their detailed study of the autokinetic illusion in relation to night flying. This phenomenon is an illusory perception of movement of a fixed object in the visual field when other visual references are inadequate or absent. The classic means of observing this is to gaze at a small light in an otherwise darkened room or at a dark spot on a plain white or gray background. After a short period of time the spot appears to move in various directions.

Graybiel and Clark found that, under laboratory conditions simulating certain features of flying in formation at night, that the subject is frequently confused inasmuch as he cannot always tell when a particular movement of the target begins or ends and often cannot distinguish real from apparent movement. This same thing was observed under actual formation flying at night if the lead plane displayed only one running light. As more lights were switched on by the lead plane the autokinetic illusion tended to disappear owing to the improvement in the visual frame of reference. It was also observed that the illusion was decreased by rapid relative movement of the target and by periodically withdrawing the subject's attention from the target for at least 10 seconds. As a result of these findings it was concluded that, although the autokinetic illusion does not constitute a hazard to flying under most circumstances, it could cause difficulty under certain conditions during formation flying at night and probably offers an explanation for some aircraft accidents which have otherwise been unexplained.

Fascination in Flying

The term fascination is used in aviation to describe a state of narrowed attention associated with excessive concentration on one portion of the task to the extent that the pilot fails to respond to clearly defined stimuli regarding the situation as a whole. An example of this is the student who has had difficulty making proper approaches during landing practice and resolves that on the next attempt he will concentrate on this difficulty. He does so and as a consequence lands with his wheels retracted even though the wheels-up warning horn was blowing and he recalls later that he distinctly heard it during his approach. A more familiar example is the pilot on low level bombing practice who concentrates so hard on hitting the target that he becomes oblivious to the excessive loss of altitude and flys into the ground. This latter is referred to as target fascination. Other examples of fascination are seen in formation flying where the attention is fixed on maintaining position with the leader to the exclusion of all else and in blind flying where the attention is riveted on one instrument instead of the whole instrument panel being regularly scanned. Numerous other similar situations could be cited but the above should be adequate to give the reader a clear picture of what fascination is and, in addition, suggests when and why the condition develops.

Fascination is seen most frequently in students and becomes less as flying experience reaches a point where the pilot's reaction to situations become largely automatic. In other words, it is most apt to develop where the pilot is overwhelmed with too many details and he elects to deal exclusively or largely with one or a few of them.

This should not be taken to mean that the highest incidence of fascination occurs in new students and decreases as training progresses for this is not the case. The reason is that the student is continuously being taught new and more complicated procedures and, thus, he may find that his span of attention has been exceeded at any point in his training and not necessarily just at the beginning. Although the frequency is not as great, graduate pilots also may experience fascination and here again it is usually associated with a new experience or one in which practice is needed. Included in this is checking out on new type aircraft, refresher training in blind or formation flying and gunnery or bombing training.

A majority of all pilots suffer from fascination at one time or another and unfor-tunately it is most apt to occur at a time when the consequences are the most dangerous, *i.e.*, during gunnery, bombing, formation and instrument flying and landings. The incidence of fascination can be lowered by warning all flying personnel of its existence and to the dangers of over concentration on a limited element of the task. In addition, the training rate of flyers should not exceed their ability to maintain a complete grasp of the total situation to the degree that they can and will make a correct response to to any significant stimuli.

Fascination is not peculiar to aviation and is seen frequently in every day life not only among drivers of vehicles but in the home and in the office. The suggestion, seen mostly in the lay press, that hypnotism is involved has no basis in fact. The writer is of the opinion that such things as daydreaming, a detached attitude, compulsive behavior and similar manifestations should not be considered as types of fascination as advocated by Clark, Nicholson and Graybiel (14) and prefers the more limited concept outlined above which is in close agreement with the earlier works of Graybiel (15) and Vinacke (16).

Miscellaneous

In addition to the various conditions described above, which have been given specific designations, there are a number of others which have not been labeled but are nonetheless equally important. These latter will now be described.

Certain structures and conditions in the cockpit may give the illusion of tilt if they are not exactly horizontal or vertical to the line of flight. Thus, if an instrument panel is tilted with reference to the horizontal the pilot may fly the panel straight and level and the aircraft with one wing down. Likewise side window panels of the cockpit whose upper and lower frames are tilted upward or downward may produce an illusion of the plane being in an equivalent position of climb or descent. Even rain streaming across the windshield at a slant has created the illusion of its being the vertical with a resultant tilt of the aircraft to the right or left as the case may be.

When flying between cloud layers they may not be exactly horizontal. Inasmuch as these clouds are likely to be used as a horizon there will be a tendency for the airplane to be flown with a corresponding degree of tilt to the left or the right. If one should be flying at right angles to the course mentioned above then the cloud horizon would be either above or below the true horizon and the tendency would be to fly in a shallow climb or dive respectively.

A small cluster of isolated lights on the ground on a dark night with a high overcast may lead a pilot to believe that he is observing the lights of a formation flight If he attempts to join this apparent formation it can result in his flying into the ground.

A wide scattering of lights on the ground on a dark night with a high overcast may lead to the illusion that the lights are stars and that the aircraft is flying upside down.

A small cluster of very bright stars in the sky may be mistaken for the lights of a formation resulting in the pilot making a futile effort to join up.

Illusions of relative motion may occur during formation flying when the motion of a wingman is transposed into the motion of the flight leader flying at a different speed. An extreme form of this is seen at very high altitude where essentially all sense of forward speed has been lost owing to the great distance to the earth. If then the leader should suddenly increase his speed the wingman may develop the illusion that the leader's plane is standing still and that his own plane is flying backward.

When flying at 50,000 feet altitude the horizon is about 275 to 300 miles away and, because of the curvature of the earth, it is depressed about 4 degrees below the horizontal. This tends to cause the pilot to fly left wing down 4 degrees, assuming he is watching out the left hand window. If he then looks to the right he finds that his right wing appears to be tilted upward 8 degrees and that he is in a decided bank. Four of these degrees of tilt are real, inasmuch as the pilot had previously placed the plane in that position while the remaining 4 degrees are an illusion caused by the horizon being that much below the horizontal.

At very high altitude the curvature of the earth makes it possible for a segment of the sky to appear to be beneath the level of the aircraft. This is especially noticeable when the sun, moon or scattered stars are at or near the horizon and are seen below the level of the wing. This can result in a very strong illusion of flying upside down.

On rare occasions pilots have reported vertigo immediately following the clearing of their ears. This has been seen both during ascent when the increased pressure in the middle ear corrected itself involuntarily and also during descent when the negative pressure in the tympanic cavity was relieved by a voluntary effort on the part of the pilot. The exact mechanism by which this pressure difference, or rather the relief of this difference, affects the nonauditory labyrinth is not known.

During a parachute jump the body usually slowly tumbles or spins until the parachute opens but these rotations seldom produce vertigo. However, when using the ejection seat, especially at high altitude, the body may tumble or spin at a rate of up to 465 r.p.m. during the free fall period. This rapid spinning or tumbling or a combination of the two has been known to produce severe disorientation, blurring of vision and nausea as a result of the induced vertigo. Although this vertigo is one of the lesser dangers of these high speed bodily rotations (see chapter 20) it does interfere with the subject's ability to carry out the necessary procedures for a safe landing.

DISCUSSION

In 1955 Ruffel Smith credited disorientation as being probably the most common cause of fatal accidents in the R.A.F. not caused primarily by mechanical failure. In 1956 Nuttall and Sanford (17) studied spatial disorientation in one of the U. S. Air Force overseas commands and found that it was the cause of 4 per cent of all flying accidents in that command and for 14 per cent of all fatal accidents. They also found that essentially 100 per cent of the pilots had experienced disorientation at least once and that some had had up to 20 such experiences. The disorientations reported were almost all associated with illusions of attitude and motion produced primarily by false sensations arising from the nonauditory labyrinth. These illusions of attitude and motion, in a severe form, were about five times as frequent in jet aircraft as in piston type planes.

As might be expected vertigo occurred most frequently during instrument flight conditions with those flying wing position in day weather formations having by far the highest incidence of disorientation. The various combinations of solo and formation flying on instruments during both day and night operations plus transition from visual to instrument flight rules together accounted for some 93 per cent of all cases of vertigo reported whereas the other 7 per cent were scattered among 18 other flight conditions. Although exact information is not available concerning the incidence of vertigo in civilian flying it is probably a factor in a considerable number of civilian accidents especially among private pilots flying at night or in weather on instruments.

Inasmuch as vertigo in flying is based on a normal physiologic response rather than to a pathologic condition there seems to be little that can be done directly to prevent its occurrence. Although at first glance it might seem that the discovery of a drug capable of temporarily suppressing sensory impulses from the nonauditory labyrinth would solve this problem this is not necessarily so for as Northington (18) has said, persons with total loss of vestibular reactions always have an equilibratory disturbance and compensation is never complete. He further stated that, "some of the opinions on the biologic utility of the vestibular function seem to be based on the assumption that normal stimulation of the vestibular receptor ordinarily evokes vertigo, nystagmus and forced movements rather than what seems to be the truth in the matter, that normal stimuli induce normal useful reactions, whereas (only) abnormal stimuli induce abnormal disabling reactions." When it is also remembered that man in flight is exposed to 6 degrees of freedom of which 3 are in rotational motion we are perhaps fortunate that the problem is not greater than it actually is. This is especially true when we further consider that erroneous impulses traveling over the vestibular nerve go not only to the vestibular nuclei in the brain stem but also to the eye muscle nuclei, motor nuclei at all levels of the cord, several areas of the cerebellum, reticular nuclei of the midbrain, the reticular formation of the pons and medulla and to the cerebral cortex (19).

PREVENTIVE MEASURES

In the absence of any currently known means of selecting pilots who are not normally susceptible to vertigo the approach to the problem appears to lie in the realm of improved aircraft and aircraft instrument design and better and more training of the individual. Aircraft with increased stability would be of considerable benefit as would a simplified cockpit layout and a flight instrument presentation which can be more quickly and easily grasped than that now available.

Better and more thorough indoctrination of pilots on vertigo, disorientation and related states should prove helpful and should include a demonstration in a Barany chair. The reason for this is that experienced pilots who appear to be quite familiar with vertigo in theory as well as in practice are usually quite amazed when given the Barany chair test for the first time (17). In the indoctrination of pilots special emphasis should be placed on three things. These are the dangers associated with trying to fly visually in marginal conditions or during instrument conditions, attempting to split one's attention between visual and instrument flight and waiting until the last moment to switch from visual to instrument flight. Another thing is the extreme danger of the Coriolis reaction and this should be demonstrated in the Barany chair.

There seems to be little question that instrument flight training and experience is important in reducing the incidence of vertigo and most other related states. However, great care should be exercised that the sequence and rate of training is such that the pilot is at all times operating well within his capabilities for to do do otherwise would only increase the hazards. Pilots tend to quickly lose their instrument flight ability and accordingly those who have not had recent practice should be reminded that they are especially vulnerable and need to undergo a course of graduated retraining to regain their former proficiency.

Since World War I (2) a series of attempts have been made to lessen or abolish the normal vestibular sequelae following rapid rotation based on repeated laboratory exposures of subjects to such rotations. The results in all cases were negative until the recent work of McCabe and Lawrence (20) who demonstrated that figure skaters develop remarkable skill in performing rapid spins exceeding 10 seconds in duration with rates as high as 5 revolutions per second (300 r.p.m.). Following a sudden stop from these spins the skilled skater has no dizziness, no nystagmus and is perfectly coordinated with no unsteadiness. During the spinning the skaters' eyes can be observed to be either closed or to have wandering autogenous movements but no nystagmus. This feat is accomplished without using the "spotting technique" which ballet dancers are trained to use.

These skilled skaters, when tested on the Barany chair by the usual technique, exhibit no nystagmus, have no sensation of dizziness, no past pointing and can immediately step from the Barany chair and walk a straight line. After-reaction is absent in testing both the horizontal canals and the vertical canals. Although in performance of the skaters' spins the major component of stimulation is in the horizontal canals it appears that central suppression of both horizontal and vertical canal effects is learned. Stimulation of both horizontal and vertical canals by use of the Caloric test is also without after-effect. During early training these skaters have severe dizziness and disorientation as a result of spinning but gradually through training are able to suppress the sensation and develop the ability to maintain a steady posture following a sudden stop.

A skilled skater will lose this ability with a long layoff period and when returning to the practice of spins will suffer dizziness and disorientation. However, they are able to regain their ability in a relatively short time with practice. This phenomenon is considered by the authors to be a central suppression of normal labyrinthine sensations. The central nervous system pathways involved in the supression are not known. However, there are numerous interconnecting pathways between the vestibular nuclei and the cerebellum and cortex and between cortex and cerebellum. It is presumed that cortical control is exerted upon this complex system.

In aviation, from the practical viewpoint, it seems unlikely that the average pilot could be expected to spend the time and effort necessary to attain and maintain a state of vestibular suppression. However, for special situations it appears that a pilot could be trained to accomplish this and thus become, as it were, immune to vertigo.

REFERENCES

(1) Webster's New International Dictionary of the English Language, Ed. 2. Springfield, Massachusetts, G. and C. Merriam Co., 1950.
(2) Anon. Air Service Medical. Washington, D.C., Government Printing Office, 1919.
(3) Anon. Aviation Medicine in the A.E.F. Washington, D. C. Government Printing Office, 1920.
(4) MYERS, D. A.: The medical contribution to the development of blind flying. Army M. Bull., 36: 18–37, 1936.
(5) TER BRAAK, J. W. G.: Ueber die Empfindlichkeit des Bogengangsapparates für Winkelbeschleunligungen. Arch. ges. Physiol., 238: 319–326, 1936.
(6) TUMARKIN, J. A.: Some observations on the function of the labyrinth. Proc. Roy. Soc. Med., 30: 599–610, 1937.
(7) CORIOLIS, G.: Traite de mechanique des corps solides et du calcul de l'effet des machines, Ed. 2. Paris, deutsch von C. H. Schnuse, Braunschweig, 1846.
(8) ARMSTRONG, H. G.: Principles and Practice of Aviation Medicine. Ed. 1. Baltimore, The Williams & Wilkins Co., 1939.
(9) GRAYBIEL, A., AND HUPP, H.: The oculogyral illusion. J. Aviation Med., 17: 3–27, 1946.
(10) COLLAR, A. R.: On an aspect of the accident history of aircraft taking off at night. R.A.F. Reports and Memoranda, No. 227, 1946.
(11) GRAYBIEL, A.: Oculogravic illusion. A.M.A. Arch. Ophth., 48: 605–615, 1952.
(12) GERATHEWOHL, S. J., AND STALLINGS, H. D.: A Study of the Oculo-Agravic Illusion. Research Report No. 58-105. Randolph Air Force Base Texas, Air University, School of Aviation Medicine, USAF, 1958.
(13) GRAYBIEL, A., AND CLARK, B.: The autokinetic illusions and its significance in night flying. J. Aviation Med., 16: 111–151, 1945.
(14) CLARK, B., NICHOLSON, M., AND GRAYBIEL, A.: Fascination: a cause of pilot error. J. Aviation Med., 24: 429–440, 1953.
(15) GRAYBIEL, A.: Disorientation in pilots. Contact, 5: 412–425, 1945.
(16) VINACKE, W.: Fascination in Flight. U. S.

Naval School of Aviation Medicine. Research Report No. N.M. 001059.01.13 (X-148-AV-4-3). Pensacola, Florida, U. S. Naval School of Aviation Medicine, 1946.

(17) NUTTALL, J. B., AND SANFORD, W. G.: Spatial disorientation in operational flying. Publication M-27-56, U. S. Air Force Directorate of Flight Safety Research, 1956.

(18) NORTHINGTON, P. O.: Discussion of paper, Aerial equilibration. J. Aviation Med., 5: 103–106, 1934.

(19) NUTTALL, J. B.: The problem of spatial disorientation. J. A. M. A., 166: 431–438, 1958.

(20) McCABE, B. F., AND LAWRENCE, M.: Suppression of vestibular sequelae following rapid rotation. Presented at the 30th Annual Meeting of the Aeromedical Association, April 1959.

16

EFFECTS OF RADIAL AND ANGULAR ACCELERATIONS

Ralph L. Christy, M.D

Man is exposed to the forces of acceleration in one form or another almost constantly throughout flight. Acceleration may be defined as change of velocity, or the rate of such change, either as regards speed or direction or both. The principal kinds of acceleration commonly referred to in aviation medicine are:

Linear

Radial (centripetal)

Angular

Radial (centripetal) accelerations are, strictly speaking, also angular accelerations, but by common usage in aviation medicine, both terms are used, largely as a result of the differences in magnitude and effects on the pilot or aircrewman. Angular accelerations involve rotation about an axis which axis may be through the pilot's body or distant to him. If the axis of rotation is through the pilot's body (or close to it), it is spoken of as angular acceleration, whereas acceleration of the body with the axis external to the pilot's body, as on a human centrifuge or in an aircraft making a turn, is spoken of as radial acceleration.

This chapter will concentrate on the effects of radial acceleration and also of certain angular accelerations (exclusive of purely disorientation effects). However, inasmuch as accelerative forces usually act in combination and inasmuch as it is the effect of combined stresses on the man which are

so important, certain references to other types of accelerative or other physiologic stress will be necessary. The pilot, aircrewman or passenger is exposed to linear acceleration on takeoff, during an increase in speed, during a catapult launching from an aircraft carrier and is exposed to linear deceleration on landing, during decreases in speed and during arrested carrier landings. Linear acceleration is also involved during ejection from an aircraft and deceleration in the windstream as he slows to terminal velocity. If during any of these linear accelerations or decelerations, or at a constant linear velocity, a change in direction is introduced, centripetal or radial accelerations are produced, and if in the course of this change of direction the aircraft is banked or rolled, angular accelerations are produced about the long axis of the aircraft. The effects of angular acceleration are principally those of stimulating the vestibular system with possible resultant vertigo, confusion and disorientation of the pilot or passenger. Linear accelerations of major interest in aviation are those of high magnitude and short duration such as occur in crashes, ejection from aircraft or, occasionally, in high altitude or high speed parachute opening, as they tend to exceed the strength limitations of the skeletal structure of the body. Radial accelerations, on the other hand, are generally of lower magnitude and longer duration and are of importance principally because of their effects on the cardiovascular system of the body. However, the physiologic problems typical of radial acceleration can also occur with prolonged linear accelerations such as in rocket aircraft and will be increasingly important in orbital or space flight. Escape at very high speeds with relatively long deceleration times can also produce cardiovascular physiologic reactions and fluid shifts that are more commonly identified with radial acceleration. It thus can be seen that the effects of acceleration cannot be completely separated into the categories resulting from linear, radial and angular acceleration and yet, for purposes of discussion, it is preferable to deal with each type of acceleration in relation to its more usual and typical effects.

RADIAL ACCELERATION

Terminology and Definitions

When an aircraft changes direction, a centripetal acceleration results directed toward the axis of the turn along the radius and this in turn produces an inertial (centrifugal) force in the opposite direction.

In considering the effects of radial acceleration on the body the duration and the magnitude of the force must be considered as well as the direction of the resultant force on the body, whether it be head to foot or positive; foot to head or negative; or transverse at right angles to the long axis of the body.

Inasmuch as from Newton's law $F = ma$ then $a = F/m$, i.e., linear acceleration is proportional to force and inversely proportional to mass. In curved flight acceleration depends on the rate of change of direction and the velocity and is expressed by the equation $F = mV^2/r$, where V is the velocity, m equals the mass, and r the radius of rotation. Also, inasmuch as weight constitutes a measure of the force of gravity and is proportional to the mass of a body, it is both logical and convenient to use the acceleration due to gravity as the unit of measure for acceleration. This unit of measure is denoted by the symbol g. Forces generated in linear accelerations are those required to overcome the inertia of the body acted upon whereas centripetal accelera-

tions are those required to constrain a body to move in a curved path.

An airplane in flight is influenced by gravity and by forces which are independent of, and in addition to, both the amount and direction of the pull of gravity. These independent forces arise from the ability of the airplane to rotate about its three axes, from the positive and negative lift of its wings and also from its propellant and braking forces. The lines of these forces in an airplane are along its three coordinate axes and are independent of the aircraft's position in space. The total force acting on the aircraft or the pilot is the resultant of the centripetal acceleration and gravity.

By common usage, accelerations acting upward on the airplane perpendicular to its line of flight are called "positive" accelerations, and those acting downward are called "negative" accelerations. They are denoted by the symbols $+$ and $-$, respectively. It must be remembered, however, that a force applied in one direction by the airplane produces an equal but opposite force in the occupant. Thus, when the airplane acts on a body in the direction seat to head, the inertia of the body acts in the direction head to seat, and the body may be said to be exposed to positive g. Conversely, a footward or downward acceleration on the aircraft results in an opposite force on the body, seat to head, tending to force body fluids toward the head, and the body is exposed to negative g.

The positive and negative accelerations mentioned above apply only to forces applied perpendicularly through the body and do not take into consideration forces applied transversely. These latter are termed "transverse" accelerations.

Accelerations Attained in Flight

The accelerations to be encountered in flight vary greatly dependent upon the maneuverability of the aircraft, its wing loading, power and the speed and altitude at which the maneuver is performed. For example, the aircraft of the 1930's and early 1940's had a lower wing loading and less power than the modern jet fighters; however, they generally flew at lower altitudes where the air density is greater and high accelerations were, therefore, possible. These earlier aircraft, including fighters and dive bombers, were able to attain accelerations of as much as nine times the pull of gravity, or 9 g. The higher accelerations were generally of very short duration—from a fraction of a second to 1 or 2 seconds—as high accelerations tend to slow the aircraft and the g drops rapidly, as it is proportional to the square of the velocity. However, in loops or diving power spirals, accelerations of 4 to 6 g lasting as long as 5 or 10 seconds or more are possible. Jet fighter aircraft with their greater power can sustain even higher accelerations (6 to 7 g) for longer times in prolonged turns at altitudes around 10,000 to 15,000 feet. However, at more usual operating altitudes of 30,000 feet or higher the decreased air density tends to cause the wing to stall as a result of inadequate lift and accelerations of 3 to not more than 5 g are the rule. With sufficient power from jet or rocket engines and properly designed wings higher accelerations would be possible at these altitudes. As a practical matter, most fighter aircraft are not designed for flight

stresses over 7.0 or 7.5 g as the greater strength requirement increases aircraft weight and wing loading which, of itself, limits maneuverability and resultant g. This level of g also coincides with upper g-tolerance levels of pilots wearing antiblackout (anti-g) suits. Table 41 (1–3) provides some additional information as to the duration and magnitude of accelerations with typical maneuvers in certain aircraft.

GENERAL CONSIDERATIONS

When the body is exposed to accelerative forces, the resulting effects manifest themselves principally in four different tissues of the body; namely, the soft supporting tissues, the bony tissues, the organs suspended within the body cavities and the body fluids. The effects vary with the magnitude, direction and duration of the force applied. Radial accelerations, as a result of the longer times of exposure, principally involve the body fluids and the organs suspended within the body cavities as contrasted with high linear accelerations of short time duration

TABLE 41

Some Typical Acceleration-Time Patterns in Aircraft

Maneuver	F6C-4 Average g	F6C-4 Time	F6C-4 Maximum g	F6C-4 Time	F6C-4 Minimum g	F6C-4 Time	AD-1 Average g	AD-1 Time	AD-1 Maximum g	AD-1 Time	AD-1 Minimum g	AD-1 Time	F6F-5 Average g	F6F-5 Time	F6F-5 Maximum g	F6F-5 Time	F6F-5 Minimum g	F6F-5 Time	F9F-8 g	F9F-8 Time
		sec.		sec.		sec.		sec.		sec.		sec.		sec.		sec.		sec.		sec.
Loop																				
1. First phase			5	1.75	4	9.75	3.6	2.1	4.6	2.4	2.7	2.9	3.9	2.8	6.4	1.0	2.8	2.5		
2. Second phase							3.5	2.0	4.3	1.5	2.5	1.2	3.5	2.7	4.3	2.6	4.3	2.6		
	140 m.p.h.		175 m.p.h.		130 m.p.h.														5000 feet pull-up	
Dive; pull-up from 40 degree dive	7.6	0.87	9.3	0.82	6.4	0.8	4.0	2.3	5.2	1.5	2.6	1.5	4.1	2.4	5.7	1.0	3.0	3.6	4.5	5.0
Immelman							4.8	1.8	5.8	1.2	4.2	2.4	3.9	3.9	4.5	3.2	2.9	4.5		
High side gunnery							4.8	1.9	6.3	0.6	3.4	1.5	3.9	1.2	5.5	0.6	2.5	4.2		
Wing over roll																				
1. First phase							2.3	2.5	3.0	2.8	1.7	3.0	2.5	3.4	2.8	4.2	2.2	1.7		
2. Second phase							2.6	1.9	3.9	1.7	2.0	2.2	2.9	3.6	3.4	4.4	2.4	7.0		
Split S													4.4	2.7	5.8	0.8	2.8	6.0		
Barrel roll																				
1			5.15	1.0	4.05	0.85	2.1	2.0	2.7	2.4	1.5	3.7	3.0	2.1	3.8	2.0	2.4	2.5		
2							2.7	1.7	3.4	1.8	2.1	0.5	2.7	2.8	3.6	5.8	2.0	5.8		
Slow roll																				
1													2.0	1.0	2.9	1.3	1.2	1.5		
2													2.7	1.0	4.4	0.8	1.9	1.3		
Turn																				
20,000 feet																			3.0	30
40,000 feet																			2.1	122

which more typically affect the structural elements of the body.

During centrifugalization, organs of considerable mass contained within the abdominal, thoracic or cranial cavities and their supporting attachments are subject to stress caused either by their displacement from their normal positions or by pressure against some unyielding part of the skeleton. Temporary disturbance of function may arise from this cause. Thus, under negative acceleration (reactive forces on the body acting seat to head), crowding of the abdominal viscera against the diaphragm may act to embarrass respiratory movement and heart action. Gell and Cranmore (4) froze rats with liquid nitrogen while exposed to accelerative stress. Figure 83 clearly illustrates the resulting displacement of the diaphragm and the abdominal and thoracic viscera.

With respect to the fluids within the body, only the blood need be considered. Here we are dealing with a large mass of fluid contained within distensible vessels and, thus, easily influenced by acceleration forces. The direction of the force with respect to the anatomy of the cardiovascular system has a decided bearing on the magnitude of the disturbance. The largest columns of blood occur in the great vessels running lengthwise through the body so that forces acting in that direction will produce the most marked effects. These effects consist of an alteration in distribution and pressure relations within these vessels and their tributaries.

The sequence of events in the cardiovascular system caused by a centrifugal force acting along the long axis of the body in a head to seat direction as a result of a headward acceleration (positive g) is as follows. A direct hydrostatic action on the blood within the large vessels tends to force the blood into the lower parts of the body. This will result in an accumulation of blood particularly in the abdominal region at the

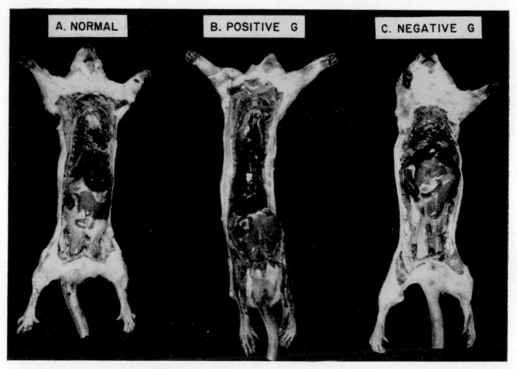

FIG. 83. Rats frozen in liquid nitrogen. A is a frozen control not exposed to accelerative stress. B and C were frozen during exposures to accelerative stress of positive and negative g, respectively, on a centrifuge. Note the differences between the normal position and relationships of the viscera in A as compared to the visceral displacement footward in B and headward in C. (From *Navy Aviation Medicine Practice*, fig. 3.7, p. 36.)

expense of the head with reduced venous return to the heart. Thus, the initial fall in pressure in the vessels of the head region is further augmented by a decreased cardiac output. The net action is a marked fall in intracranial blood pressure with a resulting secondary anoxemia of the brain and sensory organs of the head. Reflex compensatory mechanisms, such as those initiated through reduced blood pressure in the carotid sinus, will tend to counteract the fall in pressure through increased heart action and vasoconstriction. The visual mechanism, the retinas, optic nerves and cerebral optic centers are particularly sensitive to hypoxia and when a marked reduction in blood pressure in the vessels supplying these areas occurs disturbances of visual function are a natural consequence. As discussed below, visual changes usually precede loss of consciousness as the intraocular pressure causes failure of the blood supply to the retina before that to the brain. With increased fall in blood pressure the cerebral circulation may become so reduced that loss of consciousness results.

Negative g with reactive forces in the opposite direction, i.e., in the long axis of the body from seat to head, will produce changes in a reverse order. Under these circumstances, blood will be forced into the head region causing a rise in the pressure in the cerebral vessels.

Forces acting at right angles to the long axis of the body will, in general, produce effects which are sufficiently alike to permit discussing them as a group. In this case, the viscera will be subjected to pressure by displacement although, owing to the restricted extent of movements by the viscera in these planes, the amount of stress to supporting attachments is not great. Forces acting against the ventral surface of the body affect respiration and some distress is encountered as a result of pressure of the viscera against the abdominal wall. Because of the absence of large columns of blood directed along the transverse axes of the body the effect on the circulatory system is not as great as where the force acts in the long axis of the body.

Symptoms that are produced by accelerations vary markedly depending on the direction in which the forces are applied to the body. As a consequence, it is necessary to discuss positive, negative and transverse accelerations separately.

POSITIVE ACCELERATION

SUBJECTIVE SYMPTOMS. Positive accelerations acting in the direction of the long axis of the body from seat to head produce reactive forces head to seat and effects which vary with the magnitude of the acceleration, the rate with which it is increased and decreased and the duration of its action. One + g is that normally experienced by the body in the upright position by the pull of gravity and is too familiar an experience to require description here. At 2 + g's the principal subjective sensation is an awareness of the increased pressure of the body on the seat and heaviness of the hands and feet. Three and 4 + g's produce an exaggeration of the sensation of heaviness of the body and limbs and movement of the latter is accomplished only with great effort as demonstrated by Code, et al. (5). Parachute donning time was increased from 17 seconds at 1 g to 75 seconds at 3 g. The skeletal musculature involuntarily becomes tense, resisting the tendency for the body to be compressed in the vertical dimension. The trunk and head, unless well supported or maintained in a line parallel to the line of force, are held erect with difficulty. The body is almost beyond the control of the muscles except for limited movements of the arms and head and one becomes progressively more helpless physically. It is with considerable difficulty that pilots can reach canopy releases at about 6 g or ejection seat face curtain firing handles under sustained accelerations above about 6 to 7 + g's. On the other hand, with negative or irregular oscillating accelerations, pre-ejection or arm rest firing controls located on the seat may be difficult to reach. At a level of 3 or 4 g there is a distinct dragging sensation in the thorax from the heavy traction on the attachments of the thoracic viscera. The lower facial area feels pulled down and as the blood pressure falls there is a distinct diminution of vision ("veiling," "gray out" or "tunnel vision") or a complete loss of vision commonly known as "blacking out." The lower parts of the legs feel congested and there may be cramping of the calf muscles. Inspiration becomes difficult probably the result of a lowering of the diaphragm from the pull of the liver from below and the pressure of the heart and lungs from above. Generally, as a defense against a mechanically forced expiration, the glottis is closed and the breath is held in mid-inspiration.

As acceleration increases, there is an exaggeration of the above mentioned symptoms as a result of the increasing hypoxemia of the brain with its accompanying loss of sensory functions. Loss of consciousness appears between 3 and 5 + g's depending on individual tolerances. As the acceleration is decreased consciousness returns quickly followed by a return of vision and there are seldom any after effects except a few moments of slight mental confusion. There is no actual pain or even marked physical discomfort connected with positive accelerations and yet they are unpleasant as a result of the physical and psychic stress induced. No permanent effects of repeated exposure to positive accelerations have been noted in studies by Wood et al. (6).

OBJECTIVE SYMPTOMS. *Respiration and Pulse.* The anticipation of undergoing high accelerations causes the respiration, pulse and blood pressure of the test subject to fluctuate widely from the normal and it is very difficult to obtain true readings free from psychic influences. With accelerations of 2 to 4 + g's, the respiration becomes slightly increased in rate and the inhalation-exhalation ratio is also increased. At 4 to 5 + g's and above, either the breathing becomes very irregular with long, slow labored inspirations and rapid mechanically forced expirations or the breathing is stopped at midinspiration as a defense against the traction downward on the diaphragm.

Blood Pressure. The effects of positive accelerations are reflected principally in the shifting of the blood from the upper to the lower portions of the body. This shifting of the blood is manifested by a change in the blood pressure which is decreased above and increased below the level of the heart. This change in blood pressure was first studied in detail by Jongbloed and Noyons (7), Armstrong and Heim (8), Poppen (9) and Ranke (10). Of particular interest were the studies which were done on experimental animals where continuous blood pressure tracing was recorded and roentgenograms of the heart obtained during acceleration.

Schubert (11) and others (8, 9) have explained the behavior of the blood pressure during accelerations to be the result of the hydrostatic pressure and the decreased filling of the heart. This latter has been beautifully demonstrated by Ranke (10) by means of roentgenograms of the hearts of monkeys while they were being exposed to various accelerations. One series of his pictures is reproduced here as figure 84 and as can be seen the greater the acceleration the fainter the heart shadow and, hence, the less the venous return to, and filling of, the heart.

Although the principal symptoms and effects of positive accelerations are manifested by a depletion of blood and a drop in blood pressure above the level of the

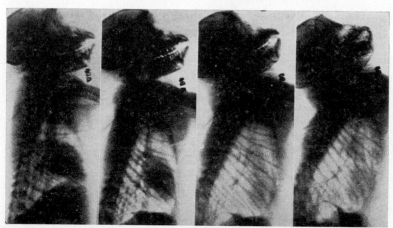

FIG. 84. Roentgenogram of a normal monkey heart (at left) and during exposure to 2,2, 5.5 and 7.7 + g's. (After Ranke.)

heart, it must be remembered that this is accompanied by an accumulation of blood and an increase of blood pressure below the level of the heart. In the lower portions of the body during positive accelerations the blood pressure in both the arteries and veins rises considerably above normal. In high accelerations this rise is sufficient to cause petechial hemorrhages about the legs and feet.

It is apparent that in each individual the ultimate effect is dependent on the tone and the resiliency of the vascular bed such that a given acceleration meets with a given increasing resistance and when the latter is sufficient to overcome the shifting of the blood mass the maximum effect has been attained. Thus, one with a poor vascular tone suffers a much worse effect than one with a good vascular tone and the former "blacks out" and suffers loss of consciousness much earlier than the latter.

Another factor which has an important influence is the reflex effect of the arterial blood pressure decrease on the carotid sinus. In the vicinity of the bifurcation of the carotid vessels and also in the vicinity of the aortic arch there are pressure receptors which cause peripheral vasoconstriction and cardio-acceleration when the blood pressure falls. As a consequence of this reflex mechanism there is a tendency for the fall in blood pressure to be checked. The more gradual the onset of positive g the less the fall in blood pressure inasmuch as it takes approximately 5 seconds before this compensation comes into full play. Thus, the mode of onset of acceleration will determine to some extent the tolerance of the individual and, on the average, a gradual onset will increase the blackout threshold by 1 g. On the other hand, if the acceleration comes on abruptly this compensatory mechanism will not have time to exert its influence.

If the acceleration is great enough and prolonged over a period of several seconds, the lack of venous return to the heart will finally result in the heart chambers becoming empty before the systolic cycle is completed. This will allow the internal walls of the heart chambers to become tightly opposed resulting in trauma and subendocardial hemorrhages may occur as a result or possibly because of increased pressure dif-ferentials between coronary vessels or owing to myocardial ischemia. There is no evidence that this trauma is dangerous to life or leads to any serious consequences.

The above work has been confirmed and extended by researchers on human and animal centrifuges throughout the world. The principal human centrifuges include: in the United States, the Mayo Clinic, Rochester, Minnesota; the Wright-Patterson Air Force Base, Dayton, Ohio; the University of Southern California; the Naval Air Station, Pensacola, Florida; the Naval Air Development Center, Johnsville, Pennsylvania; in Canada, the Royal Canadian Air Force, Toronto; in England, the Royal Air Force, Farnborough; in France, the French Air Force, Brettigny Flight Test Base; in Germany, the Institute of Aviation Medicine, Bad Nauheim; and in Sweden, the Swedish Air Force, Stockholm. There is also a centrifuge in Japan and centrifuges are under construction in Rome, Italy, and in Holland at their respective aviation medical centers.

Figure 85 is an illustration of the large centrifuge at the Naval Air Development Center, Johnsville, Pennsylvania, which has a 50 foot radius, a rate of change of acceleration of 10 g per second with a maximum of 40 g and an enclosed gondola capable of atmospheric evacuation to a pressure altitude of 60,000 feet. The gondola has power gimbals that permit it to be oriented in the resultant of normal gravity, centrifugal g and tangential acceleration (as the centrifuge changes velocity) and to be tumbled to simulate aircraft escape problems.

The Johnsville centrifuge may be controlled (1) by manual controls available to the centrifuge operator, (2) by three bakelite cams shaped to provide the desired arm angular velocity and the two gimbal angles, (3) by a punched tape which can be made more rapidly and can control for longer durations than the mechanical cams, (4) by an analog computer which generates the desired driving functions or (5) by a pilot operating flight controls from within the centrifuge gondola and controlling the centrifuge through a large analog computer. Methods 1 through 4 are called "open loop" controls in which the centrifuge subject receives prearranged acceleration patterns, unaffected by his own actions, as if he were

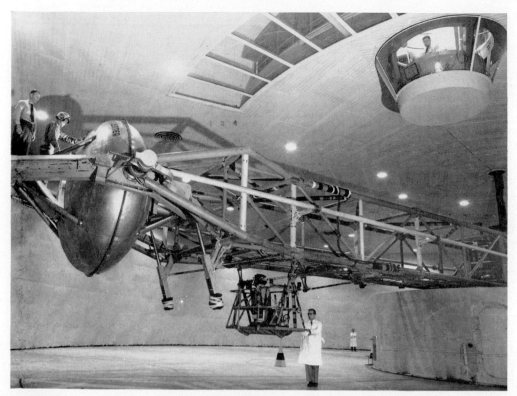

Fig. 85. Human centrifuge at the Aviation Medical Acceleration Laboratory, Naval Air Development Center, Johnsville, Pennsylvania. (From *Navy Aviation Medicine Practice*, fig. 3.4, p. 34.)

a passenger in an aircraft. Method 5 is called "closed loop" pilot computer control of the centrifuge or centrifuge dynamic control flight simulation. This method, developed for the Aviation Medical Acceleration Laboratory by the Navy's Aeronautical Computer Laboratory and their University of Pennsylvania consultants and first used in July 1957, allows the simulation of piloted flight. In this method, voltages representing pilot control motions pass from the centrifuge to a large analog computer which contains the equations of motion of a particular aircraft or space vehicle being simulated. This computer then generates the centrifuge drive signals to give to the pilot the same accelerations he would have received had he made the same control motions in actual flight in the particular aircraft. The computer also drives the cockpit instruments, to show to the pilot the changing conditions of the flight (see fig. 86). An initial application of this new technique has been the simulation of the X-15 research aircraft be-

fore the actual aircraft was flown using the test pilots scheduled to fly the X-15 as the centrifuge subjects.

Studies on human centrifuges in general have been accomplished utilizing the subjects' responses to the peripheral and central light signals and buzzer signals which are activated intermittently and responded to by the subject in a manner dependent upon his reactions to the level of g stress. In this manner the physiologic factors previously described act to cause loss of peripheral vision first, then central vision and finally unconsciousness thus providing a bioassay technique. However, the considerable stress and the undesirable episodes of unconsciousness that occasionally follow closely upon blackout have recently evoked more concentrated efforts on developing a bioassay technique which would not require the higher levels of g. Browne and Howard at Farnborough, England, have modified the technique using a red light filter and have thus reduced the g level required to produce loss

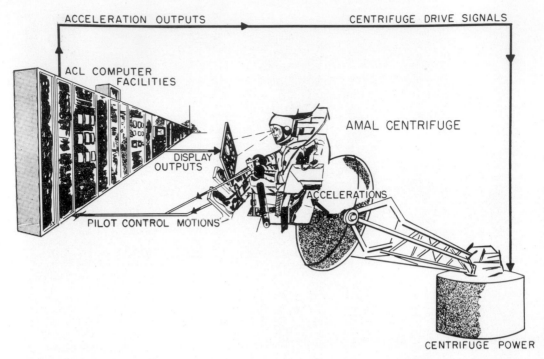

FIG. 86. Schematic drawing of Naval Air Development Center control systems. (Official U. S. Navy photograph.)

of a central red light by 1 to 3 *g*'s below levels required utilizing the white light method. This matter is under extensive study by the majority of the centrifuge groups in the hopes of achieving a modified bioassay technique of lower stress and reduced tendency to unconscious episodes.

Particular effort has been made using the centrifuges to correlate the subjective symptoms in man of dimming of vision and "blackout" with the physiologic changes. Code, *et al.* (12) of the Mayo Clinic, in a series of studies, described the changes in man and pointed out that there is a definite sequence to the physiologic events that occur in the comfortably seated human being during exposure to positive acceleration. This sequence is divided into two distinct periods: the period of progressive failure and the period of compensation.

During the period of progressive failure the pulse rate progressively increases, the amount of blood in the ear is progressively reduced, the pulse in the ear may be gradually reduced or abruptly lost, the blood pressure at the level of the base of the brain declines and reductions of vision and con-

sciousness, if they occur, become evident. As accelerations of greater magnitude are experienced the extent of these changes is increased. The period of progressive failure is usually terminated by compensatory reactions which become effective about 6 to 11 seconds after the onset of acceleration.

During the period of compensation the blood pressure rises, the ear pulse may return or increase, the amount of blood in the ear increases, the pulse rate increase is checked and the pulse may slow and, if these compensatory changes are sufficiently effective, recovery from symptoms (both loss of vision and consciousness) will occur. Figure 87 illustrates the effects of acceleration on the heart rate and blood pressure as demonstrated by ear pulse and ear opacity (blood content) changes.

Lambert and Wood (13), by direct blood pressure readings in man, showed that at the level of the eyes the decrease in blood pressure per *g* increase in positive acceleration averaged 32 mm. of Hg systolic and 20 mm. of Hg diastolic. During maintained acceleration the lowest pressure occurred in about 7 seconds and was followed by some recovery.

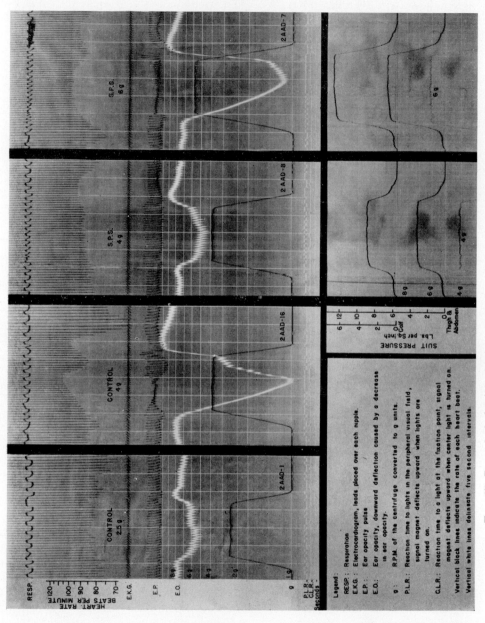

FIG. 87. Record of physiologic changes on a centrifuge. (From the Mayo Clinic)

In general, with unimpaired vision the systolic pressure at eye level remained above 50 mm. of Hg and with a complete loss of vision, it was less than 20 mm. of Hg. At the level of the heart (third interspace) the average decrease in pressure per g increase in acceleration was 4 mm. of Hg systolic and 0 mm. of Hg diastolic. During reduction in g, the pressure at heart level rose 20 to 70 mm. of Hg above the control value.

Lambert (14) conducted studies to determine the role of the retina in the causation of the temporary loss of vision or "blackout" without disturbance of consciousness in aviators exposed to high positive acceleration. He found that at 1 g (normal gravity) temporary loss of vision was produced by application of air pressure to the eyeball using special masks. The effective systolic arterial pressure to the eye (systolic pressure at head level minus the applied eye pressure) at which symptoms occurred was, in mm. of Hg; vision dim, 49 to 30; peripheral vision lost, 32 to 20; and vision completely lost, 21 to 0. These visual changes were the same in latent period and progress of development and occurred at the same level of effective blood pressure as the visual changes that occur at high positive accelerations on the human centrifuge.

On the centrifuge, application of 20 to 30 mm. of Hg pressure to the eyeball lowered by 1 g the acceleration threshold at which visual changes occurred. This pressure corresponds to the fall in systolic arterial pressure per g found to occur at head level during exposure to acceleration. The application of 30 to 40 mm. of Hg suction to the eyeball prevented the occurrence of blackout during exposure to high accelerations. When suction is applied to only one, that eye maintains clear vision while the other "blacks out." These experiments support the inference that the loss of vision (blackout) occurring without loss of consciousness during exposure to high acceleration is of retinal origin.

At the Aviation Medical Acceleration Laboratory, Johnsville, Pennsylvania, the theory of retinal ischemia as the prime factor in blackout has been further substantiated. In the work of Duane (15) a swinging car was constructed so that a seated subject's retina could be observed by an investigator using an ophthalmoscope while lying on his side.

In these positions the subject would black out at 4 to 5 g whereas the observer retained normal vision. In this manner serial illustrations were made showing the retinal changes of a subject undergoing blackout (fig. 88). Three stages of blackout were observed as illustrated in these figures. During the first stage the retinal arterioles began to pulsate as illustrated by the beadlike structure. In stage II the arterioles are completely blanched out. This is the period of blackout when the intraocular pressure equals or exceeds the arteriolar pressure of the retina. Stage III demonstrates the recovery from blackout by the refilling of the arterioles. Direct blood pressure measurements made with the ophthalmoscopic studies indicate that blackout is a direct result of reduction of blood pressure in the head.

At blackout level the ringing of a bell, which the subject turns off in a manner similar to the lights, serves as further evidence that the subject's only failing is one of sight, that he still has adequate circulation for hearing, motor control and consciousness in general. Still higher g levels will, obviously, eliminate even this last bit of circulation to the head. Unconsciousness then ensues. The bell is left ringing, the hands drop from the wheel and the head slumps forward on the chest.

It must be remembered that spinal fluid is also subjected to a dependent pooling force. The rigid character of the cranial cavity, however, prevents the general collapse of all intracranial vessels and spaces so that fluid is maintained in these areas at pressures below atmospheric. This has been well demonstrated by pressure measurements done in studies on goats and cats under accelerative stress.

Studies by Beckman et al. (16) indicated that there was a limit to the displacement of blood from the head. These studies reported that the duration of stress required to produce signs of unconsciousness did not vary significantly for magnitudes of 8 to 15 + g. The authors interpreted their data as suggesting that up to 8 g the amount of blood entrapped within the brain varies inversely with the accelerative stress and at this level the maximum displacement of blood from within the semirigid skull case has occurred. In addition, 16 g as the maximum of a (1

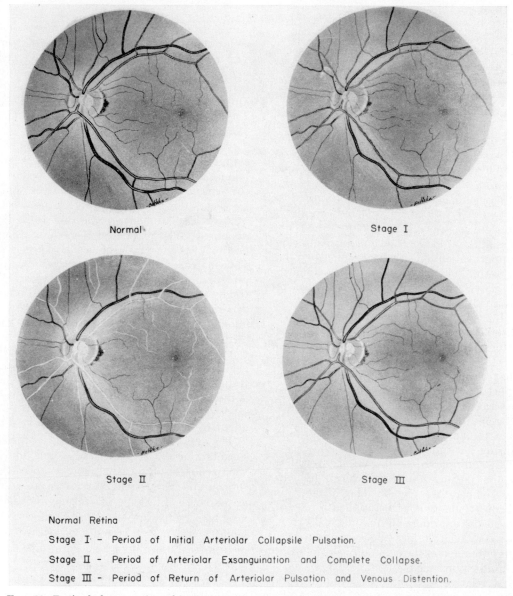

Normal

Stage I

Stage II

Stage III

Normal Retina

Stage I – Period of Initial Arteriolar Collapsile Pulsation.

Stage II – Period of Arteriolar Exsanguination and Complete Collapse.

Stage III – Period of Return of Arteriolar Pulsation and Venous Distention.

Fig. 88. Retinal changes of a subject undergoing blackout. (From *Navy Aviation Medicine Practice*, fig 3.8, p. 38.)

cosine) wave form with a period 25 seconds, which involved 10.5 seconds at over 10 g, was sustained by Gray at Johnsville in April 1958 in the seated upright position immersed in water to eye level (see below). The water immersion does not affect brain distortion within the skull yet no abnormalities were noted.

Studies by Lambert and Slaughter (17, 18) also confirmed the degree of venous pooling in the legs by means of plethysmograph and venous pressure studies. Plethysmography was used to determine to what extent pooling of blood occurs in the lower legs of subjects in a sitting position (heels 7 inches below buttocks) during exposures to positive acceleration causing impairment or loss of vision.

During 15 seconds at accelerations of 2.5 to 4.0 g the increase in leg volume averaged 31 to 42 cc. and the venous pressure in the greater saphenous vein increased by 42 to

60 mm. of Hg. This was 1.3 cc. per 100 cc. of leg tissue at the average blackout threshold (3.7 g). Compensatory recovery of arterial blood pressure began after 5 seconds and recovery of vision after 10 seconds' exposure to acceleration, although, if acceleration was continued the increase in leg volume continued for 45 to 60 seconds. The increase in volume of the lower leg was more closely correlated with the magnitude of acceleration than with the severity of symptoms which an individual experienced. No correlation was demonstrated between increase of leg volume and g tolerance of individuals.

Generally, 45 to 60 seconds' exposure to acceleration was required before venous pressure at the ankle reached a plateau and would support a column of blood sufficiently high to return blood to the heart. A somewhat similar circumstance pertained in measurements of venous pressure in the arm.

Inasmuch as compensatory recovery of arterial pressure and recovery of vision begin after the fifth and 10th seconds of exposure to acceleration, respectively, it is evident that cardiovascular compensation becomes effective despite lack of venous return from at least the more dependent parts of the extremities. This is in harmony with the fact that the amount of blood pooled in the legs during this time is relatively small.

In addition to the degree of arterial and venous pooling, g tolerance can be influenced by temperature effects. The Mayo Clinic group (Code et al. (19)) studied g tolerance in a cool environment (average: 63° F., 72 per cent relative humidity) contrasted with that obtained in the same subjects in a warm humid environment (average: 98° F., 77 per cent relative humidity) and found that in the warmer environment, the over-all g tolerance was lower on the average by 0.8 g. U. S. Navy studies at Pensacola show that sunburn has similar adverse effects on g tolerance.

Lambert (20) confirmed that the physiologic effects produced on a human centrifuge were comparable to those produced in aircraft under similar conditions although the g tolerance of subjects was higher in the aircraft owing to such factors as the excitement of flying, slightly crouched posture, effort of controlling the aircraft when piloting and cooler temperatures.

NEGATIVE ACCELERATIONS

Negative accelerations in aircraft are encountered in certain acrobatic maneuvers such as inverted spins, outside loops, push overs and inverted flight. The human body, being adapted for the upright position, is for all practical purposes normal for $1 + g$. Therefore, $1 - g$ represents a change of 2 g's from the normal.

SUBJECTIVE SYMPTOMS. The subjective symptoms of negative accelerations in the human are successively as follows: At $1 - g$ the sensation is equivalent to that of hanging head downward; namely, a moderate upward displacement of the organs in the abdomen and thorax and a moderate congestion of the face. As the negative acceleration increases there is an increase in the pressure of the restraining belt across the thighs and shoulders but this sensation is generally ignored because of the distress about the head and face. At between 2 and $3 - g$'s the face feels highly congested and there is a throbbing pain throughout the head. Between 3 and $4.5 - g$'s, the congested feeling of the face becomes intense. At this point, there is a sensation of greatly increased intracranial pressure and the skull feels as if about to burst.

The eyes feel as though shoved from their sockets and there is a gritty feeling under the eyelids resulting from congestion of the subconjunctival vessels. Most subjects suffer excessive lacrimation. Occasionally there may be a temporary loss of vision and there have been a few scattered reports that objects appear red and produce the phenomenon commonly referred to as "redding out." There have been some differences of opinion as to whether or not this latter occurs and, if so, its cause. It has been suggested that inasmuch as in negative g there is a tendency for the lower lid to gravitate over the cornea this might cut off vision. This might also explain "redding out" as the result of sunlight filtering through the palpebral tissues. Another possibility is that in very high negative accelerations there may be a staining of the lacrimal fluid with blood as a result of the rupturing of the conjunctival vessels. There is no evidence that this phenomenon is of intraocular or central origin although hemorrhages into the anterior chambers of the eyes have been observed.

Mental confusion develops at these higher accelerations and, in some instances, experimental subjects and pilots in flight have lost consciousness. Following such exposures there is a temporary state of cerebral dysfunction manifested by confusion and the gait may be staggering.

It must be kept in mind that the symptoms described above are influenced not only by the magnitude of negative acceleration, but also by the rate of onset and also the duration of acceleration. Thus, a negative acceleration of 10 g's which lasts only a fraction of a second will result in nothing more than the sensation of severe jolt to the body and a rush of air from the mouth as the viscera of the abdomen compresses the lungs.

OBJECTIVE SYMPTOMS. With negative accelerations of 2 to 3 or more g's of several seconds' duration the skin of the face becomes markedly red and congested and the blood vessels of the nose and cheeks become plainly visible. Numerous small petechial hemorrhages develop beneath the skin of this area and the face and neck appear puffy from an edema which will pit on pressure. The vessels of the conjunctiva stand out prominently, there is lacrimation and small conjunctival hemorrhages may occur.

Jongbloed and Noyons were the first to systematically study the effect of negative accelerations on the circulation and included a determination of the blood pressure changes, electrocardiographic findings, heart volume changes and changes in the volume flow through the major vessels. They noted a great increase in the pressure in the carotid artery and their electrocardiograms showed gross changes including ventricular extrasystoles and a marked bradycardia. By denervating the carotid sinus bilaterally they proved that this reflex was responsible for the slowing of the heart. By x-rays they found that the heart shadow was much smaller during accelerations and that the volume of flow through the carotids was so greatly reduced that some cerebral ischemia resulted in spite of the greatly increased vascular pressure. The work of Jongbloed and Noyons has been confirmed by many others the most recent being the studies by

Henry (21) and Gamble et al. (22, 23). Figure 89 shows extrasystoles, bradycardia, asystoles and other signs of vagal heart block. These observations plus the effect of negative accelerations on the respiration, venous pressure and arterial pressure, as indicated in figure 90, support the theory that disturbances of consciousness in high negative accelerations may be caused by a mechanism similar to the carotid sinus syncope. The work of Beckman and Wechsler (24) suggested that the effects were caused by an inadequate pressure drop across the brain so that stasis occurred with a resultant anoxemia and disturbance of consciousness.

In negative accelerations, the blood pressure rises and the mechanism at work here is apparently as follows: The hydrostatic force produced in the carotid arteries acts in the same direction as the force of the heart and, consequently, there is little inertia to be overcome and both forces contribute to a high pressure. As the arterial blood circulates through the brain within its bony cavity there is no space for free expansion of the vessels and a high intracranial pressure results. The normal tendency for this high pressure to be relieved by an increased velocity of the blood flow downward through the cerebral veins is prevented by the hydrostatic back pressure in these vessels between the brain and heart. At the same time, there is an overstimulation of the carotid sinus owing to the high arterial pressures which induces bradycardia with a fall in the cerebral arteriovenous pressure differential.

Humans at $3 - g$ for 10 to 15 seconds have shown, by an electrocardiogram, a bradycardia of 4 to 6 beats per minute. Rabbits and goats at $5 - g$ have shown temporary cardiac arrest during 30 second centrifuge runs. Respiration is also markedly impaired under negative g. The increased effective weight of the abdomen is thrown onto the diaphragm making adequate inspiration that much more difficult.

Whereas in positive g it seems possible to pool all the blood below the heart, under negative g it appears that the cephalad loop of circulation cannot hold the entire blood volume. This results in a residual venous column of blood acting on the right heart. Enough pressure may be thus produced to

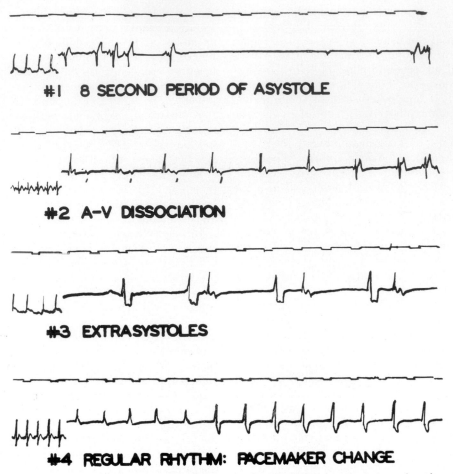

#1 8 SECOND PERIOD OF ASYSTOLE

#2 A-V DISSOCIATION

#3 EXTRASYSTOLES

#4 REGULAR RHYTHM: PACEMAKER CHANGE

FIG. 89. Inkwriter records of electrocardiograms of dogs exposed to negative acceleration showing extrasystoles, bradycardia, asystoles and other signs of vagal heart block. (After Henry.)

precipitate cardiac failure in experimental animals subjected to prolonged negative g.

It was originally assumed that these high pressures in the cerebral vessels would lead to local hemorrhages, however, more recent work has not supported this theory. It has been shown that the skull offers complete support to the blood vessels of the brain and, in addition, that the cerebrospinal fluid pressure also gives support by rising to a corresponding degree.

The rise of the venous pressure in the head correlates very closely with the degree of discomfort and the appearance of capillary hemorrhages about the face. It is this discomfort, or rather the extreme pain suffered, which normally determines the tolerance of an individual to negative accelerations. This usually amounts to 2.5 to 3 g's for a period of several seconds.

Rather recent flight tests of voluntary tolerance for negative g have been reported by Beckman and Wechsler. Maneuvers which developed a maximum stress of $5 - g$ for short periods, $4.5 - g$ for 15 seconds or $3 - g$ for periods of up to 32 seconds were tolerated without difficulty by Rod Jocelyn and other stunt fliers.

TRANSVERSE ACCELERATIONS

Accelerations directed through the antero-posterior axis of the body and through the lateral axis of the body in both the positive and negative directions produce effects which are essentially identical and, for convenience, will be discussed together.

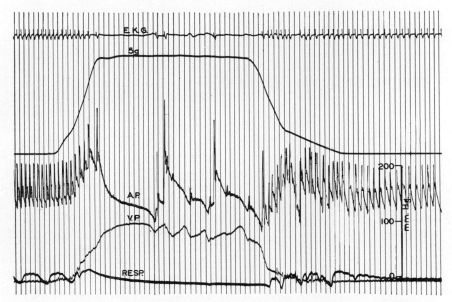

FIG. 90. Simultaneous electrocardiographic arterial and venous pressure recordings, electrocardiogram and respiration in a dog under chloralose anesthesia exposed to $5 - g$. Vertical timing lines indicate ½ second intervals. (After Gamble *et al.*)

SUBJECTIVE SYMPTOMS. Accelerations up to 6 *g*'s, directed across the body, generally produce no subjective effect except for the sensation of increased pressure on the part of the body which supports the weight although an occasional subject will report chest pain at this level. This pressure being distributed over a wide area (all of one surface of the body) does not produce as great a pressure effect as an equivalent acceleration in the long axis of the body inasmuch as in the latter the whole pressure is borne by the seat.

At about 6 to 8 *g*'s inspiration becomes increasingly difficult because of the tendency for the thorax and abdomen to be compressed in a plane perpendicular to the line of force. This compression causes the diaphragm to be displaced upward by the increased intra-abdominal pressure and for the lungs to be crowded by compression of the chest wall. As a defense against this respiratory difficulty the breath is usually held with the thorax in the midinspiratory position. Accelerations up to 12 *g*'s produce no disturbance of vision or of the other senses and the pressure on the well supported body is not unusually uncomfortable.

The point at which breathing becomes difficult varies somewhat according to the direction of force owing to the arrangement of the bony framework of the trunk. The greatest effect is produced when the centrifugal force is directed through the body from back to front (prone position) for in this position the abdomen, with no bony covering and the thorax protected only by elastic ribs, has to support the load of the bony pelvis and the spinal column in addition to that of the viscera. The next greatest effect is produced with the body in the position where the force is directed from before backward (supine position) and the pressure exerted on the spine. Here the abdomen and thorax are compressed in the anteroposterior direction from their own mass.

Although the least effect might be expected in the lateral positions because of the almost complete wall of bone on each side of the abdomen preventing its collapse and the shape of the ribs laterally which resist compression of the thorax considerable discomfort results, particularly at higher *g* levels where the weight of the thoracic spine and upper half of the thorax and shoulder girdle must be borne by the ribs, arm and shoulder on the dependent side.

OBJECTIVE SYMPTOMS. *Respiration and Pulse.* As noted above, voluntary respiration is possible up to 6 or 8 *g*'s after which more inspiratory difficulty is experienced and the breathing may cease involuntarily in the midinspiratory position as a defense against the compression of the abdomen and chest; however, it is possible to continue to breathe at levels of 12 g. The pulse increases a moderate amount proportional to the amount of acceleration but seldom rises above 100 beats per minute.

Blood Pressure. Blood pressure changes generally correspond to those found in positive or negative acceleration except that the distance of a particular part of the body above or below the heart level is considerably reduced and the effects are, therefore, correspondingly modified. In both the prone and supine position the head is at a level above the heart in order to permit forward vision in an aircraft and under positive g blood pressure increases are necessary to compensate. Vision can be maintained at levels of 12 g or more.

TUMBLING AND SPINNING

As previously indicated, accelerative forces usually tend to act in combinations of linear, radial and angular accelerations. This is particularly exemplified in escape from a high speed aircraft where ejection seat stabilization is not achieved. If the seat-man combination tumbles during the deceleration period in the windstream following escape, high alternating positive and negative accelerations can be produced. As the man tumbles the decelerative force will be directed alternately to the opposite end of his body.

Detailed studies of the effects of tumbling and spinning have been accomplished by Beckman and Lambert *et al.* in the Office of Naval Research technical reports, by workers at the U. S. Navy's Johnsville centrifuge and by the U. S. Air Force, notably Edelberg and Weiss.

Another problem involving angular and centrifugal accelerations results when the man is subject to spinning following escape. During spinning the pilot is, of course, subjected to high angular accelerations that can produce vertigo and resultant nausea and vomiting. If at high altitudes, where the pilot is required to use an oxygen mask or is wearing a pressure suit, such an event could

have particularly disturbing if not disastrous results.

In a recent escape from a British Canberra bomber at some 56,000 feet one of the pilots was subjected to a high degree of spinning because of damage of the seat upon ejection. The rate of spinning was sufficiently great that his arms and legs were forced into an extended position and the blood was, in effect, centrifuged into his extremities to a degree so as to cause pain in his arms and hands with some petechial hemorrhages, according to information obtained from the Royal Air Force.

The other effects of angular accelerations which, by stimulation of the semicircular canals, act to produce disorientation in the pilot has been discussed in chapter 15.

PROTECTIVE DEVICES

With positive accelerations, inasmuch as the principal deleterious effects are caused by a drop in blood pressure and a depletion of blood to the brain, anything that would tend to maintain or increase this pressure would act to neutralize these effects. It has been found that tensing the abdominal muscles produces a slight rise of blood pressure in the carotid artery which, however, is not constant and the pressure usually returns to normal in a few seconds. Wood and Lambert (25), of the Mayo Clinic, conducted extensive investigations to evaluate some of the factors that influence g protection. They found that tensing the abdominal muscles or performing a Valsalvan maneuver (fig. 91) would act to temporarily raise the blood pressure. However, these procedures, if continued, tend to greatly reduce venous return to the heart and as a result act adversely in protecting against the forces of acceleration. They found that by tensing of the muscles and straining with forced expiration through a partially closed glottis (M-1 maneuver, fig. 92) that some increased protection could be obtained. This varied from subject to subject and with the skill of performance of the maneuver. The difficulties of the maneuver and the fatigue effects do not make this ideal for use in combat or in gunnery exercises. In the 1930's an abdominal belt was developed by Poppen to aid in increasing the intra-abdominal pressure. This was found

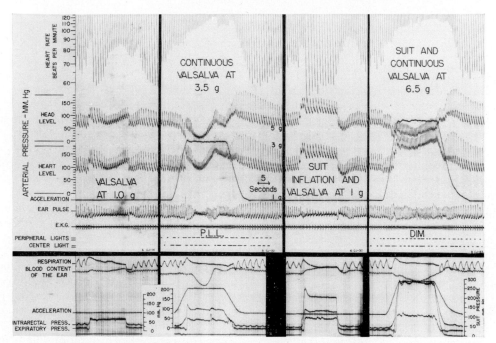

Fig. 91. Comparison of the cardiovascular reactions produced in the same subject by: (*panel 1*) performance of the Valsalvan maneuver while seated at 1 *g*, (*panel 2*) combined performance of the Valsalvan maneuver and exposure to 3.5 *g*, (*panel 3*) combined performance of Valsalvan maneuver and inflation of an antiblackout suit while subject is seated at 1 *g*; and (*panel 4*) combined Valsalvan maneuver, suit inflation and exposure to a positive acceleration of 6.5 *g*. To perform the Valsalvan maneuver, the subject blew against a slowly leaking manometer. The expiratory pressure is an index to intrathoracic pressure. (From Wood and Lambert.)

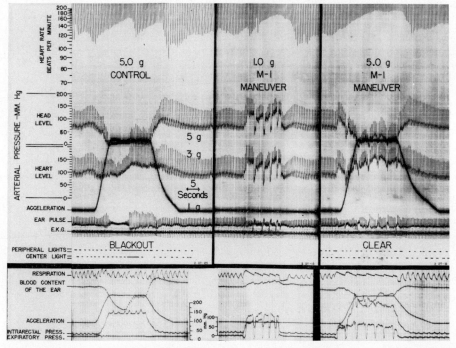

Fig. 92. Comparison of the cardiovascular reactions produced in the same subject by: (*panel 1*) exposure to a positive acceleration of 5*g*, (*panel 2*) performance of the M-1 maneuver when seated at 1 *g*, and (*panel 3*) combined performance of the M-1 maneuver and exposure to 5 *g*. The M-1 maneuver is a series of brief Valsalvan-like maneuvers with tensing of the abdominal muscles and periodically taking a breath to aid return of venous blood to the heart. (From Wood and Lambert.)

to be of value in dive bombing maneuvers as it aided in straining; however, for prolonged accelerations, it would have similar disadvantages to the other straining techniques. The Mayo Clinic group found that application of pressure to the legs as well as to the abdomen was essential in preventing venous pooling and in supporting adequate venous return to the heart. Although application of pressure to the lower extremities alone afforded a barely perceptible amount of protection (average of 0.2 g), this leg pressure combined with pressure from an abdominal bladder increased by a factor of (approximately) two the protection afforded by application of pressure to the abdomen alone.

The present antiblackout suit acts to provide support to the circulation by applying pressure to the legs and abdomen so as to prevent venous pooling and promote venous return to the heart. Various types of anti-g suits were developed and used during World War II by the various air forces. These included the Franks water suit, the gradient pressure suit and the simplified single pressure bladder system in cut-away or cover-all type of suits. These anti-g suits raised the tolerance of pilots to blackout by about 1.5 to 2 g varying with the fit of the suit, the amount of pressure used in the bladders and with the pilot's individual g tolerance. Beyond the actual protection afforded by the suits against visual changes and blackout the suits proved to be even more effective in preventing unconscious episodes. Furthermore, as emphasized by Clark and Christy (26), Navy pilots tested on both the centrifuge and in aircraft reported that the suit reduced their need to strain under g and, as a result, they were able to fly two to three times as much in combat tactics and gunnery practice as formerly because of the antifatigue benefits of the suit. The antifatigue factor should not be overlooked, particularly in modern jet aircraft flying at high altitudes where g maneuvers and turns are generally below blackout levels.

It is most important to realize that sub-blackout g stress, when combined with high altitude effects such as a mild hypoxia, carboxyhemoglobin levels from smoking, possible hypoglycemia, fatigue and other stresses can result in a combined stress of a degree that would interfere with pilot judgment and alertness and, thus, can contribute to subsequent flying or landing accidents. Pilots should, therefore, be encouraged or required to wear anti-g suits whenever possible. This is particularly true for test pilots or pilots of very high speed aircraft as control malfunctions or damage to the aircraft can produce high accelerations unexpectedly.

In aircraft not equipped with anti-g equipment but capable of producing radial accelerations of the order of 3 to 5 g, the factors favorably affecting individual g tolerance, such as a full stomach and good physical condition, should not be overlooked. In addition, the straining maneuvers as outlined above or the assuming of a forward crouch position may be used to protect a pilot in an emergency in the event that a relatively high g maneuver is required.

The forward crouch position, first pioneered by the Germans, is assumed while in the sitting position by raising the knees and feet and bending the trunk forward from the hips. The benefit derived from raising the feet is 2-fold. First, it decreases the vertical distance between the lower limbs and the heart, and second, causes the acceleration force to drive the blood in the thighs toward the heart instead of away from it.

The effect of bending the trunk forward is also 2-fold. By so doing, the vertical distance between the heart and the brain is decreased and second, the acceleration force is directed diagonally across the great vessels of the head and trunk rather than parallel to them.

As indicated above, the crouch maneuver aids in protection against blackout by reducing the height of the hydrostatic column of blood to be supported. As reported by Downey et al. (27), a crouch position that lowered the eye level 11 cm. increased the tolerance of centrifuge subjects to positive acceleration by an average of 1.2 g and this position increased the protective value of an antiblackout suit by some 50 per cent. Similarly, the use of anti-g suits with straining maneuvers can provide increased protection against positive acceleration; however, the protective effects are generally less than simply additive to the protection provided by each device or maneuver separately.

The "water suit," also pioneered by the Germans, is based on the fact that if the body is surrounded by a fluid enclosed in an inelastic container and this fluid has a specific gravity equal to that of the body, then during positive accelerations the hydrostatic pressure in the fluid and that in the body would balance each other; no shifting of the blood in the body would take place and, hence, no blacking out or unconsciousness would occur. The German "water suit" has been described as consisting of a double walled suit enclosing the body up to the level of the neck. The outer layer of the suit is made of inelastic and the inner layer of elastic water proof fabric and the space between filled with water. Test of such a suit was reported by the Germans as being capable of completely counteracting the effects of very high positive accelerations but because of its weight and its hindrance to the movements of the wearer, they concluded that its practical usefulness was doubtful.

Additional efforts to increase the amount of protection by suits include the development of the half full pressure g suit which provided protection of 2.4 to 3 g when tested on the centrifuges at Pensacola and Johnsville (28). This suit, by application of pressure uniformly over a greater area, would be expected to provide increased protection; however, it has not been used in practice as yet owing to problems of valving and of filling times of the suit. Provision of additional protection beyond the level of 3 g by applying pressure to the lower part of the body has been viewed with caution both from the structural limitations of the aircraft and from the potential dangers to the individual as a result of high arterial pressures which might damage the heart or the aortic valves. If anti-g protection were sufficient to prevent the pooling of all the blood below the heart the effects could be similar to those of negative g.

Approaches to additional protection have, therefore, been concerned with utilization of the prone and supine positions which considerably eliminate the hydrostatic column of blood which must be supported under g in the seated position. The body is thus exposed to transverse accelerations. In the prone position, 12 g's can be tolerated without any undue effect. However, in this position with the head elevated sufficiently to provide for forward vision which would be required to operate the aircraft, blackout is experienced within 15 seconds at the 12 g level. In this situation, the distance of the head above the heart, although short, will reduce the arterial pressure at head level sufficient to produce blackout but not unconsciousness. The prone position has the general disadvantage of requiring the pilot, at least in a fighter aircraft, to remain in this position throughout the flight. However, the comfort and head support problems have been considerably improved as a result of work done by the University of Southern California centrifuge group and the U. S. Air Force Aeromedical Laboratory. The Royal Air Force Institute of Aviation Medicine evaluated the prone position in a modified Meteor. The U. S. Air Force developed an experimental prone position fighter and conducted further in-flight studies in other type aircraft.

In the supine position, it is possible for healthy aviators to tolerate 12 g for 1 minute as reported by Stauffer of Pensacola (29). German investigators (30) defined man's tolerance to the supine position at 12 g for 3 minutes and 17 g for 5 seconds in a single experiment performed by Buhrlen. The supine position had been considered to be unsuited for aircraft crews inasmuch as forward visibility would not be possible without the use of such devices as periscopes; however, work by the U. S. Navy at Pensacola and Johnsville (31) utilizing a modified supine position seat which permits an upright position for takeoff and landing and a supine position for high g maneuvers, may offer some advantages. It was demonstrated that a backward tilt position of greater than 77 degrees was required to equal or exceed the protection afforded by anti-g suits. For possible future rocket flights into space where high accelerations must be maintained for considerable periods of time, the use of the transverse positions offer considerable advantage as special suits would not be required and the main limiting factor at 12 to 15 g would appear to be that of difficulty in respiration. Recent work at the Naval Air Development Center, Johnsville, has indicated that levels of a little over 20 g can be tolerated using the combined procedures of

TABLE 42

Chart of Comparative Effects and Tolerances to Various Types and Combinations of Acceleration*

Type of g	Direction of Body Movement	Aircraft Maneuver	Experimental Human Exposures (Maximum)	Physiological Limits, Human	Activities†	AMAL† Centrifuge, Animal Exposures	Animal Pathology
Positive	Head to foot	Pull out or tight turn	8 g for 15 sec. 4.5 g for 5 min. with g suit	Blackout to unconsciousness Pain in legs and blackout	All centrifuges	40 g for 15 sec., chimpanzee	Slight damage with venous congestion, intravascular thrombosis, and leg muscle hemorrhage
		Controlled escape deceleration	15 g for 1.75 sec.	Unconsciousness	AMAL centrifuge	15 g for 60 sec., chimpanzee	Unconsciousness at 9 g on build-up and unconsciousness then confused after run
		Ejection escape (upward)	20 g for 0.1 sec. with face curtain and arm rest	Skeletal damage (spine)	AMEL and WADC ejection tower	40 g for 30 sec., monkey	Slight damage
Negative	Foot to head	Push over	4.5 g for 5 sec. 3 g for 32 sec. with special helmet	Subjective pain Fullness of neck and head, bradycardia	Rod Jocelyn‡ WADC centrifuge	40 g for 30 sec., monkey	Intracranial damage; subcutaneous hematomas about the head
		Ejection escape (downward)	10 g for 0.1 sec. with leg support	Pain	WADC ejection tower	40 g for 15 sec., chimpanzee	Severe damage with hematomas in periorbital tissues, tongue and thyroid gland; venous congestion and intravascular thrombosis with intracranial damage
Transverse supine	Chest to back	Catapult launching	5 g for 2 sec.	No damage	Carrier takeoffs and AMAL centrifuge		
		Escape deceleration or higher launching stress	3 g for 9 min. 31 sec. lying flat	Monotony and giddiness Surface petechial hemorrhage and pain in chest	WADC centrifuge AMAL centrifuge	40 g for 60 sec., chimpanzee	Slight damage with small tear in right tympanum, dulling of patellar reflexes, bruising internally along vertebral column and some clotting along the bronchial blood vessels; no petechiae or hemorrhages
		Crash (facing aft)	55 g for 0.01 sec.; 35 g for 0.12 sec.	Skeletal damage	WADC deceleration track (Col. Stapp)		

Type	Direction	Situation	Human tolerance	Human effects	Facility	Animal tolerance	Animal effects
Transverse prone	Back to chest	Arrested landing	5 g for 2 sec.	No damage	Carrier landings and AMAL centrifuge		
		Escape deceleration or higher landing stress	15 g for 5 sec. with special chest and leg support	Surface petechial hemorrhage and pain in chest	AMAL centrifuge	40 g for 15 sec., chimpanzee	No damage
		Crash (facing forward)	60 g for 0.01 sec. with special harness; 38 g for 0.12 sec. with special harness	Skeletal damage	WADC deceleration track (Col. Stapp)		
Fluctuating positive	Alternating positive and transverse	Uncontrolled aircraft "jostle"	1.5 to 6.5 g for 20 sec. combined with 72 degrees pitch and roll	Additional support required other than conventional lap belt and shoulder harness	AMAL centrifuge	No animal exposures; this type was investigated to determine pilot's ability to actuate controls	
Cyclic	Alternating positive, transverse prone, negative, transverse supine	Uncontrolled escape device "tumbling"	No human experimentation due to severe damage in animal exposures		AMAL centrifuge	15 g and 20 r.p.m., chimpanzee	Fatal: cerebral hemorrhage—3 min. exposure; severe damage with hematoma and hemorrhage—15 sec. exposure
						35 g and 10 to 110 r.p.m. for 10 sec., monkey	Fatal: severe damage with hemorrhage in lungs, spleen and other organs; Necrosis of liver cells and intravascular clotting in all organs; increasing damage with increase in r.p.m.

* Note: g refers to the force on the body in multiples of body weight. Wearing g-suit increases human tolerance to blackout and fatigue. The types of g, transverse lateral and fluctuating negative have not been studied and are not included in this chart.

† AMAL, Aviation Medical Acceleration Laboratory, Johnsville, Pennsylvania; AMEL, Aviation Medical Equipment Laboratory, Philadelphia, Pennsylvania; and WADC, Wright Air Development Center, Dayton, Ohio.

‡ Rod Jocelyn was a stunt pilot contracted by AMAL for negative g maneuvers.

supination to 17 degrees or 10 degrees depending on the individual, plus a *g* suit, plus straining, plus support against sidewise spread of the chest walls. The particular contribution of each of these procedures has not yet been determined. During these studies a sinusoidal variation of *g* as a function of time was utilized. Total time for the run was 54 seconds. Time over 10 *g* was about 28 seconds, over 19 *g* was 10 seconds and between 20 and 20.7 *g* was 6.7 seconds.

If it is essential that an upright position be maintained under such conditions recent work at the Naval Air Development Center, Johnsville, using immersion in water up to eye level, may offer additional possibilities. Under such conditions the circulatory system is fully supported so that the danger of unbalanced pressure above and below heart level is sufficiently reduced provided equalization of pressure in the lungs is also achieved through pressure breathing. Their studies indicated the possibility that air pressure in the respiratory system can be utilized to aid the heart in pumping blood to the eyes and brain against the increased hydrostatic head of the blood brought about by increased acceleration. On the 1 subject tested, holding the breath in this tank of water increased positive *g* tolerance by 13 *g*. The subject's vision was good at the highest levels of acceleration attained (16 *g*). Slight contusions of the pharynx and soft palate owing to rapid and sudden passage of air by these structures limited the *g* level attained.

To protect against negative *g*, air pressure on the head and neck while the subject held his breath has been used at Wright Field (Henry *et al.*). The symptoms of fullness of the face, headache and bradycardia were considerably alleviated by this procedure. No attempt was made to endure more than 5 negative *g* but there is no reason to expect that more could not have been endured.

Recent trends in development of *g* protective devices are mainly concerned with developing mechanical systems to solve the physiologic problems brought to light by research during the period from 1936 to 1956. As the levels of acceleration go higher it becomes impossible for physiologic responses of the body to exert the necessary pressures. Protective procedures, then, are coming more and more to involve mechanical devices. An example of this trend is called the *g* capsule, a prototype protective device now being tested at the Naval Air Development Center, Johnsville. In this device very high pressures are used in the respiratory system to keep blood from intruding into the chest. The subject is kept from expanding by the rigid walls of the capsule. Water between the subject and the walls of the capsule provides for perfect "fit" of the subject within the capsule. Air pressure within the respiratory system not only provides for limiting the amount of blood within the respiratory system but also aids the heart in pumping blood despite increases of hydrostatic head during periods of high acceleration. Between periods of high acceleration respiration is somewhat like that of SCUBA equipped swimmers. During periods of acceleration, a unique automatic system of pumping air in and out of the chest is used wherein the subject and his respiratory system are maintained at constant volume. This procedure is used in order to avoid the interference with circulation which would occur if changes in the volume of the container were permitted during respiration. Special equipment is worn by the subject within the *g* capsule to prevent distorting of his gas filled spaces as the gradient of hydrostatic pressure changes in the water with changes in acceleration. Special glasses permit water pressure to act to support the subject's eyes and yet permit proper vision. Flotation of the subject does not change substantially with acceleration so that he can move quite well at all levels of acceleration.

Future rocket flights from the atmosphere and back offer considerable challenge to the ingenuity of persons developing equipment to protect against acceleration. For example, re-entry into the atmosphere at 2 degrees from the horizontal may limit a vehicle returning from orbit to a maximum level of 9 *g* during a period of acceleration lasting for about 2 minutes. The landing point of such a vehicle can be predicted with an accuracy of a few hundred miles. If the same vehicle were to come straight down through the atmosphere, levels of about 32 *g* would be reached during periods of acceleration lasting for less than a minute. The landing point with a straight down re-entry into atmosphere at escape velocity (about 26,000 miles per hour) would require re-entry accelerations of over 300 g for periods of about 10 seconds. Escape velocity would be attained by a vehicle falling from a practically infinite distance.

First manned space vehicles will most probably use low angle re-entries because of extreme weight limitations which limit structural strength. The acceleration in this situation is caused by a change in speed of the aircraft. Usual positioning of the crew in such an aircraft would provide for transverse acceleration in the prone or supine position. Although in terms of g tolerance there is not much reason to prefer either prone or supine position, the present tendency is to turn the crew around during re-entry so that they will face the rear of the re-entry vehicle. Therefore, during re-entry the crew is expected to be in the supine position. The advantage of supination in this instance is that it is easier to adequately support the crew member in this position than to support him in the prone position. An extreme forward crouch position may also prove to be a satisfactory solution. Gell and Gard (32) and Bondurant *et al.* (33) provide additional information on acceleration in general and to be anticipated in space flight.

Table 42, compiled by the U. S. Navy Aviation Medical Acceleration Laboratory at the Naval Air Development Center, Johnsville, provides comparative information on effects and tolerances to various types and combinations of acceleration.

REFERENCES

(1) DEARBORN, C. H., AND KIRCHBAUM, H. W.: Maneuverability Investigation of an F6C-4 Fighter Airplane. N.A.C.A. Report No. 386 1931.

(2) COCHRAN, L. B., GARD, P. W., AND NORSWORTHY, M. E.: U. S. Naval School of Aviation Medicine Report N.M. 001100.103.03 Pensacola, Florida, 1955.

(3) AUSTIN, F. H.: Unpublished Report to the Aero Medical Association.

(4) GELL, C. F., AND CRANMORE, D.: The effects of acceleration on small animals utilizing a quick-freeze technique. J. Aviation Med., 24: 48–56, 1953.

(5) CODE, C. F., WOOD, E. H., AND LAMBERT, E. H.: The limiting effect of centripetal acceleration on man's ability to move. J. Aeronautical Sc., 14: 117–123, 1947.

(6) WOOD, E. H., LAMBERT, E. H., AND CODE, C. F.: Do permanent effects result from repeated blackouts caused by positive acceleration? J. Aviation Med., 18: 471–481, 1947.

(7) JONGBLOED, J., AND NOYONS, A. K.: Influence of Acceleration upon the Circulation. Arch. ges. Physiol., 233: 67–97, 1933.

(8) ARMSTRONG, H. G., AND HEIM, J. W.: The effect of acceleration on the living organism. J. Aviation Med., 9: 199–214, 1938.

(9) POPPEN, J. R.: Discussion of paper, The effect of acceleration on the living organism. J. Aviation Med., 9: 214–215, 1938.

(10) RANKE, O. F.: Kreislauf unter Beschleunigung. Versuche über die Wirkung der Beschleunigung auf der Zentrifuge an Menchen und Tier. In Deutsche Luftfahrtforschung Jahrbuch. Müchen und Berlin, R. Oldenbourg, 1937.

(11) SCHUBERT, G.: Physiologic des Menchen in Flugzeng. Julius Springer, Berlin, 1935.

(12) CODE, C. F., WOOD, E. H., STURM, R. E., LAMBERT, E. H., AND BALDES, E. J.: The sequence of physiologic events in man during exposure to positive acceleration. Fed. Proc., 4: 14–15, 1945.

(13) LAMBERT, E. H., AND WOOD, E. H.: Direct determination of man's blood pressure on the human centrifuge during positive acceleration. Fed. Proc., 5: 59, 1946.

(14) LAMBERT, E. H.: The physiologic basis of "blackout" as it occurs in aviators. Fed. Proc., 4: 43, 1945.

(15) DUANE, T. D.: Preliminary Investigation into the Study of the Fundus Oculi of Human Subjects Under Positive Acceleration. Naval Air Development Center Report No. NADC-MA-5303, Johnsville, Pa., 1953.

(16) BECKMAN, E. L., DUANE, T. D., ZIEGLER, J. E., AND HUNTER, H. N.: Some observations on human tolerance to acceleration stress. Phase IV. Human tolerance to high positive g applied at a rate of 5 to 10 g per second. J. Aviation Med., 25: 50–66, 1953.

(17) SLAUGHTER, O. L., AND LAMBERT, E. H.: Plethysmographic study of leg volume changes in man during positive acceleration on a centrifuge. Fed. Proc., 6: 203, 1947.

(18) LAMBERT, E. H., AND SLAUGHTER, O. L.: Venous pressure in the extremities of man during positive acceleration on a centrifuge. Fed. Proc., 6: 146, 1947.

(19) CODE, C. F., BALDES, E. J., WOOD, E. H., AND LAMBERT, E. H.: The effect of environmental temperature upon man's G tolerance. Fed. Proc., 5: 18, 1946.

(20) LAMBERT, E. H.: Effects of positive acceleration on pilots in flight with a comparison of the responses of pilots and passengers in an airplane and subjects on a human centrifuge. J. Aviation Med., 21: 195–220, 1954.

(21) HENRY, J.: Personal communication.

(22) GAMBLE, J. L., JR., SHAW, R. S., HENRY, J. P., AND GAUER, O. H.: Physiological changes during negative acceleration. USAF Engineering Division Memorandum

Report No. MCREXD - 695 - 74L, Wright-
Patterson Air Force Base, Ohio, 1948.

(23) GAMBLE, J. L., JR., SHAW, R. S., HENRY,
J. P., AND GAUER, O. H.: Cerebral dysfunc-
tion during negative acceleration. J. Appl.
Physiol., 2: 133–140, 1949.

(24) BECKMAN, E. L., AND WECHSLER, R. L.: Effects of acceleration upon the cerebral
metabolism and cerebral blood flow. Phase
IV. Some observations on negative g developed in aerobatics. Naval Air Development Center. Report No. NADC-MA-5203,
Johnsville, Pa., 1952.

(25) WOOD, E. H., AND LAMBERT, E. H.: Some
factors which influence the protection afforded by pneumatic anti-g suits. J. Aviation Med., 23: 218–228, 1952.

(26) CLARK, W. G., AND CHRISTY, R. L.: Use of
the human centrifuge in the indoctrination of a Navy fighter squadron in the use
of anti-blackout equipment. J. Aviation
Med., 17: 394–398, 1946.

(27) DOWNEY, V. M., LORENTZEN, F. V., AND
LAMBERT, E. H.: Effect of the crouch position on the increase in tolerance to positive

acceleration afforded by an anti-blackout
suit. J. Aviation Med., 20: 289–299, 1949.

(28) LEWIS, D. H.: The g-protection provided by
the full pressure half suit. Naval Air Development Center Report NADC-MA-5511,
Johnsville, Pa., 1955.

(29) STAUFFER, F. R.: Personal communication.

(30) RUFF, S., AND STRUGHOLD, H.: Compendium
of Aviation Medicine. Leipzig, Johann
Ambrosius Barth, 1939.

(31) GELL, C. F., AND HUNTER, H. N.: Physiological investigation of increasing resistance to
blackout by progressive backward tilting
to the supine position. Naval Air Development Center Report No. NADC-MA-5406,
Johnsville, Pa., 30 June 1954.

(32) GELL, C. F., AND GARD, P. W.: Problem of acceleration. In U. S. Navy Aviation Medicine Practice (NAVPERS 10839-A), Navy
Department, Wash., D. C., 1955.

(33) BONDURANT, S., CLARKE, N. P., BLANCHARD,
W. G., MILLER, H., HESSBERG, R. R., AND
HIATT, E. P.: Human tolerance to some of
the accelerations anticipated in space
flight. U. S. Armed Forces M. J., 9: 1093–
1105, 1958.

17

EFFECTS OF LINEAR ACCELERATION

John P. Stapp, M.D.

The orientation of the universe in time and space was first formulated by Isaac Newton in terms of two mathematic correlations derived from observations of the solar system and from experiments with falling bodies. Reasoning from the primitive concepts of time and of a geometric point of origin for generating linear displacement he arrived at a universal principle known as the inverse square law for gravitational forces which states that: Every particle in the universe attracts every other particle with a force that is proportional to the product of the masses and inversely proportional to the square of the distance between the particles.

This means that any two particles free to move in space are drawn toward each other by a force that is an inherent property of their masses and varies directly with mass. This mutual attraction is, therefore, expressed as the product of the masses of the two particles. As the particles approach each other, their speed of motion increase as the attractive force becomes stronger. This attractive or gravitational force varies inversely to the square of the remaining distance between the particles. Expressed as an equation, where f equals gravitational force, m_1 and m_2 are the masses of the respective particles and r represents the remaining distance between the particles,

$$f = \frac{m_1 \cdot m_2}{r^2}.$$

Appropriate units of measurement for force, mass and length are substituted in the terms of this equation when it is used to express real quantities. For spheres of uniform density, the mass is assumed to be at the center. How did Newton arrive at this great concept for explaining the behavior of masses of every dimension, from atomic to solar?

In an experiment with a falling body the time and distance traveled are measured as it drops toward the center of the earth. If the time is measured in seconds and distance in feet while it drops for 5 seconds and assuming that it falls in a frictionless vacuum, the results are as shown in table 43. If the body had fallen at constant speed the distance fallen would be through equal increments per second. This obviously is not the case. To determine by what factor the speed changes from second to second take the distance for the first second and divide it successively into the distances at the end of each second. By inspection of table 44 it can be seen that this factor is the square of the time in seconds for each second of free fall.

We now know that the speed of the falling body changes uniformly through each second of fall because the distance covered per second increases as the seconds squared.

TABLE 43
*Illustration of Falling Body Experiment**

Time (T)	Falling Distance (S)
sec.	feet
0	0
1	16.1
2	64.4
3	144.9
4	253.6
5	402.5

* See text.

TABLE 44
*Illustration of Falling Body Experiment**

Time (T)	Falling Distance (S)	Falling Distance Divided by 16.1 (T^2)
sec.	feet	
0	0	0
1	16.1	1
2	64.4	4
3	144.9	9
4	253.6	16
5	402.5	25

* See text.

TABLE 45
*Illustration of Falling Body Experiment**

Time (T)	Time Squared (T^2)	Distance Fallen (S)	Speed (V)	Acceleration (g)
sec.		feet	feet per sec.	
0	0	0	0	
1	1	16.1	32.2	32.2
2	4	64.4	64.4	32.2
3	9	144.9	96.6	32.2
4	16	253.6	128.8	32.2
5	25	402.5	161.0	32.2

* See text.

Now add a measurement—the instantaneous speed at the end of each second. By inspection of table 45 it is apparent that the speed is increasing by a factor of 32.2 feet per second with each succeeding second. We now know that the acceleration of a falling body is a constant, which is called the acceleration of gravity, designated as g; and that it is 32.2 feet per second per second or change of free fall velocity of 32.2 feet per second squared.

The two constant factors that have ap-peared so far are the distance fallen in the first second and this acceleration constant; they are respectively 16.1 and 32.2 or a ratio of ½ to 1. Looking across the columns of table 45 equations can be formed of the relationships of variables and constants. They can be generalized by using letters to represent the factors.

Let acceleration equal g; distance dropped equal S (it bears a relation of ½ S to 1 g in the free fall data); time equal T (it bears a relation of T^2 to S as noted before); and velocity equal V (it bears a direct relation to the time inasmuch as it increases by a factor of 1 g for each second that passes. Using the letter symbols, the relationships of T, T^2, S, V and g emerge in the following equations:

$$V = g\,T \qquad \text{equation 1}$$

This can be verified by taking any elapsed time in the first column of table 45 and multiplying by g and comparing with measured velocity in the fourth column of the same table.

$$S = \tfrac{1}{2}\, g\, T^2 \qquad \text{equation 2}$$

This can be verified by multiplying any unit under T^2 by ½ g = 16.1 and comparing the result with the third column of table 45 in the same line.

$$g = \frac{V}{T} \qquad \text{equation 3}$$

This of course, is the rearrangement of equation 1 above.
Similarly:

$$T = \frac{V}{g} \qquad \text{equation 4}$$

Each term has been expressed as the relation of the other two terms in this equation. By substituting the value for T in equation 4 into the independent equation 2, it becomes

$$S = 1/2\, g \left(\frac{V}{g}\right)^2 \quad \text{or} \quad S = \frac{V^2}{2\,g} \qquad \text{equation 5}$$

The distance between two points V_2 and V_1 of known velocity measured in free fall can be expressed as:

$$S = \frac{V_2^2 - V_1^2}{2\,g} \qquad \text{equation 6}$$

These equations assumed a constant value for the acceleration of gravity. The measured values vary slightly with differences in local density of the earth. At an altitude of 20 miles from the earth's surface the value diminishes by only 1 per cent in accordance with the inverse square law. The same kind of reasoning regarding the relations of mass, time and distance led Newton to his three laws of motion. These are:

1. Every body continues in its state of rest or of uniform motion in a straight line except insofar as it is compelled by force to change that state.

2. The reaction of a body to a force is directly proportional to it and in the same direction as the force.

3. To every action there is an equal and opposite reaction; or the mutual actions of any two bodies are always equal and oppositely directed along the same straight line.

The resistance of a mass to being moved is termed the inertia, and the resistance of a moving mass to being stopped is the momentum. This momentum is measured by the mass times the square of the velocity. Speed is linear velocity per unit time whereas velocity includes both speed and direction of motion. Change in speed or in direction, or both, is called acceleration.

Acceleration in free fall toward the earth's center is measured in units of 32.2 feet per second per second called g. At right angles to the line of free fall the same unit is used to describe acceleration of a mass by a force. Here the force required to accelerate a body at 32.2 feet per second per second in a straight line is termed 1 g.

This unit measures both the increase and the decrease of linear speed. Decrease of linear speed is called deceleration. In either case the force equals the product of mass times acceleration according to Newton's third law of motion.

1. Velocity equals distance per time unit (feet per second).

2. Acceleration equals velocity per time unit (feet per second squared or g).

3. Jolt equals acceleration per time unit (feet per second cubed or g per second).

Jolt is defined as the rate of change of acceleration or the rate of onset of accelerative force. In a graph of acceleration *versus* time, the slope of increasing acceleration,

or jolt, can attain a spike or a plateau of acceleration (fig. 93). The acceleration curve decays to constant velocity, or in the case of a deceleration, to a stop. In the analysis of a typical deceleration such as is shown in figure 93 the factors defining the event quantitatively are (1) rate of onset, (2) peak or plateau of deceleration, (3) the duration of the peak or plateau and the total duration, from beginning of onset through the end of decay, and (4) the direction or axis of application of force which determines whether acceleration or deceleration occurs. The force, as determined from the product of the known mass and measured acceleration completes the analysis.

In addition to these factors, in the case of a living body the direction and area of force applied and the viscoelastic properties of tissues also play a part in determining the total effect. When reversible limits of these properties have been exceeded structural failure occurs, and in case of living bodies injury and even death may result.

For survival of accidental exposures it is important to correlate these factors with physiologic or anatomic effects of deceleration and to determine what body positions and protective restraints offer optimum safety. Both the analysis of accidents and the carefully instrumented simulation of controlled accidental exposures to decelerative force in experimental increments are essential to answer several important questions. These questions include determination of the voluntary tolerance limit of exposure, finding lethal and injurious limits with animal subjects and most favorable orientation of the body to the axis of applied force. The most favorable orientation as well as the other factors must be determined for every position of the body applicable to vehicular collisions, impacts with the earth or other objects; wind ram decelerations effects of emergency inflight exit from aircraft by ejection seat or capsule; and numerous other situations where uncontrolled decelerations are dangerously high.

A well executed emergency ditching in calm water, where both the speed and the angle of impingement of the aircraft are kept low, will result in a deceleration of less than 10 g's, entirely harmless to the well braced occupants. In a recent accident

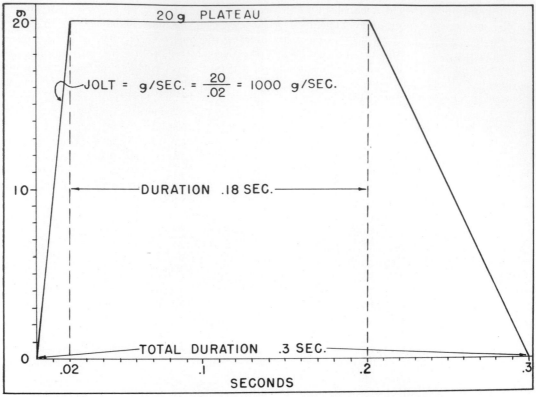

FIG. 93. Diagrammatic representation of jolt (g per second), plateau (g) and duration (second) as they would relate in an accelerometer recording of a crash type decceleration.

a jet bomber nosed in from low altitude at more than 500 m.p.h. Only 19,000 pounds of fragments, none bigger than one man could carry, were all that could be found of the 193,000 pound aircraft. The unidentifiable remains of the three crew members totaled $9\frac{1}{2}$ pounds. Between these extremes are the majority of aircraft crashes, in which, excluding the effects of fire, survivors diminish in number toward the vanishing point as the estimated decelerative forces approach 50 g's. Yet, as will be revealed presently, abrupt decelerations of 50 g's can be sustained without loss of consciousness or injury and impacts of more than 100 g's can be survived. This becomes increasingly important as airplanes fly faster and inevitably crash harder.

Based on observations of accidents and on experimental evidence it can be assumed that the dissipation of kinetic energy in an aircraft crash occurs in $\frac{1}{2}$ second or less. Crash forces are determined by the mass and velocity of the aircraft; their direction is a resultant of the horizontal and vertical components of its angle of impingement against the terrain. The subsequent irregular pattern of deceleration corresponds to the diminishing momentum of the aircraft as its structure fails and the terrain resists its motion by collision and friction. Decelerative forces can be analyzed by determining the following factors: (1) rate of change of deceleration, (2) peak or plateau deceleration, (3) direction of the forces, (4) area of distribution, (5) time displacement and (6) duration.

The forces transmitted to occupants of the aircraft are determined by: (1) their attenuation and absorption by structures intervening between the occupant and areas of the aircraft impinging against the ground, (2) distance and direction of displacement of the occupant, (3) area, configuration and resistance of objects against which the occupant is decelerated, (4) attenuation and absorption of force by the body of the occupant, (5) rate of application of the forces, (6) frequency characteristics and (7) duration.

The problem of evaluating the effect of these factors requires controlled experimental exposure of human, animal and anthropomorphic dummy subjects to crash type decelerations. Progressively augmented combinations of these variables will determine tolerance and survival limits. Simultaneously, the efficacy of various restraint configurations and development of basic principles of crash protection can be explored.

Progress in this field has been limited by the formidable mechanical problems, the difficulties of developing, maintaining and operating experimental apparatus subjected to high impact forces and the hazardous nature of the experiments for human subjects.

In 1946 a competitive design study resulted in the development of a machine to produce abrupt linear decclerations similar to those encountered in crashes, ditchings, parachute opening shocks and rocket power escape capsules. The device consisted of a 1500 pound tubular steel sled slipper mounted on a 2000 foot standard gage track and propelled by one to four solid fuel rockets, each having 1000 pounds of thrust for 5 seconds duration. After accelerating to the required velocity, the sled entered a section of fixed mechanical friction brakes located between the rails in a 50 foot length at a point 1250 feet from the beginning of the track. These brakes were preset in a predetermined sequence and were tripped by cams on the sled. Two parallel keels beneath the chassis were clasped by the closing brakes with an action similar to pulling a knife blade through a vise causing the sled to lose momentum in a controlled reproducible pattern.

The controlled range of operation was from 10 to 60 g by 5 g increments, with durations of 0.08 to 0.42 second, at rates of change of acceleration from 280 to 3400 g per second. The sled could be stopped in less than 20 feet from a velocity of 180 m.p.h., with peak decelerations exceeding 100 g's. Dummy, chimpanzee or human

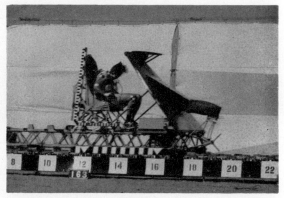

Fig. 94. Rocket powered linear decelerator during full stop in mechanical friction brakes, exposing human subject to 32 g during deceleration from 88.9 miles per hour to a stop in 18 feet. Edwards Air Force Base, 18 October 1950.

subjects, restrained in the configuration and plane of orientation required for a given experiment, were suitably instrumented with accelerometers and strain gages recording through telemetering and were photographed during deceleration by high speed motion pictures and ribbon frame cameras.

Between April 1947 and June 1951 the linear decelerator was operated by its designers, Northrop Aircraft, Inc., for the Aero Medical Laboratory of Wright Air Development Center at Edwards Flight Test Center where a suitable track was available. Seventy-two tests with parachute dummies, 73 human experiments and 88 experiments with chimpanzees were accomplished.

The volunteer human subjects included 3 flight surgeons, 1 pilot, 2 parachutists, 2 harness makers, a medical technician, an aerial photographer, an aerial gunner and an ordnance specialist. One of the flight surgeons was also a pilot. Ages ranged from 25 to 41 years, weights from 142 to 206 pounds and heights from 66.5 to 72 inches. The range of body sizes and somatotypes usually encountered in the Air Force was well represented, considering that only 12 subjects were used in the 73 experiments. The maximum number of exposures to decelerative forces sustained by any 1 subject was 26, including the most severe tests of the series. No sedation or medication of any sort was used with human subjects either before or after tests.

Eighty-eight experiments were accomplished with chimpanzee subjects to explore the performance range of the decelerator and to establish safe parameters for human experimentation with the same equipment. The use of animals of the size and ferocity of chimpanzees was justified by the close approximation to human masses, dimensions and reactions. Subjects were presented to linear decelerations while seated facing forward, seated facing backward, seated facing sidewise, lying supine feet first, lying supine head first and lying transversely across the sled while facing to the rear with the back against the bulkhead.

Human subjects were exposed in the forward facing and backward facing seated positions only. Concurrently with the evaluation of tolerance limits, development of harness configurations was accomplished.

Optimum restraint configuration for the forward facing seated position was proved to be the shoulder straps, lap belt in 3 inch width nylon webbing, with a pair of tie-down straps known as the "inverted V" to hold the belt and shoulder straps down against the bottom of the seat.

It was established conclusively that very high decelerative force can be sustained by primates provided there is adequate protection from collision with solid objects. The maximum deceleration sustained by a chimpanzee in this series was from 174 miles per hour to a stop in 27.5 feet in the supine, head first position. This could have been survived with some temporary disability by a human being. It is many times what would be encountered in any automobile collision or plane crash short of complete demolition of the vehicle.

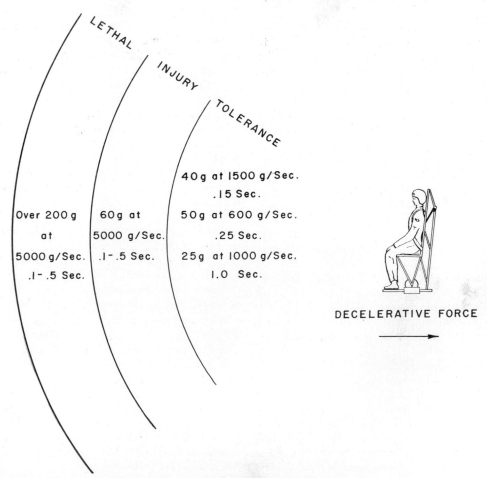

LETHAL

INJURY

TOLERANCE

Over 200 g at 5000 g/Sec. .1 - .5 Sec.	60 g at 5000 g/Sec. .1 - .5 Sec.	40 g at 1500 g/Sec. .15 Sec.
		50 g at 600 g/Sec. .25 Sec.
		25 g at 1000 g/Sec. 1.0 Sec.

DECELERATIVE FORCE

FIG. 95. Lethal, injurious and tolerable limits of linear deceleration with respect to jolt, peak force and duration for man in the forward facing seated position.

In order to evaluate the effects of impacts of high rate of onset and short duration, capable of lethal effects, a device known as a monorail decelerator was developed. The monorail decelerator consists of a welded steel carriage, sliding on and suspended from a lubricated horizontal rail. Propulsion is derived from an aircraft seat ejection catapult. Velocities varying from 15 to 47 feet per second were provided in these experiments by varying the powder charge in the catapault cartridges.

The carriage was decelerated by striking a lead cone attached to a frame welded to the rail. The coefficient of restitution of lead is sufficiently low to result in almost complete absorption of the energy of the carriage, thus minimizing rebound. Variations in the deceleration pattern were obtained by using different sizes of cones.

Electronic chronographs recorded velocity at time of impact. Motion studies were made by high speed cameras. Accelerometers and strain gages on the seat and subject recorded directly through trailing wires to an oscillograph during the 30 foot displacement of the carriage from catapult to impact point.

Experiments were performed with anesthetized hogs as subjects. One series determined the effect of impinging the subject against simulated sections of instrument panel, simulated control wheel surface and control stick. A second series evaluated the protection afforded by lap belt alone, lap belt plus shoulder straps and lap belt combined with shoulder straps and inverted V tie-down straps. Uninjured survival of anesthetized hogs occurred in all experiments up to 80 g in the backward facing seated position and to 125 g in the forward facing seated position.

The comparative vulnerability of chest,

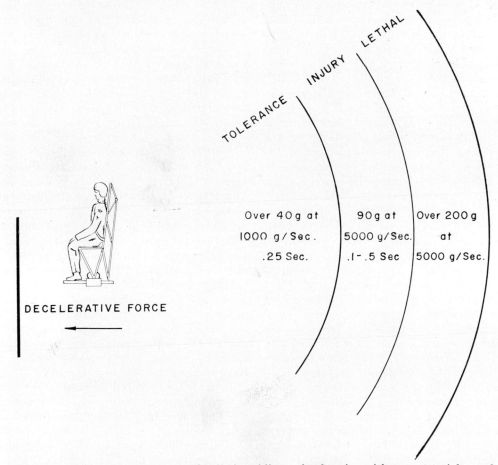

FIG. 96. Lethal, injurious and tolerable limits of linear deceleration with respect to jolt, peak and duration for man in the backward facing seated position.

midriff and abdomen to impingement by the simulated instrument panel section, control wheel and stick were determined in lethal experiments. Forces that could easily be sustained without injury while the subject was restrained with webbing caused death when the subject was impinged against the solid test objects. A total of 52 experiments have been performed with this device.

A more elaborate short track impact type decelerator having the same performance range has been activated at Holloman Air Force Base. It consists of a track 120 feet long with two rails 5 feet apart on concrete piers 3 feet high. A chrome-molybdenum steel sled is slipper mounted between the cylindrical rails and can carry up to 350 pounds of payload at a maximum deceleration of 200 g. Maximum velocity is 150 feet per second. Deceleration can be either with the lead cone method of the previously described monorail decelerator or with a braking piston carried on the front of the sled entering a water filled cylinder by rupturing a frangible stopper and displacing water through orifices in the walls of the cylinder. The orifices can be changed in size or completely closed according to the desired deceleration time pattern. A trailing cable permits direct recording of a large variety of sensing devices. In other respects, the instrumentation is similar to that used in the monorail decelerator. To date over 250 tests have been performed with this device.

Two types of experiments have been carried out at Holloman Air Development Center with a pendulum type decelerator, consisting of a weighted seat suspended like a garden swing, so that it can be elevated and allowed to drop against a test object or to swing until arrested by a snubbing cable. Anesthetized hogs were used in lethal experiments to determine impact damage to the chest and abdomen on collision with a variety of steering wheels; human experiments were done to determine tolerance to deceleration in the forward facing seated position, restrained by a lap belt.

With respect to transverse decelerative forces, accident data on human beings compared with experiments on both hogs and chimpanzees indicate that structural failure points on the chest and abdomen impinged

against a solid hard surface are practically identical. Aortas can be ruptured by a 2000 foot pound impingement of a hog's chest against a conventional steering wheel. Transverse deceleration against a webbing harness that distributes the load on the four quarters of the body indicates very little variation in tolerance, probably less than 10 per cent. It would be a conservative estimate to say that human survival of serious injury begins at two and one-half times the transverse reversible incapacitation point for either forward or backward deceleration. The rate of onset is a potent factor in determining tolerance limit for transverse deceleration. At 6000 g per second and 70 g peak in a 0.13 second duration 1 chimpanzee sustained lung injuries similar to those found in explosion blast. The calculated rate of onset and maximum force of impingement against the harness was 15 msec. to reach 75 pounds per square inch. With rates of onset of less than 1000 g per second up to 150 g peaks have been sustained without injury by chimpanzees.

Lethal experiments with anesthetized hogs indicate that at rates of onset between 5000 and 15,000 g per second, for durations between 0.04 and 0.08 second, up to 125 g could be sustained with reversible injuries, ranging to 220 g for serious to fatal injuries.

With respect to orientation, the human body is almost equally tolerant to deceleration in the backward facing position provided an even, firm backing of energy absorbing material such as a half inch of felt against sheet steel is used. Experiments did not exceed 35 g in this orientation because no higher exposure was required to provide criteria for backward facing passenger seats.

In the vertical axis, human limits of tolerance vary with the alignment and position of the vertebral column. With the column in the erect position and maximum area at apposition impinging between vertebrae forces exceeding 30 g at 500 g per second have been sustained without injury.

If the body is bowed forward to the limit of curving the spine, wedge fractures have been produced by 9 to 14 g at less than 500 g per second in the first and second lumbar vertebrae. They were tilted forward until only the front rims of the vertebral bodies carried the concentrated loading.

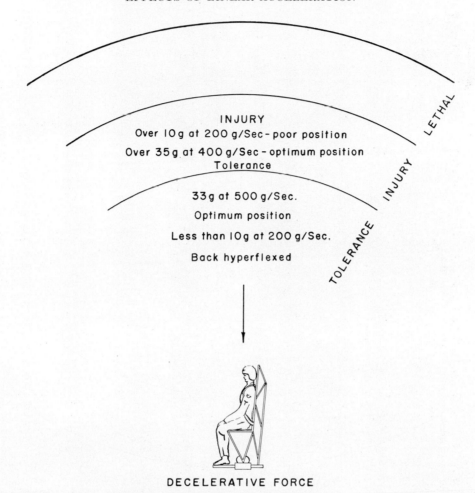

INJURY
Over 10g at 200 g/Sec-poor position
Over 35g at 400 g/Sec-optimum position
Tolerance

33g at 500 g/Sec.

Optimum position

Less than 10g at 200 g/Sec.

Back hyperflexed

LETHAL

INJURY

TOLERANCE

DECELERATIVE FORCE

FIG. 97. Lethal, injurious and tolerable limits of linear deceleration with respect to jolt, peak and duration for man in the upward ejection position.

Human tolerance to linear decelerative force in the forward facing seated position for exposures of less than 0.2 second is primarily determined by the rate of application of force (the third derivative of motion or rate of change of deceleration) and, secondarily, by the magnitude of force provided that the force is applied to the solid quarters of the body through webbing restraints.

In the range of less than 0.2 second duration, tissues react to application of mechanical force by structural damage or failure with no gradients of fluid displacement. Below 0.2 second duration is a refractory period with respect to tissue elasticity and viscosity. This is the time-g area in which tissues behave like inert materials under conditions of mechanical stress analysis where structural damage and failure are independent of displacement effects in the sense of gradients of fluid displacement or tissue deformation. In this area it is the physiologic response to injury that has a tendency to lag and develop progressively long after the application of forces has ceased.

Here the thresholds for reaction to rate of onset and magnitude of forces are related to the physical properties of tissues such as elasticity, viscosity, frequency response, tensile and shearing strength and compressibility and are very high in comparison to centrifuge exposures to forces requiring more than a second for just the build-up to peak magnitude.

By keeping durations below 0.2 second of exposure and varying the rate of applica-

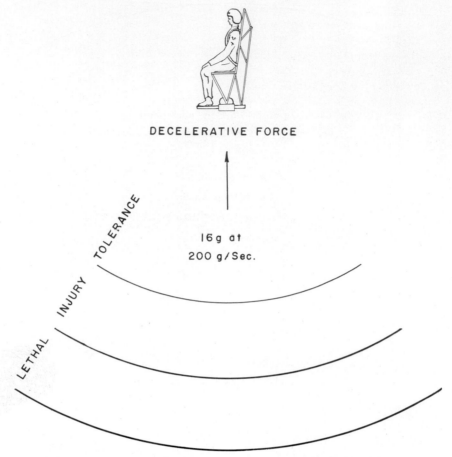

DECELERATIVE FORCE

16g at
200 g/Sec.

LETHAL   INJURY   TOLERANCE

FIG. 98. Tolerable limit of linear deceleration with respect to jolt, peak and duration for man in the downward ejection position.

tion of deceleration up to peak magnitude for a sequence of stepwise increments of force magnitude it was possible to demonstrate a threshold for shock manifested by momentary fall in blood pressure, rise in pulse rate and weakness and pallor, comparable to the reaction of a boxer to a mildly staggering blow. This threshold occurred at the 30 *g* plateau with rate of change of deceleration of 1000 *g* per second. In round figures, a limit of human endurance was reached at 1500 *g* per second and 40 *g* where syncope comparable to a knockout in boxing occurred.

With the rate of application of force at 500 *g* per second or less and durations of less than 0.25 second, the limit of human tolerance for magnitude of force was sought in stepwise increments. Such a limit, de-

noted by moderate shock and signs of concussion during the subsequent 48 hours was attained at more than 45 *g*. The duration was sufficient to produce petechiae of the scleras and a retinal hemorrhage. Consequently, in round figures, 50 *g* at 500 *g* per second rate of onset without exceeding 0.2 second duration can be taken as a magnitude of force limit of endurance.

Hydrostatic pressure effects resulting from displacement of body fluids, have a latent period of 0.2 second before they are appreciable; they are definitely evident at 0.4 to 0.6 second of exposure to as low as 10 *g* at 500 *g* per second rate of application.

Displacement effects are manifested in negative *g* congestion of the head and carotid sinus reflex stimulation at about 15 *g* maintained during 0.6 second. It is possible thus to elicit centrifuge type reactions in about half a second of linear force application.

Human subjects who were accelerated up to 14 g on the centrifuge in the positive g position in less than 3 seconds and promptly decelerated to a stop went through the usual hydrostatic reactions without the gray out or blackout phenomena because duration of arrested circulation to the brain was below threshold for diminishing consciousness by withholding oxygen. The latent period for blackout is no less than 3 seconds.

The duration *versus* g spectrum of the decelerator overlaps that of the human centrifuge in the range above 0.5 second for the decelerator and below 3 seconds for the centrifuge.

This disposes of the no man's land of g time effects previously existing between the centrifuge and the decelerator performance ranges. It becomes evident from the high levels of tolerance found with human volunteers and the extremely high forces survived without injury by animal subjects, chosen for their approximation of human dimensions and weights, that protection of human occupants of aircraft from abrupt crash forces is determined not by human limitations but by airframe dynamic stress limitations.

To evaluate the effectiveness of the passenger safety belt for crash protection and to determine human tolerance limits to abrupt impingement against the belt during deceleration, progressive exposures were made of human volunteer subjects, decelerated while restrained with a lap belt 3 inches in width. They were seated facing forward in three different experimental devices:

1. An aircraft seat hanging by 20 foot cables forming a swing pendulum which could be raised and dropped through a measured vertical component and arrested by a steel cable;

2. A sled, on a 120 foot track, propelled by an ejection seat M1-A1 catapult and decelerated by water inertia brakes; and

3. A catapult accelerating a seat by means of rubber shock cords in an 18 foot distance and decelerating it with mechanical friction brakes in 30 inches or less.

Subjects varied in weight from 128 to 187 pounds, in age from 19 to 45 years and in height from 5 feet 4 inches to 6 feet 2 inches. Physical condition was controlled throughout the study by frequent examinations by the flight surgeon. Therefore, subject selection, which excludes females, children and old people, and the number of tests performed necessarily imposes limits in applying the data on human tolerance to lap belt deceleration.

Decelerative force exceeding 10 g, at a rate of onset of 300 g per second and duration of 0.002 second resulted in minimal contusions over the hip region at lap belt impingement areas. This type of injury is of a minor nature and would not incapacitate the subject or prevent his immediate recovery from the experimental exposure.

In the 13 g range at 300 g per second onset and duration of 0.002 second, in addition to contusions, there may be strain of abdominal muscles with resultant tenderness and soreness. The degree of this injury will vary with the pain threshold and physical condition of individual subjects. Slight injury was produced during these experiments at the 26 g peak at 850 g per second onset with a duration of 0.002 second.

The subject of this test complained of severe epigastric pain persisting for about 30 seconds. Soreness was evident over the thoracic vertebrae which persisted for 48 hours. Roentgenograms revealed no fractures. This deceleration was tolerable for this subject. The force calculated from the weight of the subject times the deceleration is 165 pounds times 26 g equals 4290 pounds of force. Impingement area on the belt was 48 square inches (16 inches in length by 3 inches in width); therefore, average impingement pressure was 89.3 pounds per square inch.

Most air transports are equipped with forward facing seats stressed to about 6 to 9 g and a 2 inch wide lap belt of between 2000 and 4000 pounds break strength. The lap belt alone, used in the forward facing seated position, can permit uninjured survival of exposure to decelerations up to 20 g at a 1000 g per second rate of onset and possibly of higher forces with some degree of injury, if the following conditions can be met:

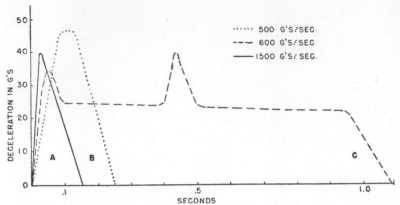

FIG. 99. Human tolerance to linear deceleration limit for reversible incapacitation with respect to jolt, peak and duration in the forward facing seated position. From accelerometer recordings.

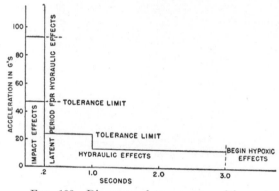

FIG. 100. Diagram of parameters of impact, hydraulic and hypoxic effects of acceleration on man.

1. Belt, seat and all attachments to seat and to aircraft floor are of 20 g strength with adequate safety factor for brief overloads.

2. A minimum clearance of 44 inches between seats is provided so that the passenger does not strike his head on the back of the seat in front of him.

3. The 20 g deceleration must be in the long axis of the cabin and free from violent gyrations and lateral or vertical components that might throw the passenger out of the belt loop or against arm rests.

4. The belt must be tightened properly into the crease of the hips, leaving no slack to apply abrupt overloads to seat attachments.

For all of these conditions to be met simultaneously would indeed be fortuitous, even though 20 g seats, lap belts and at-

tachments with adequate spacing between seats were provided. The tightness or looseness and the position of the lap belt are at the discretion of the passenger as well as his attitude and posture in the seat.

The final requirement, of course, is that the passenger be a young athletic adult, preferably male. Pregnant women, infants, small children, the obese, the elderly and the infirm are not anatomically and physiologically adapted to such violent protection.

The answer is in the use of high strength backward facing seats for which the present lap belt is adequate restraint. In such seats the reclining feature for the back can be retained provided the pivot point is above the center of gravity of the occupant so that crash forces would return the back to the near vertical posture. Head rests should extend above the passengers' heads so that the roof is held away in case the aircraft overturns and caves in.

In the case of a 175 pound occupant applying 300 square inches of back surface to a rear facing seat during deceleration at 40 g, the loading pressure will be $175 \times (40/300) = 23.3$ pounds per square inch. In contrast, consider the case of a 175 pound occupant of a forward facing seat restrained by a 2 inch wide lap belt impinging approximately 20 inches of its length across the anterior aspect of his trunk. Against 40 square inches of belt surface, the occupant will sustain 87.5 pounds per square inch of pressure at 20 g; at 40 g deceleration, 175 pounds per square inch. There is no question that 23.3 pounds per square inch can be sustained against the back surface of the body; 26.7 pounds per square inch has been sustained by a human subject on the decelerator without ill effects.

A high strength, backward facing seat that can be folded out of the way has been designed by the Aircraft Laboratory of Wright Air Development Center and is installed in all aircraft of the Military Air Transport Service. The British have installed high strength, backward facing seats not only in RAF transports but in some domestic airliners. It has been reported that more than 150 passengers have survived uninjured in about half a dozen crashes of aircraft with rear facing seats. Cornell Crash Injury Research published a careful analysis of two RAF crashes of aircraft with rear facing seats, one of a four engine transport in December 1950 and the other of a twin engine plane in February 1951, in which 39 survived, all of them occupants of rear facing seats.

These experimental results and their correlation with the protection afforded in accidents where strength and configuration of seats, belts and attachments were designed to human tolerance specifications indicate the way to prevention of injury and death in aircraft crashes.

Wind Drag Deceleration and Wind Blast

Loss of the canopy or seat ejection at supersonic speed exposes the victim to wind blast and wind drag deceleration which are functions of the air density and the speed, whose combined action is measured as ram pressure. Some conception of ram pressure in relation to speed and altitude is provided by the data compiled by the National Advisory Committee for Aeronautics in table 46.

From this table it is evident that the higher the speed and the lower the altitude, the greater the ram pressure that will be encountered during escape from high performance aircraft. It is evident that one factor over which the pilot can exercise a certain degree of control is that of the altitude at which an attempt to escape is initiated. Ram pressures will be more than four

TABLE 46
Ram Pressure versus Air Speed*

Altitude	Ram Pressure		Total Pressure to 4 Square Feet Drag Area of Man
feet	*p.s.i.*	*p.s.f.*	*pounds*
50,000	1.1	158.5	634
40,000	2.0	288.0	1152
30,000	3.0	432.0	1728
20,000	4.8	692.0	2768
15,000	5.9	850.0	3400
10,000	7.0	1010.0	4040
5,000	8.6	1240.0	4960
Sea level	10.0	1440.0	5760

* Speed = Mach. 0.9 (1000 feet per second or 600 knots per hour at 60° F.).

times as great at 5000 feet altitude as they are at 40,000 feet altitude for the same velocity. Inasmuch as both the deceleration and wind blast experienced in the first second of escape are a direct function of ram pressure, a margin of safety of several hundred per cent can be provided by prompt decision and well drilled reflexes to take advantage of all the altitude possible.

Several emergency escapes and the experiments of Neilson and Sperry have demonstrated that ram pressures of 650 pounds per square foot or better are capable of flailing the arms, legs and head in spite of all muscular effort to oppose the ram pressures. German experiments in World War II with human subjects dipped into wind tunnels demonstrated that exposure of the bare face to wind blast exceeding 400 knots for several seconds can be sustained with slight but reversible injuries to eyelids, nostrils, lips and ears. It is conceivable that supersonic wind blast could apply damaging counter pressure to the lungs or inflate the stomach by pressure through the esophagus.

Another potential hazard of canopy jettisoning at supersonic speeds could be the organ pipe effects of turbulent flow over the cockpit opening and perhaps shock waves of high intermittency with concomitant pressure changes of perhaps 10 per cent of the total ram pressure.

During ejection from a high performance aircraft at 1600 knots and 40,000 feet, a drag force of 1200 pounds per square foot is encountered as the seat and occupant emerge into the supersonic air stream. Assuming a weight of 360 pounds for man and seat and an equivalent drag area of 10 square feet (allowing for a supersonic halo of turbulence increasing drag by 40 per cent of actual area) the initial ram force encountered will be 1200 pounds per square foot times 10 square feet, or 12,000 pounds; this divided by the 360 pounds of weight gives 33.3 g initial deceleration. The decay of wind drag deceleration from such a peak requires 1.5 seconds to values below 5 g. This is in the order of 10 times the duration of a crash deceleration.

In order to achieve velocities in air of ground level density that would be comparable to Mach 1.0 to 3.0 range of velocities at altitudes of 30,000 to 50,000 feet against the thin atmosphere, with respect to wind ram pressures between 1000 and 2500 pounds per square foot; and at the same time, to store enough kinetic energy to permit decelerations in the order of 20 to 40 g for 2.0 to 0.5 seconds duration, duplicating wind drag decelerations of ejection seats in supersonic escape, a new high performance decelerator was developed. Friction brakes were out of the question at the required 500 to 900 miles an hour sled speeds. A track 3500 feet long with rails 7 feet apart, to accommodate a 5 foot wide ditch 14 inches deep formed in the concrete bed between them was available at Holloman Air Force Base. It was designed for a high speed sled braking system consisting of a deflecting scoop under the sled to retard it by inertia of water picked up between impounding frangible dams in the ditch over which the sled passed. A new high performance decelerator to make use of this braking system in order to accomplish the desired performance range was developed.

The high performance decelerator consists of a test sled weighing 2000 pounds carrying the subject and instrumentation, pushed by a propulsion sled on which solid fuel rockets are mounted. The test unit is separable from the propulsion vehicle to reduce the weight considerably and, consequently, the drag required of its water brake in attaining desired high inertia force levels.

Both vehicles are mounted on dural slip-pers with stellite bearings, surrounding the rail head. The two units are propelled along the track by solid fuel rockets and, subsequent to rocket burnout, are retarded by water brakes. The chrome-molybdenum steel tubing test sled is of sufficient size to accommodate a single test subject in one of several configurations, an onboard telemetry system, high speed cameras and the water brake.

Both sleds have fixed scoop water brakes mounted under the chassis. Water entering the scoops on the test sled is turned 90 degrees through conduits and ejected to the sides. A retarding force of approximately 1 pound for each pound of water passing through the conduit is applied to the sled. The propulsion sled also has fixed scoops but of lower clearance so that braking begins at a shallower depth of water. The U-shaped conduits on this sled turn 180 degrees, throwing water forward during deceleration. About 2 pounds of retarding force results from each pound of water passing through them. The lower clearance scoops and higher retarding forces provided by the 180 degree turn in the ducts on the propulsion sled insure its immediate separation and retardation apart from the test sled, which enters water brakes at a safe interval beyond the propulsion sled and is decelerated in the predetermined inertia force pattern required for the subject or article being tested.

The sled instrumentation consists of inboard high speed motion picture cameras aimed at the subject, and a maximum of 12 channels of Bendix FM-FM telemetering adaptable to appropriate sensing devices such as strain gauge accelerometers, bonded strain gauge tensiometers, wind pressure pickups, electrocardiograph pickups and electroencephalograph leads.

Stationary instrumentation includes the Sleran time-distance recorder, consisting of parallel units each 10 feet along the track. Each unit is a tuned circuit triggered by a focused radio frequency source mounted on the sled as it passes over the Sleran unit actuating it in 1 msec. Velocities are determined with an accuracy of plus or minus 1 foot per second at 1000 feet per second.

An optical method of slightly lower accuracy is used as a secondary check on velocity. This consists of a sequence of ribbon frame cameras at fixed stations with overlapping coverage parallel to the track. High speed motion picture cameras at 750 frames per second are available to record events in particular positions along the track, such as the water brakes.

Propulsion power is obtained by use of from 1 to 12 solid fuel rockets of 4500 pounds thrust and 5 second duration. Following acceptance tests during which the high performance decelerator successfully withstood 110 g at 5000 g per second rate of onset during 0.1 second exposure to 300,000 pounds of water brake force while going from 273 knots to 43 knots in 30 feet, chimpanzee and human experiments on simultaneous exposure to wind blast and simulated wind drag deceleration were performed.

The culminating human experiment was accomplished at the maximum performance possible with 5 seconds of acceleration to still leave sufficient track distance for water brakes to maintain deceleration over 25 g for more than 1.0 second. The sled was actually stopped only 32 feet from the far end of the track.

In order to provide some insight into the reactions and effects encountered in a combined wind blast and wind drag deceleration simulation of an escape by ejection seat at 1600 knots and 40,000 feet, this experiment is reported in detail. It was accomplished on 10 December 1954. Wind blast exposure was obtained by mounting the subject on a seat on the front deck of the sled, using no windshield. The subject's head was inclosed in a wind-proof fiber glass helmet with plexiglass visor, secured to the headrest. Teeth were protected with a bite block of plastic formed to the dental impression. A standard wool flying coveralls, flying gloves and low quarter shoes completed the equippage. Six thousand pound test mylon, 3 inch wide webbing in double thickness was used for shoulder straps, chest belt, lap belt and inverted-V tie down. One thousand pound test 1 inch webbing was used to lash the feet to the foot rest, hands to the subject's knees and elbows to the back of the seat. These restraints were to prevent flailing of head and extremities. A pitot tube was mounted on the platform of the sled im-

mediately in front of the subject's knees and two motion picture cameras were mounted at the front, pointing back toward the subject. Propulsion was by nine rockets totalling approximately 40,000 pounds thrust for 5 seconds.

Upon reaching maximum velocity of 937 feet per second (562 knots) 0.1 second was allowed after burnout before the sleds were separated by entry of the propulsion vehicle into water brakes. In 0.3 seconds from burnout the test sled entered the first water brake after being decelerated by wind drag and rail friction from a speed of 937 feet per second (562 knots) to 857 feet per second (508 knots) in a distance of 310 feet, at between 5.5 and 16.8 g. Water brakes were entered by the test sled 3080 feet from the start of the track. The rate of onset was 600 g per second, going from 12.9 to 35 g as recorded by the accelerometer over the sternum of the subject. A plateau oscillating at values above or below a mean of 25 g occurred immediately after the initial spike of 35 g in 0.4 seconds from the start of deceleration, a second spike of 40 g with 0.08 seconds, returning to the plateau of 25 to 27 g for a total duration of a little more than 1 second, with decay to a stop in a total of 1.1 seconds during deceleration from 857 feet per second (508 knots) in a distance of 380 feet. The total stopping distance from point of maximum velocity of 937 feet per second (562 knots) was 690 feet; the test sled went from maximum velocity to a stop in 690 feet and 1.4 seconds. For 1.1 seconds of this time, deceleration was a value greater than 25 g, including two peaks of 35 and 40 g, respectively.

Immediately after the run (see table 47) the face of the subject was flushed a bright red. Respiratory effects were gasping, occurring approximately every 5 to 8 seconds. When the face piece was opened (approximately 20 seconds after the run) the subject's face began to turn cyanotic, then a deep purple. He first removed the mouth piece. There was a marked, bilateral exophthalmos.

When asked how he was, he replied weakly: "I'm all right." When not spoken to, the subject's head would fall forward as if there was a temporary loss of conscious-

TABLE 47

*Physical Examination Data for Run No. 21,
10 December 1954*

	Before	After
Temperature	99.0° F.	98.4° F.
Blood pressure	134/80	Shock levels
Pulse	110/ min.	80 to 100/min.
Respiration	20/min.	6 to 8/min.; in 1 minute, 18
Ophthalmo-scopic	Normal	See text
Neurologic	Mildly hyper-active	See text
Urinalysis	See text	See text

ness. During the period of several minutes required to remove the straps it was noted that on the exterior surface of the upper left eyelid there was a hematosis bleb. Both upper and lower conjuctivas were covered with large and small petechiae. At this point the subject complained that he could see only light, and had serious difficulty opening his eyelids, apparently because of edema. With the release of the right chest strap the marked facial cyanosis subsided and the subject's respiration increased with a normal pattern of one each 2 to 3 seconds.

Upon release of the harness it was noticed that the subject was quite limp. Inasmuch as an obvious cyanosis remained an effort was made to give him oxygen. The subject refused to accept it, mumbling, "I'm all right." He was apparently still confused and was unable to support his own weight owing to marked skeletal-muscular weakness and relaxation. He insisted upon attempting to walk to the stretcher from the sled. Approximately 5 minutes after the run the subject was placed in the ambulance on a stretcher.

At this time, the facial cyanosis had reduced to about normal color. The finger nails showed a normal color and the subject talked more freely. Some confusion remained, however, inasmuch as he was unable to recount the events of the run in proper sequence. Vision check showed that he was capable of counting fingers; he claimed that he had normal vision when he opened his eyelids. By this time the marked exophthalmus had been replaced by a periocular edema which was increasing.

When the subject was examined at the hospital, about 30 minutes following the run, the lateral half of the bulbar conjunctiva of both eyes showed massive quill hemorrhages. The palpebral conjunctival petechiae had coalesced to a form of almost complete ecchymotic coverage of the palpebral conjunctival surfaces. Examination of the right fundus shortly after arrival at the hospital showed a normal disc with no evidence of retinal hemorrhage within the quill area or hemorrhage in the anterior chamber. The subject stated at this time that the retinal areas felt as if the discs choked immediately after the run.

There were areas of ecchymosis across the shoulders and strap bruises across the thighs. There were numerous fine petechiae above a line sharply demarcated by the upper border of the tight chest strap. These extended across the antero-posterior chest, shoulders, neck and face. The tip of the nose showed marked edema; ecchymosis of the periorbital tissues began to become apparent. There was no noticeable vascular trauma of the buccal mucosa.

The subject mentioned later in the afternoon that bright red blood passed from the nose, presumably from the frontal sinuses. He also stated that there was no headache following the run; however, a sense of fullness and congestion in the anterior cerebral areas and the front of the face were noted.

Examination of the eye grounds the following day revealed normal retinal areas with some cloudiness of the anterior chamber.

Reflexes remained hyperactive during the day after the run. Within 5 days after the incident, the patient was discharged and returned to duty.

The subjective report records the following:

An hour and 20 minutes was required to fasten all harness components and adjust the helmet. The straps were pulled unusually tight. The chest strap was tightened in the last 20 minutes of this time, and was pulled tight enough to restrain all rib motion and breathing. The diaphragm only was used in breathing from that time until the chest belt was removed at the end of the run. The subject recalls taking in about half a breath and holding it from the count down of 5 until the end of the run, or for about 12 seconds. Allowing for the absence of a windshield, which would heighten the impression of speed, the acceleration was noticeably greater and the thrust of the seat against the subject's back more violent than in any previous run. The concrete ditch, which was clearly in focus between the rails before motion began, became a blurred image owing to inability to focus and perhaps to vibration of the head rest and helmet. At about the count of 2 vision narrowed to the central fields only and by the count of 3 there was a visual blackout. This was strictly confined to the eyes with no decrease in consciousness or feeling at this point.

At the instant of burnout the pressure of acceleration against the back instantly disappeared as forces were reversed, and the wind drag and rail friction effects decelerated the sled in the power off phase at about 5.5 to 16.8 g. The instant that forces reversed and harness pressure could be felt on strap impingement areas, there was a very rapid transition from black to yellow in visual perception, followed by a brief view of the track and water brakes, somewhat like a stroboscopic flash, before entry into the water brakes threw the subject's body violently forward against the harness. Up to this point there is a vague recollection of wind pressure being felt as a fluttering of the shoulders of the coveralls but without buffeting or unpleasant sensation.

On entry into the water brakes, the face immediately felt congested with severe pain around the eyes, as though they were being pulled from the sockets. Vision became a shimmering salmon colored field with no images—evidently the pupils were impinged against the stretched upper eyelids and the visual sensation was caused by light coming through the lids. The congestion and pain increased noticeably during the exposure to more than 25 g for more than 1 second. Sensation in the eyes was somewhat like the extraction of a molar without an anesthetic. This pain was sufficient to over-ride sensations caused by impingement on harness straps even though later abrasions and contusions were visible at all strap pressure areas.

When the sled stopped the visual impression of shimmering salmon color not only persisted but was present when the eyes were forced open. There was a marked exophthalmos which made it difficult to open the eyes without using the fingers. The chest strap was so tight that it was extremely difficult to breathe. Mental confusion like that of struggling against the onset of anesthesia was present. As soon as the chest strap was loosened and the bite block removed, normal respirations were possible and the confusion diminished. There was no loss of consciousness at any time. A piece of cotton, apparently soaked with spirits of ammonia, was rubbed on the nose but the nasal passages were blocked and there was no sensation of smell. An oxygen mask was pressed on the subject's face but was rejected with the request that the attendants hasten to loosen the straps. The subject insisted that he was all right merely wanting to get out of the seat.

After the straps were removed the subject stood up but could not see to get off the sled. He was picked up by attendants and put on a stretcher. The congestion of the eyes then receded sufficiently to permit return of vision in an estimated $8\frac{1}{2}$ minutes after the run. Central vision returned first, then peripheral, by glimpses of intermittent patches of the sky which gradually persisted and coalesced into normal visual fields. There was diplopia on moving the eyes with gradual convergence if they were fixed on an object. This persisted for about 3 hours. Enroute to the hospital there was pain in the eyeballs that was at first considered to be caused by increased intraocular tension but this responded later to treatment with cold packs. There was no fuzziness of vision or sensations of retinal spasms as had been experienced in 1951 following a run in which a retinal hemorrhage occurred. Aside from congestion of the nasal passages and blocking of paranasal sinuses, hoarseness and occasional coughing from congestion of the larynx and the usual burning sensation from strap abrasions, there was a feeling of relief and elation in completing the run and in knowing that vision was unimpaired.

A wind pressure of 1108 pounds per square foot was encountered at the maximum velocity attained during approximately 6 seconds of exposure; deceleration of 600 g per second rate of onset, peaks respectively of 35 and 40 g, rising from a plateau of 25 g, was sustained during 1.1 seconds of a total 1.4 seconds from rocket burnout.

Verification of this simulated ejection occurred on 26 February 1955, when production test pilot George Smith of North American Aviation, escaped by ejection seat from an F-100 fighter in a vertical dive at 670 knots and 6500 feet altitude. At Mach 1.1, wind ram of 1240 pounds per square foot subjected him to more than 50 g initial deceleration. Intense shock wave bombardment following jettisoning the canopy caused him to loosen shoulder harness and bend over as he ejected. Subsequent flailing and prolonged negative deceleration as he emerged with chest pressed to his knees caused congestion and conjunctival hemorrhages comparable to but much more severe than the signs and symptoms elicited during the experiment reported above. No fractures were sustained. Shock was profound and prognosis grave for 18 hours following the ejection. Subsequently surgery was required for adhesions and perforation of the distal ileum. Six months after the accident he was able to return to test flying F-100 production models.

Using a small, streamlined sled especially designed for wind blast exposures at speeds above 900 miles per hour, anesthetized chimpanzees were subjected to wind ram of more than 2000 pounds per square foot. Exposure in 50 msec. was obtained by jettisoning a windshield at maximum speed, for comparison with continuous exposure during the run.

At a ram pressure of 2040 pounds per square foot, the anesthetized chimpanzee subject with head and face inclosed in a windproof protective helmet and body protected by one layer of cotton, canvas coverall suit, suffered no consequences. Sonic booms were heard as the sled traversed the speed of sound and shock wave patterns were impinged in the sand on either side of the track at the point of transonic speed. The velocity of Mach 1.2 at ground altitude of 4000 feet which resulted in the 2040 pounds per square foot exposure corresponds to Mach 2.3 at 40,000 feet and Mach 2.9 at 50,000 feet. This caused no injury to chimpanzees either during abrupt exposure

in 50 msec. or with continuous exposure during the run.

These experiments indicate that with adequate restraints to prevent flailing and exclusion of wind by an inclosing helmet to protect facial openings, abrupt, or buffeting, or continuous wind pressures can all be sustained without injury provided the wind drag deceleration curve can be mitigated by attenuating onset and peaks with corresponding increase of duration, for ejections in the performance range of Mach 1.0 to Mach 3.0 at 40,000 feet. It is important to note that the wind drag deceleration problem is changed only in degree by inclosing the crew member in a capsule which affords over-all protection from exposure to wind blast.

SPACE FLIGHT ACCELERATIONS

The feasibility of manned space flight in ballistic missile vehicles is dependent on human tolerance to prolonged linear accelerations of magnitudes comparable to the highest radial accelerations briefly sustained in aerodynamic flight. Some conception of the required linear time g programs for reaching orbital or escape velocities can be gained from current experience with artificial unmanned satellites put into orbit by ballistic trajectories.

An artificial satellite must be accelerated to approximately 8 kilometers per second (4.97 miles per second) before centrifugal force comes into equilibrium with the mass of the satellite to attain a circular orbit 200 to 250 kilometers (125 to 155 miles) above the earth. A constant linear acceleration of 828 g seconds is required to reach this velocity. Escape velocity of 11 kilometers per second (6.83 miles per second) can be attained in 1152 g seconds of constant linear acceleration.

These two calculated constant g second acceleration values can be divided by any chosen duration to give the corresponding acceleration required for that duration. For example, 2, 4, 6 or 8 minutes of acceleration, respectively, would require constant values of g as shown in table 48. Human tolerance to combinations of time g have been investigated on the human centrifuge. It was found that front to back application of force

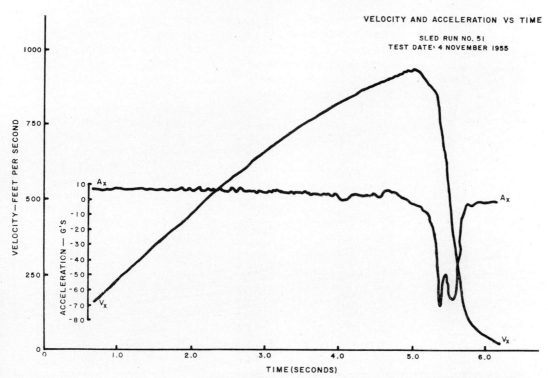

FIG. 101. Typical velocity and acceleration-deceleration record from a high performance decelerator experiment exposing a chimpanzee subject to more than 50 g.

with the knees bent and head elevated slightly in a seated subject positioned to face the center of the centrifuge offered the optimum orientation for prolonged exposure.

The most efficient trajectories for attaining orbital or escape velocity make use of three or more stages of rocket propulsion. Each stage accelerates at a constantly increasing rate as fuel burns off diminishing the mass to be accelerated and as distance diminishes the pull of gravity. The result is a succession of accelerations to maximum at burnout followed by abrupt decay in the pauses between stages.

A family of curves for three stage rocket accelerations corresponding to time g patterns of existing missiles capable of orbital or escape velocity were simulated on the centrifuge to determine tolerance of optimally positioned human volunteers by Bondurant and Clarke in 1958. Rate of build-up of acceleration varied from 0.1 to 8 g per second in reaching three successive peaks of 8, 10 or 12 g, with duration of each simulated stage adjusted to obtain a final

TABLE 48

Time Acceleration for Orbital Escape Velocities

Minutes	g to Orbit	g to Escape
2	6.90	9.6
4	3.45	4.8
6	2.30	3.2
8	1.73	2.4

velocity of 8000 meters per second (18,000 feet per second), allowing 15 to 25 per cent excess exposure to acceleration owing to mechanical lag in stopping the centrifuge.

Tolerance limits were determined subjectively when volunteers lost peripheral vision, were unable to breath or felt pain of an intensity that impaired judgment or performance. Within these limits a subject would be expected to see, think and exercise finger control, although accuracy and competence of coordination and judgement remain to be evaluated. Experience with the centrifuge and motivation were appreciable factors. Continuous acceleration of 8 g or

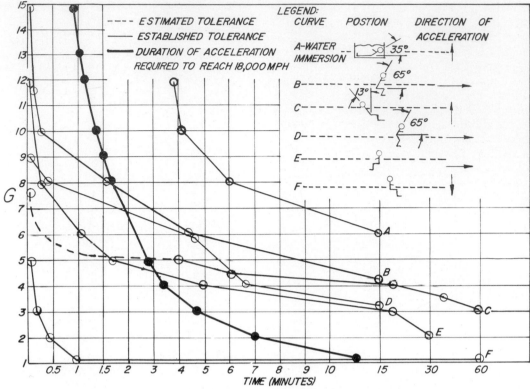

Fig. 102. Time-*g* tolerance to simulated space flight accelerations on the centrifuge. (From Bondurant and Clarke)

more is limited by blackout or dyspnea. Three *g* could be sustained for 1 hour if the rate of build up to 3 *g* is gradual enough to allow reflex cardiovascular compensatory mechanisms to adjust incrementally. With semisupine subjects immersed in a water tank on the centrifuge, tolerance to duration of maintained accelerations of 6, 8, 10 and 12 *g* were reported by Bondurant and Clarke. A skin diver's valve mounted under water at chest level delivered air for respiration at a pressure equal to the hydrostatic pressure against the chest wall. For the immersed subject, a 35 degree angle of the trunk to the line of force was optimal. Tolerance to acceleration was definitely greater, both for duration and magnitude of exposure to acceleration, than in air. The most significant difference was in the ability to move extremities freely under water compared to limiting movement to wrists and fingers during corresponding acceleration in air. Petechiae on feet occasionally observed during acceleration in air were absent even at 12 *g* during submerged exposure.

In the optimally positioned subject even the three successive peaks of 12 *g* sustained for durations to attain orbital velocity can be withstood in air; submerged protection need not be resorted to unless protection from much higher inadvertent accelerations, as in steep re-entry from orbit is required.

Accelerations up to 4 *g* can be tolerated in chest to back, back to chest or foot to head directions for durations that would reach escape velocity.

One recent unreported experiment exposed a human volunteer to 2 *g* for 24 hours during which he was able to eat, sleep and accomplish tasks. The physiologic, psychologic and anatomical adaptability of man to accelerative force encompasses the conditions of space flight adequately. Two *g* sustained linear acceleration for 24 hours would attain a velocity of 3,795,757 miles per hour. At the opposite end of the spectrum is man's endurance to 50 *g* for ¼ second of abrupt linear deceleration.

The viscous-elastic properties of living tissues react to abruptly applied force by deformation against the inertia of the portion still at rest. Tissue distortion against accelerative force relates to resonant frequency response of elastic masses to rate of application of force. Reversible limits of deformation in living tissues and related disturbance of their vital functions determine injurious or lethal effects of accelerative force factors of rate of application, magnitude and duration along a given axis.

Human survival of the hazards of high velocity transportation in ground, air or space vehicles depends on statistical probabilities of exposure to these factors and the effectiveness of protective measures against them.

REFERENCES

(1) BONDURANT, S., CLARKE, N. P., BLANCHARD, W. G., MILLER, H., HESSBERG, R. R., JR., AND HIATT, E. P.: Human tolerance to some of the accelerations anticipated in space flight. U. S. Armed Forces M. J., **9**: 1093–1105, 1958.

(2) EIBAND, A. M., SIMPKINSON, S. H., AND BLACK, D. O.: Accelerations and Passenger Harness Loads Measured in Full-Scale Light Airplane Crashes. Lewis Flight Propulsion Laboratory, Cleveland, Ohio. Washington, D. C., NACA Tech Note 2991, 1953.

(3) FERENCE, M., JR., LEMON, H. B., AND STEPHENSON, R. J.: Analytical Experimental Physics, Ed. 2. Chicago, University of Chicago Press, 1957.

(4) LEWIS, S. T., AND STAPP, J. P.: Human tolerance to aircraft seat belt restraint. J. Aviation Med., **29**: 187–196, 1958.

(5) RUFF, S.: Brief acceleration, less than one second. German Aviation Medicine, In World War II, pp. 584–586. Washington, D. C., U. S. Government Printing Office, 1950.

(6) STAPP, J. P.: Effects of mechanical force on living tissues. I. Abrupt deceleration and windblast. J. Aviation Med., **26**: 268–288, 1955.

(7) STAPP, J. P., AND HUGHES, C. D.: Effects of mechanical force on living tissues. II. Supersonic deceleration and windblast. J. Aviation Med. **27**: 407–413, 1956.

(8) STAPP, J. P.: Crash protection in air transports. Aeronautical Engineering Rev., **12**: 71–78, 1953.

(9) STAPP, J. P.: Human tolerance to deceleration. Am. J. Surg. **93**: 734, 1957.

(10) STOLL, A. M., AND MOSELY, J. D.: Physiologic and pathologic effects in chimpanzees during prolonged exposure to 40 transverse. g. J. Aviation Med., **29**: 575, 1958.

18

EFFECTS OF ACOUSTIC ENERGY

Horace O. Parrack, Ph.D

The primary tools of aviation, aircraft, propulsion systems, ground maintenance equipment and facilities, have produced acoustic energy (sound waves, noise and mechanical vibrations) since the first airplane flight was made. However, it was the World War II demand for large numbers of high performance aircraft that focused attention upon the adverse effects of aviation noise upon personnel. During World War II the effect of noise on communication was the primary concern. Noise interference to communication is still a major problem for personnel operating aircraft, riding as passengers, performing aircraft maintenance or conducting business near a busy airport.

Following World War II, the rapid development of larger, more speedy aircraft with their more powerful propulsion systems increased the adverse effects of noise on man. Damage to the ear, interference to communication, disturbance to movement, nausea and other nonauditory effects are pressing problems today. Parrack (1–3) has analyzed these problems and suggests a program to obtain solutions for the problems that is based upon the interactions among these components of a functional system: (1) acoustic energy sources, (2) acoustic energy transfer media (paths) and (3) men as receivers of acoustic energy. This approach emphasizes the fact that relief from the adverse effects of aircraft noise on man must be sought by an integrated attack made by a scientific and technical team consisting of aviation medicine specialists, acoustical engineers, physicists, aircraft and engine design specialists and many other specialists.

Inasmuch as one primary responsibility of the aviation medicine specialist is to insure that aviation work environments are compatible with good health, effective performance, comfort and general well being, this specialist must assume leadership of the necessary technical team and initiate a program to reduce or to control the adverse effects of aviation noise on the men who conduct the operations. Thus, the aviation medical specialist becomes responsible for developing a broad, integrated program in preventive occupational medicine. This chapter should provide an insight into the problems and furnish data for use in organizing and carrying out the required preventive medicine program.

It is convenient to use certain symbols when discussing effects of noise on man. Certain of these may not be familiar to all readers and accordingly, an alphabetical list of the symbols used in this chapter is given immediately below. All symbols are defined in the text except the three which are defined in the list.

List of Symbols Used in Text

db = decibel.
EPS = equivalent point source.
HTS = hearing threshold shift.

284

IL = intensity level or sound intensity level.

MAF = minimum audible field. This term is applied when describing the sound pressure level for threshold hearing when the tests are made in a free field. The pressure is measured when the listener is out of the sound field. Listening may be by one or both ears. The sound field may be described as a random field, sound waves coming from all directions simultaneously, or as a directional field where the sound comes to the ear from some specified direction.

MAP = minimum audible pressure. This term is applied when describing the sound pressure level for threshold hearing when the signal is presented using an earphone and earphone cover. Tests are usually made on one ear at a time.

OASPL = over-all sound pressure level.

OBSPL = octave band sound pressure level.

PTS = persistent threshold shift.

PWL = power level.

SAM = standard air mass.

SC = speech communication. The symbol for these words is usually used with the word criteria or criterion as, for example, SC criteria. The symbol is also used with numbers as, for example, SC-40, to denote, as in this case, an application of SIL-40 as speech communication criterion.

SIL = speech interference level.

SMS = standard measurement sphere.

SPL = sound pressure level.

TS = threshold shift.

TTS = temporary threshold shift.

Measuring and Describing Acoustic Energy Fields

Solid bodies executing oscillatory motions (mechanical vibrations) force nearby air particles to make similar oscillations (sound waves). The amplitude of such motions may be constant or highly variable in time. The energy contained in these oscillatory motions, either mechanical vibrations or sound waves, is *acoustic energy*. Acoustic energy produced by aviation equipment must be measured and quantitatively described before one can predict man's responses to it. One must be familiar with certain acoustic principles to interpret the descriptions of acoustic energy fields or to measure and de-scribe them. First, let us learn how to measure sound waves.

Sound Fields of Simple Sources

A simple source of acoustic energy, here-after called an "equivalent point source" (EPS), is used to explain essential acoustic principles. The "equivalent point source" (EPS) is a tiny sphere (balloon) that can pulsate, that is, expand and contract so that its surface moves, first outward and then inward, through a constant small distance from a position of rest. The movements of the sphere's surface, from its position of rest to the position of maximum outward displacement and then to the position of maximum inward displacement followed by a return to its position of rest, constitute one complete cycle of motion. The EPS repeats this cycle of motion any desired number of times each second. Now, locate the EPS in the center of a large body of air, hereafter called the "standard air mass" (SAM). The SAM is, at a constant pressure, equal to the mean atmospheric pressure at sea level and its temperature and water vapor content are constant, at specified values. Now, the acoustic impedance (resistance to organizing the motions of air particles into sound waves) of the SAM is constant and the EPS is far enough from solid surfaces to avoid reflections of sound waves.

Generation of Sound. As the surface of the EPS expands, the air particles touching it are pushed against other, nearby air particles. The pressure in a small volume of air near the EPS rises above the mean pressure of the SAM. As the surface of the EPS contracts, air particles near it spring apart and the pressure in the same small volume of air falls below the mean pressure of the SAM. The movements of the surface of the EPS have produced small, alternating motions of the air particles first in one direction then in the opposite direction. These motions of the air particles are accompanied by a local rise and fall in pressure (above and then below the mean pressure). These moving air particles strike adjacent air particles and force them to make corresponding motions. These motions are also accompanied by local pressure oscillations. By these processes a sound wave is generated and is then propagated throughout the total volume of air.

FREQUENCY. Inasmuch as the EPS can make any desired number of cycles of motion in 1 second let it complete 500 such cycles. Each cycle of motion of its surface induces a cycle of rarefaction and compression in the air and 500 such cycles occur each second. The frequency of the sound wave generated by the EPS is 500 cycles per second (c.p.s.).

SPEED OF SOUND. The sound wave, consisting of local and very short, oscillatory motions of air particles accompanied by alternating compressions and rarefactions of the air, spreads outward from the EPS at a specific speed. At sea level air pressure and room temperature this speed is about 1100 feet per second. One second after the EPS initiates a sound wave it can be detected 1100 feet away. The speed of a sound wave is independent of its frequency and sound waves of 100, 1000 or 10,000 c.p.s. travel at the same speed.

WAVELENGTH. The relations between the speed of a sound wave and its frequency give rise to the concept of wavelength. Wavelength equals the speed of sound divided by the frequency; the wavelength of a 100 c.p.s. sound wave is $1100/100 = 11$ feet and that of a 1000 c.p.s. sound wave is $1100/1000 = 1.1$ feet. The wavelength is the distance between the peaks of two successive waves or it is the distance the wave travels in the time required to complete one cycle of motion or pressure variation.

STRENGTH OF THE SOUND WAVE. As the surface of the EPS moves about its position of rest nearby air particles move back and forth. The total distance they move (the amplitude of their motion) is one measure of the strength of the sound wave. The motions of the air particles are accompanied by an alternate rise and fall of pressure of the adjacent air. The total pressure variation, above and below the mean air pressure (the pressure amplitude), also is a measure of the strength of the sound wave. Points on the surface of the EPS follow a specific velocity pattern which is imparted to the air particles touching the surface. The air particle velocity is another measure of the strength of the sound wave.

ENERGY IN A SOUND WAVE. If the strength of a sound wave is measured farther and farther from the center of the EPS the more distant measures are smaller. To explain this, another measure of sound wave strength is introduced, namely, energy. If force is applied to a body at rest and the body remains at rest, no work is done. If the body moves, work is done and an equivalent amount of energy is expended. Work is measured in terms of force times the distance through which it acts.

Work (ergs) = force (dynes) × distance (cm.)

Energy, the capacity for doing work, is numerically and dimensionally identical with work.

The sound wave set up by the EPS moves away from it in all radial directions. The first condensation is itself a sphere just slightly larger than the EPS. As the sound wave moves farther away, the spherical surfaces that are the sites of successive condensations and rarefactions of the air become larger and larger. If the energy remains constant, the energy density or the energy per unit area must decrease because the same energy is spread more and more thinly over larger and larger surfaces. The surface area of a sphere is related directly to the square of its radius. This rule coupled with the notion of constant energy is the basis of the inverse square law. The law states that sound intensity decreases inversely as the square of the distance from the sound source. The intensity is simply the energy that flows through a unit area per unit of time, but energy (joules) per time (seconds) is power in watts. Intensity, expressed in watts per square centimeter, is equal to the power (watts) per area (square centimeter). Sound intensity decreases as the surface of the sphere on which it is measured is located farther and farther from the source. If we measure intensity at a point on the surface of a sphere and multiply it by the area of this surface, we obtain the total power passing through the spheric surface. This power is the rate at which work is done—energy per unit time. The surface of a sphere, hereafter called the "standard measurement sphere" (SMS), is used whenever the total acoustic power output of the EPS is measured. The surface area of the SMS is 1000 sq. cm. (approximately 1 square foot) and its radius is 8.9 cm. (approximately 0.282 foot). When the EPS generates sound in the

SAM (acoustic impedance is constant) the power flow per unit area (watts per square centimeter) is directly proportional to the square of the sound pressure per unit area (dyne per square centimeter) and the acoustic power flow per unit area can be computed by squaring the measured sound pressure.

DIRECTIONAL RADIATION. Sound waves generated by the EPS propagate outward in all directions. Sound pressures measured at all points the same distance from the center of the EPS are identical. The EPS is a "nondirectional" source; that is, it radiates acoustic energy uniformly in all directions within the SAM. Now, let a very rigid, hemispheric, steel case enclose one-half of the EPS (sphere). Let the free edge of the steel hemisphere coincide with a vertical plane that passes through the center of the EPS. Now, only the free (nonenclosed) hemispheric surface of the EPS can pulsate because the steel case prevents motions of the encased part. Face the EPS so that its moving surface lies to your right. The free, right half of the EPS generates sound waves which travel out into the space to your right but no sound waves are present in the space opposite the rigid steel case. This modified EPS is "directional" because more sound energy is radiated in some directions than is radiated in other directions.

The total acoustic power radiated by the "nondirectional" EPS can be computed from one measurement by multiplying the power per unit area by the area of the SMS. Likewise, the total acoustic power radiated by the "directional" modified EPS can be computed (approximately) from one measurement because it is known that exactly one-half of the surface of the EPS generates sound. The total acoustic power output of the modified EPS is the product of the power per unit area and one-half the area of the SMS.

Measuring the Sound Fields of Simple Sources

Sound fields usually are measured by pressure sensitive microphones that have been calibrated by applying known pressures to their diaphragms and recording the resulting electrical outputs. These calibrations are made for the desired range of pressures and frequencies and entered on a calibration chart. Unknown sound pressures are meas-

ured by recording the responses of the calibrated microphone to them and reading the pressure values from the calibration chart. Standard commercial sound measuring instruments usually are designed to include the calibration factors and to indicate sound pressures directly. Their calibration must be checked frequently.

SOUND PRESSURE. Let the EPS generate a 500 c.p.s. sound wave and also let it generate this wave at five different arbitrary sound pressure levels. Measure the sound pressure, for each step, using a calibrated microphone located at any point on the SMS. By your measurements these five sound pressures (in dynes per square centimeter) were found: 0.0002, 0.0004, 0.0008, 0.002 and 200. They are uniform over the entire SMS.

SOUND PRESSURE LEVEL. The sound pressures of interest in aviation may range from 0.00002 to more than 200,000 dynes per sq. cm., a total pressure variation greater than 10 billion to one. Therefore, the numbers used to record either the sound pressures or their ratios are large and hard to manage. To reduce these difficulties engineers have developed a special notation, the decibel (db), to describe sound pressures. When this notation is used the term "sound pressure level" (SPL) is used instead of sound pressure. Let us see how db units are used to describe sound pressure in terms of SPL.

When using db, the observed (measured) sound pressure is always compared to a specific, known pressure called the "reference pressure." The SPL in db is equal to 20 times the logarithm (to the base 10) of the ratio of the observed sound pressure to the reference sound pressure. This relation is expressed as follows:

$$SPL \text{ (in db)} = 20 \log_{10} \frac{p \text{ (observed)}}{p \text{ (reference)}}$$

$$= 20 \log_{10} \frac{p \text{ (observed)}}{0.0002 \text{ dyne}} \text{ per sq. cm.}$$

The reference pressure, 0.0002 dyne per sq. cm., used in the formula above is frequently used in acoustics and is the one used for all SPL computations in this chapter. Let us describe five measured sound pressures as

SPL in db. For the first measurement (0.0002 dyne per sq. cm.):

$$\text{SPL (db)} = 20 \log_{10} \frac{0.0002}{0.0002}$$

$$= 20 \log_{10} 1 = 0: \qquad \text{SPL} = 0 \text{ db}$$

For the second measurement (0.0004 dyne per sq. cm.):

$$\text{SPL (db)} = 20 \log_{10} \frac{0.0004}{0.0002}$$

$$= 20 \log_{10} 2 = 6: \qquad \text{SPL} = 6 \text{ db}$$

For the third measurement (0.0008 dyne per sq. cm.):

$$\text{SPL (db)} = 20 \log_{10} \frac{0.0008}{0.0002}$$

$$= 20 \log_{10} 4 = 12: \qquad \text{SPL} = 12 \text{ db}$$

For the fourth measurement (0.002 dyne per sq. cm.):

$$\text{SPL (db)} = 20 \log_{10} \frac{0.002}{0.0002}$$

$$= 20 \log_{10} 10 = 20: \qquad \text{SPL} = 20 \text{ db}$$

For the fifth measurement (200 dynes per sq. cm.):

$$\text{SPL (db)} = 20 \log_{10} \frac{200}{0.0002}$$

$$= 20 \log_{10} 10^6 = 120: \qquad \text{SPL} = 120 \text{ db}$$

The SPL in db is not always positive, for example, the smallest sound pressure of interest was given as 0.00002 dyne per sq. cm. and we have:

$$\text{SPL (db)} = 20 \log_{10} \frac{0.00002}{0.0002}$$

$$= 20 \log_{10} \frac{1}{10} = -20: \quad \text{SPL} = -20 \text{ db}$$

Let us examine the sample computations of SPL for general relations. When the ratio, measured pressure to reference pressure, is 1, the SPL is zero db; when it is 2, the SPL is 6 db; when it is 4, the SPL is 12 db; when it is 10, the SPL is 20 db; when it is 10^6, the SPL is 120 db; and when it is $\frac{1}{10}$, the SPL is -20 db. In general, if two sound pressures are equal the difference between their SPLs is zero. If one sound pressure is two times another the SPL of the higher pressure is 6 db greater than that of the lower, for example, a sound pressure of 200 dynes per sq. cm. = 120 bd and one of 400 (2 × 200) dynes per sq. cm. = 126 db. Likewise, when one sound pressure is one-half another pressure, the SPL of the lower pressure is 6 db less than that of the higher pressure. Similar relations hold for the other pressure ratios and the corresponding SPLs, for example, when one SPL is 20 db greater than another the higher sound pressure is 10 times the lower. These relations hold throughout the db scale.

One further generalization, any pressure may be used as a "reference" and the relations above hold, however, the selected *reference pressure must be stated*. Also, a particular SPL can be used as a reference SPL and other measured SPLs referred to it. The SPL at three positions, near a sound source, are measured and they are: position 1 = 125 db, position 2 = 100 db and position 3 = 140 db. Then relative to position 1, position 2 is −25 db and position 3 is +15 db; or relative to position 3, position 1 is −15 db and position 2 is −40 db. (Additional information on measuring sound fields has been published (4–7) and tables for computing the SPL in db are also available (4).)

SOUND INTENSITY. When a sound wave is generated by the EPS in the SAM, the sound intensity (in watts per square centimeter) is directly proportional to the square of the sound pressure per unit area. Applying this relation to five measured sound pressures gives the five sound intensities shown below:

Sound pressure = 0.0002 dyne per sq. cm.; sound intensity = 10^{-16} watt per sq. cm.
Sound pressure = 0.0004 dyne per sq. cm.; sound intensity = 4×10^{-16} watt per sq. cm.
Sound pressure = 0.0008 dyne per sq. cm.; sound intensity = 16×10^{-16} watt per sq. cm. = 1.6×10^{15} watts per sq. cm.
Sound pressure = 0.002 dyne per sq. cm.; sound intensity = 100×10^{-16} watt per sq. cm. = 10^{-14} watt per sq. cm.
Sound pressure = 200 dynes per sq. cm.; sound intensity = $10^{12} \times 10^{-16}$ watt per sq. cm. = 10^{-4} watt per sq. cm.

SOUND INTENSITY LEVEL. Sometimes db are used when comparing sound intensities. When the db notation is used the term "sound intensity level" (IL) is also used. The IL in db is equal to 10 times the logarithm (to the base 10) of the ratio of the unknown sound intensity to a reference sound intensity. This relation is expressed as follows:

$$\text{IL (in db)} = 10 \log_{10} \frac{I \text{ (observed)}}{I \text{ (reference)}}$$

$$= 10 \log_{10} \frac{I \text{ (observed)}}{10^{-16} \text{ watt}} \text{ per sq. cm.}$$

The reference intensity, 10^{-16} watt per sq. cm., used in the formula above, is one standard reference intensity used in acoustics. Under many practical conditions it is equivalent to the reference pressure employed to compute the SPL in db. Let us express the five sound intensities given in the preceding section as IL in db.

$$\text{IL (db)} = 10 \log_{10} \frac{10^{-16} \text{ watt per sq. cm.}}{10^{-16} \text{ watt per sq. cm.}}$$

$$= 10 \log_{10} 1 = 0: \qquad \text{IL} = 0 \text{ db.}$$

$$\text{IL (db)} = 10 \log_{10} \frac{4 \times 10^{-16} \text{ watt per sq. cm.}}{10^{-16} \text{ watt per sq. cm.}}$$

$$= 10 \log_{10} 4 = 6: \qquad \text{IL} = 6 \text{ db.}$$

$$\text{IL (db)} = 10 \log_{10} \frac{16 \times 10^{-16} \text{ watt per sq. cm.}}{10^{-16} \text{ watt per sq. cm.}}$$

$$= 10 \log_{10} 16 = 12: \qquad \text{IL} = 12 \text{ db}$$

$$\text{IL (db)} = 10 \log_{10} \frac{100 \times 10^{-16} \text{ watt per sq. cm.}}{10^{-16} \text{ watt per sq. cm.}}$$

$$= 10 \log_{10} 100 = 20: \qquad \text{IL} = 20 \text{ db}$$

$$\text{IL (db)} = 10 \log_{10} \frac{10^{12} \times 10^{-16} \text{ watt per sq. cm.}}{10^{-16} \text{ watt per sq. cm.}}$$

$$= 10 \log_{10} 10^{12} = 120: \qquad \text{IL} = 120 \text{ db}$$

Examination of the computations above and those of the section on "Sound Pressure Level" shows the SPLs and ILs expressed in db are the same when the power flow per unit area corresponds to the square of the pressure per unit area. The coefficient of the logarithm for computing SPL is "20" and that for computing IL is "10." Let us see why this is so. The power flow per unit area is directly proportional to the square of the pressure per unit area and the formula for computing SPL may be written:

$$\text{SPL (db)} = 10 \log_{10} \frac{(p \text{ observed})^2}{(p \text{ reference})^2}$$

and using a numerical example;

$$\text{SPL (db)} = 10 \log_{10} \frac{(200)^2}{(0.0002)^2}$$

$$= 10 \log_{10} \frac{40,000}{0.00000004}$$

$$= 10 \log_{10} 10^{12} = 120: \qquad \text{SPL} = 120 \text{ db}$$

This SPL is the same as that obtained by the original computation. Now, the logarithm of any *number squared* is equal to *two times* the logarithm of the number. We then, remove "2" from its exponent position after the pressure ratio and multiply the coefficient "10" by the "2" to give,

$$\text{SPL (db)} = 20 \log_{10} \frac{p \text{ (observed)}}{0.0002 \text{ (reference)}}$$

ACOUSTIC (SOUND) POWER. The sound intensity of the EPS is expressed as power per unit area (watts per sq. cm.). To measure the total power radiated into space by the EPS the power per unit area is multiplied by the surface area of the SMS, that is, 1000 sq. cm. The total power radiated by the EPS for each of five intensities is, therefore:

1×10^{-16} watt per sq. cm. $\times 10^3$ sq. cm.

$$= 10^3 \times 10^{-16} \text{ watt} = 10^{-13} \text{ watt}$$

4×10^{-16} watt per sq. cm. $\times 10^3$ sq. cm.

$$= 4 \times 10^3 \times 10^{-16} \text{ watt} = 4 \times 10^{-13} \text{ watt}$$

16×10^{-16} watt per sq. cm. $\times 10^3$ sq. cm.

$$= 16 \times 10^3 \times 10^{-16} \text{ watt} = 16 \times 10^{-13} \text{ watt}$$

100×10^{-16} watt per sq. cm. $\times 10^3$ sq. cm.

$$= 100 \times 10^3 \times 10^{-16} \text{ watt} = 100 \times 10^{-13} \text{ watt}$$

$10^{12} \times 10^{-16}$ watt per sq. cm. $\times 10^3$ sq. cm.

$$= 10^{12} \times 10^3 \times 10^{-16} \text{ watt} = 10^{12} \times 10^{-13} \text{ watt}$$

Power is a measure of the rate at which work is being done (energy per unit time). The powers computed above are measures of the rate at which work is done by the EPS in organizing the air into sound waves. These sound powers also are available to act upon receivers (either men or equipment).

ACOUSTIC POWER LEVEL. The total acoustic power generated by a source is frequently expressed in decibels (db), and then the term "power level" (PWL) is used instead of acoustic power. The PWL in db is equal to 10 times the logarithm (to the base 10) of the observed acoustic power to a specified, "reference" acoustic power. The relation is expressed as follows:

$$PWL \text{ (in db)} = 10 \log_{10} \frac{W \text{ (observed)}}{W \text{ (reference)}}$$

$$= 10 \log_{10} \frac{W \text{ (observed)}}{10^{-13} \text{ watt}}$$

where W is the acoustic power in watts. The PWLs in db for five total power outputs are:

$$PWL \text{ (db)} = 10 \log_{10} \frac{10^{-13} \text{ watt}}{10^{-13} \text{ watt}}$$

$$= 10 \log_{10} 1 = 0: \qquad PWL = 0 \text{ db}$$

$$PWL \text{ (db)} = 10 \log_{10} \frac{4 \times 10^{-13} \text{ watt}}{10^{-13} \text{ watt}}$$

$$= 10 \log_{10} 4 = 6: \qquad PWL = 6 \text{ db}$$

$$PWL \text{ (db)} = 10 \log_{10} \frac{16 \times 10^{-13} \text{ watt}}{10^{-13} \text{ watt}}$$

$$= 10 \log_{10} 16 = 12: \qquad PWL = 12 \text{ db}$$

$$PWL \text{ (db)} = 10 \log_{10} \frac{100 \times 10^{-13} \text{ watt}}{10^{-13} \text{ watt}}$$

$$= 10 \log_{10} 100 = 20: \qquad PWL = 20 \text{ db}$$

$$PWL \text{ (db)} = 10 \log_{10} \frac{10^{12} \times 10^{-13} \text{ watt}}{10^{-13} \text{ watt}}$$

$$= 10 \log_{10} 10^{12} = 120: PWL = 120 \text{ db}$$

RELATIONS AMONG MEASURES OF THE SOUND FIELDS OF SIMPLE SOURCES. The total acoustic power output of practical, acoustic energy sources is frequently expressed as PWL. However, the sound pressure or the SPL at a particular position near the practical source, usually are the measures desired. These measures can be obtained from the PWL only when specific relations exist. Let us examine certain relations among the measures of the sound fields of simple sound sources. The sound pressure generated by the EPS was 0.0002 dyne per sq. cm. at the surface of the SMS. The corresponding sound intensity was 10^{-16} watt per sq. cm. The total radiated acoustic power, obtained by multiplying the intensity (10^{-16} watt per sq. cm.) by the surface area of the SMS, 10^3 sq. cm., was $10^{-16} \times 10^3$ watt or 10^{-13} watt. The computed SPL, IL, and PWL were zero

db. In another case the computed SPL, IL, and PWL all were 120 db. When the acoustic measures are made on the surface of the SMS the SPL, the IL and the PWL (in db) always are identical.

When the radius of a measurement sphere differs from that of the SMS the SPL and the IL (db) are not equal to the PWL. For example, let the radius of a measurement sphere be 89 cm. (2.82 feet). The ratio of this radius to that of the SMS is 10, and in accord with the "inverse square rule" the intensity decreases by the factor "10^2" to 10^{-18} watt per sq. cm. and the sound pressure decreases by the factor "10" to 0.00002 dyne per sq. cm. and the IL and SPL are -20 db. The total acoustic power still is 10^{-13} watt and the PWL is zero db. The SPL and IL are identical but their value differs from that of the PWL. Now, retain the same measurement sphere (radius length 89 cm. or 2.82 feet) and allow the EPS to increase its output to 20 dynes per sq. cm. The SPL is now 100 db. The intensity is $10^{10} \times 10^{-16}$ watt per sq. cm. and the IL is 100 db. The SPL and the IL are identical. The total acoustic power is $10^{10} \times 10^{-16}$ watt per sq. cm. $\times 10^5$ sq. cm. (area of sphere) = 0.1 watt and the corresponding PWL is 120 db. Note that the PWL differs from both the SPL and IL. Usually the PWL differs from both the SPL and the IL, as these examples show.

If an EPS radiates sound into the SAM the difference between the SPLs for two positions, at different distances from the EPS, equals 20 $\log_{10}$ distance to position 1 divided by distance to position 2. This relation combined with the relation of identity of SPL and PWL on the surface of the SMS provides a formula for computing SPL from PWL and *vice versa*. When the PWL is given, the SPL at any distant position is computed as follows:

$$SPL = PWL - 20 \log_{10} \frac{d}{0.282}$$

where d is the distance in feet from the EPS to the position for which the SPL is to be computed and 0.282 is the radius in feet of the SMS. Assume, for example, a PWL from an EPS of 160 db and compute the SPL at a position 282 feet from the EPS. Then,

$$SPL = 160 - 20 \log_{10} \frac{282}{0.282} \text{ or } SPL = 160$$

$-20 \log_{10} 1000 = 160 - 60 = 100$ db; the desired SPL. In another case, the PWL is 170 db and the SPL is desired for a position 2820 feet from the EPS. Then, SPL $= 170 - 20 \log_{10} \dfrac{2820}{0.282}$ or SPL $= 170 - 20 \log_{10} 10,000 = 170 - 80 = 90$ db; the desired SPL. When the SPL is given for a position separated from the EPS by a specified distance the PWL is computed as follows:

$$ PWL = SPL + 20 \log_{10} \frac{d}{0.282} $$

Assume, for example, an SPL of 70 db at a position 2820 feet from an EPS. Then PWL $= 70 + 20 \log_{10} \dfrac{2820}{0.282}$ or PWL $= 70 + 20 \log_{10} 10,000 = 70 + 80 = 150$ db; the desired PWL. In another case the SPL at a position 282 feet from an EPS is 120 db. Then PWL $= 120 + 20 \log_{10} \dfrac{282}{0.282}$ or PWL $= 120 + 20 \log_{10} 1000 = 120 + 60 = 180$ db; the desired PWL. Some results of additional calculation, using these two formulas, are given in table 49. These relations and computations are valid when the sound source is an EPS. Later, methods for applying them to sound fields from complex practical sources of acoustic energy will be described.

Complex Sounds

Our study of acoustic principles has been based upon simple sound waves in which the acoustic power was carried by one frequency. The over-all sound pressure level (OASPL) of the total wave and the SPL of the one frequency component were the same. However, sound waves of practical sources usually contain many frequency components and the SPL of each component contributes its pressure to the combined larger SPL of the complex wave. Let us examine a complex sound wave, produced by a "modified" EPS to learn how complex waves from practical sources are analyzed and described.

FREQUENCY ANALYSIS OF COMPLEX SOUNDS. The complex sound wave to be studied is produced by a "modified" EPS consisting of a large number of EPSs, grouped together in a very small space. Each EPS generates one frequency at a particular SPL and all frequencies from 15

TABLE 49

Relationships between Sound Pressure Level (SPL) and Power Level (PWL) for an Equivalent Point Source (EPS)*

Measured SPL	Distance from Center of EPS	Radius of Measurement; Radius of SMS	Computed PWL
db	*feet*		*db*
80	282	$\dfrac{282}{0.282} = 1000$	140
100	282	$\dfrac{282}{0.282} = 1000$	160
120	282	$\dfrac{282}{0.282} = 1000$	180
120	28.2	$\dfrac{28.2}{0.282} = 100$	160
120	2.82	$\dfrac{2.82}{0.282} = 10$	140
120	0.282	$\dfrac{0.282}{0.282} = 1$	120

* *Note:* The ratios of the radii at the points of measurement to the radius of SMS are whole numbers in these examples. In practical work these ratios are frequently not by whole numbers.

to at least 15,000 c.p.s. are present in the complex sound wave. A calibrated microphone is placed in the sound field and the electrical copy of the sound wave which results is applied to a frequency analyzing instrument.

More than one frequency analyzer may be required to make the analyses desired. First, let us use an analyzer that detects and records the SPL of one frequency at a time but which can be switched, in turn, to each frequency component of the sound field. Each frequency component from 20 to 10,000 c.p.s. is measured successively and the SPL of each is found to be 50 db. This is a very detailed analysis of the sound field and it requires much time. In addition, the detailed information may be more than we need. Therefore, let us try analyzers that combine the SPLs of several frequency components. Now, we lead the output of the microphone to an analyzer that combines (sums) the pressures of each frequency component into a single pressure reading for

TABLE 50

Octave Band Sound Pressure Levels (OBSPL) of a Sound Field Containing All Frequencies from 20 to 20,000 c.p.s. When Each Freqeuncy Component is at a Constant Sound Pressure Level of 50 db

Octave Band		OBSPL	Geometric Mean Frequency of the Band
c.p.s.		*db*	*cycles*
20 to	75	68	39
75 to	150	69	106
150 to	300	72	212
300 to	600	75	425
600 to	1200	78	850
1200 to	2400	81	1700
2400 to	4800	84	3400
4800 to	10,000	88	6900

the complex wave. This is the over-all sound pressure level (OASPL) of the wave and for the complex wave we are using it is 90 db. The OASPL of the complex wave usually is not enough information for estimating the effects of a sound wave on man. Therefore, an analyzer that combines the pressures of selected bands of adjacent frequencies is frequently used. One much used analyzing system combines the pressures of frequency groups 1 octave wide. The octave bands used in this analysis are: 20 to 75 c.p.s., 75 to 150 c.p.s., 150 to 300 c.p.s., 300 to 600 c.p.s., 600 to 1200 c.p.s., 1200 to 2400 c.p.s., 2400 to 4800 c.p.s. and 4800 to 10,000 c.p.s. The octave band sound pressure level (OBSPL) for each of these bands of the complex sound field from our "modified" EPS are given in table 50. The center (geometric mean) frequency of each octave is also shown in table 50 because it is used when converting OBSPLs to SPLs of bands 1 cycle wide.

Sometimes frequency analyses providing more detail than is obtained by octave band analyses are needed. Then analyzers that combine the sound pressures of groups of frequencies in bands $\frac{1}{2}$ or $\frac{1}{3}$ octave wide are used. Other analyzers that combine the pressures of a specific number of frequencies, for example, 50 or 200 cycles, are used occasionally. These analyzers may be switched to any part of the audible frequency range to measure any desired group of frequencies 50 or 200 cycles wide.

Any one or all of the different frequency analyses are performed, as required, to obtain the information needed for making specific decisions. Frequency analyses tell us how the total energy of a complex sound wave is partitioned among the frequencies in the complex wave; that is, the spectrum of the complex sound field. Although any of these analyses are used for special purposes the data used in this chapter will usually be given as OASPLs or as OBSPLs.

Applying the Acoustic Principles to Practical Sources

An EPS and its sound field were used to study the generation, the frequency, the speed, the wavelength and the strength of a sound wave. The EPS also was used to study the various methods of defining the strength of a sound wave. One modified EPS (directional) was used to define "directivity" of a sound source and another modified EPS was used to generate a complex sound wave for use in describing the means for analyzing complex sound waves into their frequency components. The next step is to apply these principles and methods to the analysis and description of the sound fields of practical sources.

PWL AND SPL OF PRACTICAL SOURCES. The total acoustic power radiated by a practical source frequently is stated in terms of a "power level" relative to an arbitrary reference power of 10^{-13} watt, as shown by the following formula:

$$PWL = 10 \log \frac{W}{10^{-13}} \text{ db re } 10^{-13} \text{ watt}$$

where W is the acoustic power in watts, the logarithm is to the base 10 and "re" means referred to. Specifying the acoustic power output as an arbitrary "power level" allows one to determine the relative strengths of sources but PWL is not the only information needed. Essential data on the sound field, as for example, the sound pressure at an arbitrary distance and direction from the source, cannot be obtained from PWL without using additional information.

How, then, do we obtain desired SPLs when the PWL of a source is given? To do this, an EPS, radiating at the same PWL, is substituted for the real, practical source and it is placed at the center of the practical source. Then using the identity of SPL and PWL on the SMS around an EPS and the ratio of radii, we calculate the SPL at the specified distance from the substituted EPS using the formula given in the section on "Relations Among Measures of Sound Fields of Simple Sources." This computation gives the OASPL at the desired distance from the EPS, and in any direction from the EPS. It is called the "space average OASPL," when dealing with a practical source, because this OASPL is for a nondirectional source and must be corrected for the directional characteristics of the real source to obtain the actual OASPL at the specified distance and direction from it.

As an example, let us compute the SPL 282 feet from an afterburning turbojet engine radiating acoustic energy at a power level of 180 db. The "jet stream" is the principal acoustic energy generator of this source. We substitute for this "real" source an EPS producing the same PWL (180 db). The "substituted EPS" is placed at the jet nozzle of the engine. The necessary data, the formulas, the computation and the resulting *space average OASPL* are given in table 51. Note that the *space average OASPL* is the same in all directions as it must be around an EPS. However, the turbojet engine is a directional radiator and the space average OASPL must be corrected for this directivity. This correction is made, using the generalized, average directivity factors for jet engines given in table 51, as shown in the formula in the same table. As a result, we have many different "position" OASPLs, 282 feet from the jet nozzle, and the actual OASPL at each position depends on its direction from the jet nozzle. These relations are shown in table 51. The OASPL for positions located in directions from the jet that do not appear in table 51 can be obtained by interpolation. If the same directions, relative to the jet nozzle, are used the directivity factors given in table 51 can be used to compute the OASPLs from the PWL of any jet engine because their directivity patterns are almost identical.

The PWL of an engine also can be computed from the OASPL. If a position 282 feet from the center of the jet nozzle lies on the 145 degree radius and the OASPL is 135

TABLE 51

Computation of "Space Average OASPL"* and Position OASPL from PWL of "Real Engine" Sound Source by Substitution of EPS for "Real Engine" Source

Data:

PWL of real engine is 180 db

PWL of "substituted EPS" is 180 db

Radius of "measurement circle" around real engine is 282 feet

Radius of SMS around EPS is 0.282 foot

Computation:

Space average OASPL is computed as follows:

$$\text{space average OASPL} = \text{PWL} - 20 \log \frac{282}{0.282};$$

or space average OASPL = 180 − 20 log 1000 = 180 − 60 = 120 db.

"Position" OASPL is obtained as follows: position OASPL = space average OASPL + directivity factor. For 90 degree position: position OASPL = 120 + (−6) = 114 db. For 145 degree position: position OASPL = 120 + (+8) = 128 db.

Angle from Forward End of Engine and Positions of Directions of Measurement	Directivity Factor	Position OASPL
degrees	*db*	*db*
0 and 360	−14	106
20 and 340	−13	107
40 and 320	−12	108
60 and 300	−10	110
80 and 280	−8	112
90 and 270	−6	114
100 and 260	−4	116
120 and 240	+2	122
130 and 230	+5.5	125.5
140 and 220	+7.5	127.5
145 and 215	+8	128
150 and 210	+7	127
155 and 205	+4.5	124.5
160 and 200	+1.5	121.5
180 and 180	−13	107

* The space average OASPL is 120 db for all angles in this table.

db, the PWL may be obtained as follows: the space average OASPL is 135 db − 8 db = 127 db; then, PWL = 127 + 10 log $\frac{282}{0.282}$ = 127 + 10 log 1000 = 127 + 60 = 187 db, the desired PWL (see section on the relations between SPL and PWL).

After an OASPL for a position is calculated from the PWL of an engine, one usually needs the octave band sound pressure levels

294   AEROSPACE MEDICINE

(OBSPL) in addition. The OBSPL can be computed from the OASPL by subtracting an appropriate number of db from the OASPL to obtain OBSPL of each octave band. The relation of the OBSPL to the OASPL varies with position around the engine. However, many measurements show that two sets of relations are adequate for practical problems. One set of relations applies to all positions from 0 to 125 degrees around the engine. Another set applies to all positions from 125 to 160 degrees around the engine. The computational procedure, the band factors and results of sample computations are given in table 52.

The methods we have examined apply to jet engine sources, operated at high power settings, where the jet stream is the principal sound generator. The principles apply to any practical source, but directivity factors, octave band factors and other needed factors must be determined if not known. The methods discussed and the examples given should enable one to understand and in-

TABLE 52

Computation of OBSPL from "Position OASPL" for Varying Positions (Direction in Degrees) around a Turbojet Engine

Computation:

The position OASPL for the applicable direction from the jet nozzle is obtained from table 51. As determined by the direction of the position from the jet nozzle, the factors shown below are subtracted from the OASPL to obtain the OBSPL of each octave (see sample results in columns 4 and 5)

Octave Bands	Number to be Subtracted from Position OASPL for Each Band		Computed OBSPL for Sample Position Using OASPLs from Table 51	
	Any position between 0 and 125 degrees	Any position between 125 and 180 degrees	Position 90 degrees; OASPL = 114 db	Position 145 degrees; OASPL = 128 db
c.p.s.	db	db	db	db
20 to 75	13	12	101	116
75 to 100	11	7	103	121
150 to 300	4	4	110	124
300 to 600	6	6	108	122
600 to 1200	8	12	106	114
1200 to 2400	9	16	105	112
2400 to 4800	12	21	102	107
4800 to 9600	16	26	98	102

terpret published data on practical acoustic energy sources used in aviation operations. However, many simplifications have been employed and more detailed and exact data or procedures are required for making acoustic measurements (4, 7). In addition, specific techniques and their limitations must be thoroughly mastered before actually making measurements on practical sources of acoustic energy.

THE HUMAN EAR

The human ear is a specialized structure, "a sense organ," uniquely adapted for the detection of sound waves. It is one of several essential body structures that together perform the general human function called hearing. Davis (8), Stevens and Davis (9) and Sataloff (6) give good descriptions of the anatomy of the sense organ and these authors, as well as Hirsh (5), discuss the function of hearing including the participation of the neural elements. The ears of young adults can detect sounds throughout the frequency range 15 to 15,000 c.p.s. or perhaps 20,000 c.p.s. The ear's response to high frequencies decreases with age and many persons more than 40 years old detect no frequencies above 4000 to 6000 c.p.s. For the frequencies to which it is most sensitive, the ear detects sound pressures less than 0.0002 dyne per sq. cm. and remains sensitive to sound of any pressure level up to 2000 dynes per sq. cm. or more. However, the listener gives special responses to the higher sound pressures and when the pressure is approximately 200 dynes per sq. cm. (OASPL = 120 db) it evokes a sensation of discomfort localized in the ear. Furthermore, a sound pressure of about 2000 dynes per sq. cm. (OASPL = 140 db) elicits a sensation of pain in the middle ear and when the sound pressure is about 20,000 dynes per sq. cm. (OASPL = 160 db) rupture (mechanical breakage) of the ear drum or of a component of the inner ear occurs in some individuals. The localized sensations, discomfort and pain and the potential for mechanical damage are dependent only on the sound pressure and are independent of the type of sound wave.

Hearing

When a sound wave of adequate strength is present at the human ear, it initiates a complex mechanical and neural process that produces a sensation, which the listener describes by saying, "I hear." The word "hearing" is used to identify and describe the entire complex process. The mechanical structures of the outer, middle and inner ear and the neural elements of the inner ear participate in this process together with the nerve cells and fibers of the auditory nerve and numerous additional nerve cells and fibers in the brain. The individual knows that he hears a sound when he is aware of the sensation it evokes. However, we, as observers, do not know that he hears the sound (perceives the sensation) until he says "I hear." That is, we cannot share the listener's sensation and we become aware of it only by observing his response. The individual's response, correlated with the presence of the sound, is our only indicator that he hears the sound.

THRESHOLD HEARING LEVELS FOR PURE TONES. Seat a listener comfortably in a quiet room and place a calibrated headphone tightly but comfortably over his ear. Now connect the headphone to a generator of sinusoidal electrical voltages that can be controlled in amplitude and adjusted to any desired frequency. The headphone, now, will produce a sinusoidal sound wave (pure tone) of the frequency selected and at any desired pressure. Instruct the listener to signal "I hear" by raising the index finger of his right hand whenever he hears the tone. Now select a frequency of 1000 c.p.s. and starting

with a very weak sound wave, so weak that it is not heard, and slowly increase the strength of the sound until the listener signals "I hear." This is the listeners "threshold hearing level" for the 1000 c.p.s. sound wave. That is, the sound pressure in the ear at this time is the smallest sound pressure of a 1000 c.p.s. wave that can initiate the complex process which gives rise to the sensation, which the listener describes by saying "I hear!" The actual sound pressure at the ear drum can be determined from the data for the calibrated headphone. This sound pressure, expressed in db, is the listener's "threshold sound pressure level" for hearing a sound wave of 1000 c.p.s.

If the process is repeated for each frequency to which the human ear responds, a "threshold sound pressure level" for hearing each frequency is obtained. This has been done many times by many investigators using large numbers of listeners. Average "threshold sound pressure levels" for hearing the important audible frequencies are available from these studies (10). The average threshold sound pressure levels (minimum audible pressure, MAP) for selected frequencies are given in table 53, row 2. The "threshold hearing level" for each frequency, given in the table, is expressed as sound pressure level; that is, in db above the reference pressure of 0.0002 dyne per sq. cm. Comparing the data (row 2, table 53) for several frequencies shows that the sound pressure level of a tone, when it is "just heard,"

TABLE 53

Threshold Hearing Levels—Obtained for Several Different Listening Conditions

Row Number*	Frequency in Cycles per Second											Comments
	60	250	500	750	1000	1500	2000	3000	4000	6000	10000	
	db	db	db	db	db	db	db	db	db	db	db	
1	44	16	6	0	−1	−5	−7	−8	−7	−6	1	Binaural, threshold random MAF
2	60	24	14	11	8	5	5	6	8	14	26	Monaural, threshold MAP
3		20	8		4		3		4			Monaural, MAP "tonality"
4		17	4		−1		−1		−3			Monaural, MAP just detectable
5		38	25		17		17		15	18		Threshold, "0" for audiometers

* See text for an explanation of each row.

varies with frequency. A sound wave of 60 c.p.s. is 53 db higher in level (pressure 450 times greater) than a 1000 c.p.s. sound wave when it is just audible. Similarly, the pressure of a 250 c.p.s. sound wave is seven times greater and that of a 500 c.p.s. wave two times greater than the pressure of a 1000 c.p.s. wave when just detected by the ear.

If an individual listens with both ears while seated in a quiet room where no reflections occur, the "threshold hearing levels" given in row 1, table 53, will be obtained when the sound waves come to the ear from all directions. These binaural (two ears) thresholds are lower; that is, the ears detect the sound waves when their pressures are lower than the pressures required for listening with one ear. Again, the sound pressures at "threshold hearing level" vary as the frequency is changed and these variations are approximately the same as those for one ear listening (see row 1, table 53).

PURE TONE AUDIOMETRY. The data just given on threshold hearing levels for pure tones were obtained using experimental equipment. Information on threshold hearing levels for tones is required to evaluate the "normal" hearing ability of an individual and later to evaluate changes in his threshold hearing level that may have been caused by exposure to industrial noise. To obtain the information on threshold hearing levels and their changes, measurements are made using the audiometer; an instrument designed to generate sound waves (in the ear canal) at an agreed, standard pressure for each frequency. This standard pressure is marked "0 db" on the "Hearing Loss" dial of the audiometer and it corresponds to the average of the sound pressures for each frequency that are detected by a large sample of adult American people. This standard, normal "threshold hearing level" is given in row 5, table 53. The actual sound pressure of each frequency at the agreed, standard "threshold hearing level" is greater than the pressures shown in rows 1 and 2, table 53, because they are the average threshold hearing levels of a representative sample of a population rather than the average threshold hearing levels of a selected sample of young individuals with no known deficiencies of hearing.

Hirsh (5) discusses the basic principles underlying applied pure tone audiometry. Glorig (11) and Sataloff (6) discuss the selection of instruments, their standardization or calibration and techniques for using pure tone audiometers in evaluating the hearing of personnel working in industrial noise. In programs designed to determine the possible effects of exposure to industrial noise on the ears of workmen, a special form of pure tone audiometry called "monitoring audiometry" is employed. The medical principles underlying monitoring audiometry are discussed by Davis *et al.* (12) and guides for its application have been prepared by the "Subcommittee on Noise in Industry" (13). This specialized form of pure tone audiometry is a tool of major importance in assuring adequate protection for the ears of personnel exposed to aviation noise.

THE PITCH SENSATION. When an individual listens to pure tones at pressures above the threshold hearing level he becomes aware of a quality of the sound, a sensation, identified by the term "pitch." This sensation, the pitch, changes as the frequency of the sound is changed. Pitch is, primarily, related to frequency but is also affected to a small extent by the pressure of the sound wave. Complex sound waves usually do not evoke a sensation of "pitch" but if high level single frequency components are present a rough pitch sensation may be perceived. The sensation of pitch may affect the determination of the threshold hearing level (by pure tone audiometry) for a pure tone in a curious way. If, for example, the listener is instructed to signal "I hear" the moment he perceives a sound having a tonal quality, a pitch quality, the threshold hearing level obtained for each frequency will be similar to that shown in row 3, table 53. If, in contrast, he is instructed to signal "I hear" the moment he just detects the presence of a sound, the threshold hearing level for each frequency will be similar to that shown in row 4, table 53. Comparing the data in row 3 with those in row 4, table 53, shows that the threshold hearing level for each frequency has been raised by 3 to 7 db (pressure is increased 1.5 to 2.25 times) simply by instructing the listener to signal "I hear" only when he perceives a pitch sensation evoked by the test frequency. The perception and discrimination of pitch may be altered by exposure to high level noise and they may be used for evaluating the effects of noise on men's hearing.

LOUDNESS SENSATION. When determining the threshold hearing level, the listener signaled "I hear" as soon as he was aware of a specific sensation. When he gave his signal, the sound pressure had attained a particular value. This sound pressure level is the "zero loudness level" for the frequency under test and it is identical with the threshold hearing level. If the sound pressure level of the tone increases, the sensation grows stronger and the "loudness" of the tone increases. The sensation, "loudness," is primarily related to the sound pressure level of a sound wave. However, the loudness of a sound wave of one frequency may differ from that of another frequency when the sound pressure levels are identical. Near the hearing threshold, the differences in sound pressure level required to arouse equally strong sensations of loudness for the audible frequencies are essentially the same as the pressure differences required for their detection by the ear. As the sound pressure level and the loudness of each tone increases, the difference in the absolute pressure required to produce an equal sensation of loudness becomes smaller. These relations are shown in table 54. In row 1 the pressures of selected frequencies, at zero loudness level or threshold hearing level are given. To obtain the data shown in row 2, table 54, the pressure of the 1000 c.p.s. sound wave was raised 40 db above threshold (or zero loudness) to a sound pressure level of 48 db. The listener then compared a sound of another frequency with the 1000 c.p.s. tone and varied the sound pressure level of the test tone until he judged its loudness to equal that of the 1000 c.p.s. tone. An examination of the data in row 2 shows that both low frequency and high frequency sounds which are judged equal to the 1000 c.p.s. tone in loudness are at higher sound pressure levels. Similar data are shown in row 3, table 54, for tests in which the 1000 c.p.s. tone was adjusted to a pressure level 70 db above threshold. The data in this row show that high and low frequency tones still must be higher in pressure in order to equal the 1000 c.p.s. tone in loudness, but that the amount by which their pressure must be increased is less than that required when the 1000 c.p.s. tone is 40 db above threshold. The data in row 4, table 54, were obtained when the pressure of the 1000 c.p.s. tone was raised 110 db above threshold. These data show that at this loudness level any frequency is essentially equal to any other frequency in loudness when their sound pressure levels are the same. The data given in table 54 pertain to pure tones, but complex sound waves containing many frequencies also evoke a sensation of loudness which increases as their sound pressure levels increase. The ear responds in the same way to spoken words; that is, human voice signals. These relations between the pressure level of a sound and the loudness sensation it evokes are important because they apply to voice communication and the interference to communication that aviation noise produces.

AUDITORY MASKING. A tone produces auditory masking when it raises the threshold hearing level of a second tone. The measure of masking is the number of db that the hearing threshold level of the masked tone is raised because the masking tone is pres-

TABLE 54

Equal Loudness Contours—Sound Pressure Levels of Various Frequencies that Appear to be Equally Loud

Row Number*	Frequency in Cycles per Second							Comments
	60	250	500	1000	2000	4000	6000	
	db	db	db	db	db	db	db	
1	60	24	14	8	5	8	14	0 db equal loudness contour
2	80	57	50	48	49	52	60	40 db equal loudness contour
3	91	79	78	78	78	81	88	70 db equal loudness contour
4	120	118	118	118	118	118	119	110 db equal loudness contour

* See text for an explanation of each row.

ent. Masking is measured by turning on the masking sound at the desired level and then gradually increasing the pressure level of the masked tone until it is just detectable. The difference in db between the sound pressure level of the masked tone, at the time it is just detected in the presence of the masking tone, and its sound pressure level when just detected, in the absence of the masking tone, is the auditory masking value. The masking effect of a single frequency is greatest for frequencies very close to it. However, a tone may exert a reduced masking effect on frequencies as much as 2 or 3 octaves above it in the frequency scale. The farther the masked tone is removed from the masking tone, the smaller is the masking effect. The masking effects of pure tones are less important to us than are the masking effects of broad band noise because the masking action of pure tones is restricted to frequencies near it. In contrast, a wide band noise contains all audible frequencies and, therefore, masks any other signal made up of frequencies contained in the masking noise.

To examine the masking action of broad band noise, let us use the complex noise (produced by the modified EPS) used in our earlier study of methods of analyzing complex sound waves. This complex sound (noise) field contained all frequencies from 20 to 10,000 c.p.s. The SPL of each frequency was 50 db. Now, compare the SPL of each of these components with the SPL of the same frequency at hearing threshold (row 1, table 53) to obtain an estimate of the masking effect of the complex noise. In a quiet, outside space a 1000 c.p.s. speech component can be detected when its SPL is −1 db. The SPL of the 1000 c.p.s. component of the complex noise is 50 db. The masking value of this noise component on the 1000 c.p.s. component of the speech is 51 db. Therefore, the pressure of the 1000 c.p.s. voice component must be increased more than 300 times before it is just detectable in the presence of the masking noise. Similarly, the SPL of other voice frequencies must be raised before they are detected in the presence of the masking noise. If the SPL of the complex noise increases until the level of each frequency is 60 db, the speaker must again raise his voice until the SPL of each essential speech frequency is at

least 60 db. The practical effects of the first noise (SPL = 50 db per 1 cycle) is to force the speaker to stand about 6 inches from the listener and speak very loudly in order to be understood. In the second noise (SPL = 60 db per 1 cycle) the speaker must shout at the top of his voice to be understood when 6 inches from the listener. These two examples show the practical significance of the masking effect of broad band noise in situations where effective voice communication is essential to effective job performance.

THRESHOLD HEARING LEVELS FOR SPEECH. Let us return to our listener, seated in the same environment and furnished with the same equipment he used for determining threshold hearing levels of pure tones. Now, replace the source of controlled pure tones by a source of controlled recorded speech. Instruct the listener to signal "I hear" whenever he hears a sound from his headphone. Now, apply selected short samples of speech to the headphone, starting with a speech SPL that is too low to be heard. Slowly increase the SPL of the speech while counting the number of speech samples presented and recording the number of times the listener signals "I hear." Soon a speech SPL is reached at which the listener reports "I hear" for 50 per cent of the speech samples presented to him. This is the threshold of detectibility for speech. The OASPL of the speech signal at this threshold is about 12 db. The listener does not understand any word presented but he knows that a sound is present and he may be able to state that it is a speech sound.

Now, using the same selected short samples of speech and the same equipment, let us perform a new experiment. The listener is now instructed to repeat to us each short speech sample that is presented to him. Again, starting with a low SPL of the speech signals slowly increase the SPL of these signals until the listener correctly repeats 50 per cent of the words in the speech samples presented to him. This is the threshold of intelligibility for speech. The OASPL of the speech signals at this threshold is about 23 db. In this experiment the speaker has heard and identified the speech samples and is able to correctly repeat 50 per cent of them. If instead of slowly increasing the strength of the speech signals we present a selected speech sample at a fixed sound pressure level comparable to the levels used in every-day conversation and asked the listener to repeat back to us each speech sample he hears, we obtain another measure of his ability to understand speech. This measure is called the "speech discrimination score" and is recorded as the actual percentage of speech samples correctly repeated by the listener.

SPEECH AUDIOMETRY. The techniques discussed above suggest another means of evaluating hearing for speech which is called speech audiometry. Because we are primarily interested in an individual's ability to hear speech, when evaluating the effects of industrial noise exposure, speech audiometry would appear to be a useful measuring technique. However, speech audiometry has not been completely evaluated and standardized as has pure tone audiometry. Hirsh (5) describes the basic principles underlying speech audiometry and Sataloff (6) discusses briefly techniques and materials. Davis (14) discusses the applications of the several measures of the capability of the hearing function that can be obtained by speech audiometry and shows how they may be applied to the practical evaluation of the adequacy of an individual's capacity for hearing everyday speech. Although speech audiometry is not recommended now for the evaluation of the effects of aviation noise on hearing, it is reasonable to expect that, with further study and standardization, it may, in the future, replace pure tone audiometry for this purpose.

STANDARDS OF HEARING. The average threshold of hearing for a sample of the American population is shown in row 5, table 53, and the standard pure tone audiometers used in the U. S. A. are calibrated to deliver this pressure to the ear when the "hearing loss" dial is set to zero. These standard sound pressure levels for the several test frequencies are usually referred to as "normal hearing threshold" which is equivalent to the term "threshold hearing level" we have used. It is generally agreed that an individual's hearing is within the normal range when he hears each test frequency at a sound pressure level that is not more than 15 db higher than that for the "zero setting" of the audiometer. This means that upper limit for the actual SPLs for

normal hearing at each test frequency is: 250 c.p.s. = 53 db; 500 c.p.s. = 40 db; 1000 c.p.s. = 32 db; 2000 c.p.s. = 32 db; 4000 c.p.s. = 30 db; and 6000 c.p.s. = 33 db.

A group of selected individuals may have better hearing than that corresponding to the "normal hearing" for which the audiometer is calibrated. An example of the average hearing of a group of this kind is shown in row 2, table 53. In addition, young individuals and a fair number of older individuals may hear frequencies above 6000 c.p.s.; perhaps frequencies as high as 15,000 to 20,000 c.p.s. Thus, the maximum hearing capacity of the ears of young persons may be much better than the "normal hearing" specified by the zero setting of the audiometer. Naturally, it is the desire of members of the medical profession to preserve the physiologic hearing function at its maximum capacity. However, this maximum capacity does change with age and the change is in the direction of a reduced capacity. In addition, illnesses, exposures to chemical agents and a variety of other incidents that an individual may experience during his lifetime also tend to reduce the maximum capacity of the hearing function, particularly in the direction of a reduction of sensitivity for the higher frequencies. Now, exposures to industrial noise may also induce a decrement in the hearing function and this decrement frequently will be indistinguishable from that caused by aging and other factors. Because of these factors, the only reasonable and economically feasible approach to be used, where persons are exposed to industrial noise, is to concern ourselves with the preservation of the ears sensitivity for those frequencies which are essential to understanding human speech under everyday working and living conditions. The frequencies essential for understanding human speech range from about 200 to 2000 c.p.s. At present the test frequencies, 500, 1000 and 2000 c.p.s., are used in pure tone audiometry to evaluate the functional capability of the ear for those frequencies essential to understanding human speech. Frequencies above 2000 c.p.s., including 3000, 4000 and 6000 c.p.s., are used in audiometric tests. Changes in threshold hearing level for these frequencies occur earlier, when an individual is exposed to industrial noise,

TABLE 55
Suggested Threshold Hearing Levels (Standards)

	Frequencies in Cycles per Second						Comments
	500	1000	2000	3000	4000	5000	
	db	db	db				
Both ears	15	15	15	Average of 35 db for these three frequencies			New employment or beginning of training
Both ears or	20	20	20	No requirement			Continue on duty or employment if skilled
Better ear	15	15	15	No requirement			
Worse ear	No requirement			No requirement			
Better ear	20	20	20	No requirement			Continue in employment if skilled
Worse ear	20	40	40	No requirement			

than do the changes in threshold hearing level for 500, 1000 and 2000 c.p.s. Changes in these higher test frequencies, 3000, 4000 and 6000 c.p.s., can serve as a warning that changes in the hearing function are taking place which ultimately may lead to disability for understanding human speech. Based on these considerations, the requirements for the functional status of the human ear are usually stated in terms of requirements for 500, 1000 and 2000 c.p.s. Some suggested requirements to guide personnel in making up their own criteria are given in table 55. When establishing criteria for taking on new workmen, particularly young workmen who are to begin their training, it is suggested that the requirements stated in the top row of the table are satisfactory. This requirement states that the threshold hearing level should be within "normal limits" for the frequencies 500, 1000 and 2000 c.p.s. Hearing for the frequencies, 3000, 4000 and 6000 c.p.s., may be below these "normal limits" as indicated by the chart. Hearing of the quality indicated is essential for both ears. After an individual has been trained and especially if he is skilled, criteria for continued employment may be similar to those shown in the second row of table 55. If the employee is especially skilled, or if he has a strong desire to continue to perform the duty for which he is skilled, then the requirements indicated in the last row of table 55 are suggested as satisfactory. The requirements given in table 55 are suggestions only. Each individual organization must establish its own specific criteria or requirements for the quality of hearing performance that is essential to the performance of the duties required of their employees. Likewise, they must establish their own criteria for the decrement in the hearing function that will be permitted before an individual is given an assignment free of noise exposure or other hazards to his hearing. Sometimes there are special duties that require hearing for frequencies above those required for understanding speech. In this case the organization must specify the quality of hearing performance for the frequencies which are essential to the particular job.

Effects of Noise on Hearing

Aviation acoustic energy (noise) impairs hearing by two distinct actions on the end organ, namely: (1) auditory masking or interference to the detection of desired sound signals, particularly human speech signals and (2) the reduction of end organ sensitivity as evidenced by temporary or persistent shifts of hearing level and permanent elevations of threshold hearing level. It is convenient to evaluate the two effects separately and develop independent criteria for their significance.

EFFECT OF NOISE ON COMMUNICATION BY SPEECH. Here, we shall consider only those effects of noise on speech communication that disappear as soon as the noise stops or the listener moves out of the noise. They are the masking effects of the noise and they make the ear insensitive to desired

TABLE 56

Sound Pressure Level per Cycle, for 500, 1000, 2000, 3000, 4000 and 6000 c.p.s., for Threshold of Hearing Sample of Speech, Communication Criteria and Samples of Noise

Row Number*	Frequencies Tested in Cycles per Seccond						Comments (Source, etc.)
	500	1000	2000	3000	4000	6000	
	db	db	db	db	db	db	
1	15	7	7	6	5	8	Minimum (−10 db) reading of audiometer
2	25	17	17	16	15	18	Average "normal" threshold (approximate)
3	40	32	32	31	30	33	Upper limit of "normal" hearing (+15 db) reading of audiometer
4	41	37	28	20	17	8	Normal speech—long time average pressure 3 feet from speakers mouth
5	41	34	26.5	22	19	14	Residential community—traffic noise background
6	54	42	39	38	36	29	Garbage disposer
7	69	59	49	46	42	35	Inside jet aircraft—cruising at 30,000 feet
8	86	70	57	51	46	37	Inside jet aircraft—takeoff
9	84	75	69	65	61	55	Jet aircraft with A/B on ground in operation 90 degrees to long axis of airplane, at 1000 feet
10	21	14	7.5	4	−3	−6	SC-40 communication criterion
11	36	29	22.5	19	12	9	SC-55-communication criterion
12	56	49	42.5	39	32	29	SC-75-communication criterion

* See text for an explanation of each row.

speech sounds, our most used means of communication. Let us use the data in table 56 to gain some understanding of the practical significance of the auditory masking produced by noises. First, let us examine rows 1, 2 and 3 of table 56. In row 2 the (approximate) reference "normal" hearing threshold sound pressures produced by audiometers are shown for recommended test frequencies. Some persons hear better than this and the threshold sound pressure levels for persons whose hearing threshold level is 10 db better is shown in row 1. Other person's ears are less sensitive than the average of the group and the threshold sound pressure levels for persons whose threshold hearing level is 15 db higher are shown in row 3.

Now, let us compare the data in row 4, table 56, with that in rows 1, 2 and 3. The long time average sound pressure levels of selected frequencies from speech are shown in row 4. The pressures were measured 3 feet from the speakers' lips when speaking levels were monitored and held 6 db below the level that could be maintained indefinitely. The frequencies selected from the speech are those used in audiometric testing, so their pressure may be compared with those representing threshold hearing level.

If the pressure levels of these speech frequencies are compared with the pressures at average threshold hearing level, the pressure levels of the speech signals are found to exceed threshold hearing for all frequencies except 6000 c.p.s. The pressure levels of the speech components exceed the threshold levels of all frequency components for the more sensitive ears (compare row 4 with row 1). However, the pressure levels of the "average speech" components are lower than the threshold pressure levels required by less sensitive ears, except for frequencies 500 and 1000 c.p.s. Now, recall that ability to detect and recognize the words used in everyday conversations is evaluated in terms of the *average threshold hearing level* for frequencies 500, 1000 and 2000 c.p.s. The data in rows 1 to 4, table 56, show that the pressure levels of these components of average speech exceed threshold hearing levels by a larger amount and more often than does the pressure levels of the 3000, 4000 and 6000 c.p.s. components. Apparently there is good reason for the fact that ones ability in everyday speech communication is correlated with the sensitivity of the ear for 500, 1000 and 2000 c.p.s. The speakers talked at a comfortable level, 6 db below the level they could maintain indefinitely, while producing the average speech samples. Now, increasing the strength of the speech signals 6 db improves hearing conditions for listeners, especially those with less sensitive ears. In fact, the speakers could raise the level of the speech signal 18 db and maintain this speaking level for some time, and for a limited time the speakers could raise the level of the speech signal as much as 24 db.

Speech contains frequency components of much higher frequency than 2000 c.p.s. These higher frequencies, up to about 6800 c.p.s., do contribute to the recognition of some English words. However, words in everyday use under everyday circumstances are detected and recognized adequately when the listener can hear all frequency components up to 2000 c.p.s. at pressure levels produced by speakers using moderate to loud voice levels. Ability to detect frequencies above 2000 c.p.s. is desirable but not essential to everyday conversation and communication.

Now let us see what effects noise has on communication by speech signals. To do so let us first examine the composition of some noises frequently present in our environments. In row 5, table 56, the pressure levels of selected components of traffic noise in a community are shown. By comparing these pressure levels with the threshold hearing levels (row 2) we observe that they are well above those of "average hearing." These noises will be heard, but, in addition, they will raise the "effective" threshold hearing level to their pressure level. This is auditory masking by noise, and the "noise masked" threshold hearing level for 500 and 1000 c.p.s. is higher than the poorest hearing that falls within the accepted normal hearing range. The effect of this noise is to make all ears of average and better than average sensitivity equivalent to ears having sensitivities reduced beyond the normal hearing range for 500, 1000 and 2000 c.p.s. This effect lasts only while the noise is present; the masking disappears when the noise ceases. If the pressure levels of these sample frequencies of the noise are compared with the same frequencies of speech (row 4, table 56) it is seen that raising the voice level 6 db and, thereby, the pressure level

of the speech signals overcomes the masking effect of this noise.

Data on the sound pressure levels of other noises are shown in rows 6, 7, 8 and 9, table 56. These noises are produced by: a garbage disposer in operation (row 6); a jet aircraft in flight, at 30,000 feet—noise levels inside (row 7); inside noise level at "takeoff" in the same jet aircraft, (row 8); and a jet aircraft operated on the ground with afterburner (measurement site 90 degrees to the long axis of aircraft and 1000 feet from the jet nozzle, row 9). Let us evaluate the practical significance of these noises for speech communication among those exposed to them. To do this we shall use the average SPL for average "normal" hearing threshold for frequencies 500, 1000 and 2000 c.p.s., which is 20 db, the SPL of the long time average of speech signals (frequencies 500, 1000 and 2000 c.p.s.), which is 36 db and the average SPLs of these same frequencies in each of the noises. The average SPL of 500, 1000 and 2000 c.p.s. in the garbage disposer noise is 45 db and exceeds the SPL for average threshold hearing level; an "effective" loss in hearing sensitivity of 25 db is produced by the noise. Now, the average SPL of 500, 1000 and 2000 c.p.s. in our speech sample was 36 db and the level of these frequencies in the noise (45 db) is 9 db higher; the speaker can make himself heard by increasing his speaking effort four times to increase the SPL about 12 db. A similar analysis of the noise conditions in the aircraft cruising at 30,000 feet altitude (row 7) shows the average threshold for the frequencies, essential for understanding everyday speech (500, 1000 and 2000 c.p.s.), to be increased 39 db by the noise. The speaker will need to increase the level of his speech signal 23 db to make himself heard. During takeoff of the same aircraft (row 8, table 56) the noise elevates the threshold hearing level by 51 db and the speech signal level must be increased 35 db for the listener to recognize the words. The last noise sample, an aircraft on the ground with its afterburner in operation (row 9, table 56), elevates the threshold hearing level (average for 500, 1000 and 2000 c.p.s.) by 56 db and its average SPL (500, 1000 and 2000 c.p.s.) is 40 db above the average of SPL of the same frequencies in the sample speech (row 4, table

56). In this case, the speaker will need to increase the SPL of his speech about 100 times in order to bring the level up to that of the noise. This the speaker cannot do, but he might raise his speech level about 30 times for short intervals and move up to about 3 inches from the listener's ear. Then he could probably make himself understood. Special, simplified vocabularies might also be used to improve the communication. If the listener could anticipate the context of the speaker message, the communication could also be improved. All of the factors mentioned above influence "speech communication" in noise and must be considered in estimating the quality of communication that can be maintained under exposure to aviation noise.

Three additional sets of data are given in table 56 (rows 10, 11 and 12). These three sets of data are derived from "speech communication" (SC) criteria that we shall use later; data from the SC-40 criterion, the SC-55 criterion and the SC-75 criterion appear in rows 10, 11 and 12, respectively. Analysis of the SC-40 criterion shows that the average SPL for 500, 1000 and 2000 c.p.s. is 14 db. This is 6 db below the average SPL for the same frequencies at threshold hearing level and 22 db below the SPL of these frequencies in the speech sample. Speech communication between persons 3 feet apart should be excellent. The average SPL for 500, 1000 and 2000 c.p.s. in the SC-55 criterion is 29 db and this is 9 db above the average SPL of these frequencies at threshold hearing level but 7 db below the average SPL of these frequencies in the speech sample. Communication in this noise should be completely adequate, although there is an "effective" elevation of hearing threshold for ears of average sensitivity. The average SPL for 500, 1000 and 2000 c.p.s. in the SC-75 criterion is 49 db or 29 db above the average SPL of these frequencies at threshold hearing level and 13 db above the average SPL of the same frequencies in our average speech sample. To achieve satisfactory communication, the voice level must be raised more than four times.

This method of evaluating the effects of noise on capacity to communicate in noise by speech signals has been used to emphasize (1) that auditory masking is an "effective" elevation of threshold hearing level which lasts only as long as the noise is present, (2) the importance of the frequencies, 500, 1000 and 2000 c.p.s., for detecting and recognizing everyday speech signals and (3) that noise interference to speech communication can be estimated from the "effective" increase in threshold hearing level that it produces.

Some persons would say that the aviation medical practitioner is unlikely to be asked to estimate the effects of noise on communication. However, experience indicates that he is often expected to give guidance in this area. In addition, these effects of noise may be rather closely related to his responsibility for maintaining the general health and effectiveness of personnel because the annoyances and stresses induced by the effort to communicate in noise are related to general health and over-all effectiveness of performance. There are more detailed standard methods for evaluating the effects of noise on communication. The basic principles underlying these methods and some of their applications are discussed by Hirsh (5), Rosenblith and Stevens (24), Kryter (15) and Hawley and Kryter (16). However, a simplified method for making approximate estimates of the effects of aviation noise is outlined here for use by the aviation medical specialist when he needs to determine whether more detailed analyses are required for specific operational problems.

CRITERIA FOR SPEECH COMMUNICATION IN NOISE. Beranek (17), Beranek and Newman (18) and Beranek (19) proposed the use of the "speech interference level" (SIL) for predicting the effects of noise on speech communication and for expressing permissible noise interference to speech communication. Rosenblith and Stevens (24) discuss these criteria and their applications in detail. Peterson and Beranek (4) furnish charts and tables to facilitate their application and von Gierke and Pietrasanta (20) show how the SIL may be used to state criteria for the effect of noise on communication in critical areas of an air base.

The "speech interference level" (SIL) of a noise is a number, obtained by averaging (arithmetically) the SPLs, in db, of three octave bands, the 600 to 1200 c.p.s., the 1200 to 2400 c.p.s., and the 2400 to 4800

TABLE 57

Sample Communication (SC) Criteria, SC-40, SC-55 and SC-75 for Comparison with Octave Band Levels of Speech Sample and Several Different Noises

Row Number*	Octave Bands of Fequency in Cycles per Second								Remarks
	20 to 75	75 to 150	150 to 300	300 to 600	600 to 1200	1200 to 2400	2400 to 4800	4800 to 9600	
	db	db	db	db	db	db	db	db	
1				52	47	48	49	57	SPL for octave band containing test frequencies at average threshold SPL
2		56	61	65	65	61	54	43	SPL for octave bands for long time average speech sample
3	73	63	55	48	43	40	37	36	SC-40 curve (SIL = 40 db)
4	88	78	70	63	58	55	52	51	SC-55 curve (SIL = 55 db)
5	108	98	90	83	78	75	72	71	SC-75 curve (SIL = 75 db)
6	71	75	65	68	64	62	59	53	Dishwasher noise (SIL = 62 db)
7	72	72	80	82	71	70	72	65	Garbage disposer noise (SIL = 71 db)
8	71	70	69	67	64	59	55	50	Community noise from traffic (SIL = 59 db)
9		88	92	96	90	81	79	71	Noise inside jet aircraft—cruising at 30,000 fect (SIL = 83 db)
10		108	107	115	100	91	83	72	Noise inside jet aircraft—Takeoff (SIL = 91 db)
11	109	114	115	111	104	102	98	91	Jet aircraft with A/B on ground in operation 90 degrees to long axis of airplane, at 1000 feet (SIL = 101 db)

* See text for an explanation of each row.

c.p.s. bands. The precision with which this number, the SIL, predicts the noise interference to speech communication also depends on certain inter-relations among the pressure levels of the octave bands (the octave band spectrum shape). If these interoctave relations are similar to those of the spectrum of human speech the predictions are more accurate. These interoctave pressure level relations are shown in rows 3, 4 and 5, table 57, where the band pressure levels for each octave are given for the SC-40, the SC-55 and the SC-75 criteria. Examination of the SC criteria show that the interoctave pressure differences are the same regardless of the absolute pressure level of the several octaves of the criterion. When the interoctave pressure relations of the noise spectrum (octave band spectrum) are similar to those of the criteria, the SIL gives its best prediction of noise interference to speech communication. The greater the interoctave pressure level relations of the noise differ from those of the criteria the poorer is the prediction of communication interference derived from the SIL.

Table 57 also contains additional data to be compared with the SC criteria data. The frequencies normally used for audiometric tests have been selected and the octave band pressure level of the octave containing each selected frequency has been computed for the condition; that the pressure of the test frequency is that required by the "normal" average hearing threshold. These computed octave band sound pressure levels (OBSPL) are given in row 1, table 57. The octave band SPLs of the speech sample, used in previous discussions, are given in row 2 of this table. By comparing data from row 2 with those of rows 3, 4 and 5, one can see the extent to which the interoctave pressure relations of speech spectra are matched to those of the SC criteria. Rows 6 through 11, table 57, contain data on the octave band SPLs of several different noises, together with the computed SIL of each noise. We now know how to compute the SIL and we also know how SC criteria are derived from the SIL. Let us find out how to translate SIL values and SC criteria into estimates of the quality of communication that can be maintained in the presence of a given noise.

In table 58 the SIL in db is shown in rela-

TABLE 58

Speech Interference Levels (SIL) as Related to Distance and Voice Level

Distance	Normal	Raised	Very Loud	Shouting
feet	*bd*	*db*	*db*	*db*
0.5	71	77	83	89
1	65	71	77	83
2	59	65	71	77
3	55	61	67	73
4	53	59	65	71
5	41	57	63	69
6	49	55	59	65
8	57	53	59	65
10	45	51	57	63
12	43	49	55	61
16	41	47	53	59
20	39	45	51	57
24	37	43	49	55
40	33	39	45	51

tion to distance between speaker and listener and in relation to the speaker's voice level. In order to have reliable communication, SILs should be lower than the numbers shown for the distances and voice levels tabulated. The other conditions assumed are (1) no reflecting surfaces, (2) speaker is facing listener, (3) the spoken material is unfamiliar to the listener and (4) the speech material is difficult. If the vocabulary is limited and selected or if the listener can anticipate the general context of the speakers message the communication will be improved; perhaps the distances shown could be doubled or the indicated voice level reduced one step. The relation between SC criteria expressed by SILs and the communication conditions for a degree of speech recognition that is *marginal* with a conventional vocabulary and *good* with a selected vocabulary are given in table 59. In using these criteria one must remember that the more the actual measured noise deviates from the general interoctave relations of the SC criteria the poorer will be the predictions given by the SC criteria.

Use of the telephone is satisfactory when the SIL is below 60 db, it is difficult when the SIL is 60 to 75 db and impossible when the SIL is above 75 db. The SIL, measured when the space is not in use, should not exceed (1) 40 db for a small private office, (2) 30 db for a conference room for 20, (3) 55 db for secretarial offices (typing), (4) 25 db for sleeping areas of homes and (5) 25 db for school rooms (20).

Now refer to table 57 where data are given for the OBSPL and the SIL of each of several

TABLE 59

Relation between SIL and Communication Conditions

SIL	Voice Level and Distance	Nature of Possible Communication	Type of Working Area
db			
45	Normal voice at 10 feet	Relaxed conversation	Private offices, conference rooms
55	Normal voice at 3 feet	Continuous communication in work areas	Business, secretarial, test cell, control rooms, etc.
55	Raised voice at 6 feet	Continuous communication in work areas	Business secretarial, test cell, control rooms, etc.
55	Very loud voice at 12 feet	Continuous communication in work areas	Business, secretarial, test cell, control room., etc.
65	Raised voice at 2 feet	Intermittent communication	
65	Very loud voice at 4 feet	Intermittent communication	
65	Shouting at 8 feet	Intermittent communication	
75	Very loud voice at 1 foot	Minimal communication (danger signals; restricted prearranged vocabulary desirable)	
75	Shouting at 2 to 3 feet	Minimal communication (danger signals; restricted prearranged vocabulary desirable)	

noises. The noise inside the jet aircraft cruising at 30,000 feet gives an SIL of 83 db (row 9). If the listener is to recognize the words in a speaker's message, when both are in this noise, the speaker must shout and must not be more than 1 foot from the listener. If a limited vocabulary of simple words were used perhaps the speaker could stand 2 feet away from the listener. The OBSPLs and the SIL for traffic noise penetrating into a residential community are given in the same table (table 57, row 8). The SIL is 59 db. In this noise a conversation can be carried on, using a normal voice level, if the speakers are about 2 feet apart. The speaker-listener separation may be increased to 4 feet if a raised voice level is used. These examples show how to use the SIL and the SC criteria to estimate the adverse effect of noise on communication. Such estimates will permit the aviation medical specialist to determine the order of magnitude of disturbance and decide whether more detailed evaluations are required. If detailed methods are required, it is best that qualified specialists be employed to perform these analyses.

EFFECTS OF NOISE ON THE INNER EAR. The auditory masking and the interference to speech communication (discussed in the last section) disappear as soon as exposure to noise is terminated. However, there are effects of the noise exposure that persist well beyond the exposure period. Measure an individual's threshold hearing level, using a standard audiometer, immediately after he has been exposed for 1 hour to the noise produced by an aircraft engine. These measurements provide the SPL, for each test frequency, that corresponds to the individual's post noise exposure threshold hearing level. When this post noise exposure hearing level is compared with the threshold hearing level of the same individual before the noise exposure, the sound pressure levels required to reach hearing threshold are found to be higher after the noise exposure. This elevation of the threshold hearing level (or reduction of the detection sensitivity of the ear) is called a "threshold shift" (TS) or a hearing threshold shift (HTS). When these threshold shifts disappear in a few hours they are called "temporary threshold shifts" (TTS) and when they last for a longer period, several hours to 2 or more days, they are

called "persistent threshold shifts" (PTS). After an individual has incurred noise exposures repeatedly, over a period of years, the hearing threshold shift may become permanent; that is, he has a permanent elevation of his threshold hearing level which is called a noise induced hearing loss.

TEMPORARY HEARING THRESHOLD SHIFT (TTS). Shifts of the threshold hearing level produced by varying times of exposure to several different types of noise and the recovery from these hearing threshold shifts are illustrated in table 60. One individual (W.D.N.) exposed his ears for 15 minutes to the noise field of a turbojet engine when the OASPL varied between 125 and 140 db. The shifts of his hearing thresholds (measured 2 hours after exposure) for the test frequencies of a standard audiometer are shown in row 1 for the right ear and row 2 for the left ear. The recovery of his threshold hearing levels, measured $19\frac{1}{2}$ hours after the exposure, are shown in row 1a for the right ear and row 2a for the left ear. Two hours after the exposure was terminated a maximum threshold shift of 35 db was measured for 4000 c.p.s. in the right ear and for 8000 c.p.s. in the left ear. A recovery of 10 db for the hearing thresholds at 4000 c.p.s. had occurred after $19\frac{1}{2}$ hours leaving a residual threshold shift for this frequency of 25 db. In the left ear the recovery at 8000 c.p.s. was 20 db and the residual threshold shift was 15 db $19\frac{1}{2}$ hours post exposure. Similar data for another individual exposed to the same noise field for the same length of time are shown in rows 3, 3a, 4 and 4a, table 60. The threshold shifts for this individual were greater, especially at 3000 c.p.s. for the right ear and 2000 c.p.s. for the left ear. The residual threshold shifts, $19\frac{1}{2}$ hours after the noise exposure, were 35 db for 4000 c.p.s. (right ear) and 20 db for 8000 c.p.s. (left ear). The threshold shifts, shown by both these individuals, are classified as temporary threshold shifts because they lasted more than 15 but less than 40 hours. These threshold shifts were not permanent because the individual's threshold hearing levels later returned to normal. The results of another exposure for one of the individuals (W. D. N.) are shown in rows 5 and 5a, table 60. This exposure lasted 2 minutes and the noise levels were the same as in the previous ex-

AVIATION NOISE ENVIRONMENTS *VERSUS* HUMAN TOLERANCE CRITERIA

In this section we shall present samples of the noise fields characteristic of the environments in which aviation operations are conducted. A comprehensive description of all environments is not intended, but it is the intent to show the general characteristics of such noise fields and to indicate the principal sources of the noise. The noise fields are then compared with human tolerance criteria to identify the need for noise reduction or noise control.

Noise Environments Inside Aircraft

The acoustic energy (noise) fields inside airplanes are composite; that is, they contain energy contributed by several different sources. The relative importance of the contributions by each of these sources varies with the phase of operation, as for example, taxiing, ground roll, climb out, cruise, etc.

SOURCES OF NOISE INSIDE AIRCRAFT. The noise inside an airplane is made up of components generated by (1) the propulsion system (engine), (2) the flow of air over the outside surface of the airplane, (3) the flow of air inside ducts and over louvers of the heating, ventilating, and pressurizing systems and (4) noise generated by mechanical equipment, pumps, generators, motors, etc. The sources and the mechanisms of sound generation relevant to each one is discussed in detail by von Gierke (25) and also by Bolt *et al.* (26).

CHARACTERISTICS OF NOISE FIELDS INSIDE AIRCRAFT. Typical noise fields inside military jet aircraft are shown in table 57 where the inside noise field during takeoff is shown in row 10 and that during cruise at 30,000 feet altitude is shown in row 9. Additional discussions, data and reference to sources of information on noise inside aircraft are given by von Gierke (27). The OASPL at one station inside the aircraft (from which the data of table 57 was obtained) varied from 120 db, during takeoff at maximum power, through 109 db down to 102 db, during climb to altitude, to 99 db, during cruise at 30,000 ft altitude; the octave band SPLs varied proportionately. At any power setting the OASPL varies with position along the long dimension of the aircraft and the range of variation is of the order of 6 to 10 db, with the SPLs tending to be lower in the forward part of the airplane (crew compartment). Past civilian transport aircraft have tended to have lower noise levels than the corresponding military aircraft and the difference in SPL has been of the order of 20 db. It is reasonable to expect future jet transports to have lower inside noise levels than military aircraft and again the difference in SPL may range from about 6 db in certain interior spaces to 20 db in other spaces.

INSIDE SPL *VERSUS* CRITERIA. The typical noise fields inside a jet aircraft were compared with the communication criteria (see table 57, rows 9 and 10). During cruise at 30,000 feet the SIL is 83 db and adequate communication is possible using a "shouting" voice level over a distance of about 1 foot. If this SIL were reduced (20 db) to 63 db the same voice level would permit communication over a distance of about 10 feet or over a distance of 2 to 3 feet when using a "raised" voice level. These levels may be acceptable to passengers in terms of ability to converse. During the "takeoff" the SIL was 91 db. No real conversation is possible, but if the SIL is lowered 20 db to 71 db, conversation, using a "raised" voice would be possible for persons seated about 2 feet apart. The flight crew uses headphones fitted with ear cups, and, in addition, can control the output of the voice signal from the communication system. The necessary communication is possible, at the higher SIL values, but lower noise levels are highly desirable.

The summed level of the 300 to 600 and 600 to 1200 c.p.s. bands for cruise operation is 97 db. When this SPL is compared with the two band long time exposure criterion (98 ± 2 db) it is found to be within the allowable range and no unusual risk to the inner ear is indicated for exposures up to 8 hours in any 1 work day. Passengers usually do not spend 8 hours each day in flight so they are not subjected to a risk of inner ear damage from cruise noise levels. Using the same procedure, we find during "takeoff" a two band SPL of 115 db. When this is compared with the two band short time exposure criterion (100 db), the criterion is exceeded by 15 db and the "allowable exposure" is about 15 minutes each 8 hour work day. If the exposure to the "takeoff" noise level does not exceed 8 minutes, each 8 hour work day, then this exposure can be combined with 7 hours, 52 minutes of exposure to the "cruise" level without exceeding the limits established by the two band short time noise exposure criterion. In military aircraft, this might be achieved and in commercial aircraft noise levels will be lower so there appears to be no significant risks to the inner ear for either aircrew or passengers. In military operations the use of ear protection is desirable. Actually the noise levels of the flight crew station were about 6 db below those of the station used in the preceding analysis, therefore, the flight crew could be exposed 30 minutes to takeoff noise and 7½ hours to cruise noise levels without exceeding the two band criterion.

Noise Environments Outside Aircraft

The noise fields outside aircraft (particularly on the airport or air base) are composed of contributions from a larger number of sources than contributed to the noise fields inside aircraft. Furthermore, there are a great many more operations that may be affected by the noise fields and, therefore, a greater range of personnel categories which one must consider.

SOURCES OF NOISE OUTSIDE AIRCRAFT. The propulsion systems of aircraft in flight operation, in taxiing operation and under maintenance test on the ground constitute one major group of airport noise sources. Data on these and other sources have been published (25–27). Ground support facilities and equipment also add to the noise of the airport environment. Ground support equipment is of particular importance for maintenance personnel because of their relatively long periods of continuous operation. Not all noise sources can be described in detail here so certain selected sources are used to illustrate the general characteristics of airport acoustic energy (noise) fields.

CHARACTERISTICS OF NOISE FIELDS OUTSIDE AIRCRAFT. Because the propulsion system of aircraft is the most powerful source of airport noise we shall examine the characteristics of the noise field from a modern turbojet propulsion system (fig. 104) in some detail. Figure 104 is a plot of the OASPLs for positions around a modern single engine aircraft 100 feet from the jet nozzle. The most striking feature of this noise field is the variation in SPL with engine power setting (compare idle power with afterburner operation). Multiengine aircraft usually do not employ afterburning but the SPL shown in the figure for afterburning are about the same as those from an aircraft equipped with 6 to 8 engines. The range of OASPLs is about 45 db from idle power to afterburner power. The second striking characteristic of these noise fields is the variation of the SPL with direction from the nozzle (compare levels at zero degrees, straight ahead of aircraft, with those at 135 degrees) where the range of SPLs is about 25 db. The directional radiation of these sources is more strikingly illustrated by figure 105 when a constant OASPL of 120 db was selected and the distance from the "jet nozzle" at which this OASPL would be obtained was computed for all directions from the nozzle. Three engine power settings were used; "cruise", "military" and "afterburner." Note that in afterburner operation these distances range from about 50 to about 750 feet depending on direction from the "jet nozzle." Data on the characteristics of the noise fields of a variety of jet aircraft have been assembled by Eldred and Kyrazis (28). The octave band SPLs needed for comparison with communication and damage risk criteria can be obtained using data from figure 104 and from table 52. For example, the OASPL at "cruise" power 100 feet from the jet nozzle on the 135 degree radial is 130 db (fig. 104). Subtracting from this OASPL (130 db) the number of db for each octave band given in table 52 (125 to 180 degree radials) results in OBSPLs as follows: 20 to 75 c.p.s. = 118 db; 75 to 150 c.p.s. = 123 db; 150 to 300 c.p.s. = 126 db; 300 to 600 c.p.s. = 124 db; 600 to 1200 c.p.s. = 118 db; 1200 to 2400 c.p.s. = 114 db; 2400 to 4800 c.p.s. = 109 db; and 4800 to 9600 c.p.s. = 104 db. Similar computations can be made for other positions and directions. These propulsion systems produce the same noise field in low altitude flight, when installed on test stands or when operated during "pretakeoff" or "postmaintenance" tests while installed in aircraft. Many of these operations go on

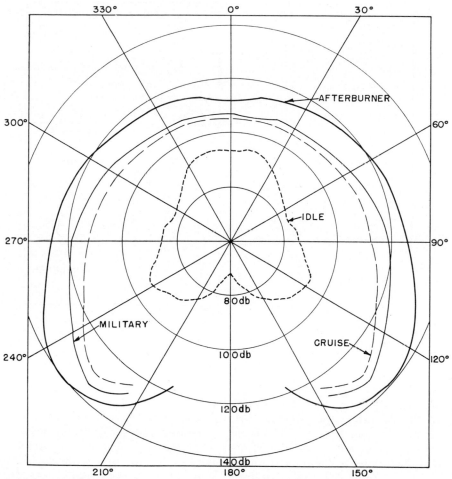

FIG. 104. Over-all sound pressure levels at measurement positions 100 feet away from the jet nozzle of a modern single engine aircraft. Data are given for engine power settings of "idle," "cruise," "military" and "military with afterburner." See text for discussion.

simultaneously and, of course, the more aircraft operating on, into and out of an airport, the greater the amount of noise contributed by propulsion sources.

Items of equipment (on the flight line) used in support of aircraft are also sources of airport noise. This noise is less intense than propulsion system noise (the OASPLs range from about 90 to 107 db at positions 25 feet from the center of these support units) but they are operated more continuously and provide nearly continuous noise exposure to maintenance personnel. The OASPLs at the "operators position," beside this equipment, range from about 105 to 125 db. Sample OBSPLs at the operators position are given, for four different equipment items, in table 61, and more detailed information is avail-

able from a study by Cole (29). Support facilities, such as hangars and shops, contribute noise to the airport environment; the noise characteristics will depend on the equipment in operation or the process being carried out. Data on noise in areas around industrial machines and at the operators positions beside these machines are given by Karplus and Bonvallet (30) and additional data may be obtained from several chapters of the book by Harris (7).

NOISE OUTSIDE AIRCRAFT VERSUS CRITERIA. The two band SPL 100 feet from the jet nozzle (engine at cruise power setting) on the 135 degree radial (see subsection on characteristics of noise fields outside aircraft) is 125 db. This is 25 db above two band criterion level for an 8 hour work day. Nearer

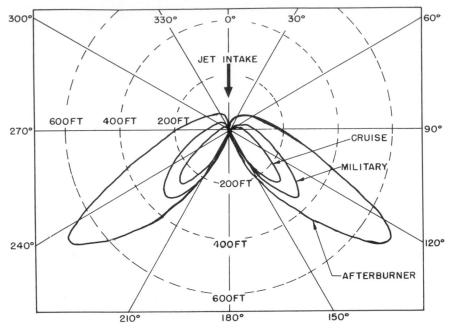

F‌IG. 105. This figure shows the distances from the jet nozzle of a modern single engined turbojet aircraft at which an OASPL of 120 db would be measured when the engine is operated at "cruise," "military" and "military with afterburner" power settings. See text for discussion.

the jet nozzle and at higher power settings, the two band SPL will be still higher. In row 5, table 61, the data show the two band SPL to be 112 db 1000 feet from the jet nozzle (on the 90 degree radial) when the afterburner is in operation. At the same distance on the 135 degree radial the two band level might be 122 db. These numbers clearly show that in terms of the two band damage risk criterion the SPLs must be reduced by 12 to 25 db depending on distance and direction from the jet nozzle. Similar comparisons show a requirement for noise reductions for the criterion bands of 35 to 40 db at positions occupied by maintenance personnel if these positions are occupied 8 hours each day. Similar reductions are required to reduce the SIL to levels compatible with essential communication at distances of 500 to 1500 feet from operating propulsion systems.

Support equipment requires smaller noise reduction to satisfy criteria for risk of damage to the inner ear. These reductions range from a few db to about 20 db to satisfy the two band criterion. Greater noise reduction is desirable to maintain adequate communications near this equipment; reductions of the SIL ranging from 30 to more than 50

db are desirable depending on the specific piece of equipment.

MEANS FOR CONTROLLING AVIATION NOISE

Examination of the acoustic energy fields in aircraft and in the work areas of an airport, in comparison with criteria for communication in noise and criteria for risk of damage to the inner ear, shows a need for reduction of the acoustic energy (noise) generated by most equipment used in the various operations of the aviation industry. In this section the procedures, equipment and facilities that may be employed to reduce or to control aviation acoustic energy (noise) are described.

Noise Suppressors

Noise suppressors are devices, attached to or made a part of a particular noise source, for preventing generation of noise or for absorbing or dissipating it immediately adjacent to the source and before it propagates into areas around receivers (men or equipment) that may be injured or caused to perform inadequately by the noise.

IN-FLIGHT NOISE SUPPRESSORS. In-flight noise suppressors are designed for use primarily with the propulsion system. They have been considered for turbojet engines but have not been used on military equipment. They are planned for use on commercial transport aircraft, primarily to reduce noise disturbance in communities near airports and under regular flight paths. It is estimated that devices can be produced to reduce the total acoustic power output to about one-tenth of that produced by unsuppressed engines. The reduction of the OASPL, in the direction of maximum radiation, might be 18 to 24 db under these conditions. However, equipment for immediate use will be less effective, reducing the total acoustic power by about 6 to 8 db and the OASPL, in the direction of maximum radiation, by 8 to 12 db. A corresponding reduction of the "propulsion" component of the noise inside the aircraft would result and under present operational plans, would be used during "takeoff" where needed most. Outside noise would be reduced by the factors estimated and would be a major improvement of the maintenance environment; but not enough to remove risk of damage to the inner ear. Communication, particularly at moderate distances from the aircraft, would be improved. These noise suppressors usually make the engine a more nearly nondirectional source so that the SPLs of some positions, forward and to either side of the engine, may be just as high or perhaps higher than without the suppressor.

Little has been done to date, but suppressors can be applied to airborne equipment. This has been necessary, in some military equipment, to maintain satisfactory inside noise fields and it may become essential for commercial transport vehicles.

GROUND USE NOISE SUPPRESSORS. Suppressors considered to date have been intended primarily for use with turbojet propulsion systems. Several types have been used or have been proposed. One type is used with engines under test; after removal from the aircraft. Noise reducing treatments for engine test cells are in this category, and almost any amount of noise reduction can be obtained if there is no limit on costs. Reductions of noise levels to values that permit adequate communication in outside areas around the test facility are possible at moderately high costs.

Recently, portable "engine test" stands, equipped with portable "noise control" equipment, have been proposed. These control units can provide noise reductions that "on the average" will assure SPLs below the long exposure time damage risk criterion for hearing in any area outside a rectangle about 100 feet wide and 200 feet long centered about the long axis of the engine and treatment; with the middle of the long side of the treatment placed near a plane through the engine nozzle. Similar treatments or devices can be made for use with engines installed in the airframe and can provide equal performance. Equipment to provide any lesser amount of noise reduction can be built; the primary problem is to provide an optimum compromise between noise reduction and cost. If cost is not considered then the highest performance possible now does not remove all hazards to the ear and still leaves noise levels which cause significant disturbance to communication in all areas closer to the engine than 1000 feet.

Noise suppressors can be provided for nearly all items of ground support equipment. If initially designed into the equipment, the cost need not be unreasonable and noise reductions that remove nearly all risk of damage to the unprotected ear should be possible. Users of this equipment must demand "noise control" or "noise reduction" for this equipment or the manufacturer will nelgect the problem.

DESIGN OF SOURCES TO REDUCE NOISE OUTPUT. Appropriate attack on noise generation during engine design will produce the most effective, least penalizing in-flight suppressor for gas turbines, although it may still be effectively an engine accessory. Users of the equipment, the aircraft operator, must apply pressure on engine manufacturers before an adequate application of this approach is made for aircraft engines.

Design of airborne equipment to prevent or minimize noise generation can reduce the noise output of nearly all items of airborne accessories. The work of design and application is yet to be accomplished. Essentially, the same state of affairs exists relative to ground support equipment although some effort has been made, and with reasonable success, to reduce noise of ground power supplies, engine starting units, etc.

Personal Protective Equipment

Inasmuch as neither the design of equipment which produces aviation acoustic energy (noise) nor the design and application of noise suppressors has reached a stage where acoustic energy levels are below the damage risk criteria for the human inner ear, personal protective equipment must be relied upon to provide the necessary additional noise reduction when suppressors are used or all of the noise reduction when suppressors are not used. These devices are usually made in the following forms: (1) ear plugs, (2) ear muffs or coverings, (3) combinations of plugs and muffs and (4) helmets (head gear) incorporating muffs or plugs or both combined.

Ear plugs have been used longer in modern noise fields. If carefully fitted and used with care by the wearer, especially when care is taken to maintain a good seal, they are quite effective. For the 300 to 600 c.p.s. octave ear plugs reduce the noise level in the ear canal 14 to 20 db; they reduce the level of the 600 to 1200 c.p.s. band 18 to 24 db; the noise level of the 1200 to 2400 c.p.s. band 25 to 31 db and the noise level of the 2400 to 4800 c.p.s. band 30 to 36 db. The variation of noise level reduction depends primarily on the fit of the plug and the care used in retaining a good fit. In applying these factors to determine whether exposure criteria are satisfied you will recall that the measured octave band SPL is reduced by the attenuation factor of the protector and then compared with the risk criterion.

Ear muffs can be equal to ear plugs in performance. However, the better designs must be used to attain this amount of noise attenuation. Inasmuch as practical situations require as much noise attenuation as can be obtained, it is assumed the best muffs will be used, then the attenuation factors given for ear plugs are applicable.

Combinations of ear plugs and ear muffs give more protection than either alone; however, the combination does not give attenuations in db equal to the sum of the individual attenuations provided by each device. The better ear plugs combined with the better ear muffs give noise attenuations as follows: 300 to 600 c.p.s. band, 24 to 30 db; 600 to 1200 c.p.s. band, 28 to 34 db; 1200 to 2400 c.p.s. band, 36 to 42 db; and 2400 to 4800 c.p.s. band, 40 to 45 db.

Ear muffs in particular can be combined with hard hats or helmets. The performance of these combinations is essentially that of the muffs alone. If ear muffs are combined with flying helmets, the helmet may provide some additional noise attenuation.

Flight crews frequently use headsets with earphone covers. These devices afford some noise attenuation but not as much as ear plugs or ear muffs. Attenuations as shown below may be expected from these devices: 300 to 600 c.p.s. band, 7 to 10 db; 600 to 1200 c.p.s. band, 13 to 16 db; 1200 to 2400 c.p.s. band, 20 to 23 db; and 2400 to 4800 c.p.s. band, 30 to 33 db.

All personally worn devices, except headphone covers and flight helmets, are worn primarily to protect the inner ear from the damaging effects of noise. Headphone covers were designed to exclude noise to improve communication by interphone and radio equipment. Flight helmets are primarily for head protection. Any of the noise attenuating devices will improve communication by voice signals, if communication is at all possible, in comparison with the communication in the noise without ear protection. Where communication equipment such as headphones is used, the signal level can be controlled and communication can be greatly improved by using noise attenuating devices unless the signal originally contained noise.

One of the major problems in securing appropriate use of personal protective equipment is that of convincing the wearer of its value. All such devices are somewhat uncomfortable and their use then depends on the user's evaluation of the importance of "comfort" in contrast to "good hearing." Comfort frequently wins unless the benefits of protection are convincingly presented to the persons who must work in noise.

Special Procedures for Noise Control

When noise sources produce noise levels that exceed criteria, improvements can often be obtained by controlling the use or operation of the noise producing equipment. Controlled flight patterns can reduce noise in specific areas near the flight path. Selection of run-up sites and control of the run-up operations can also reduce noise disturbances. If one recalls the greatly reduced noise output at "idle" power settings of turbojet engines, one must immediately recognize that when maintenance tests can be performed at low power settings, major reductions in noise levels are obtained. Development of test procedures appropriate for use at low engine powers would be a major contribution to noise control on any and all airports. Similar control of the operation of support facilities can be used to control noise where other means are not available.

Finally, if the risks to personnel cannot be reduced sufficiently by other means of noise control already discussed, controlled personnel assignments may be used. That is, the time individuals spend in a given high noise level area is limited to a time of exposure that assures compliance with the criteria for risk of damage. Frequently this can be done by appropriate scheduling of daily work activities without any significant loss of the services of the personnel so scheduled.

An Occupational Medicine Program to Protect Man from Aviation Noise

If man is the primary recipient of the adverse effects of aviation noise, the specialist in aviation medicine has the primary responsibility for taking action to reduce or remove the adverse effects. He must utilize other technical specialists in his program. However, he himself must take the initiative in developing and maintaining an appropriate preventive, occupational medicine program.

Evaluation of Hazards of Environmental Noise

The first step of the program is the evaluation of the noise exposure hazards of work areas. Noise sources which produce noise levels in work areas that result in hazardous noise exposures when workmen occupy these areas during normal working hours must be identified. Then their operational schedule must be examined and their acoustic energy (noise) output determined. Detailed specifications of the noise fields may be obtained from published material or by a measurement program as

required. In addition, work schedules of personnel are studied to estimate the probability of hazardous noise exposure. The medical specialist will use the technical capabilities of physicists, acoustical engineers and other specialists in this phase of the program.

Applying Noise Control Equipment and Procedures

The second step of the program is to take action to control the noise levels in work areas so that desired safety, comfort and performance capability of personnel is maintained. Here, the medical specialist will require the assistance of management personnel and will undoubtedly call upon acoustical engineering specialists as consultants in selecting and installing the appropriate noise control procedures and equipment. The medical specialist and his assistants have the following methods of noise control to consider, evaluate and apply: (1) noise suppressors, (2) personal protective equipment, (3) controlled procedures and operational techniques and (4) controlled assignment of the noise exposed personnel. The significant responsibility of the medical staff is to recognize the need and see that appropriate action is taken.

Monitoring the Effects of Noise on Personnel

This phase of the program requires the application of medical knowledge and is the sole responsibility of the medical staff. Inasmuch as the significant adverse effects of noise exposure are usually the effects on the human ear, this phase of the program consists of two major parts: (1) the determination of the functional capability of employees ears at the time they start working and (2) monitoring the hearing capability of employees who work in areas where hazardous noise exposure may occur.

General Audiometry Program. This program is to determine the capability of the employee's hearing function at the time he starts and terminates employment. Audiometric tests are given to determine how well he hears. Emphasis is placed upon hearing for speech signals. The minimum requirements in this phase of the program are (1) a service entry audiometric examination and (2) a service termination audiometric examination. The service entry audiometric examination is done before the employee starts work and specifies the capabilities of his hearing function at the time he begins his employment. The service termination audiometric examination indicates any change in the employee's hearing function that has occurred during his employment. In the aviation industry, these two audiometric examinations should be given to all employees regardless of their potential for incurring hazardous noise exposure.

MONITORING AUDIOMETRY PROGRAM. This program applies to all personnel who may reasonably be expected to incur hazardous noise exposure. The first step is to make an audiogram before the employee actually starts performing duties where hazardous noise exposure is probable. This audiogram is identified as a *reference audiogram*. A classification must be established for these reference audiograms because an individual whose hearing capability is slightly deficient should not be allowed to incur as large an elevation of hearing threshold as is permissible for an individual whose threshold hearing level is within normal range. For each class of reference audiograms a "monitor limit" for permissible threshold shift (TS) must be established. This monitor limit states the amount of TS that is permitted before the individual receives special diagnostic attention or is assigned to work that does not involve hazardous noise exposure.

The remaining elements of this program consist of establishing a schedule or routine audiometric checks to determine whether an individual's threshold hearing level has shifted to or beyond the "monitor limits" applicable to his reference audiogram. In this monitoring program, criteria should be established for taking specific action on a routine basis as noise exposed individuals exhibit shifts in the threshold of hearing in the course of working in the noise environment.

Basic principles for establishing the monitoring audiometry program have been previously published (12). The essential elements of the program may be summarized as follows: (1) making reference audiograms, (2) defining classes of reference audiograms and specifying how much threshold shift will be permitted for each class before special action is initiated, (3) stating criterion threshold shifts (from the reference audiogram) that require specific steps of the monitoring procedure, (4) conducting routine follow-up audiometric tests at specified intervals to determine any changes of hearing from the reference audiogram, (5) carrying out the routine procedures of the monitoring audiometry program until threshold shifts (changes in threshold hearing level), properly verified, dictate a specific, complete diagnostic examination and (6) making every effort, through indoctrination in the use of personal equipment and personal control of exposure, to prevent excessive noise exposure, to utilize, trained, skilled men until unavoidable, excessive elevation of hearing threshold dictates assignment to other work or other appropriate action.

Special emphasis is placed on the monitoring audiometry program because it is the only means for adequate assessment of the effectiveness of the entire "noise control" program, and even more important, it is the means by which each individual can be assured maximum protection for his hearing while working at duties for which he has greatest skill.

REFERENCES

(1) PARRACK, H. O.: Noise and vibration control in the U. S. Air Force. J. Aviation Med., **26**: 146–155, 1955.

(2) PARRACK, H. O.: Protection from aircraft noise. A. M. A. Arch. Indust. Hyg., **10**: 273–287, 1954.

(3) PARRACK, H. O.: Noise, vibration, and people. Noise Control, **2**: No. 6, 10–24, 1956.

(4) PETERSON, A. P. G., AND BERANEK, L. L.: Handbook of Noise Measurement, Ed. 3. Cambridge, General Radio Co., 1956.

(5) HIRSH, I. J.: The Measurement of Hearing. New York, McGraw-Hill Book Co., 1952.

(6) SATALOFF, J.: Industrial Deafness. New York, Blakiston Division, McGraw-Hill Book Co., 1957.

(7) HARRIS, C. M.: Handbook of Noise Control. New York, McGraw-Hill Book Co., 1957.

(8) DAVIS, H.: The hearing mechanism. In HARRIS, C. M.: Handbook of Noise Control, Chapter 4. New York, McGraw-Hill Book Co., 1957.

(9) STEVENS, S. S., AND DAVIS, H.: Hearing: Its Psychology and Physiology, New York, John Wiley & Sons, Inc., 1938.

(10) SIVIAN, L. J., AND WHITE, S. D.: On minimum audible sound fields. J. Acoustical Soc. Am., **4**: 288–321, 1933.

(11) GLORIG, A.: Audiometric testing in industry.

In Harris, C. M.: Handbook of Noise Control, Chapter 6. New York, McGraw-Hill Book Co., 1957.

(12) Davis, H., Hoople, G., and Parrack, H. O.: The medical principles of monitoring audiometry. A. M. A. Arch. Indust. Health, 16: 1–20, 1958.

(13) Research Center, Subcommittee on Noise in Industry: Guide for Conservation of Hearing in Noise. Los Angeles, American Academy of Ophthalmology and Otolaryngology, 1957.

(14) Davis, H.: The articulation area and the social adequacy index for hearing. Laryngoscope, 58: 761–778, 1948.

(15) Kryter, K. D.: The effects of noise on man. J. Speech & Hearing Disorders, Monograph Suppl. 1, 1950.

(16) Hawley, M. E., and Kryter, K. D.: Effects of noise on speech. In Harris, C. M.: Handbook of Noise Control, Chapter 9. New York, McGraw-Hill Book Co., 1957.

(17) Beranek, L. L.: Airplane quieting. II. Specification of acceptable noise levels. Tr. Am. Soc. Mechanical Engineers, 69: 97–100, 1947.

(18) Beranek, L. L., and Newman, R. B.: Speech interference levels as criteria for rating background noise in offices. J. Acoustical Soc. Am, 22: 671, 1950.

(19) Beranek, L. L.: Noise control in office and factory spaces. In Transactions of the Chemical Engineering Conferences, Second Hygeine Foundation of America, 1950.

(20) von Gierke, H. E., and Pietrasanta, A. C.: Acoustical Criteria for Work Spaces, Living Quarters and other Areas on Air Bases. WADC Technical Note 57–248. Dayton, Ohio, Wright Air Development Center 1957.

(21) Davis, H., Morgan, C. T., Hawkins, J. E., Galanbos, R., and Smith, F. W.: Temporary Deafness following Exposure to Loud Tones and Noise. Acta oto-laryng., Suppl. LXXXVIII, 1950.

(22) Rosenblith, W. A., and Committee: The Relation of Hearing Loss to Noise Exposure. New York, American Standards Association, 1954.

(23) Eldred, K. M., Gannon, W. J., and von Gierke, H. E.: Criteria for Short Time Exposure of Personnel to High Intensity Jet Aircraft Noise. WADC Technical Note 55-355. Dayton, Ohio, Wright Air Development Center, 1955.

(24) Rosenblith, W. A., and Stevens, K. N.: Noise and Man, Handbook of Acoustic Noise Control, Vol. II. WADC Technical Report 52-204. Dayton, Ohio, Wright Air Development Center, 1953.

(25) von Gierke, H. E.: Aircraft noise sources. In Harris, C. M.: Handbook of Noise Control, Chapter 33. New York, McGraw-Hill Book Co., 1957.

(26) Bolt, R. H., Beranek, L. L., and Newman, R. B.: Physical Acoustics, Handbook of Acoustic Noise Control, Vol. I. WADC Technical Report 52-204. Dayton, Ohio, Wright Air Development Center, 1952.

(27) von Gierke, H. E.: Aircraft noise control. In Harris, C. M.: Handbook of Noise Control, Chapter 34. New York, McGraw-Hill Book Co., 1957.

(28) Eldred, K. M., and Kyrazis, D. T.: Noise Characteristics of Air Force Turbojet Aircraft. WADC Technical Report 56-280. Dayton, Ohio, Wright Air Development Center, 1956.

(29) Cole, J. N.: Noise Evaluation of Air Force Ground Support Units. WADC Technical Note 56-335. Dayton, Ohio, Wright Air Development Center, 1956.

(30) Karplus, H. B., and Bonvallet, G. L.: A noise survey of manufacturing industries. Am. Indust. Hyg. A. Quart., 14: 235–263, 1953.

19

TEMPERATURE STRESSES

Paul Webb, M.D.

Heat and cold are dominant factors in aviation today. Our military and civilian bases are located throughout the world and climatic temperature extremes are experienced by the flying population. Further, the upper atmosphere is constantly cold and, paradoxically, high speed flight through the atmosphere can be a source of tremendous heat.

In this chapter the sources of heat and cold related to aviation will be examined and the regulation of body temperature will be reviewed. The physiologic reaction to extremes of heat and cold and the tolerance limits for extreme thermal exposure are discussed. Finally, we shall consider the means which have been devised for protecting the flyer against the effects of temperature extremes.

TEMPERATURE EXTREMES IN AVIATION

Sources of Cold

The major source of cold in aviation is the low temperature of the atmosphere at altitudes above 10,000 feet. Commercial and military jet powered aircraft normally operate at levels between 30,000 and 40,000 feet. At this altitude the air temperature is consistently between −40 and −70° F. Air temperature falls progressively to a height of about 50,000 feet. Here a constant temperature of about −70° F. is maintained to over 80,000 feet. Above this level there is a progressive increase in air temperature; however, the air is so thin that temperature in

the ordinary sense begins to lose its meaning. At extreme altitudes, "temperature" means the kinetic energy of an air molecule, or more properly, of a gas particle. An ordinary thermometer suspended in the rarified air of 150,000 feet would register a temperature which is the result of the air particles around it and of the radiation temperature of the earth, the sun and the void of space. These latter two influences would be more important to the final reading of the thermometer bulb. A number of curves of temperature versus altitude have been derived and in figure 106 a standardized curve is presented, with a range of common deviations from it.

Several problems arise from the coldness of the atmosphere where most flying is done. The aircraft must have supplementary heating unless it is flying at supersonic speed. The pilot must be clothed appropriately to protect him from the direct effects of windblast. Wind screens and other transparencies, such as the faceplate of a protective helmet, are subject to frosting from the cold of the atmosphere and the moisture generated by the man.

Windblast was a particular problem during World War II when bomber aircraft were designed with open stations for gunners. Frostbite of the exposed areas (fingers, nose and ears) was common. Windblast and cold air are also difficult problems during bailout at high altitude. High altitude bailout is usually accomplished by free falling from initial altitude to a level of 10,000 or

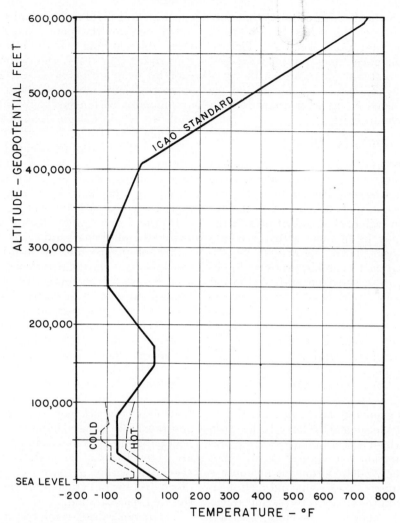

FIG. 106. The standard atmosphere of the International Civil Aviation Organization (consistent with and extended by the ARDC standard atmosphere). Below 100,000 feet two added curves represent the hot and cold variations from the standard atmosphere.

12,000 feet to avoid severe opening shock when the parachute canopy deploys. During the free fall through cold air, windblast leads to frostbite of exposed parts. Cold air with high air movement cools much more rapidly than common experience leads one to expect. The effect has been termed "windchill" and is caused by the greatly increased convective transfer coefficient. It is, therefore, essential to cover the skin to avoid injury.

Not all cold exposure is associated with high altitude. Many air bases are located in the sub-Arctic and Arctic. Not only are air bases located in cold parts of the world

but often global flights originate in warm zones and traverse a frigid zone to reach their destination. If an emergency occurs while the aircraft is over the polar region, and landing or ditching is required, then cold exposure is a major problem in survival.

Frequently an aircraft emergency requires ditching in cold water. The special problem of cold water immersion has led to many casualties. Water temperatures near the freezing point are not uncommon in the North Atlantic, Arctic and sub-Arctic waters. Survival times for an unprotected man are in the order of minutes. Loss of life has been so serious, especially during Navy operations in the Korean conflict, that special protective clothing has been devised and experimental work has been done to establish tolerance times for men exposed to different water temperatures with varying amounts of protection. These findings will be discussed in the section on "Human Thermal Tolerance."

Sources of Heat

On the ground heat is a familiar problem in tropic, subtropic and desert areas. Inasmuch as air bases are located in such areas and inasmuch as global flights may traverse any climatic region, the student of aviation medicine must be familiar with the effects of climatic heat. There is a distinct physiologic adaptation to chronic exposure to climatic heat, thus, personnel stationed in hot areas must be given time to grow accustomed to their new surroundings. Consideration must also be given to the problem of survival when an emergency landing occurs in desert or tropical terrain.

A most important new feature in aviation medicine is the extensive use of protective clothing which strongly aggravates the effect of a mild or moderate heat exposure. Heavy arctic flight clothing may have to be worn in flights which either originate in or traverse cold terrain but also extend over hot climatic zones. Such clothing is not only a burden because of its weight and high insulation value but is also effectively impermeable to water vapor and, therefore, a serious limitation when sweating is called upon to dissipate body heat. This feature of impermeability is found in other protective clothing used in modern flying. The anti-exposure suit which has been developed to protect the flyer against cold water immersion is a coverall made of rubberized cloth which will not pass water vapor. Pressure suits to protect the flyer against the effects of explosive decompression and low barometric pressure contain layers of impermeable material. The effect of such material is to intensify even a mild heat exposure. When the body surface produces water for cooling, and that water cannot evaporate, there is no cooling effect. A man completely enclosed in an impermeable garment will suffer from the effects of heat exposure at temperatures of 80° F. There have been experimental flights which had to be terminated because the pilot was wearing impermeable clothing and the cabin temperature rose to 95° F. Without the ability to cool by evaporation of sweat, in a warm space the man's metabolic heat production accumulates within his body. This quickly leads to a physiologic tolerance limit resembling heat stroke.

Intense heat exposure occurs in flash fires and in the blast of a nuclear explosion. The rate of heat flux is so great that serious burning of the body surface occurs before there is significant body heating.

In the future, when flights at extreme altitudes and in space are achieved, another source of intense radiant heating will be from the sun. On the earth's surface we are accustomed to the protective effect of our atmosphere which absorbs much of the sun's energy. However, at altitudes above 100,000 feet the heating effect of this radiant source is considerably greater; it must be considered when designing high altitude and space vehicles.

Actually the thermal environment of space is a radiation environment rather than one in which convection, conduction and radiation all have important roles. Both heat gain and heat loss from a space vehicle are through radiation pathways. The heat generated within a space vehicle must be dissipated by radiation from the vehicle to the cold space around.

The major cause for interest in the effects of heat in modern flying is the phenomenon of aerodynamic heating. In supersonic aircraft flying within the atmosphere there is heating of the surface or skin of the vehicle. A simple way of expressing this is that a body passing through the atmosphere with great velocity becomes hot from the friction between the body and the air. This is the reason meteors burn up when they come into the earth's atmosphere.

A more precise concept of aerodynamic heating involves the boundary layer, the layer of still air next to the surface, in which the temperature and pressure become higher and higher as velocity increases. The high temperature in the boundary layer heats the aircraft structure but there is simultaneous loss of heat through radiation to sky and earth and through conduction along the

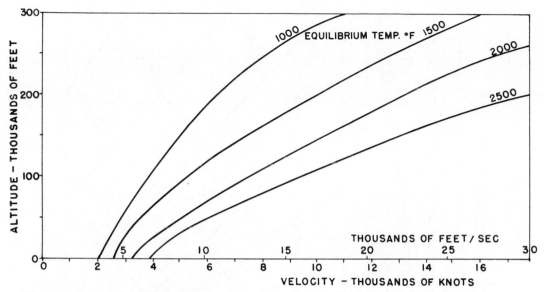

FIG. 107. Curves of equilibrium temperature at a point 1 foot back from the stagnation points at the leading edges or nose of a supersonic vehicle.

boundary layer until an equilibrium temperature is reached. At the stagnation areas directly ahead of the leading edges of the wings and the nose of the aircraft this heating is greatest. In figure 107 plots of equilibrium temperatures at a point 1 foot back from the leading edges of the aircraft are shown as functions of the velocity of the vehicle and of altitude.

This phenomenon of aerodynamic heating is of great importance not only to supersonic flight of jet powered vehicles within the atmosphere, it is also a limiting factor in the design of vehicles which are intended to escape from and re-enter the earth's atmosphere. Designers have had to include larger and larger cooling units in high performance aircraft. Although it may be desirable for the aircraft to protect the man from extremes of heat and cold, and the burden of protection has always been placed on the aircraft designer, nevertheless, research in aviation medicine must encompass the effects of exposure to extreme heat and cold. There is no doubt that sufficient heating or cooling can be provided in aircraft to afford comfort conditions. However, in some very new and advanced aircraft it may be that the high performance sought may be compromised by the power and weight of the air conditioning unit required to produce comfort. In military aviation,

where the margin of performance over a potential enemy may be small, it might be important that the aircrew withstand a certain amount of heat or cold stress to gain an extra margin of power, speed or altitude.

HUMAN THERMOREGULATION

In the first section of this chapter the reader may have received the impression that in aviation medicine we are concerned only with the dramatic or extreme situation. Actually, under normal conditions in commercial and military flying we are first of all interested in what constitutes comfort and what extensions beyond comfort are compensable by the normal body mechanisms. A lightly clothed man is comfortable within a range of temperatures from approximately 65 to 85° F. at moderate to low humidities. In figure 108 a graphic representation of the comfort zone and the compensable zones on either side of it are presented. In these regions the normal thermoregulatory processes maintain thermal balance for hours at a time. The limits of such cool and warm exposures are more from fatigue than from any failure of thermoregulation.

The major topic of this section is a brief description of the thermoregulatory responses in man to heat and cold. These are

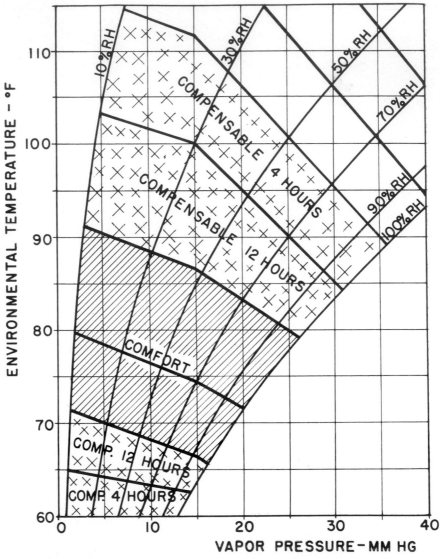

FIG. 108. Allowable ranges of temperature and humidity for aircraft cabins. (Redrawn from Air Force Memorandum Report TSEAL 3-695-56.)

the responses which maintain thermal balance in the compensable zones shown in figure 108. These same responses are also called for in the more extreme exposures which are described in the next section. Although the responses to heat and cold in extreme cases are the same, we distinguish between compensable and extreme exposure by whether or not these responses succeed in maintaining thermal balance.

The regulation of body temperature is like any control system. There are sensors, computers and active responses used to achieve a thermal balance. The sensors in thermoregulation are located on the body surface and are very probably located centrally as well. The computer in this case is the hypothalamus, where integration of sensory information is accomplished and decisions made as to what responses are called for. The responses are four in number, possibly five in man. Each of these major parts of the control system will be discussed.

SENSORS. The sensation of heat or cold on the skin is familiar to everyone and medical students are familiar with the process of mapping hot and cold spots on skin. There are even special end organs described for receiving sensations of both hot and cold. These are the familiar end bulbs of Krause and the end organs of Ruffini. However, recent research in temperature reception indicates that bare nerve endings of unmyelinated fibers play a major role in temperature reception. Some doubt has been cast on the function and perhaps of the existence of the special end organs described in classic histology. The student who wishes to pursue this subject further may start with the excellent bibliographic summary prepared by the Environmental Protection Division of the Army Quartermaster Research Laboratories (1).

The important consideration in the description of temperature receptors in the skin is the ability of these receptors, whatever they may be histologically, to detect thermal gradients. The temperature receptors in the skin respond not to an absolute level of temperature but rather to the direction of heat flow or the direction of the thermal gradient and its magnitude as well. Anatomically then, one has to think in terms of receptors located in depth from the skin surface. The sensation of cold is one of an increasing flow of heat from inside out. Conversely, the sensation of warmth is caused by a change in the thermal gradient from the previous condition to one of lesser flow of heat from inside out or a reversal of the gradient with a flow of heat from outside in.

The existence of central temperature receptors has been postulated for some time but so far these receptors have not been located and described anatomically. Heating and cooling of the blood which goes to the brain causes classic thermoregulatory responses in the absence of peripheral sensations of heat or cold. Direct heating of the hypothalamus and direct cooling of the same area also cause thermoregulatory responses similar to those observed when heating or cooling at the skin surface occurs. This is strong evidence in support of either discrete thermoreceptors in the brain or perhaps a certain temperature sensitivity of brain tissue.

Inasmuch as there is apparently both a central and peripheral set of receptors to inform the computer of heat or cold, the next question concerns which plays the dominant role in various situations? Is peripheral information more important than central? At present there is no clear answer. All of the responses can be elicited by stimulating either the peripheral or the central receptors alone. Under ordinary climatic conditions it seems that the cutaneous receptors play a dominant role. Thermoregulatory responses occur in the absence of any measurable change in internal temperature. On the other hand, it can be argued that the central receptors are being stimulated by extremely small variations in internal temperatures which are so small as to be nearly undetectable. Answers to these questions are one facet of present research in temperature regulation.

REGULATORY RESPONSES. There are four or perhaps five responses to heat and cold exposure in man. In cold the cutaneous blood vessels constrict in order to reduce the amount of heat lost from the skin surface. The effect is to allow the skin surface to cool rapidly to cold air making the gradient from skin to air smaller. In heat the opposite effect occurs, namely, vasodilation. Opening of cutaneous blood vessels serves to increase the rate of loss from the skin surface. As long as the ambient temperature is lower than the skin surface temperature, an increase in circulating blood will mean increased transfer of heat from the interior to the surface, where it can be lost to the air. However, the same mechanism of vasodilation occurs even when the air temperature is higher than the surface temperature, and this would result in a gain in heat were it not for sweating.

In cold exposure the second response, which occurs later than vasoconstriction, is increase in the activity of skeletal muscle. This is first an increase in muscle tension which can be detected with an electromyograph, followed by clonic movements or shivering. A related muscular response is the increase in voluntary activity, such as running, stamping and beating of arms, a natural activity in cold. All of these increase the heat production of the body by the most readily mobilized source of heat, namely the skeletal muscles. Inasmuch as the muscles are doing no measurable physical work the energy expended in muscle contraction appears as heat.

The fourth major response to temperature change is sweating. Under ordinary circumstances sweating occurs whenever skin temperatures go above approximately 93° F. There are some experimental situations, however, in which sweating does not begin until much higher skin temperatures are reached so that it would be incorrect to say a certain level of skin temperature is the initiating cause for sweat production. The subject of sweating in man has received a good deal of experimental attention, and important reviews of the subject have been written by Kuno (2) and Ferguson et al. (3).

Another response to cold exposure, and this is the fifth major response, is the possibility of an increase in the nonshivering level of heat production. This chemical production of heat, also called "nonshivering thermogenesis," is easily demonstrated in rats and other experimental animals. Recent work has also shown evidence for the same process in man. This mechanism is important if there is a real adaptation in homeotherms to cold, although it would not be expected to be of much importance in acute exposure to cold, which is the more common or more troublesome problem in aviation.

In homeotherms other than man there are two additional thermoregulatory responses which are important. These are panting, a means of increasing heat loss by rapid exchange of respiratory air over the moist lining of the upper respiratory tract, and piloerection, which is a response in cold, effective in animals with fur coats. Erection of hair in the fur increases the thickness of the still layer of air trapped between the hair fibers and, therefore, increases the insulation in the animal's coat. Piloerection in man is commonly called goose flesh.

HYPOTHALAMIC CONTROL CENTERS. In the central nervous system, information from the thermal receptors is received and interpreted, then decisions are taken on the need for regulatory responses. The nature of the decision is a somewhat complex one. The body is basically a heat engine; there is an irreducible amount of heat being produced all the time. This metabolic heat production is lowest with sleep and increases in the waking states up through various stages of physical activity. At the same time the ambient or environmental conditions may be changing. The computer, therefore, must somehow achieve a temperature balance between the varying levels of heat production and the heat loss or heat gain from the environment. The object is to maintain a certain reasonably constant heat content of the mass of the human body. Changes in heat content, which are measured by changes in internal and surface temperature, are allowable within certain limits. This is true at least for short periods of time. In the long run, of course, the thermal balance must be such that the over-all heat content of the body does not change from day to day. Heat balance can be obtained, then, either by varying the level of heat production or varying the level of heat loss and gain through the body surface.

The principal means of changing the heat production of the body is by varying the activity level of the skeletal muscles. The most familiar response is that of shivering during cold exposure. The other response is the increase in heat production not related to shivering, referred to above. The mechanism and the pathway for its initiation have not been defined. During exposure to heat there does not seem to be any mechanism for reducing the level of internal heat production.

The rest of the thermoregulatory responses employed by the hypothalamic centers are ways of changing the rate of heat loss or heat gain at the body surface. Vasoconstriction, vasodilation and sweating are the important responses for varying loss of heat. The hypothalamus influences the vasomotor centers. Sweating is controlled through the sympathetic nerve fibers although at the sweat glands the response is characterized pharmacologically as cholinergic.

The change in caliber of cutaneous blood vessels is the first mechanism employed by the hypothalamus when environmental temperatures change from the comfort zone, or when there is an increased need for heat loss during increased muscular activity. If these changes in the skin surface are not sufficient to restore thermal balance then shivering or sweating is called upon to increase the magnitude of the response. Both shivering and sweating are more powerful regulatory responses than vasomotor changes. During exposure to heat the sweating mechanism is effective regardless of environmental temperatures which may be higher than the skin surface temperature. Evaporative heat loss continues to be effective as long as there is dry air to remove water vapor.

The hypothalamus has been explored to locate the site of the control of thermoregulatory responses. The responses which are used during cold exposure (the heat conserving responses) are controlled in the posterior portion of the hypothalamus. Those responses which are used during heat exposure are located in the anterior hypothalamus. By direct and indirect heating or cooling through an extracorporeal circuit of the blood leading to the head an experimental animal can be made to pant or shiver or increase his metabolic heat production.

An excellent summary of the subject of temperature regulation has been published in a monograph edited by Newburgh (4). More recent information is summarized periodically in the yearly volumes of the *Annual Review of Physiology*.

CLIMATIC ADAPTATIONS. The subject of adaptation has received extensive investigation by environmental physiologists. There is a clear-cut acclimatization to climatic heat. This consists principally of an improved sweating response, meaning a fuller and earlier sweating response in heat, and the acquisition of the ability to produce a more dilute sweat secretion with a consequent lessening of the loss of mineral solutes. This acclimatization takes place over a period of about 5 days in men who are active and are exposed to desert or tropical heat. The acclimatization is useful in chronic exposure to heat such as might be experienced by troops stationed at an air base located in a hot climate.

Adaptation or acclimatization to cold is harder to demonstrate in humans despite considerable effort to prove or disprove the existence of such a mechanism. In man, at least, there is no significant increase in metabolic level during a prolonged exposure to cold. Some, however, believe that when the

cold exposure is truly effective in terms of keeping the men cold for days at a time that there is an increase in the nonshivering level of heat production. Another mechanism which has been described by Carlson *et al.* (5) consists of the change in response to a limited cold exposure, that is, one which will be of only a few hours duration followed by rewarming. This response consists of a lessening of the vasoconstrictor response in the skin with subsequent increased cooling of the central body core. The effect is to prevent extreme cooling of peripheral areas especially the tips of the extremities, but of course at the expense of lowering the total body heat content. Evidence of a similar kind has been collected by Scholander *et al.* (6) in a study of the responses of primitive people, the Australian aborigines, who habitually sleep almost unprotected on the ground during uncomfortably cold nights. They too permit a remarkable degree of cooling of the body surface and of the internal temperature as well. These people are able to withstand a much greater degree of cooling without shivering or without being uncomfortable or awakening during the night. This apparent adaptation to cold exposure would not seem to be of much use to personnel who are stationed in sub-Arctic and Arctic climates.

The thermoregulatory responses which have been described in this section are employed successfully to maintain thermal balance in the comfort zone and in the compensable zones of warm and cold. When the heat exposure or the cold exposure exceeds the limits of the compensable zone then the responses are inadequate to maintain a uniform heat content of the body mass. These exposures are necessarily limited. The time that such exposures can be tolerated depends upon the amount of heat storage or heat deficit. In the next section these noncompensable exposures will be discussed in terms of heat and cold levels required to produce heat storage and heat deficit and the tolerance limits in terms of time for given exposures.

HUMAN THERMAL TOLERANCE

Tolerance to heat exposure is defined in terms of performance and in terms of the ability or inability to adjust physiologically. The tolerability of environmental conditions covers the whole range from comfort to thermal injury.

There is a range of thermal conditions in which tolerance is time limited to increasingly short intervals. Tolerance to compensable environmental conditions may last for many hours. Exposures to more severe heat or cold beyond the compensable zones lead to a deterioration of performance and to physiologic failure. Tolerances to extremely intense heat or cold are very short because of injury from burning or freezing of the body surface. In this section tolerance will be described in these various terms: *comfort*, which means indefinite tolerance, *limited tolerance* in the compensable zone, *more limited tolerance* in the noncompensable zone and *very brief tolerance* to high intensity thermal exposure. In these four ranges of tolerance the two most pertinent to the subject of aviation medicine are comfort with indefinite tolerance and the noncompensable zone leading to performance decrement and collapse.

Comfort, Indefinite Tolerance

Individual choice plays an important role in thermal comfort. However, considerable progress has been made in the air conditioning industry in defining statistically averaged, acceptable values of comfort. Standards have been defined for comfort conditions under the two major seasonal influences of summer and winter. Adjustment has also been made in terms of regional preferences, that is comfort as defined by a person living in the northern sections of this country as opposed to that defined by inhabitants of the extreme south. This material is summarized in the *Heating, Ventilating, Air Conditioning Guide* which is published with yearly revisions by the American Society of Heating and Air Conditioning Engineers.

Based on the data published in the most recent edition of the *Heating, Ventilating, Air Conditioning Guide* (7), the summer comfort zone for most individuals is a combined air and wall temperature of $76 \pm 5°$ F. and 50 per cent relative humidity. The winter comfort zone for most individuals is approximately $72 \pm 3°$ F. and 50 per cent relative humidity. Although there has been no special study made of comfort under conditions of low barometric pressure it may be as-

sumed that these same figures will apply for most commercial aircraft.

The studies on comfort have not included the effects of special clothing as worn in military aviation. Neither have they included the possible effects of noise, vibration, acceleration, low pressure, etc., on comfort. From a strictly thermal standpoint tolerance to comfort conditions as defined here should be indefinite. However, a fatigue limit may be reached in aircraft because of the various other stresses which are imposed.

Compensable Conditions, Extended Tolerance

If comfort conditions cannot be provided in an aircraft then there are acceptable levels of warmth or coolness which can be easily compensated for by physiologic adjustment. With proper motivation an individual will have a prolonged tolerance to such conditions. However, a limit is reached eventually because of the fatiguing effects of making the physiologic adjustment.

Added to the fatiguing effects of adjusting to a temperature just beyond the comfort zone are the various other stresses of flying. Inasmuch as the tolerance limit is basically set by a fatigue reaction there are no clear physiologic indications of this limit. Relatively little experimental work has been done in this area. Such tests would have to be conducted using a number of stresses as they occur in aviation.

Experimental work has begun in the areas of combined stresses and fatigue. Other experiments described in current literature are being undertaken to discern the physiologic effects of prolonged exposure to low levels of heat stress. Although the goal in aircraft design should be to remove all low level stress, such has proved unrealistic in the past. It is perhaps unreasonable to expect the internal environment of the airplane, a highly specialized machine, to duplicate ideal working conditions on the ground.

Severe Exposures, Limited Tolerance

Severe exposures to cold or heat are a necessary accompaniment of military flying and occasionally civilian aircraft operation. The importance of this subject is attested to by the large volume of experimental work and published information during the past 10 or 12 years.

The subject of severe exposures is a difficult one because the heating load or the cooling load is the result of many different variables. One must consider the environmental variables of air temperature, wall temperature, humidity, air density and air movement. There may be an added amount of heating from direct solar radiation. There are also the variables which relate to the man's metabolic rate or activity level and the preceding state of thermal balance. Intermediate between the man and the environment are a set of variables which relate to his clothing. These are reflectivity and absorptivity of the clothing surface, clothing insulation and permeability of the clothing assembly to water vapor. This formidable list of important variables has prevented environmental physiologists from finding any simple way to express human thermal tolerance limits in terms of heating load or tolerance in terms of the physiologic effects of these variables which, taken together, make a certain heating or cooling load.

LIMITED EXPOSURES TO COLD. There are very few flying situations today in which the man is exposed to severe cold during flight. Protective clothing and cabin heating, as discussed in the next section, are thoroughly worked out and reliable. Cold exposure in the atmosphere from loss of canopy or during the free fall of a bailout is not of sufficient duration to lead to a tolerance limit from body cooling. However, surface injury or frostbite is a problem in these cases. The only common exposure which leads to a tolerance limit from general body cooling is cold water immersion.

Cold water immersion has been studied in both Navy and Air Force laboratories with the result that today there are prediction curves for survival, an extreme expression of tolerance, in various temperatures of water. Because of the multiplicity of important variables even in this fairly simple type of cold exposure a number of technical reports have been written discussing various aspects of the problem. For example, the man subjected to cold water immersion may be exposed to water temperatures ranging from near freezing to fairly warm water around 70 or 80° F. At the same time his clothing

may be anything from light summer flying clothing to heavily insulated clothing with a waterproof cover, this latter suit being the antiexposure suit. The clothing may contain various amounts of water which influence the insulation value. Finally, the man may stay in the water or he may be immersed for a brief period and then climb out into a life raft but still be subjected to low air temperature. References to reports on this subject are found in the reference section at the end of this chapter (8–11).

Experiments and actual experience have shown that a lightly clothed man in very cold water, near the freezing point, has a survival time of only a few minutes. Although there is some individual variability, most people can survive in freezing water for 5 minutes, but not longer than 10 or 15 minutes. With heavier clothing, even though wet, the survival times in the same freezing water begin to increase. A man who wears heavy clothing which is covered by the impermeable shell of the antiexposure suit may be expected to survive for longer than 2 hours although discomfort in the extremities and other unprotected areas will be severe. Figure 109 shows a prediction curve for tolerance time at two cold water temperatures for a man wearing heavy clothing and the antiexposure suit shell but containing various amounts of water from leakage or perhaps from accumulation of perspiration prior to the exposure. Both the presence of water and the compression of the insulation by hydrostatic pressure reduce the insulation value of the clothing and lead to a faster cooling. The limit is related to a given amount of body cooling. This lower limit of heat loss amounts to approximately 100 kcal. per square meter of body surface. Continued exposure to the conditions which have produced this amount of cooling will be lethal. Another prediction curve is shown in figure 110. Here experimental evidence and actual experience in cold water immersion are summarized as tolerance time *versus* water temperature. The curve shown in the chart is from experimental work conducted at the Aero Medical Laboratory, Wright Air Development Center, in which subjects were clothed in exposure suits which had a wetness of 1.6 liters of water. The bars show the range of variability based on Navy

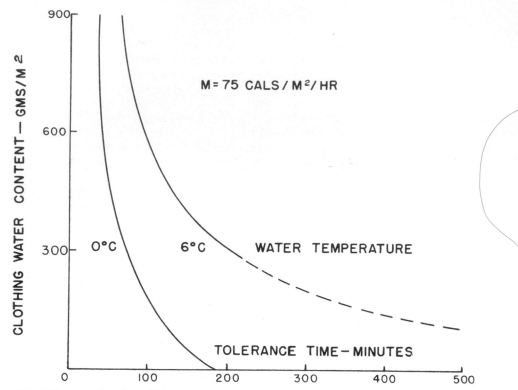

FIG. 109. Tolerance time in cold water for a man wearing an antiexposure suit containing various amounts of water. Metabolic rate is taken as 75 kcal. per square meter per hour (10).

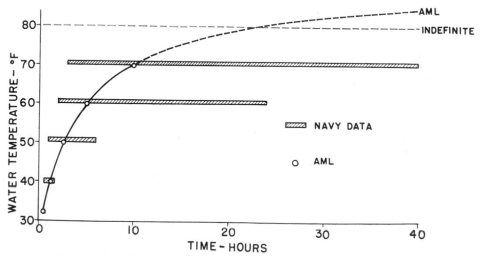

FIG. 110. Prediction for survival at various water temperatures wearing antiexposure suits. AML data (10) is valid for a man whose antiexposure suit contains about 1.6 liters of water. Navy data are for experience in many real situations, described in the *Navy Medical News Letter*, Vol. 31, June 1958.

experience for survival times at various water temperatures. Notice that the variability between individuals is greatest at the higher water temperatures and least at the very low water temperatures.

These severe exposures to cold are characterized physiologically by vasoconstriction and shivering which begins almost at once and is continuous and severe. Measurements of surface temperatures show a steady decrease toward the water temperature with average skin surface temperatures decreasing by perhaps 20° F. Individual temperatures on fingers and toes may drop to as low as 40° F. At the same time, the internal body temperature decreases. The limit of cooling is set by the average body temperature, a combination of rectal temperature and skin surface temperature multiplied by the body weight and the specific heat of the body, which is 0.83. A change in body temperature of 100 kcal. per square meter is critical. Cooling beyond this point is lethal. Prior to this extreme degree of cooling there are symptoms of extreme, painful coldness in fingers and toes and severe shivering, followed by a sense of lethargy.

The terminal event in cold water immersion is considered to be ventricular fibrillation as seen in experimental hypothermia. A review of the subject of induced hypothermia (12) summarizes much of the current knowledge of this subject.

LIMITED EXPOSURES TO HEAT. Human tolerance to levels of heat far above those experienced under normal climatic conditions has been studied intensively in the Air Force for the past 10 years. This interest has arisen from the potential problem of heat exposure in supersonic aircraft which fly within the atmosphere. The study has been complicated by all of the variables which were mentioned above, namely, numerous environmental variables, variation in activity level and variables related to clothing worn by the man. Nevertheless, a large amount of information has been compiled to predict tolerance for many common situations in flying.

The majority of the basic work was done at the University of California at Los Angeles under the direction of the late Dr. Craig Taylor. This work concerned exposure of test subjects to temperatures ranging from 160 to 240° F. at ground level and altitude. A number of clothing assemblies were also used in order to explore the range of insulation values common to Air Force clothing. However, the important variables relating to impermeability and to ventilation of clothing were not explored in this early work. Tolerances for this level of heat exposure were expressed both in terms of performance and a physiologic tolerance limit.

In order to bring together the numerous variables with which the experimental work was done at U. C. L. A., a single physiologic index was employed which was simply the rate of storage of body heat. These exposures were to levels of heating so severe that the normal physiologic adjustments of vasodilation and sweating had relatively small effect. In other words, heat exposures were so severe that compensation was not possible. The body storage index as used by these workers was an expression of the unsteady state. A summarizing description of this work is briefly presented by Blockley et al. (13), and more extensively summarized by them in a Wright Air Development Center Technical Report (14). This work has also been condensed and put in graphic form for inclusion in the Air Force Manual entitled *Handbook of Instructions for Aircraft Designers*. Figure 111 shows the graphic summary which is used to predict performance and physiologic tolerance limits to various environmental conditions with different clothing weights and different activity levels. This graphic solution while complex in appearance represents a great simplification and distillation of the original work. It has been useful in many design situations.

The effect of the work by Taylor et al. has been to show aircraft designers what permissible levels of heat exposure could be tolerated for certain periods of time without undue penalty to the flight crew. Exposures to heat of this variety are obviously beyond the comfort level. The argument has been that providing comfort conditions under all circumstances might result in penalizing the aircraft performance. Secondly, a knowledge of human tolerance to such heat exposures has set limits on what can be expected of a flight crew when an emergency occurs during supersonic flight.

Performance has been tested under heat exposure but more needs to be done in order to clarify the relationship between a performance limit and a physiologic tolerance limit. At the moment a general rule of thumb has been that performance begins to deteriorate in any given condition at about three-fourths of the physiologic tolerance limit. In other words, if the heat exposure is predicted to bring the tolerance point at the end of 1

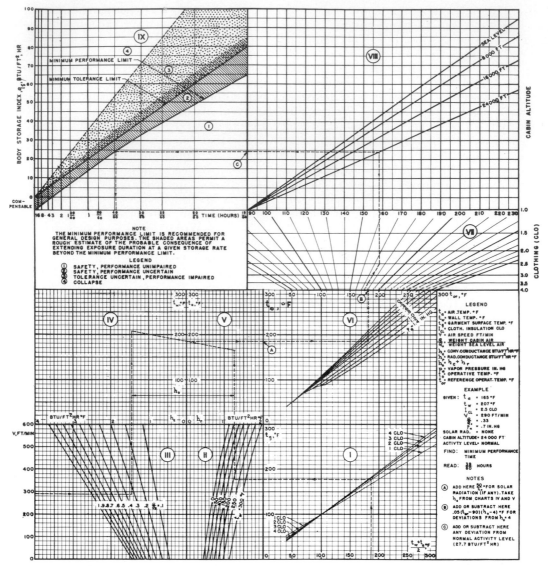

Fig. 111. Hot zone requirements for crew positions in aircraft—from the H.I.A.D. A graphic method for predicting the result of exposure to various conditions typical of flying in high performance aircraft.

hour then performance is expected to fall off at approximately 45 minutes.

Permeability of clothing is an extremely important factor in heat exposure. Although this fact was recognized by the group at U. C. L. A., they did not have experimental equipment to define the point clearly. Later work at the Aero Medical Laboratory (15) shows that while permeability is related to the weight of insulation of the clothing, it is also a separable and important variable. In heat exposure, heavy clothing is probably a burden as much because it is relatively im-

permeable to water vapor as because of its insulation value. In fact, the insulation value when the external temperature is high may be a factor in improving thermal tolerance inasmuch as the effect is to reduce the transfer of heat from outside in. The worst clothing to wear in heat would be impermeable clothing which is light in weight and of poor insulation value. In figure 112 tolerance time, in terms of the physiologic tolerance limit, is plotted against chamber temperature for a series of flight clothing assemblies, both permeable and impermeable and light

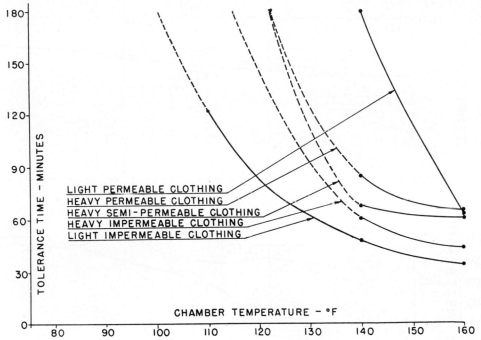

FIG. 112. Time to reach the physiologic tolerance limit *versus* chamber temperature (air and wall equal) in different types of clothing.

and heavy in insulation. At rather mild chamber temperatures around 130° F. the tolerance limit is 1 hour for light impermeable clothing whereas wearing heavy impermeable clothing allows another ½ hour before the tolerance point is reached.

All of this predictive information for tolerance to heat exposure is completely altered when ventilation of clothing is undertaken. This method of relieving the effects of heat exposure is extremely effective. Its value will be seen in the next section when protective measures will be discussed.

The heat exposures employed in establishing the data presented here are steady state levels of air and wall temperature, usually with air and wall temperature being equal. Some exploration of the effects of various air densities has been included and a limited amount of information has been gained on the effects of variation in air motion and air humidity. This has served to establish basic information in the area of severe heat exposure to which physiologic compensation is not possible. However, in the actual aircraft situation transient or dynamic changes in thermal conditions will be more characteristic.

Experimental work using temperature transients, that is, changing temperature levels, heat pulses and repeated brief exposures to heat, has only just begun. At the time of this writing a very preliminary statement can be made that man's tolerance to extremely high temperatures, for example 400° F. air and wall, is surprisingly good for very brief periods. It is expected that further work of this sort will result in tolerance limits similar to those which have been set for lower temperatures under steady state conditions.

DEFINITION OF THE PHYSIOLOGIC TOLERANCE LIMIT. The end point which has been used in experimental work in heat exposure has the following characteristics. There is a high and rapidly rising internal temperature. The pulse rate is high, generally 140 beats per minute and above. Sweating, which has been heavy during the exposure up to this time, decreases abruptly and the skin appears dry. The blood pressure is normal or above normal with a widened pulse pressure. There may be an increase in the depth and rate of respiration. The skin surface is flushed. The subject will be restless and unable to fix his attention. Various other

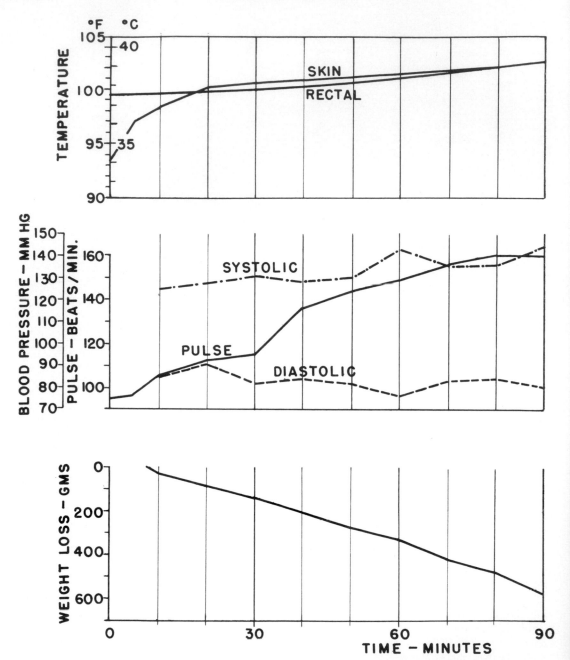

FIG. 113. Data from a severe heat exposure for a lightly clothed man. Conditions are chamber air-wall temperature, 140° F.; clothing, one piece cotton underwear; and sitting activity. The tolerance limit is reached in 90 minutes.

symptoms may appear, such as headache, nausea, disorientation and faintness. Measurements of the cardiac output at this point indicate that it is high. Figure 113 shows graphically the course of events during a typical severe exposure to heat in which physiologic adjustments are ineffective. At the end of 90 minutes the subject has reached the physiologic end point.

Inasmuch as the rapid pulse, high rectal temperature, dry flushed skin and mental changes are characteristic findings in heat stroke, this condition has been termed "impending heat stroke." Experience in the experimental chambers has shown that if a heat exposure is continued beyond this point unconsciousness occurs and the subject can be revived only by vigorous cooling of his body surface. Notice that this condition is by no means similar to what has been termed heat exhaustion or heat prostration. A clear distinction can be made between clinical heat stroke and heat exhaustion. In clinical practice heat exhaustion is characterized by faintness, a cool moist skin, a very rapid but thready pulse and other symptoms which suggest a vasomotor collapse or shock syndrome.

The measured rectal temperature when the physiologic end point has been reached is not alarmingly high. The subjects used in the experiments described here are sitting quietly or doing a light performance task during the course of the heat exposure. When tolerance is reached their rectal temperatures have risen to 102 or perhaps 103° F. In clinical practice, of course, it is not uncommon to see rectal temperatures of 105 or 106° F. in febrile disease. However, the conditions are in reality quite similar. A calculation of the actual heat content of the body depends not only on the measured rectal temperature, but also on the measured average skin temperature. In the kind of heat exposures used in these experiments, skin temperatures averaged over the body surface go as high as 104° F. When skin and rectal temperatures are combined and multiplied by body weight and specific heat, the heat content of the body is found to be increased by 80 to 100 kcal. per square meter. This increase in heat content seems to be some sort of physiologic limit, whether acquired through external heating or through increase in metabolic rate with retention of metabolic heat as seen in fever. Notice that the figure 100 kcal. per square meter is similar in this area of positive heat storage to the figure of negative storage or heat loss discussed under the subject of cold water immersion. The significance of this upper limit of heat storage was recognized in the work of Blockley et al. (13) and has been further verified in the experimental work conducted at the Aero Medical Laboratory, Wright Air Development Center.

MEDICAL HAZARDS IN EXTREME COLD AND HEAT. Very briefly, the medical hazard of cold exposure is described under cold water immersion. In homeotherms death seems to occur from ventricular fibrillation. A search for prophylactic and preventive measures for ventricular fibrillation has begun with the hope of reducing death during rewarming. The subject of rewarming following a cold exposure has been debated in the literature; in general, the methods for rapid rewarming find most favor.

A patient who has been exposed to severe heat and is in a state of impending or actual heat stroke requires immediate attention lest the condition become irreversible with a runaway increase in internal temperature. Death in hyperthermia is poorly defined experimentally but immediate cooling is the only treatment of value. Cooling can be accomplished by immersion in cool water, cold showers, wet towels or direct cooling from a fan, especially if the skin is moistened. The important point is to begin whatever cooling is easiest. Removal of the patient from the heat exposure takes precedence over all else.

In the most severe heating and cooling situations, which produce frostbite or burns, respectively, on the body surface, medical treatment is well described in the medical literature.

PROTECTIVE MEASURES

In aviation the first line of defense against exposure to heat and cold is the aircraft air conditioning system, a well developed specialty in the aircraft industry. Cooling systems for supersonic aircraft are also well developed and effective. With 100 per cent reliability there would be no reason to explore the subject of human thermal tolerance and protective measures. However, experience has shown that 100 per cent reliability is unrealistic even with today's advanced technology. Furthermore, and this is openly a matter of debate, adequate cooling systems for the most advanced military aircraft and for early space vehicles may be excessively costly in weight, power and volume.

Currently the air conditioning groups responsible for cooling and heating in advanced aircraft have shown that under nearly all operating conditions temperature can be held within the comfort range or very near it. In commercial and military aviation, aircraft designers are required to provide comfort conditions for most circumstances. Only a little leeway is granted for the designers of advanced military systems and this leeway is defined in the graph shown as figure 111. On the other side of the debate are those who argue for increased knowledge in human thermal tolerance and protective measures, when the air conditioning fails and when other emergencies occur such as ditching in cold water.

It is clear that aeromedical research should explore further tolerance limits as they may apply to future aircraft. A rapid high temperature transient, or heat pulse, might be permissible to save weight and power. If tolerance limits for this kind of exposure are not known the aircraft designer may be unnecessarily restricted in his choice of systems. The designer of future advanced vehicles is constantly making trade studies for the best possible compromise between conflicting requirements, limits and other parameters in the design of his vehicle. One function of research in aviation medicine is to provide clearly defined limits to all possible kinds of conditions which might occur in flight. Intolerable conditions must be defined before they can be declared unallowable.

The strongest argument in favor of the so-called "shirt sleeve environment," in which the environmental conditions in the aircraft are maintained within the comfort zone, concerns the difficulty of devising personal equipment for the aircrew which is unrestrictive in every respect. It may be possible to protect a man with an unrestrictive garment for one or two flight stresses at a time. When, however, the protective equipment must provide primary protection against low pressure, low oxygen tension, g forces, heat and cold, and in addition, be able to cope with many kinds of emergency situations, then the protective equipment the man must wear becomes unreasonably bulky and unmanageable.

This section will describe the several useful protective measures which have been devised to protect the aircrew against the effects of heat and cold. The extent to which any of these is used will be decided at the time the aircraft is flown. Without going further into the arguments on using or not using protective equipment, the remainder of this section will present the equipment which has been devised and which is available for use when necessary.

Clothing Insulation and Reflective Coatings

The primary means of protection against cold exposure is by use of heavy insulated clothing. Familiar examples are Arctic clothing and the heavy flight clothing developed during World War II and still in use in military aviation.

The insulation of clothing is defined quantitatively in units called "clo." One clo is the amount of clothing required to maintain comfort for a sitting person in a normally vented room with a temperature of 70° F. and humidity less than 50 per cent. A more rigorous definition of clo is the unit of resistance to heat flow which will permit the passage of 1 kcal. per square meter per hour with a temperature gradient of 0.18° C. (16). A moderately heavy garment for cold weather would have an insulation value for the garment of 2 to 2.5 clo, whereas a very heavy outfit would have a value of 4 clo. Measurements of the insulation value of clothing assemblies are made on a special electrically heated copper manikin. Insulation values for many types of flying clothing have been defined and published in an Air Force technical report (17).

In addition to the protection afforded by insulation, which is a way of increasing the resistance to heat transfer through clothing, another method of altering heat gain and loss is by choice of surface materials with appropriate radiative characteristics. A clothing assembly which is covered by a reflective outer coatings reject external heat loads. Aluminized cloth and other common reflective outer coating rejects external heat loads. Aluminized cloth and other common reflective materials are effective at moderately high wall temperatures as well as for protection against fire, blast from nuclear weapons and sunlight. At wall temperatures of 150° F. the coating rejects radiant heat but at higher wall temperatures where the energy received through radiation is high the protection becomes more significant physiologically.

Layers of cloth with reflective coatings

which are included in layers below the surface of a clothing assembly have little effect in reducing heat gain or heat loss. They do in fact add to the impermeability of the clothing assembly which is a burden. They do not alter the radiative heat gain or heat loss to the clothing.

ELECTRICALLY HEATED FLYING SUITS. In aircraft where bulky clothing can be a disadvantage, clothing with electrical resistance wires wound in an inner layer has been developed. Such clothing was developed during World War II and served a useful purpose in high altitude flying of that period (see Newburgh, p. 441 (4)). Little new development has been made in this type of clothing in recent years. Some of the disadvantages of electrically heated clothing, such as the existence of hot spots under the wires and breakage of wires, could perhaps be solved by additional development, especially in view of today's improved electrically heated blankets and similar materials.

Ventilated Clothing

The most effective measure for protection against heat exposure in ordinary clothing or for improving tolerance in impermeable clothing is ventilation. The need for ventilated clothing has been recognized for many years and these needs were clearly spelled out by Fetcher et al. (18).

Many varieties of ventilating garments, devices for distributing ventilating air under the clothing, have been developed. The most effective distribution device was originated by Mauch et al. (19, 20). This basic method has been further developed in the Air Force so that it is possible now to ventilate effectively many types of clothing, from standard Air Force flight clothing to antiexposure suits, full pressure suits and partial pressure suits.

Figure 114 is a photograph of a current Air Force ventilating garment which is worn with several types of complete clothing assemblies. The ventilating garment proper is made of a double layer of plastic film. Air is distributed from a central delivery hose between the double layers so that a major portion of the body surface receives ventilating air. The supply air can escape from the double layer only by leaving tiny pinholes in the inner layer of plastic film. These pinholes

are distributed over the entire inner layer and the air flow through them is roughly equal at all points. This ventilating air then leaves the layer next to the skin and traverses both layers of the ventilating garment by coming out through the large holes visible in the photograph. This escaping air is conducted away to the outlet point or points. A recent report on the design of ventilating garments in the Air Force reviews a number of types and also stresses the principles involved in making a proper distribution system for effective ventilation (21).

Ventilated clothing is effective because direct cooling is through convective heat transfer and additional cooling results from evaporation of water produced in response to the need to lose heat. The amount of air required for proper ventilation depends on the desired result. If complete air conditioning with comfort is the object under a pressure suit or other impermeable garment and the external heat load is not high, then comfort can be achieved by using air flows of 30 to 35 cubic feet of air per minute the temperature of which is approximately 80° F. In contrast to this a more severe external heating condition can be satisfactorily met with 10 cubic feet of air per minute if instead of choosing comfort as the goal of ventilation, one permits a mild heat stress on the man and makes use of evaporative cooling through the normal sweating mechanisms evoked in response to the heat load. Evaporative cooling is a much more effective method of heat protection than convective cooling as long as it is necessary to cause the man to accept a mild degree of stress.

The protective value of ventilated clothing can best be illustrated by citing some physiologic test results. Figure 115 shows the difference in the responses of 2 subjects, 1 of whom is ventilated while the other is not, during a severe heat exposure with a heavy impermeable protective garment. In these experiments the heat load was high enough to cause the unventilated subject to reach tolerance in 1 hour. The subject who was ventilated under the same conditions with 12 cubic feet of air at 60° F. endured the heat exposure for 3 hours and showed moderate physiologic strain at the end of the experiment.

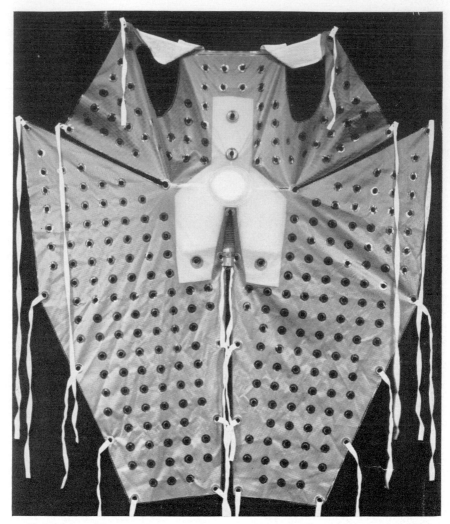

Fig. 114. Air Force ventilating garment, type MA-3. This apronlike device is tied around trunk and legs after the wearer is clothed in underwear. Other flight clothing is worn over the ventilating garment.

Experimental work has been done in Air Force and Navy laboratories aimed at defining the influence of pertinent variables, air flow, temperature and humidity of ventilating air, chamber temperature and clothing, on the physiologic effect of ventilation. Several reports (20, 22–25) have been published with the results of these investigations. When enough information has been gathered, predictive charts can be prepared to allow aircraft designers to choose proper variables in ventilated clothing for expected heat loads.

The general value of ventilation during heat exposure has been established. Actual experience under operating conditions has

been limited. However, more experience should be forthcoming as more and more the military flyer is required to wear other protective clothing which without ventilation would be limiting. Pressure suits require ventilation if worn for any period of time, or must be ventilated even for short periods of time unless the environment is kept cool.

Precooling as a Protection Against Heat

Because the physiologic tolerance limit is reached after there has been storage of a certain quantity of heat it should be possible to increase tolerance by lowering the heat content of the body prior to an expected

TABLE 60

Temporary Threshold Shift (TTS) and Recovery of Threshold Hearing Level after Exposure to Jet Engine Noise—Level Range 125 to 140 db OASPL

Row Number[a]	Test Frequencies in Cycles per Second						Ear	Descriptive Comments
	250	500	1000	2000	4000	8000		
	db	db	db	db	db	db		
1	0	10	10	15	35	15	Right	Exposure for 15 min. with ears not pro-
1a	−5	0	0	−5	25	0	Right	tected; TTS measured 2 hours after exposure in lines 1 and 2; remaining TTS measured 19½ hours after ex-
2	0	15	15	25	5	35	Left	posure in lines 1a and 2a; No other
2a	−5	5	0	0	−10	15	Left	exposure (W. D. N.).
3	5	5	15	35	35[b]	25	Right	Exposure as above; (II. J.)
3a	−5	0	−5	5	20[c]	5	Right	
4	5	0	25	40	30	35	Left	Exposure as above (H. J.)
4a	−5	−5	0	5	10	20	Left	
5	0	−5	5	0	15	0	Right	Exposure for 2 min. with no protection;
5a	5	0	10	5	15[d]	0	Left	test made 2 hours after exposure (W. D. N.)
6	−5	−10	−10	20	48[e]	10	Left	Exposure for 16 minutes to 120 db 2000 c.p.s.; TTS measured 2 minutes after
6a	5	0	−5	−5	10[f]	0	Left	exposure in line 6 and 23 hours after exposure in line 6a.
7	0	48	55	55	50[g]	50[g]	Left	Exposure to broad band noise., 130 db,
7a	5	10	20	18	0	10[h]	Left	for 8 min.

[a] See text for an explanation of each row.
[b] Loss at 3000 c.p.s. = 50 db.
[c] Loss at 3000 c.p.s. = 35 db.
[d] Loss at 3000 c.p.s. = 20 db.
[e] Loss at 3000 c.p.s. = 48 db.
[f] Loss at 2500 and 5000 c.p.s. = 28 db; recovery in 23 hours.
[g] Loss at 6000 c.p.s. = 25 db; recovery in 2 minutes.
[h] Loss at 5000 c.p.s. = −10 db; recovery in 44 hours.

posures. The audiometric test made 2 hours after the exposure showed slight threshold shifts, (maximum threshold shift 20 db at 3000 c.p.s., left ear) but the individual's threshold hearing level was within the range of normal hearing except for 3000 c.p.s., left ear. These threshold shifts are temporary because the threshold hearing level has returned, essentially, to normal limits in 2 hours. The results of the exposure of another person to another type of noise is shown in rows 6 and 6a, table 60 (see also Davis *et al.*, 21). This exposure lasted for 16 minutes and the sound was a pure tone of 2000 c.p.s. at a sound pressure level of 120 db. The effects of the exposure were measured 2 minutes after the exposure was terminated (row 6). A maximum threshold shift of 48 db was recorded for test frequencies 3000 and 4000 c.p.s. The threshold shift at 2000 c.p.s. was 20 db and the threshold hearing level for 250, 500 and 1000 c.p.s. was improved over that measured before exposure. A recovery curve for this ear was obtained 23 hours after the noise exposure and the data are shown in row 6a, table 60. The residual threshold shifts are insignificant except for 2500 and 5000 c.p.s. where the threshold shift is 28 db. Later tests showed that recovery did take place, therefore, these threshold shifts were not permanent threshold shifts. Data are given in rows 7 and 7a, table 60, for the threshold shift and its recovery from an 8 minute exposure to broad band noise at an OASPL of 130 db. Significant threshold shifts occurred at 500, 1000, 2000, 4000, 6000 and 8000 c.p.s., with a maximum shift of 55 db at 1000 and 2000 c.p.s. Further tests showed that it took approximately 72 hours for this ear to return to normal hearing threshold levels. This is another example of a persistent threshold shift which was not a permanent threshold shift because, after a sufficient rest period, the individual's hearing returned to normal levels.

Earlier in this chapter it is pointed out that the effect of auditory masking on communication is an "effective" elevation of the threshold hearing level while the individual is in the noise. Now the temporary and persistent shifts of the threshold hearing level, just described, will have effects on ability to communicate by speech signals that are similar to those produced by a masking noise which induces the same "effective" threshold shifts. Any particular value of the threshold shift will require an equivalent increase in the level of the speech signal before the listener will be able to detect and recognize the contents of the speech. One can estimate the effects of temporary and persistent shifts of the hearing threshold on communication by evaluating them in terms of an equivalent noise masked threshold of hearing.

Most of the threshold shifts discussed above were persistent; that is, they did not recover within the period of 15 to 16 hours that usually intervenes between two industrial work periods. If we move into an industrial situation where similar exposures could occur, the workman would begin a second work period, with its accompanying noise exposure, before his hearing thresholds had recovered to normal levels. Any new threshold shifts, induced by his new noise exposure would be superimposed upon the residual threshold shifts incurred during the previous work period. This sequence would be repeated each day throughout the work week and the individual would have a continuously reduced hearing sensitivity. It is presumed that these accumulated residual threshold shifts, incurred by several years of working in industrial noise, result in a permanent elevation of threshold hearing (noise induced hearing loss).

Although the varied relations between noise exposure and hearing loss are not all clearly defined (Rosenblith et al., 22), there is general agreement that (1) many noise exposures can produce a permanent elevation of threshold hearing level that may affect communication by speech, (2) the permanent elevations of the threshold hearing level result from the destruction of certain inner ear structures which cannot be replaced, (3) the degree of hearing threshold elevation produced by a given noise exposure varies from person to person, (4) noise induced elevations of threshold hearing levels first affect man's hearing of sounds higher in frequency than those necessary for communication by speech (therefore, most early noise induced elevations of threshold hearing level pass unnoticed unless they are detected by suitable hearing tests) and (5) noise exposure is characterized by (a) the noise level, (b) the composition of the noise, (c) the duration and distribution of noise exposure during a typical work day and (d) the total time of exposure during a work life.

RISK OF DAMAGE TO THE INNER EAR. The detailed relations between noise exposure and noise induced permanent elevation of threshold hearing level (noise induced hearing loss) cannot be stated quantitatively. Despite these uncertainties, operators of industrial facilities must make decisions about noise exposure limits for their personnel. Several years ago the United States Air Force developed a tentative damage risk criterion to guide its personnel in making decisions about permissible noise exposures. This tentative criterion for risk of damage to the inner ear, by wide band noise, is shown in figure 103. When used judiciously and with full knowledge of its limitations, the criterion is a valuable guide for making operational and engineering decisions relative to noise exposure and its control.

Rosenblith and Stevens (24) discuss the backgrounds of the tentative criterion. The essence of their comments on its limitations should be understood before using the criterion. The criterion of figure 103 is for wide band noise; that is, a noise containing

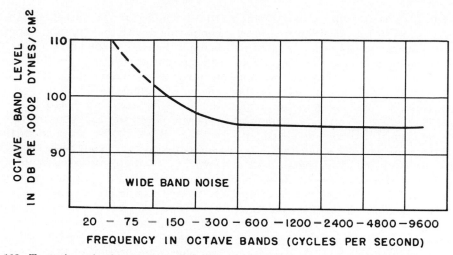

FIG. 103. Tentative criterion for risk of damage to the inner ear by long time exposure to wide band noise. The applications of this criterion are discussed in the text.

all audible frequencies. It has a reasonably continuous time character without sharp energy peaks. The specified noise levels are considered to be safe in terms of exposures during working days for durations up to a lifetime. When the SPL of any one octave band of a noise exceeds the band criterion level the criterion is exceeded. The criterion levels should not be taken too literally, deviations of the order of 1 or 2 db in either direction probably could be disregarded. The contour should be interpreted as a zone with uncertainties attending the measurement of the noise exposure and biologic variation modifying the probability of damage. However, a contour 10 db lower would involve negligible risk indeed and one 10 db higher would increase significantly the risk of permanently elevated threshold hearing levels.

A recent review of the criterion resulted in agreement that available, new data does not warrant revision of the criterion, that the new information does more clearly define the significance of the criterion expressed as pressure per octave bands for all octave bands shown in figure 103, that action to protect personnel should be mandatory when the sound pressure level of any one octave band exceeds the criterion value, that the criterion is a basic one for exposures of 25 working years when exposure recurs daily each usual work day of the working lifetime and that the criterion applies to wide band

noise, continuous in time, without any significantly large pressure peaks as a function of either time or frequency.

The basic criterion states a risk concept. It specifies noise levels in which a group of people may work and be assured that not more than a specified percentage of the group will develop a permanent elevation of the threshold hearing level equal to or in excess of a specified acceptable value. The acceptable elevation of threshold hearing level is stated in terms of hearing level for frequencies essential to understanding speech, namely, 500, 1000 and 2000 c.p.s. An elevation of threshold hearing level is acceptable, if it is less than the hearing level elevation for speech frequencies for which compensation is paid to veterans. This is the agreed limit of permissible permanent elevation of threshold hearing level. Now, a certain number of representatives of any group (population), either exposed to noise or *not* exposed to noise, will develop elevations of threshold hearing level that exceed the permissible value. Noise has no relation to the elevated threshold of hearing for these persons but their presence in a noise exposed population must be accounted for because *no* amount of protection can prevent the change of their hearing level. These persons may be separated into at least two groups. One group develops elevated hearing levels solely as a result of aging, of living the 25 work years. The second group develops elevated hearing thresholds because of dis- eases, exposure to chemical agents or a variety of other factors in no way related to noise exposure. Some information is available on the number of people that will develop elevated hearing thresholds in excess of the agreed acceptable limit because of aging processes. There is less certainty about the second group but it may include about one- tenth of the noise exposed population.

If the criterion shown in figure 103 is examined in the light of recent data, one can make an estimate of the degree of risk confronting the noise exposed population. It is estimated that about two-thirds of the noise exposed group will not develop eleva- tions of hearing threshold that exceed ac- ceptable limits. About one-tenth of the population will develop elevated hearing thresholds from aging alone (not affected by noise exposure). Perhaps another tenth (per- haps even a larger part) will develop hearing loss for *reasons other than noise exposure.* This means that about one-fifth (perhaps less) of the population (those most suscept- ible to the effects of noise) could develop elevated hearing thresholds from noise ex- posure incurred while working in the sound fields allowed by the criterion. These mem- bers of the noise exposed group incur a risk of inner ear damage. Those persons actually subjected to the risk of incurring elevated thresholds from noise exposures and, as well, those that may develop elevated hearing thresholds from other causes, should be identified. This identification is accomplished by monitoring audiometry (to be discussed later) employed in support of the criterion for risk of damage to the inner ear.

The criterion for risk of damage to the inner ear, as shown in figure 103, applies to wide band noise only. Some noise fields (turbojet engine at "idle" power, etc.) have most of their energy carried by a single frequency or a narrow band of frequencies. There is evidence that a single frequency, carrying the same energy as a wide band of frequencies, may produce more ear damage than the band. Presumably, this is caused by the concentration of the energy on a more restricted portion of the inner ear. Therefore, to apply the damage risk criterion to a single frequency or a "narrow band" of adjacent frequencies (less than 50 c.p.s. wide)

10 db is added to the measured SPL before comparing it with the criterion. For example, assume the ear is exposed to a pure tone of 900 c.p.s. at an SPL of 88 db. This frequency is in the 600 to 1200 c.p.s. octave band, and the SPL reading, 88 db, is increased by 10 db to 98 db and then compared with the criterion level for the 600 to 1200 c.p.s. octave. When it is determined that the "measured octave band SPL" of any noise field is contributed by one frequency or a "narrow band" of frequencies, 10 db is added to the measured octave band level and then the "wide band noise" criterion is applied.

In formulating the criterion for risk of damage to the inner ear, emphasis was placed on time, the duration of the exposure. The shortest interval of exposure time was 1 day (8 hours) but this daily exposure recurred regularly over a long period of time, a work- ing lifetime. The shortest time interval em- ployed in the basic criterion is *8 hours.* In many practical situations a criterion for permissible noise exposure is needed when the daily intervals of noise exposure are less than 8 hours. The octave band sound pres- sure levels specified by the long time expo- sure criterion can be interpreted as specifying for each octave band a "constant quan- tity of acoustic power per unit time" (a constant acoustic power level), available at the ear drum for a period of 8 hours each work day. Therefore, one may say that the risk of damage to the inner ear is propor- tional to the total energy or total power (acoustic power available times the time it is available) per octave band delivered to or acting upon the ear drum in the 8 hour period. Eldred *et al.* (23) applied this con- stant total power (constant energy) concept in formulating a criterion for permissible short time exposures to jet aircraft noise. They assumed that the risk of damage to the inner ear is proportional to the total power per octave band acting upon the ear drum each 8 hour interval but that this power may be delivered at any rate (power level) per unit time provided the total power delivered does not exceed that delivered to the ear drum in 8 hours at the power levels (rate of delivery) specified by the long time exposure criterion. If these relations hold, criterion SPLs for noise exposures shorter than 8 hours can be derived from the long time exposure criterion. Inasmuch as the acoustic power (power level) available at the ear drum doubles when the octave band sound pressure level increases 3 db, the exposure time must be reduced to one-half the former value to maintain constant the total power delivered to the ear drum. The SPLs for each octave band are specified for an exposure time of 8 hours in the long time exposure criterion. If, now, the SPL of one or more of these bands rises 3 db above those of the long time exposure criterion, the exposure time must be reduced to 4 hours (that is, the same total power is delivered in one-half the time when the rate of delivery is doubled). Similarly, a rise of 6 db in the SPLs of the octave bands results in the delivery of acoustic power at four times the rate per unit time specified by the long time criterion and the exposure time must be reduced to one-fourth of 8 hours or 2 hours. A 10 db rise of the SPLs above the long time criterion levels delivers acoustic power at 10 times the criterion rate and the exposure time (time during which acoustic power is delivered to the ear) must be reduced to one-tenth of 8 hours or 48 minutes. By continuing this procedure, permissible SPLs can be computed for any desired exposure time less than 8 hours. The specification of the permissible sound pressure levels per octave band, when the durations of the daily noise exposures are less than 8 hours, constitutes the short time noise exposure criterion.

PRACTICAL APPLICATION OF THE RISK CRITERIA. The long time exposure criterion (fig. 103) permits noise exposures of 8 hours each day when SPLs are 95 db for the 300 to 600 c.p.s. band and all higher octave bands. The permissible SPL for the 150 to 300 c.p.s. band is 98 db, for the 75 to 150 c.p.s. band it is 103 db, and for the 20 to 75 c.p.s. band it is 110 db. This does not mean that permanently elevated threshold hearing levels occur in all noise exposed individuals as soon as these criterion SPLs are exceeded. A realistic interpretation is that SPLs per octave band, in excess of criterion levels, create a significant risk of excessively increased hearing threshold levels for a significant part of the noise exposed population. The risk increases as the actual SPLs exceed the criterion levels by larger and larger amounts. In addition, the risk in-

creases as the number of octave bands, whose SPLs exceed the criterion values, increases. The basic criterion applies to the whole range of audible frequencies and may be applied to single frequencies and "narrow bands" of frequencies under conditions already described.

In applying the criterion, one must remember that the data upon which the criterion is based were obtained on groups of people and expressed as average effects of noise exposure. Furthermore, the measured noise levels and exposure times were subject to uncertainties or variances of measurement. These factors are the basis for the original qualification that the specified SPLs should be considered as zones of SPLs for the octave bands. The specified octave band SPL is the center value of this zone which extends about 2 db above and below the center value. Now in applying the criteria we measure noise fields and these measurements are subject to variances of ± 1.5 to ± 3 db about the central value. Exposure times may be more uncertain and the responses of the group of exposed persons also vary about a center value. These factors must be considered in applying the criterion. Therefore, it is proposed that a range of ± 2 db be used with each specified octave band SPL. In the region where the octave band SPL is specified as 95 db, this number is considered the center value of a zone of SPLs and any SPL from 93 to 97 db is within the criterion range of values. The criterion SPL does not represent an SPL at which an abrupt change takes place but a region within which the risk of elevated hearing thresholds increases as the numerical values of the SPL increase from the lowest to the highest.

The long time exposure criterion (fig. 103) applies to any sources of noise and to persons engaged in any occupation. However, our primary concern is for persons engaged in industrial activities where adequate ability to detect and recognize speech signals is essential for the work activities and for other activities of daily life. Our principal aim is to protect and preserve hearing for the sound frequencies essential for recognizing speech. These frequencies range from about 500 to about 2000 c.p.s. and test frequencies, 500. 1000 and 2000 c.p.s., are used to evaluate

TABLE 61

Sample Noise Fields of Aviation Equipment—Sound Pressure Level in db per Octave Band

Row Num- ber*	Octave Bands of Fequency in Cycles per Second								Noise Source
	20 to 75	75 to 150	150 to 300	300 to 600	600 to 1200	1200 to 2400	2400 to 4800	4800 to 9600	
	db	db	db	db	db	db	db	db	
1	96	97	97	96	93	91	85	75	Gas engine generator unit
2	96	106	111	116	116	118	121	120	Gas turbine starter unit
3	92	99	103	107	105	100	100	101	Gas turbine starter unit
4	97	106	107	96	96	91	89	91	Gas engine generator unit
5	109	114	115	111	104	102	98	91	Jet aircraft with A/B in operation, 1000 feet from engine nozzle
6		108	107	115	100	91	83	72	Inside jet aircraft—takeoff
7		88	92	97	90	81	79	71	Inside jet aircraft—cruise

hearing for speech. Now, industrial employees usually work in noise environments that have somewhat similar characteristics as is shown in table 61. Under these circumstances we may restate the long time exposure criterion in terms of the SPLs for two octave bands, namely, the 300 to 600 and the 600 to 1200 c.p.s. bands (13). The criterion now states that when the SPL of either the 300 to 600 or the 600 to 1200 c.p.s. bands (or the SPLs of both) exceed 95 ± 2 db, the risk of damage warrants action to protect the hearing of noise exposed persons. Of course the higher the SPL of these bands the greater the risk. If the sound field is very unusual or the hearing requirements for a special function warrant special consideration, the basic criterion should be used.

In many instances, it may be convenient to add SPLs of the 300 to 600 and the 600 to 1200 c.p.s. octaves to formulate a *two band criterion*. The SPLs of the two bands are added and compared with the summed pressures of the long time exposure criterion. The data which follow are used for adding the SPLs of the two bands. When the difference between the SPLs is zero to 1 db, add 3 db to the higher band level to obtain their sum; when the difference in band SPLs is 2 to 4 db, add 2 db to the higher level; when the difference in band SPLs is 5 to 8 db, add 1 db to the higher level; and when the difference in band SPLs is 9 db or more make no correction to the level of the higher band. The criterion values of the SPL

for each of the two bands is 95 ± 2 db and the difference in SPL is zero db; therefore, the sum for the two bands is 95 ± 2 db plus 3 db or 98 ± 2 db. Let us examine the data for several noise fields characteristic of the aviation industry (table 61). In row 1 the 300 to 600 c.p.s. SPL is 96 db and the 600 to 1200 c.p.s. SPL is 93 db, the difference is 3 db and the sum is 98 db, the two-band SPL. In row 4 the SPL of both bands is 96 db, the difference in SPL is zero and the sum of the bands SPL's is 99 db, the two-band SPL. If these two, two-band SPLs are compared with the criterion, we see that the criterion level is 98 ± 2 db and the upper limit is 100 db and the summed SPLs of the noise field of row 1 and row 4 are, respectively, 98 and 99 db. Both are within the limits of the two-band criterion for an 8 hour daily noise exposure. Now, for contrast, look at the data in row 6, table 61. The SPL of the 300 to 600 c.p.s. band is 115 db, that of the 600 to 1200 c.p.s. band is 100 db, the difference is 15 db and no correction is made. The two-band SPL is 115 db and when compared with the two-band criterion SPL it is 15 db above the upper limit of the criterion. Action must be taken to reduce the SPL at the ears of workmen exposed to this noise 8 hours each day. If ear plugs and ear muffs are used, the reduction for the 300 to 600 c.p.s. band is 24 db; and 115 db minus 24 db equals 91 db in the ear canal. For the 600 to 1200 c.p.s. band the reduction by the protective device is 28 db; and 100 db minus 28 db equals 72 db in the ear canal. The two-band pressure at the ear drum with protection is 91 db and this is below the lower limit of the two-band criterion SPL. With the ears protected, workmen may stay in this noise 8 hours each day.

In applying the short time noise exposure criterion, all the measurement uncertainties and variable responses of exposed personnel that affected the long time noise exposure criteria must be considered. In addition, the short, exposure time criterion may be applied in different forms. If the noise exposure is one continuous exposure less than 8 hours, then 8 hours divided by the actual exposure times gives the ratio of the permissible sound power increase. If, for example, the exposure lasts one-half hour, the ratio is $8 \div \frac{1}{2} = 16$, and the acoustic power delivered may increase 16 times. This increase, expressed in db, is 12. In the region where the octave band level of the long exposure time criterion is 95 ± 2 db the allowable band SPL is 107 ± 2 db for the $\frac{1}{2}$ hour exposure. Similar computations can be accomplished for other exposure times. If the two-band long exposure time criterion is used in the example above, and this is recommended, then the 12 db is added to the sum of the levels of the two bands (98 ± 2 db) and the allowable two band SPL is 110 ± 2 db. Now, the decreased time of exposure allows a longer recovery time than is available following an 8 hour exposure. Inasmuch as the ear has more time to recover from the effects of exposure, it is recommended that the upper limit of allowable SPL be used when computing allowable levels for short time noise exposures. Then, using the two-band criterion, 12 db is added to 100 db (98 db + 2 db for the two-band SPL of the long exposure time criterion) to give an allowable two-band SPL of 112 db for a single daily exposure of $\frac{1}{2}$ hour.

Frequently, workmen are exposed to several short time noise exposures each 8 hour work day. Then, one may wish to determine the number of exposures to a specific SPL that is equal to an 8 hour exposure or when the number of exposures are known one may desire to compute the permissible SPL or SPLs for these exposures. There are several ways of doing these computations but the one to be described is recommended for use when persons are exposed to aviation

noise fields. The two-band long time noise exposure criterion is used as the basic criterion from which to derive this short time exposure criterion. The allowable two-band SPL for 8 hour exposures is then 100 db. Now, recall that the short time exposure criterion is based on the delivery of a constant quantity of energy or constant total acoustic power to the vicinity of the ear canal or ear drum each 8 hour work period. In addition, it is assumed that this constant acoustic power may be delivered at any rate for any time period which does not result in a total acoustic power in excess of that permitted by the long exposure time criterion.

The allowable SPL for the two-band criterion is 100 db. At this SPL a power flow of 1 μw. per sq. cm. is delivered to the ear in the ear canal or near the ear drum (the area of the ear drum is about 1 sq. cm.). (This is the power per square centimeter available to do work on the ear.) This rate of power flow is maintained for 8 hours. Therefore, when the SPL corresponds to the two band criterion level (100 db) 8 μw. hours of power are available (through each square centimeter of air) to do work on the ear. It is not known how much of this power actually reaches the inner ear because the transfer characteristics (power factors) of the ear drum and middle ear structures are not known. Nevertheless, there are 8 μw. hours of power available. This power can also be expressed as 480 μw. minutes. Now assume four separate noise exposures each day to a two-band SPL of 110 db. This SPL corresponds to a power flow 10 times greater than for an SPL of 100 db and the maximal allowable exposure time at this rate of power delivery is one-tenth of 8 hours or 0.8 hour or 48 minutes. The four noise exposures can each last 12 minutes without exceeding the criterion. In addition, when the two band SPL is 110 db, any number of exposures may be permitted so long as the total exposure time (their sum) does not exceed 48 minutes. Again, if the two-band SPL of a noise is 120 db, it is 20 db above the two-band criterion level. This 20 db increase in level means that the rate of power delivery is increased 100 times. Therefore, the allowable exposure time must be reduced to one-hundredth of 8 hours or 0.08 hours or 4.8 minutes to avoid exceeding the criterion.

One exposure of 4.8 minutes can be tolerated each 8 hour day or more than one exposure to the 120 db two-band level are acceptable if their sum is not greater than 4.8 minutes. If the two-band SPL of a noise is 130 db it is 30 db above the two-band criterion level (100 db) and the rate of power flow is increased 1000 times. The exposure to this noise must not exceed one-thousandth of 8 hours or 0.008 hours or 0.48 minutes if the two-band criterion is not to be exceeded. Using this method the maximum permissible total acoustic power delivered to the air near the ear drum or ear canal is 8 μw. hours or 480 μw. minutes each 8 hour work period. Computation of allowable two-band SPLs or of maximum durations of exposure for given noise levels are relatively easy using this method. In addition, several short exposures to varying SPLs can also be computed easily. Tables or nomograms may be constructed to speed up the computations. These short exposure time criteria should not be applied to exposures shorter than 0.25 or preferably 0.5 minutes. When personal protective equipment is used the attenuation it provides is subtracted from the levels of the two octave bands used in the two-band criterion (300 to 600 and 600 to 1200 c.p.s. bands). This procedure was illustrated in the discussion of the basic, two band long exposure time criterion.

OTHER SENSORY RECEPTORS

Strong sound waves may activate several other sensory receptors in addition to the ear. The end organs of the vestibular apparatus, the pressure receptors of the skin, the stretch receptors of the muscles, joints and tendons; the heat receptors of the skin and the receptors of some internal organs may be activated by intense sound waves.

The vestibular apparatus is closely associated with the inner ear. It participates with other sensory receptors in maintaining body equilibrium and orientation in space. Sound pressure levels of the order of 135 db activate this receptor. This unusual stimulation of the vestibular apparatus may lead to loss of orientation in space. Devices that protect the ear also prevent disturbances of the vestibular apparatus until very high sound pressure levels (150 to 160 db) are attained. Stretch receptors of the muscles, joints and tendons participate with the vestibular apparatus in maintaining man's erect posture. They also participate in precision regulation of movements of the appendages (arms, hands, fingers, etc.). Low frequency sound waves at SPLs around 145 to 150 db can vibrate or move muscles of the arms and legs; this activates the stretch receptors and this may interfere with precision muscular movements. In addition, false information from these end organs, combined with erroneous information from the vestibular apparatus, may bring about disorientation and ineffective control of walking movements.

In sound waves whose SPLs are above 110 db, receptors in the skin are stimulated and the presence of the sound wave can be felt. The strength of the stimulation increases as the sound pressure levels increase and the resulting sensations create the impression that the structure on which one stands is vibrating. These sensations and impressions are reported as annoying and uncomfortable by many persons.

Low frequency sound waves having SPLs around 140 db move or vibrate the abdominal and thoracic walls of the human body. These movements, the stimulation of sensory end organs in the abdominal wall and the stimulation of some internal sense organs may cause nausea and vomiting in some persons when exposed to these sound waves. The nausea and vomiting actually may result from the combined stimulation of the abdominal and visceral sensory mechanisms and the vestibular apparatus.

In sound fields whose SPLs are about 150 db, sufficient acoustic energy is absorbed by the human skin to stimulate heat receptors located in it. The result is a sensation of "warmth" or "heat" which, under some circumstances, evokes a sensation of "heat pain."

The effects of intense sound waves that have been described in this section are known as the "nonauditory" effects of noise. The effects of long time exposures to sound levels that produce "nonauditory" effects are not known. For this reason, exposure to SPLs of 150 db and higher should be avoided where ever possible; at least until the long time effects of these intense stimulations are more clearly defined.

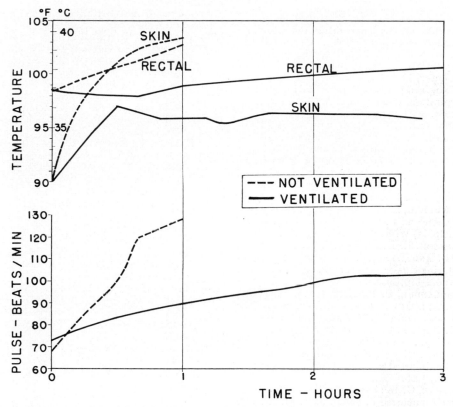

FIG. 115. Responses of a subject who is exposed to an air-wall temperature of 160° F. while wearing an impermeable antiexposure suit assembly. When ventilated with 12 cubic feet of 60° F. dry air per minute, he does not reach a tolerance limit in 3 hours. Unventilated, he is near collapse after 1 hour.

heat exposure. The assumption is that body defenses against cooling and heating will be insignificant under severe cooling and heating loads. In other words, the body would be treated as if it were a tank of water with the specific heat of 0.83 and having no physiologic defenses. It is taken that the tank of water has an upper absolute level of temperature which cannot be exceeded. Therefore, by lowering the temperature of the tank before the heat exposure a longer time is needed to reach the upper limit.

This approach to improving tolerance to heat has been tried experimentally and the results were as predicted (26). If a man lightly dressed is placed in the heat chamber at 160° F. air-wall temperature, his tolerance limit is reached in approximately 60 minutes. When the same man is cooled in a tank of water to produce a fall in skin temperature and a lowering of rectal temperature by 2° F., the man's tolerance to the same heat

exposure is increased to almost 120 minutes. The interesting thing is that the subject's physiologic responses to heat are slow in appearing at first, following the precooling. Sweating does not begin until 10 or 12 minutes after the heat exposure when the skin temperature has risen to over 100° F. The sweating response and the physiologic tolerance limit are more closely related to the average body temperature (combined skin and rectal temperature) than to levels of skin or rectal temperature alone.

Although this work is at present more a laboratory experiment than something useful, further work is being done to determine the practicality of such a method of protection when a man must be exposed to a limited heat exposure which is predictable in advance. For example, precooling might be useful during a prolonged re-entry into the earth's atmosphere when heat loads within the vehicle might be quite high.

REFERENCES

(1) SHAMBAUGH, G.: Temperature Receptors, an Annotated Bibliography. Technical Report No. EP-24, Natick, Massachusetts, Quartermaster Research and Development Center, 1956.

(2) KUNO, Y.: The Physiology of Human Perspiration. London, J. & A. Churchill, Ltd., 1934.

(3) FERGUSON, I. D., HERTZMAN, A. B., RAMPONE, A. J., AND CHRISTENSEN, M. L.: Magnitudes, Variability and Reliability of Regional Sweating Rates in Humans at Constant Ambient Temperatures. WADC Technical Report No. 56-38. Wright-Patterson Air Force Base, Ohio, 1956.

(4) NEWBURGH, L. H.: Physiology of Heat Regulation and the Science of Clothing. Philadelphia, W. B. Saunders Co., 1949.

(5) CARLSON, L. D., BURNS, H. L., HOLMES, T. H., AND WEBB, P. P.: Adaptive changes during exposure to cold. J. Appl. Physiol., 5: 672–676, 1953.

(6) SCHOLANDER, P. F., HAMMEL, H. T., HART, J. S., LeMESSURIER, D. H., AND STEEN, J.: Cold adaptation in Australian aborigines. J. Appl. Physiol., 13: 211–218, 1958.

(7) Heating, Ventilating, Air Conditioning Guide. New York, American Society of Heating and Air-Conditioning Engineers, Inc., 1958.

(8) MOLNAR, G. W.: Survival of hypothermia by men immersed in ocean. J. A. M. A., 131: 1046–1050, 1946.

(9) GLASER, E. M.: Immersion and survival in cold water. Nature, 166: 1068, 1950.

(10) HALL, J. F., AND POLTE, J. W.: Effect of water content and compression on clothing insulation. J. Appl. Physiol., 8: 539–545, 1956.

(11) HALL, J. F., KEARNY, A. P., POLTE, J. W., AND QUILLETTE, S.: Body cooling in wet and dry clothing. J. Appl. Physiol., 13: 121–128, 1958.

(12) DRIPPS, R. D.: The Physiology of Induced Hypothermia. Publication No. 451. Washington, D. C., National Research Council-National Academy of Sciences, 1956.

(13) BLOCKLEY, W. V., McCUTCHAN, J. W., LYMAN, J., AND TAYLOR, C. L.: Human tolerance for high temperature aircraft environments. J. Aviation Med., 25: 515–522, 1954.

(14) BLOCKLEY, W. V., McCUTCHAN, J. W., AND TAYLOR, C. L.: Prediction of Human Tolerance for Heat in Aircraft: a Design Guide. WADC Technical Report No. 53-346. Wright-Patterson Air Force Base, Ohio, 1954.

(15) VEGHTE, J. H., AND WEBB, P.: Clothing and Tolerance to Heat. WADC Technical Report No. 57-759. Wright-Patterson Air Force Base, Ohio, 1957.

(16) GAGGE, A. P., BURTON, A. C., AND BAZETT, H. C.: A practical system of units for the description of the heat exchange of man with his environment. Science, 94: 428–430, 1951.

(17) HALL, J. F., AND POLTE, J. W.: Thermal Insulation of Air Force Clothing. A Catalog and Part 4 of a Series. WADC Technical Report No. 56-482. Wright-Patterson Air Force Base, Ohio, 1956.

(18) FETCHER, E. S., RAPAPORT, S. I., HALL, J. F., AND SHAUB, H. G.: Biophysical requirements for the ventilation of clothing. J. Appl. Physiol., 2: 49–60, 1949.

(19) MAUCH, H. A.: Status of ventilated garments for high speed aircraft. J. Aviation Med., 26: 56–60, 1955.

(20) MAUCH, H. A., HALL, J. F., AND KLEMM, F. K.: A ventilating system for clothing. WADC Technical Report No. 55-152. Wright-Patterson Air Force Base, Ohio, 1955.

(21) WEBB, P., AND KLEMM, F. K.: Design of Ventilated Clothing. WADC Technical Report No. 58-608. Wright-Patterson Air Force Base, Ohio, 1958.

(22) WEBB, P.: Ventilated Clothing as a Protection Against Heat Exposure. Paper No. 56-AV-4. New York, The American Society of Mechanical Engineers, 1956.

(23) WEBB, P., AND VEGHTE, J. H.: Several Variables Affecting Performance of Ventilated Clothing. WADC Technical Report No. 56-43. Wright-Patterson Air Force Base, Ohio, 1956.

(24) GREIDER, H. R., AND SANTA MARIA, L. J.: Subjective thermal comfort zones of ventilated full pressure suit at altitude. J. Aviation Med., 28: 272–276, 1957.

(25) SKILLING, D. C., McCUTCHAN, J. W., AND TAYLOR, C. L.: A Quantitative Investigation of the MA-1 Ventilating Garment when Used with a Modified MK-IV Anti-Exposure Suit. WADC Technical Report No. 56-209. Wright-Patterson Air Force Base, Ohio, 1956.

(26) VEGHTE, J. H., AND WEBB, P.: Extending Human Tolerance to Heat by Prior Body Cooling. WADC Technical Report No. 58-412. Wright-Patterson Air Force Base, Ohio, 1958.

20

ESCAPE, SURVIVAL AND RESCUE

James B. Nuttall, M.D.

Emergency in-flight escape from aircraft has become one of the most critical human factors problem areas in modern aviation. This first phase of the flight emergency triad—escape, survival and rescue—is primarily associated with military aviation and its support by the aviation industry. Survival and rescue problems are applicable to both civil and military aviation although in somewhat greater degree to the latter. This discussion will have primary applicability to to the military flyer; however, many aspects will have an equal significance for his civilian counterpart. The three phases of the triad, although interdependent, will be discussed individually and in logical succession; escape, survival and rescue.

ESCAPE

The reasons for abandoning an aircraft during flight are manifold. In some instances the reason may appear to be inadequate, as for example a malfunctioning emergency warning indicator; at the other extreme there is obviously little choice for the flyer in the case of a massive fire or a disintegrative explosion. Whatever the reason, when the decision is made by or for the flyer to abandon his aircraft, it should be possible for him to carry out this decision with a reasonable chance of successful escape. This is an important concept which supports the morale and effective performance of the flyer. With

the increasing complexity of military aircraft and air operations it has become progressively difficult to meet adequately the requirements imposed by this concept. Successive eras in military aviation have marked the progress in development of escape devices. The parachute was introduced by the Germans in World War I. Marked advances in aircraft performance during World War II led to the use of the ejection seat; again, by the Germans. Escape passages or tunnels and wind stream deflectors were also employed. The Korean conflict spurred progress in the development of very high performance aircraft with the result that modified and more sophisticated ejection seats have been developed, these perhaps soon to be followed by jettisonable cockpits or ejection capsules. It is of interest to follow in a more or less chronologic order this evolution in escape devices forced by human requirements and which has today produced major fields of specialization in human factors research, developmental engineering and industrial production within the aircraft industry.

The Parachute

During the early years of aviation it was apparently not considered necessary to abandon an aircraft in trouble. It was more economical and quite convenient to land in almost any open pasture. With the advent of World War I and aerial combat the advantages of abandoning a flaming, disabled aircraft became more apparent—"to return and fight again." The German Air Force developed the parachute. Its use was soon adopted by all organized air forces and many independent flyers. Later aerial stunt artists and parachuting clubs expanded its use. Today massive airborne armies are trained in its use for vertical assault in combat. It is an effective means of transport for man and cargo as well as one of escape. It is even used as a braking device for high speed aircraft. In the escape role it is primarily used in military flying. Commercial air transports do not carry parachutes; likewise in some military transports and aeromedical evacuation flying, parachutes are not used. There are primarily two reasons for this; first, the type of emergency permitting the use of parachutes rarely occurs in transport operations, and second, it is impractical for a large number of untrained passengers to parachute successfully from an aircraft during a sudden in-flight emergency. There are also other reasons such as the adverse psychologic effect which would be produced by the wearing of parachutes by commercial passengers.

The parachute as an escape device has undergone many important developments. Although it may appear to be a relatively simple device, extensive scientific effort has been expended in configuration design and fabric development to meet the exacting requirements of rescuing the flyer from flight conditions of multivariate altitudes and velocities without exceeding man's tolerance limits to unavoidable forces. It is impractical at this time to discuss the technical details involved; however, certain practical aspects of the use of the parachute should be mentioned.

TYPES OF PARACHUTES. There are basically three types of parachutes: seat, back and attachable chest types. Each has certain advantages as well as disadvantages under specific circumstances. The seat type has been used most commonly in training and fighter type aircraft. In flight the pilot sits upon the chute pack and is relatively unencumbered; however, on the ground and in circumstances necessitating manual bailout, without benefit of ejection devices, the seat type parachute is extremely unwieldy. As

newer and better packing techniques are being developed the seat pack is being replaced by the back type parachute which is now preferred for almost all types of flying. This pack fits snugly to the back; is relatively unencumbering during bailout or escape from a crashed aircraft; and further, its location permits the use of the seat area for survival and emergency equipment. The third type of parachute, the attachable chest pack, is infrequently seen now but was used commonly by bomber and transport crews during World War II. It permitted the crewman to wear only the parachute harness while performing his duties, then if the necessity arose to abandon the aircraft the chest pack could be quickly attached to the harness by means of snap hooks and D rings. The greatest disadvantage of this parachute is that, at times of emergency, the crew member might not be able to reach the pack or attach it to the harness quickly enough for a safe bailout. At the present time the use of the chest pack is restricted almost exclusively to airborne troops who use it as an auxiliary or reserve parachute. Most sport or exhibition jumpers also use the chest pack as a reserve parachute.

PARACHUTE STRUCTURE AND KINEMATICS. All parachute assemblies consist of three main parts; the harness, pack and canopy with accessories. The suspension lines connect the canopy with the harness and each suspension line is continuous from one side of the harness across the dome of the canopy and back to the other side of the harness.

The harness consists of a series of nylon web straps arranged to fit the body by means of sewed or metal connecting devices. Its basic configuration is such that a sling is formed which supports the buttocks. This sling is designed to absorb directly the major portion of the parachute opening forces. The position of the body in this sling is secured by leg, chest, shoulder and back straps which form integral parts of the harness.

The pack protects the canopy and accessories and holds them in place for orderly sequential release when the rip cord is pulled. Parachute packing is a highly skilled procedure in which several techniques are employed to accomplish specific aims. A particular technique which should be mentioned is the use of the quarter deployment bag. The quarter bag is used to contain the lower quarter of the canopy and for orderly arrangement of the suspension lines in sequential hesitator loops. The remainder of the canopy is arranged in S shaped folds in the upper part of the pack. Main pack flaps cover the folded canopy and a small pilot chute is contained in a separate compartment on the main pack. When the rip cord is pulled the special pilot chute compartment is unlocked and the pilot chute is spring ejected into the air stream. The drag of the pilot chute extends the uninflated upper part of the canopy, pulls the quarter bag out of the pack, and permits the suspension lines to withdraw. Release of the last suspension line loop unlocks the quarter deployment bag and frees the lower quarter of the canopy permitting it to inflate. This sequence controls inflation of the canopy and reduces opening shock primarily by insuring continuous tension of the suspension lines. This provides a continuous, smooth application of drag to the individual producing a more uniform force pattern which avoids excessive rate of application of *g* forces with high peaks. The significance of this technique will be pointed out in later discussion of high altitude and high speed bailout.

Quite obviously the third main part of the parachute assembly, the canopy, is a subject unto itself. Chapters or even volumes could be devoted to various aspects of the canopy such as, type of fabric, porosity, size, configuration, venting (ribbon chutes) and special design features (slots and guide extensions). Only a few general statements will be made regarding the canopy. It is composed of triangular panels of fabric called gores which radiate from a central opening, the vent, to the circumference which is termed the skirt. The most suitable fabric is special rip resisting weave nylon of high tensile strength. The elasticity of nylon permits elongation during opening thus absorbing some of the energy of opening shock and also permitting some pressure venting during the opening. Nylon suspension lines also reduce transmission of opening shock energy to the parachutist. The most frequently employed canopy size for emergency escape from aircraft is the 28 foot diameter

canopy which permits a descent rate at sea level of 14 to 26 feet per second depending upon the load and atmospheric conditions. These rates are equivalent to jumping from platforms 3 to $10\frac{1}{2}$ feet high onto solid ground. Larger canopies may be desirable from the standpoint of reducing descent rates, however, they impose the problem of increased weight and pack size. With existing fabrics the 28 foot canopy appears to be a reasonable compromise of all factors and has reduced the rate of landing injuries associated with the 24 foot canopy. Surprisingly this increase in size from 24 to 28 foot diameter also effectively reduces the opening shock as shown in figure 116. This, according to Scheubel (1) is because the shock forces of small canopies increase as the square of the canopy radius, whereas the shock forces of very large canopies are inversely proportional to the radius. The determining dividing line as to when the switch from direct to inverse proportionality occurs is when the mass of air set in motion by the developing parachute significantly decreases the velocity of the man-parachute system before full opening of the parachute occurs. With a very small parachute canopy the ratio of the mass of air set in motion to the man's mass is small, therefore, little momentum is transferred from man to canopy and the velocity of the system practically does not change during the opening phase. When opening is complete the air resistance and, hence, opening shock is directly proportional to the surface and the square of the velocity. Inasmuch as the velocity has scarcely changed the shock will then be proportional to the square of the radius of the canopy. On the other hand, very large canopies with a large mass ratio of air set in motion to the mass of the man impart a significant momentum to this air mass. This substantially reduces the velocity of the man-parachute system during the opening phase. With a significant transfer of momentum during the opening period the filling time of the parachute becomes important. Under conditions of reduced velocity of the system the filling time of the canopy will be approximately proportional to its radius and inasmuch as the deceleration force is determined by the rate of decrease of the man's momentum divided

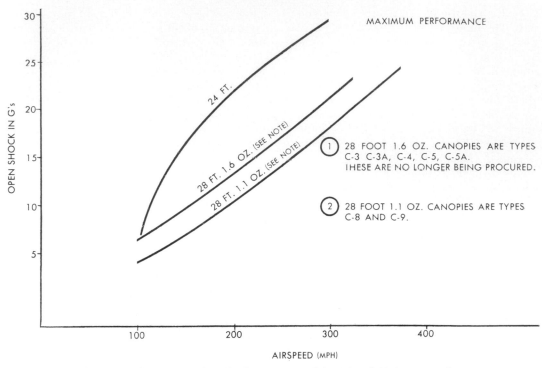

FIG. 116. Canopy opening shock *versus* speed for 24 and 28 foot canopies

by the filling time, the force will be inversely proportional to the radius. In other words, less opening shock with an increase in size of the canopy.

The most commonly used configuration is the flat, circular canopy. An improved design feature of the circular canopy particularly applicable to high altitude bailout consists of added guide extensions with slots attached at the lower rim or skirt of the canopy opposite every other gore. This design reduces the speed of opening of the canopy at high altitude thus reducing the opening shock. This has advantages but also disadvantages which will be discussed at a later point. The guide surfaces of this design also reduce parachute oscillation thus producing a stabilized descent. This prevents many injuries formerly incurred by hitting the ground during oscillatory or swinging motions which are additive to the impact velocity as well as disruptive to appropriate landing attitude.

CONVENTIONAL BAILOUT. The method of escape from a disabled aircraft is determined, for the most part, by the performance characteristics of the aircraft itself. Conventional

escape or "bailout" is unassisted by any mechanical forces other than the muscular power of the individual and the force of gravity. The probability of successful unassisted bailout is indirectly proportional to the speed of the aircraft and becomes marginal at indicated airspeeds above 180 m.p.h. Escape from high performance aircraft, therefore, requires the use of high energy devices which forcibly separate the individual from the aircraft. Such devices will be fully discussed in later paragraphs and, for the moment, the discussion will be limited to conventional escape procedures.

BAILOUT TECHNIQUES. Emergency bailout may be regarded by many as a very simple procedure; however, studies have shown that inadequate preparation and unfamiliarity with appropriate bailout procedures severely reduce the chances of successful escape. Although detailed bailout procedures cannot be covered in this limited discussion, certain general instructions will give an understanding of the problems involved. Conventional bailout is not a haphazard procedure as may be implied by the time worn phrase "open the hatch and bail out." Successful escape is largely dependent upon how well specific rules are followed by everyone involved in the emergency. The commander of an aircraft is responsible for seeing that all crew and passengers are properly fitted with parachutes and instructed in escape procedures. The parachute should be worn at all times in combat aircraft. Escape procedures vary and are specific for each type aircraft. All personnel must be familiar with the location and method of egress from emergency exits, escape hatches and escape tunnels or chutes. Improper technique in leaving the plane will often result in serious injury or even fatal outcome from striking parts of the plane. A 3 year study of emergency parachute escapes in the U. S. A. F., from 1946 to 1949, revealed 1054 attempted parachute escapes with the result that 10.2 per cent were fatal and only 52.2 per cent involved no injury. The two greatest cause factors for the deaths were (1) being struck by the aircraft, and (2) jumping too low. These two hazards accounted for 53.3 per cent of all the deaths. This study illustrates the necessity for proper procedures and for quick decisions by the aircraft commander and prompt action by every individual. These things are only attainable through knowledge, training, drill and discipline.

Although the average person may instinctively jump feet foremost this is usually dangerous in leaving an airplane. In general, it is best to dive head down as into a pool of water in order that the most vulnerable part of the body avoids striking the aircraft. This is particularly applicable when leaving belly or side hatches. There are, however, exceptions as in the KC-135 jet tanker where the individual drops feet first through an escape tunnel from a horizontal hand bar. With most belly hatches it is best to squat at the rear edge of the hatch, tuck the knees under the chin and roll forward and down into the air stream in the "cannon ball" attitude. When jumping from narrow side doors, one should crouch, hold both sides of the door and propel the body out and down with both arms and legs. If the side door is wide, the jumper should leave from the rear edge. When exiting close to tail surfaces, radomes or other protuberances it is advisable to curl into a "cannon ball" immediately upon leaving the aircraft. This reduces body drag and curtails rapid loss of forward velocity thus permitting a greater chance of avoiding the external surfaces of the aircraft. The eyes should be kept open during the bailout and it should be determined that the aircraft is cleared before pulling the rip cord.

Parachute Opening. The appropriate time for pulling the rip cord will vary with circumstances. At altitudes below 500 feet the delay should be only that necessary to clear the airplane. One second should be adequate. The minimum altitude at which it is possible to use a parachute on conventional bailout, without fatal injury, will vary considerably with speed, type of parachute and chance. It is probable that a jump from 100 feet or less will almost invariably be fatal. When it is realized that 2 seconds or more may be involved in full deployment of the parachute a glance at figure 117 will indicate that escape below 200 feet is marginal under the best of circumstances inasmuch as this amount of altitude is lost in a little over 3 seconds. In most instances at medium altitudes (2000 to 15,000 feet) it is desirable to wait 5 to 10 seconds before pulling the rip cord. The time is usually estimated by counting "one thousand one, one one thousand two," etc. This delay is particularly essential if the aircraft is traveling at speeds in excess of 200 m.p.h. The delay will permit slowing down to terminal velocity which at low altitude is approximately 120 m.p.h. This value of the terminal velocity or ultimate speed attained by a free

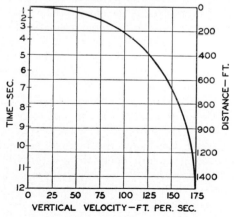

Fig. 117. Rate of vertical free fall of a human body at low altitudes.

falling body was first determined in experiments at the Army Air Corps Materiel Division (2). It was found that a man equipped with a parachute pack, not opened, will fall at a maximum rate of between 160 feet per second (109 m.p.h.) and 175 feet per second (119 m.p.h.) and that he will gain this velocity in almost 12 seconds, having fallen 1400 to 1500 feet (fig. 117). It is important to recognize that this so-called "terminal velocity" is dependent upon the ratio of aerodynamic drag to the weight of the body. This drag/weight ratio varies with the density of the atmosphere, consequently at higher altitudes the terminal velocity is greater than at lower altitudes. This "terminal velocity" is essentially that velocity which creates an air drag equal to the weight of the man. Therefore, a falling body, in the strict sense, does not attain "terminal velocity" except with regard to a given air density. The velocity will vary as the body falls through various levels of altitude. This velocity will also vary with the position and attitude of the body because the frontal area exposed to air resistance or the drag area is affected. For example, the projected frontal area of the body standing is approximately 8.4 square feet. This is reduced to about 5.0 square feet in the seated position and is considerably less in the crouched "cannon ball" attitude previously mentioned. Tumbling motion also produces variations. These factors account for the wide variation in terminal velocities and in time to fall from high altitude for different individuals.

The significance of terminal velocity limits is that on bailout if the speed of the aircraft is greater than the terminal velocity at the bailout altitude the jumper will rapidly decelerate to terminal velocity. The rate of deceleration will vary with the square of the velocity and the density of the air. At high speeds it is important that a sufficient time elapses before pulling the rip cord to permit slowing to the terminal velocity. If this does not occur, the faster the body is traveling when the parachute opens the greater will be the shock load. This will result in a greater stress on the parachute and on the jumper. For example, the opening shock load at 120 m.p.h. for an average man is about 1200 pounds; at 200 m.p.h. about 2400 pounds;

at 250 m.p.h. about 3600 pounds; at 300 m.p.h. about 5000 pounds; at 325 about 6000 pounds (3) and at still higher speeds increasingly higher increments of force. Such forces result in failure of the parachute structure and serious injury or death of the individual. The problem becomes very serious when escaping from high performance aircraft and this will be discussed under that heading. In any event, high speeds demand that opening of the parachute be delayed until velocities safe for the parachute and the jumper are reached. This problem becomes most acute at very low altitudes where the time available for slowing down is limited.

HIGH ALTITUDE BAILOUT. Another factor which imposes a requirement for delayed parachute opening is altitude. At high altitude it is desirable to delay parachute opening for several reasons. These are first, exposure to high opening shock forces; second, exposure to hypoxia; and third, exposure to low temperature. The first of these is most important. At high altitudes because of the decreased air density it takes longer to reach terminal velocity which makes an initial parachute opening delay important. Secondly, the terminal velocity at high altitudes is much greater than at lower altitudes. This makes a prolonged delay or free fall necessary to reduce the terminal velocity to levels that will not produce an intolerable opening shock. For example, at 7000 feet the parachute opening shock is approximately 9 g whereas at 40,000 feet it averages 32 g (fig. 118). This level of deceleration may cause failure in the structure of the parachute as well as serious injury or death of the parachutist. In actual experience, serious injuries and death have resulted from the impact of parachute opening at altitudes above 25,000 feet.

Strangely, it was an earlier belief that free fall was to be avoided and as late as 1943 it was believed that if the parachute were deployed at high altitude a severe opening shock would be avoided because of the less dense atmosphere. However, there was a rude awakening when Colonel W. R. Lovelace, III, MC, on 24 June 1943, made an experimental jump from 40,000 feet with immediate opening of the parachute. The

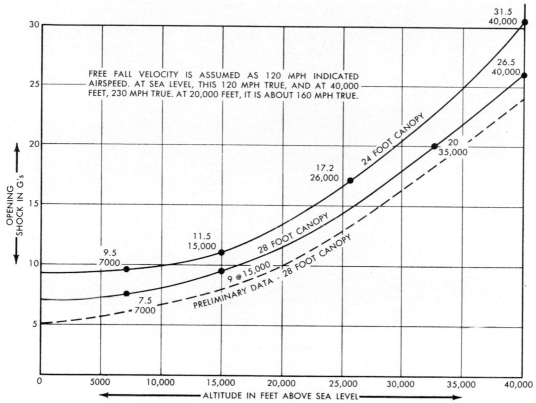

FIG. 118. Opening shock of 24 and 28 foot parachutes at various altitudes at the terminal velocity of the average crewman.

parachute opening shock was severe rendering Colonel Lovelace unconscious and causing the loss of his gloves with resulting severe frostbite injury. He suffered from shock in addition to frostbite of the left hand. His right hand was protected, remarkably, by a thin nylon liner glove which was retained. Additional evidence of the dangers of opening shock at high altitude was obtained in July 1943 when Major P. J. Ritchie made an emergency jump without oxygen from 32,000 feet. He delayed pulling the rip cord until he felt that he was losing consciousness; however, he experienced a severe opening shock at 27,000 feet, lost consciousness and sustained a lumbar vertebral dislocation. These incidents spurred experimental investigation of high altitude opening shock and a series of altitude dummy drop tests in 1944 gave data which proved that parachute opening shock is greater at high altitude. This indicated a need for free fall to a safe lower altitude if

severe trauma and injury were to be avoided. It was also obvious that free fall would minimize the hazards of exposure to cold and hypoxia. Figure 119 shows comparative times of free fall and open parachute descents. It also indicates individual variations in free fall times previously mentioned. The solid curves are accurate plots from radar data whereas the dotted curves are plotted from estimated averages from total times. The variation of terminal velocity is also indicated for different altitudes.

It is appropriate at this time to briefly explain the apparently paradoxical situation of a high parachute opening shock in the relatively thin air of high altitude *versus* a low opening shock in the more dense air of low altitude. Primarily three factors are involved; the terminal velocity, the kinematics of parachute opening and the mass ratio of air set in motion during the opening phase to the mass of the man. With regard to the first factor it has already been indicated that

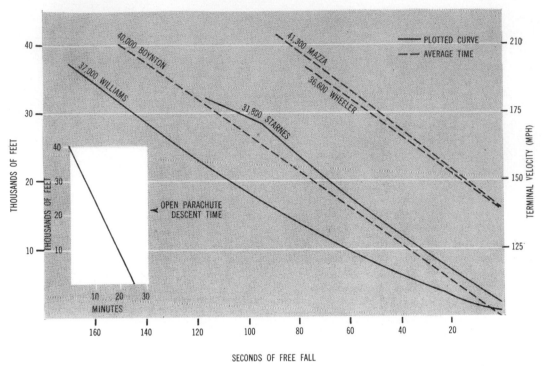

Fig. 119. Comparing the rate of descent of a free falling body and an open parachute descent

terminal velocity increases with increasing altitude and opening shock is directly proportional to the velocity at the time of opening. The study of opening kinematics has shown that in less dense air (high altitude) the parachute canopy deploys at a very high rate because of an increased rate of air inflow and more rapid lateral movement of the canopy's edge as a consequence of low density air resistance. This rapid deployment produces higher peak shock forces because less time is available for deceleration of the man-parachute system during the opening phase. Finally, the deceleration forces acting during the opening phase and prior to full canopy deployment are considerably less at high altitude than at low altitude as a function of the ratio of air mass set into motion to the mass of the man. In other words, during inflation of the canopy a large mass of air is set in motion including not only that being trapped inside but also the air around the canopy which is displaced as the canopy inflates. This air mass is calculated to be about one to one and a half times the air mass of a sphere whose radius is equal to the radius of the canopy. The ratio

of this air mass to the mass of the man is important because of its effect in decreasing the velocity of the man-parachute system during the canopy opening phase. This factor was previously discussed in relation to canopy size; it is also affected by air density. With increasing altitude this mass ratio decreases in proportion to the decrease of the air density. As a result of this, the mass ratio is only one-fourth of its ground level value at an altitude of 40,000 feet. Because of this, there is significantly less deceleration of the man-parachute system prior to full inflation of the canopy. This factor affords a significant contribution to the increased parachute opening shock peak force at high altitude.

Hypoxia Hazard. This additional factor which makes free fall descent a desirable procedure has been briefly mentioned. The prolonged period of exposure to the low partial pressure of oxygen when the parachute is opened at high altitude is readily apparent in figure 119. This hypoxia can be severe enough to be fatal in itself or it may combine with combat injury or parachute opening shock to be the determining factor in a fatal outcome. Hypoxia will also make the individual more susceptible to frostbite. It might be considered that with present day oxygen equipment this hazard can be neutralized; however, malfunction and damage may render even the best equipment ineffective. The maximum altitude from which it is safe to descend in an open parachute is not a practical consideration in view of the many variables in an escape situation including variations in individual susceptibility to hypoxia, either inherent or as a result of one's physiologic status at the time of bailout. Cold exposure and injury are additional factors. The variable rate of descent which may be seriously modified by updrafts is also of great importance. Studies in the altitude chamber (4) indicate that it is possible for a man to descend in an open parachute from 30,000 feet to the ground without using oxygen equipment and without losing consciousness. However, this is under rather ideal conditions and cannot be realistically carried over to the escape situation. Simulated free fall studies in the low pressure chamber (5) indicate that it is possible for a man to descend from altitudes up to 40,000 feet without loss of consciousness and without emergency oxygen equipment with the following provisions: (1) he is not injured, (2) he bails out immediately after using 100 per cent oxygen, (3) he free falls to lower altitude and (4) he holds his breath for 30 seconds if at 40,000 feet. It was also determined that if for some reason consciousness were lost after leaving the aircraft at 40,000 feet it is probable that the individual would regain consciousness in sufficient time to open the parachute and that he would not know consciousness had been lost. Regardless of these findings it was recommended that emergency bailout oxygen equipment be developed and it is now standard practice to supply flyers with personal emergency oxygen equipment for flights above 25,000 feet. However, with the development of the automatic parachute opening device, which will be described more fully later, the requirement for emergency oxygen is less critical than before at altitudes below 40,000 feet. At higher altitudes, emergency oxygen systems and pressure suits become absolute necessities.

Cold Hazard. Cold injury can occur in free fall descent as well as in open parachute descent if the individual does not have adequate protective clothing. At extreme altitudes and high speed, frostbite is produced very quickly, therefore, it is mandatory that the entire body be covered with protective clothing. It has been demonstrated on a number of occasions that even a thin pair of capeskin or nylon gloves will prevent an otherwise serious frostbite. Even with adequate protective clothing, however, open parachute descent magnifies the cold exposure hazard over that of free fall descent. The opening parachute shock may cause loss of protective clothing, exposure to the cold is longer and permits this stress to combine with other stresses such as physical trauma and hypoxia to produce a possibly fatal outcome.

FREE FALL DESCENT. The foregoing discussion leaves little doubt that emergency escape from altitudes above 25,000 feet should be accomplished by free fall rather than open parachute descent. Under combat conditions this is obviously even more important from the standpoint of avoiding attack in the air as well as apprehension upon landing. The free fall technique is now an accepted routine procedure. However, a great deal of pioneering effort first laid the foundation which led to the development of our present concepts and procedures.

As pointed out by Armstrong (3), not too many years have passed since it was supposed that a free fall in the atmosphere would produce unconsciousness and probably death. General Armstrong was the first to make a free fall with the specific purpose of studying its effects on the individual and dispel many of the erroneous concepts held at the time. The results of his studies can best be presented by quoting from the third edition of his *Principles and Practice of Aviation Medicine:*

" . . . just exactly what the effects of such a fall were was not generally known until described by the author in 1935. This description was based on a free fall which was made in an attempt to analyze the subjective mental and physical reactions to a free fall through space and especially to determine why most individuals who made parachute jumps either refused or were unable to follow simple specific instructions.

"With reference to the latter it was found that

most individuals failed to follow instructions principally because of mental excitement or fear and not due to any clouding of consciousness or loss of motor functions.

"The subjective mental and physical reactions which are experienced during a free fall are as follows:

"*Mental Reactions.* Throughout a free fall, all conscious mental processes seem normal. As soon as the airplane is cleared, fear and excitement tend to disappear. Consciousness is unclouded and ideation is rapid, precise, penetrating and clear.

"Visual perception is normal. The earth, objects and individuals below and the sky above are normally visible. There are no consciously perceptible heart beats or other bodily processes.

"Probably one of the most interesting features of a free fall is in regard to the perception of position and motion in space. At the moment of jumping the earth is in full view. For the first second of fall there is a velocity attained of about 16 feet per second. At the same time there may be a trembling motion of the body. Of these motions, the only one recognized is rotation of the body.

"During the second second of fall the vertical velocity is increased to about 24 feet per second and still there is no conscious realization of any movement except the body rotation.

"If the eyes are voluntarily closed all sense of motion is lost. Not only are the linear velocities and accelerations and decelerations, both horizontal and vertical, imperceptible but also the previously recognized body rotation. In short, the sensation is that of being suspended at rest in mid-air.

"At an altitude of about 1,900 feet, if the ground is watched, there is for the first time a beginning definite sensation of falling. This sense of fall increases rapidly and at an altitude of 1,000 feet, there is fully perceptible vertical velocity.

"The increased sense of motion (falling) as the ground is approached is readily explained by a normal lack of sufficient depth perception acuity at high altitude to recognize the shortening of the distance to the earth. As the fall continues, of course, the shortening of the distance becomes more readily recognizable and the sense of falling increases.

"*Physical Sensations.* The period of free fall is remarkably free from abnormal physical sensations. There is no nausea or vertigo, and the lack of a distinct sense of motion may be the controlling factor.

"There are no abnormalities noted in the cardiovascular system, there is none of the empty or 'gone' feeling in the abdomen so common in elevators and in airplanes, and the eyes, although unprotected from the high wind blast, are not irritated and vision is normal. Breathing is even, regular and undisturbed. The undisturbed breathing and the unirritated eyes lead to an interesting speculation as to the explanation for this unusual phenomena which is so contrary to expectations and previous experience. The opinions of airplane designers and wind tunnel experts differ. Some suggest a turbulent airflow about the body, producing small eddies and air currents instead of a strong blast. Others suggest that the body acts as a fairly good airfoil, the downward portion of the body acting like the leading edge and the upward part like the trailing edge of a wing with a smooth even flow of air over the surface. Still others suggest that there is a static air condition so that there is no flow of the air around the body and that the pressure in the static area is a partial vacuum.

"The last phenomenon to be described is the only positive physical finding and is difficult of accurate description. It has to do with the skin of the body. It consists of that force which restricts terminal velocity to about 119 miles per hour instead of infinity and appears in consciousness as a very gentle, evenly distributed, generalized, superficial pressure on the surface of the body toward the earth."

Although proven feasible and without ill effects, the free fall technique was not seriously considered as an essential adjunct to parachute procedure for a period of several years. Following Colonel Lovelace's high altitude jump in 1943 and the further revelation of high parachute opening shock at altitude by dummy tests in 1944, accelerated efforts were directed toward the development of free fall concepts and techniques. In August of 1944, Lt. Colonel M. W. Boynton, a flight surgeon at the Aero Medical Laboratory, attempted a free fall bailout from 40,000 feet without the use of an automatic parachute opening device. He failed to pull the rip cord and plummeted to his death, apparently miscalculating his free fall time to the altitude which he planned to open the parachute. Although he used a stop watch it has been pointed out that the free fall descent rate is variable. In figure 119 it is noted that the plotted time for Williams' free fall from 37,000 feet was considerably greater than Boynton's observed time from 40,000 feet. This time was actually about 30 seconds shorter than the time previously calculated on the basis of data from lower altitude free fall trials.

AUTOMATIC PARACHUTE OPENING. Today the use of the automatic rip cord release device has become routine. This device might be more appropriately discussed under high performance escape because it is a very essential and integral part of all high performance escape systems. However, it is also used in conventional bailout and will be briefly described at this time. This device is designed to provide automatic time and altitude delays for high speed jumps at both low and high altitude. It consists of a small, compact mechanism which is contained in a pouch of the parachute pack. A spring loaded power cable provides the force to pull the rip cord. The spring loaded cable is automatically released by two controls; one, an aneroid device which can be set for activation at preselected altitudes; the other, a timer with a mechanical release that can be preset for activation after from 1 to several seconds delay. A standard procedure for conventional bailout is to set the aneroid 5000 feet above the highest terrain to be flown over and the timer for 5 seconds delay. Escape from high performance aircraft imposes quite different requirements which will be discussed later. In using the automatic opening device the jumper pulls the automatic release arming handle when he clears the aircraft. If he is above the preset altitude the device provides a free fall delay to the selected altitude where the spring loaded power cable will automatically pull the rip cord following the 5 second delay. If the bailout is below the altitude of the aneroid setting the rip cord is automatically pulled after the 5 second time delay. If the bailout occurs at very low altitude the jumper should pull the parachute D ring and, thus, override the automatic device. The automatic release device has proved to be both accurate and reliable and has saved countless lives. Its advantages with regard to accurate free fall delay and time delay for higher speeds are quite obvious. Another advantage is that this device can be used to safely drop injured or unconscious crewmen if an emergency warrants such action.

PARACHUTE OPENING AND DESCENT. Prior to pulling the rip cord, if done manually, it is desirable to assume a particular body position. The best position is chin on the chest so that the rip cord D ring is in view. Also, with the head down it is in the best position to avoid being struck by a riser, connector link or pilot parachute. The exception to this is that the head is turned to the side when the chest pack is used. The body should be bent slightly at the waist and the feet held tightly together. This will prevent deployment of the canopy and lines

between the legs which can occur. When the rip cord handle is grasped it should actually be looked at. The right hand is always used and with the back and seat type chutes both hands may be used; however, when the chest type chute is used it is best to hold the bottom of the pack with the left hand and pull the rip cord with the right.

If the free fall and automatic parachute release procedure is used it is recommended that the same preopening position be maintained during free fall; however, the complication of tumbling and spinning may occur, in which event there appear to be no fixed set of rules which apply to control tumbling or spin. In some instances extending the foot or hand may slow or reverse a spin; at other times waving the arms and kicking the feet, as if swimming, effects some control; sometimes just relaxing with no voluntary motion will work. The effect of spinning and tumbling can be quite serious. Most commonly disorientation and nausea are produced. Sometimes vomiting occurs and the after effects of nausea and general malaise can remain for several hours after landing. If the spinning has not been controlled before the parachute opens the lines may become twisted and delay effective deployment of the canopy. Usually the spinning reverses and the lines untwist but time is required. More serious effects, including severe g force hydraulic effects may be produced by tumbling; however, this is usually associated with escape at very high altitude and will be discussed under escape from high performance aircraft.

Following canopy deployment there are occasional complications which may occur. Risers may be twisted from rotation of the body and prevent raising the head. The risers will untwist without assistance but the process can be hurried by manually spreading them apart. Infrequently an inversion of the canopy may occur when one or more of the suspension lines are whipped across the top of the canopy producing the effect of two large bulges nicknamed the "Mae West." Usually this can be corrected by pulling the suspension lines of the smaller of the two bulges and the fouled lines will slip off. If not corrected it is not a serious matter although there will be some increase in rate of descent and, consequently, a heavier landing impact.

Oscillation or pendulumlike movement of the body can occur and may present some danger during landing on the ground. This motion can be decreased by pulling down on two adjacent risers and slowly releasing them to their normal positions when the oscillation has slowed down. This of course results in a slip with marked increase in rate of descent and should, therefore, never be attempted below 200 feet.

During descent, depending upon the type of survival equipment used, certain procedures are followed. These will be discussed in later paragraphs concerning survival.

Parachute Landing

The importance of this phase of emergency escape is emphasized by studies (6, 7) which have shown that 90 per cent of nonfatal injuries resulting from emergency bailouts were incurred on landing and 60 per cent of the nonfatal major injuries were the result of poor landing technique. The relatively low incidence of landing injuries among trained parachutists points up the value of expert knowledge and training. Yet in view of the fact that the emergency jumper rarely elects the time and place of escape it is surprising that the incidence of injury is not even higher. Reports of emergency parachute jumps reveal innumerable accounts of the most hazardous landing situations with miraculous escape from injury. This leads to the supposition that the element of chance is an important consideration in any emergency bailout. This, of course, does not alter the common sense view that certain basic rules of parachute landing which have been developed through experience should be followed.

Landing conditions largely determine the degree of injury risk and these conditions have almost as many variations as the number of emergency jumps. The most serious situation occurs when the bailout is too low and insufficient time is available for full parachute deployment. Resulting injuries and death cannot correctly be ascribed to parachute failure or faulty landing technique. The seriousness of a landing is determined by atmospheric and terrain conditions. High surface winds combined with rugged, hard terrain offer the most serious hazard and this combination produces most of the major and fatal full deployment landing injuries. Some deaths occur from drowning as a result of poor technique in water landings. Under adverse conditions good landing technique pays the highest dividends although some landing hazards cannot be overcome even by the most expert parachutist.

In uncomplicated landings the rate of descent is very important and is a highly variable factor. Larger canopies produce lower rates of descent. The 24 foot canopy with a 200 pound load is generally considered to have a sea level velocity of about 24 feet per second (9 foot platform jump equivalent), whereas the velocity of the 28 foot canopy under like conditions is approximately 19 feet per second (5.6 foot platform jump equivalent). It is obvious that the descent rate will be greater for heavier persons than lighter. Parachute descent may be slowed by updrafts and is also less rapid when the barometric pressure is high and in the presence of a high relative humidity. Another important factor is the terrain altitude at the point of landing. Bailing out in mountainous regions is hazardous enough because of the ruggedness and hardness of the terrain, the elevation is an additional hazard. For example, the rate of descent for a landing in the Andes or Himalayas at the 15,000 foot level would increase the rate of descent at landing by as much as 5 or 6 feet per second over that of the sea level rate. Inasmuch as the impact force increases in proportion to the square of the impact velocity the relatively small increase in descent rate will have rather large kinetic energy effects.

Avoidance of injury from uncomplicated parachute landing is a matter of using appropriate techniques to permit attenuation and absorption of the impact forces by the proper body structure and areas. The prelanding position is an essential part of the landing technique and should be assumed at approximately 1000 feet above the ground. At this time, both arms are stretched overhead and the hands firmly grasp the risers, the knees are slightly bent and the feet are held together. The line of vision should be directed out at a 45 degree angle to the ground and not straight down. In this position the time of impact will not be anticipated thus avoiding the hazard of retracting the legs prior to impact. The landing should be on the balls of both feet and at the time of impact the body should be permitted to collapse in the direction the parachute is moving. Collapsing in this manner distributes the impact forces over a larger area of the body and avoids overstressing any one anatomical structure or point. One of the most common causes of injury is failure to keep the feet together permitting one leg to bear the brunt of the impact. Pelvic and spinal injuries may result when the legs are retracted just prior to impact; this may be prompted by looking directly down at the ground rather than at the 45 degree angle. Taking the hands off the risers in an attempt to ward off ground impact is responsible for upper limb injuries.

After landing injuries can result from being dragged by the parachute. It is, therefore, necessary to collapse the parachute as soon as the landing is made. In the absence of a quick release harness the best method is to pull the lower risers. There are several types of quick release harnesses. Earlier designs provided for quick removal of the entire harness; however, a more simple and effective device is the shoulder canopy release which provides a quick disconnect of the risers on one or both sides and is activated by pressing release buttons between the thumb and forefinger. This method is quicker than throwing off the entire harness; also, when the harness remains on it simplifies retention of survival gear which is most critical in water landings.

In ground landings at night preparations for a normal landing should be made as soon as the parachute opens so that one is prepared for contact at any time. Statistics (8) indicate that the chances of injury in an uncomplicated night landing are less than in the day. This is ascribed to less anticipatory tensing and reflex leg withdrawal just before the time of impact.

The technique for ground landing is slightly modified for landing in trees. In this situation the arms are folded over in front of the face and no attempt should be made to grasp tree limbs. This can best be assured by grasping opposite risers with arms crossed over the face. The feet should be kept together and not crossed.

Water landings require prelanding preparations primarily concerned with avoiding being dragged under the water and drowned. The landing impact is of no concern. During descent oxygen masks or the face piece of pressure helmets should be removed. Also during descent it is advisable to inflate the life preserver. If the preserver is the Mae West type which is under the harness, the chest strap should be loosened or unfastened before inflating. A new type underarm life preserver inflates external to the parachute harness. Before landing the safety guard of the canopy release should be opened and the hand held near the release in readiness to activate it when the feet hit the water. This should not be done before touching the water because depth perception over water is deceptive and it is almost impossible to judge the height. It is very essential, however, to immediately activate the canopy release upon entering the water because of the danger of being dragged underwater. Even mild surface winds will do this and once it occurs it is very difficult if not impossible to reach the release mechanism on the shoulder against the force of the water. Failure to release or collapse the canopy has caused many deaths by drowning; victims have included robust individuals who were good swimmers. As soon as the canopy has collapsed it is best to swim up wind from it to avoid entanglement in the suspension lines. The next order of action is to get into the dinghy or life raft. The problems concerned with water survival will be discussed in the survival section of this chapter.

Escape from High Performance Aircraft

Although high speed and high performance are not synonymous terms, high speed has been primarily responsible for advances in improved methods of escape from disabled aircraft. During World War II it became obvious that the speeds attained by fighter aircraft had made escape by conventional bailout impractical if not impossible. The escape fatality rate increased significantly and collision with aircraft structures on bailout was responsible for a number of deaths and injuries. It was not possible to determine how many fatalities resulted from inability to separate from the aircraft because of pressure forces of wind blast or immobilization by g forces in spins and other uncontrolled gyrations. Wind blast at 200 m.p.h. or centrifugal forces of $2\frac{1}{2}$ to 3 g may be sufficient to prevent escape. Such forces in far greater magnitude were routinely being encountered early in the war. The Germans had anticipated the need for a positive means of escape which would overcome these forces and had begun research in this area as early as 1939. By 1944 the ejection seat was being installed in German fighter aircraft and by the end of the war 60 emergency escapes by ejection seat had been made. British development of ejection seat escape proceeded rapidly after 1944 and the first live test of the Martin-Baker seat was made in the United Kingdom in July 1946. American efforts were delayed; however, progress was more rapid through the use of German and British research data and the first live ejection in the United States was made in August 1946. The development of the ejection seat was truly a milestone in the solution of the problem of escape from "high performance" aircraft; however, the criteria of high performance have been altered considerably since the introduction of this escape device. In less than a decade operational aircraft speeds have progressed from subsonic to transsonic and supersonic. Hypersonic speeds are just around the corner. Concurrently, the operational flight ceilings of aircraft have been extended to extreme altitudes. This phenomenal progress in aircraft performance capabilities has increased the magnitude and complexity of in-flight escape problems. The paragraphs which follow will indicate what progress has been made in meeting these problems; they will also indicate those escape problems which are daily encountered in routine military flying and for which solutions are being sought in an extensive and vigorous research program in the military services and industry.

PERSONNEL ESCAPE CHUTES. The use of escape chutes or tunnels has already been mentioned under conventional bailout. Escape by this means depends upon the force of gravity and the chute entrance frequently has a centered horizontal bar from which the escapee drops. The exit is usually protected from wind blast by a spoiler or wind stream deflector. This method of escape has an application in the lower part of the high speed spectrum and has been successfully employed in some multiplace, high performance aircraft. The escape chute has been flight tested by bailout of personnel at speeds up to 440 m.p.h. (9). Its usefulness at high speeds is questionable and the aerodynamic characteristics of some aircraft preclude its use at speeds in excess of 300 m.p.h.

THE EJECTION SEAT. This device has saved hundreds of lives and is considered by the Germans to be one of the most important safety developments which they have invented. In principle it is simply a rigidly constructed seat which is forcibly ejected from the airplane cockpit by means of an explosive charge. There are numerous designs but a typical ejection seat assembly consists of a rigid metal bucket type seat with a back and head rest. It usually has arm and foot rests and projecting sides which give lateral support to the legs in the region of the knees and lower thighs. An outer catapult cylinder or tube is attached to the back of the sturdy seat frame and is the part which transmits the propulsive force to the seat in the ejection process. The outer catapult tube telescopes over an inner catapult tube which is attached to the cockpit structure. The explosive cartridge is fired in the inner tube propelling the outer catapult tube and the seat from the cockpit with almost instantaneous force. Some catapult models have three telescoping tubes to increase the length of the propelling stroke. Directional control of the seat during the firing is maintained by a guide rail assembly attached to the cockpit. There are two standard directional types; an upward and a downward. A third type, the canted, has been proposed but is not in operational use.

The upward ejection seat was developed first, primarily because of the convenient exit provided by the canopy area. Downward ejection was developed later to provide a means of escape from the underside of aircraft where upward ejection is not feasible. One of the first requirements for downward ejection installations was in two deck bomber aircraft where structural design and equipment arrangement made it necessary that lower deck seats be ejected downward. In multiplace aircraft it is also desirable to use both upward and downward ejection in order to reduce the probablility of collisions which may occur if all crew members were to eject from the same surface. Sequential firing when used adds further complications to an already complex problem. A downward ejection requirement in single place aircraft also exists where external structures on the upper surface are of sufficient height to intersect the trajectory of the upward seat at speeds within the aircraft's performance range. Some very high speed aircraft (*e.g.*, F-104) have exceeded the capability of conventional cartridge catapults to provide an adequate seat trajectory and stay within human acceleration tolerance limits. In this circumstance the downward ejection seat has the distinct advantage of requiring less velocity for successful separation from the aircraft. However, among other disadvantages, the downward ejection seat requires at least 300 feet more altitude for successful escape than the upward ejection seat. In view of the large percentage of aircraft accidents during the takeoff and landing phases of flight this deficiency in low level escape capability is a serious indictment of the downward ejection system.

The sequence of events in ejection seat escape are jettisoning of the canopy or hatch; ejection of the seat; separation from the seat; free fall, if at high altitude; deployment of the parachute; prelanding activation of survival equipment; and landing. The mechanisms, procedures, stresses and hazards associated with these events are extremely variable. These variations will depend upon aircraft type, equipment and the escape environment with respect to altitude, speed, aircraft attitude and type of emergency. Some of the salient features of the various phases of ejection escape are presented in the following paragraphs.

Pre-ejection Considerations. Prior to ejection a decision must be made and circumstances may frequently delay this decision until a fatal outcome is inevitable. Studies (10) have shown that over one-third of the aircrew fatally injured experienced the emergency at an altitude sufficient to insure a high probability of survival but failed to eject or waited until too low an altitude was reached. A follow-on of this problem is the speed and accuracy of accomplishing the emergency procedures once the decision is made. Under the stress of emergency reaction is slowed, sometimes to the point of complete inaction. Both of these problems are under constant attack through the media of indoctrination and training. Ejection seat training devices which actually subject the individual to the forces of catapult ejection are in use and were particularly effective in establishing confidence in the procedure when it was first introduced. Procedure drills in simulators and in the cockpit are valuable in establishing a habit pattern which will become automatic under emergency conditions. A more effective approach to this part of the problem would be to simplify the escape procedure through more adequate and reliable equipment design. However, it should be recognized that increasing automaticity of a system increases maintenance problems and frequently encroaches on reliability. Even with the most simple push button procedure it is highly probable that fatalities resulting from delayed ejection will continue to occur. Mason (11) has made a study of this aspect of ejection escape and found that an important factor in delayed ejection is the strong motivation of the pilot to control the aircraft up to the last instant before crashing in order to avoid loss of civilian life on the ground. It is also indicated that some reluctance to use the ejection seat is fostered by "fear of the unknown" particularly by those flyers who have not received live ejection seat trainer indoctrination. Some older pilots, because of previous successful crash landing experience, have elected this more familiar procedure in preference to ejecting. Although an exceptional effort may be made to save a prototype or experimental aircraft it is apparent from pilot interviews that neither the financial aspects of total loss of an aircraft nor the possible consequences of official investigation exert any influence at all on the decision to eject. On the other hand, face saving may be a factor of some importance and in some situations delay or failure to eject may result from avoidance of a blow to professional pride incident to failure to "bring the aircraft in."

The problem of delay in escape is much more complex in multiple place aircraft because of communications and emergency warning relay factors. Consequently, it is not uncommon that just one member of a multiple man crew safely escapes, whereas one or more fail to do so. Training and simulated practice do not solve this problem. Proposals of automatic sequential operation of all crew escape devices by a master control have not yet been adopted. It appears that a completely automatic system would be necessary to overcome delayed escape problems. To be effective, such a system would necessarily include emergency sensors and evaluators as essential components of an automatic activator. It is obvious that this device would be rather complex and perhaps not as reliable as the present human counterpart.

Jettisoning the Canopy. This first action in ejection escape in some instances, depending upon time available and aircraft model, may be preceded by a host of activities such as dumping cabin pressure, stowage of loose equipment, stowage of controls or radar equipment, activating emergency oxygen, disconnecting communications, oxygen and other leads to aircraft systems, lowering of helmet visor and lowering the head to avoid being struck by a "dishing" canopy. Earlier systems located the jettison control remote from the ejection seat control thereby further complicating pre-ejection procedure. Experience has shown that these complexities combined with mechanical difficulties and maintenance errors to produce unacceptable delays and actual failure of canopies to jettison. The latter was particularly critical inasmuch as many systems depended upon canopy release to arm the ejection seat, in which case the seat would not fire unless the canopy jettisoned.

These difficulties were soon recognized and some functions were made automatic or were eliminated in order to simplify ejection procedure. More important, the canopy jettisoning controls were placed in proximity to or combined with the seat ejection control. The

jettisoning actuator mechanism was made more reliable and more simple to maintain by replacing mechanical systems of cables, bell cranks and levers and equally unreliable electrical systems with the gas initiator system. This is an entirely new principle in actuating devices and consists of firing explosive initiator cartridges into sealed flexible hoses. The pressure of the gas from the burning propellent can be transmitted by means of the flexible hose to any point in the aircraft to actuate or trigger such devices as canopy removers, control stowage thrusters and seat catapults. The control for firing such initiators is simple and reliable. Initiator cartridges can be made with variable time delays which meets certain other requirements in ejection escape systems. The gas initiator principle is one of the most important improvements in ejection systems. Another important advance was realized by eliminating successful canopy jettison as an essential part of ejection seat arming action. In case of canopy jettison failure it is now possible to eject through the canopy without delay. Many flyers have ejected through the canopy with little or no injury. There are also instances on record of ejection through "frozen" canopies on the ground after a crash and fire to escape burning to death. This is almost always attended by serious or fatal injury upon impact with the ground and is not recommended except as a last resort.

Stresses and hazards attending canopy or hatch jettisoning include danger of being struck by an erratically separating canopy, physical buffeting and loss of protective equipment by the effects of wind blast, exposure to the ambient environment which at altitude includes explosive decompression, inadequate partial pressure of oxygen, low temperature and low barometric pressure. As a matter of interest, the open cockpit pressure at high speeds can be even lower than the ambient pressure as a result of the venturi effect. These problems of the ambient flight environment are covered in other chapters. Adequate protective equipment, appropriately integrated and used in a correct manner, should overcome the environmental difficulties presented at this stage of ejection escape.

Ejection of the Seat. After the canopy has been jettisoned the correct position for ejection is assumed before actuating the seat firing mechanism. In some cases this position must be attained prior to jettisoning the canopy. There are several types of firing mechanisms and, as will be seen, one of these assists in assuring correct head and body position. The head should be back against the headrest, the body erect, the arms close to the body and on arm rests if provided, the buttocks well back and the feet firmly implanted in the foot rests. This position assists in preventing forward arching of the head and trunk which would place excessive stress on the anterior portions of the vertebrae during ejection. Leaning forward and loose or unfastened shoulder straps during ejection have been conducive to a number of anterior wedge vertebral compression fractures. The most vulnerable part of the spinal column in upward ejection is in the region T-11 to L-2. The forward bending moment during ejection is contributed to by the fact that the centers of gravity of the head and torso are considerably anterior to the spinal plane; in addition, the line of ejection thrust is at a backward angle in aircraft in which rearward inclined rails are used. Appropriate positioning also helps to avoid injury by impact of arms, knees or feet with parts of the cockpit.

The position of the feet has been shown to be of not too great importance in upward ejection, but in downward ejection it becomes a critical factor in avoiding serious injury. This is because in downward ejection there is an upward movement of the arms and legs with respect to the body. Jackknifing of the legs while passing through the escape hatch may result in injury from impact with the hatch rim. Of more serious import in high speed flight is the certainty of wind blast flail injury of both upper and lower limbs upon entry into the wind stream unless appropriately restrained in less vulnerable positions. The hazard of wind blast flail injury will be discussed more fully, suffice it to say at this point that position restraint of both upper and lower limbs must be assured in downward ejection. Various methods are used for this purpose. One design employs a pair of crescent shaped metal retainers mounted above the foot rest which automatically partially encircle the ankles when the feet are placed on the rests. Upward motion of the feet is prevented but forward motion of the ankles will permit separation from the seat. Restraint of the upper limbs is assured by a firm grip with both hands on the D ring activator which is designed as a restraining device in addition to the function of firing the hatch and the seat.

The correct position of the torso and head in downward ejection is more or less assured by the firing procedure; however, it is important that the lap belt be very tight to avoid overloading the shoulder straps. All of the ejection force is imparted to the body through the shoulder straps and lap belt. It is desirable for the lap belt to engage most of this force and it is designed for this requirement. Lap belts on downward ejection seats have an accessory inverted V, tie down strap which passes from the buckle forward beneath the front of the seat pan. This device prevents the lap belt from rising during ejection and automatically tightens the harness when the leg guards are activated prior to ejection by placing the feet on the foot rests. Experimental trials (12) with the downward ejection catapult have demonstrated the desirability of transmitting a large portion of the ejection load to the pelvis by means of the lap belt and the potential dangers of transmitting large forces to the shoulder girdle through the shoulder restraining harness. In the latter case the upper thoracic vertebrae are subject to compression fracture at acceleration levels of 13 to 18 g.

Ejection Controls. Efforts to optimize ejection procedure should eventually produce a simple standardized activator control accessible to either hand which initiates an automatic ejection sequence encompassing body positioning and restraint retention of limbs, equipment and control stowage, canopy and catapult firing and any other essential action. Unfortunately, this state of the art has not yet been achieved and procedures required of the man are not single action in many cases and vary from one aircraft to another. There are, however, two basic ejection activating methods for upward ejection and one for downward ejection. One upward method used principally by the Air Force consists of raising an armrest to fire the canopy followed by squeezing a trigger on the arm rest to fire the seat catapult. In some cases raising the opposite arm rest tightens and locks restraints. The advantage of the arm rest method lies in its ready accessibility which is important from the standpoint of time and g force factors in many emergencies. Arm rests also offer the advantage of supporting some of the weight of the arms and shoulder girdle which may reduce the ejection load on the lower spine by as much as 30 per cent. The second upward method is used principally by the British forces and the U. S. Navy. This consists of a face blind which is withdrawn from a recess at the top of the seat forward and down over the occupant's head and face. The initial travel of this face curtain fires the canopy and its completion fires the seat catapult. This method has important advantages of aiding correct positioning and of protecting the head and face against wind blast effects during both canopy jettisoning and entry into the wind stream. This latter effect helps to prevent the loss of essential equipment such as the oxygen mask and protective helmet. Holding the blind handle also supports some of the weight of the shoulder girdle although perhaps not to the same extent as the arm rests. One disadvantage of this method is its poor accessibility which can be critical under variable g force conditions of uncontrolled aircraft maneuvers and gyrations. Aircrew injury might also impose an insurmountable handicap. Although centrifuge studies (13) have shown that the seat firing curtain can be reached and actuated up to levels of 6 to 8 positive g while wearing a g suit, these forces do entail a definite delay and there are doubtless some instances of uncontrolled flight gyrations with fluctuating g forces which render this action impossible. It appears that it would be advantageous to use the face curtain as the primary method with a more accessible actuating control as an alternate.

The downward ejection seat is actuated by a D ring trigger located at the front of the seat between the legs, this is pulled upward with both hands and operates a firing cable. This single action jettisons the hatch and also fires the seat catapult. It has previously

been pointed out that the D ring trigger also serves a second and very important function of hand and arm restraint. When this firing and restraint mechanism was first tried experimentally in actual flight (14), it was found that upon ejection into the wind stream in the region of 390 knots IAS (indicated air speed) the hands were forcibly dislodged from the D ring by the impact of the wind blast on the arms. Following dislodgement, the hands and arms of two subjects ejecting at 390 knots were violently thrown back resulting in elbow dislocation and arm fracture in both subjects. Analysis revealed that each wrist was subjected to ram air loads in excess of 200 pounds for a period of four one-hundredths of a second (0.04 second) while the seat was still connected to the ejection rails during the terminal part of the ejection. Under the condition of fully extended arms and sudden preloading by the catapult thrust, the human grip cannot withstand loads of this magnitude. To avoid this rapid application of high loads for a brief instant which effectively breaks the grip, a spring device providing gradual preloading was installed on the D ring cable. This resulted in an elastic system which absorbed suddenly applied forces. This shock absorber device reduced peak loads by as much as 70 per cent. In-flight testing of this firing mechanism resulted in successful retention of the D ring to speeds as great as 425 knots IAS. With an improved D ring for effective gloved hand gripping and a lengthened cable to prevent overextension of the arms, this device has successfully proven itself in operational use.

EJECTION FORCES. During the actual ejection process, when the catapult thrust is acting on the seat, the important physiologic problem of concern in both upward and downward ejection is the maximum peak of acceleration and rate of change of acceleration (jolt) which can be sustained by the seated human body along the vertical axis of the spine. Sufficient velocity must be imparted to the seat and occupant before it leaves the aircraft to insure clean separation and clearance of all projections of the aircraft, such as, for example, a high vertical stabilizer. Because of the limited stroke distance of the catapult the thrust is applied for a very short period of time. This means that the seat and occupant must go from zero velocity to maximum velocity in the order of tenths of a second (approximately 0.2 second). This of necessity results in relatively high acceleration forces of short duration. The physiologic problem is, therefore, one of impact effects. The vulnerable anatomical structure in this case, for both upward and downward ejection, is the vertebral column. This was well demonstrated in early German experimental work in which many subjects suffered compression fractures of the vertebrae. Spinal g tolerance limits have been used by the engineers and ordnance experts as criteria for the design of safe ejection systems.

The amount of acceleration required for successful ejection of the seat and occupant depends upon a number of factors including the speed, altitude and flight path of the airplane; height of tail or other projection to be cleared and its distance from the cockpit; and the drag-over-weight ratio and lift-over-drag ratio of the occupied seat. Higher speeds at lower altitudes require greater seat acceleration. Aircrew instructions for many aircraft state the indicated airspeeds beyond which ejection should not be attempted. Unfortunately, such instructions cannot always be complied with and fatal contact with aircraft structures on ejection has occurred. If the flight path of the aircraft is resulting in positive g forces a greater catapult force may be required because of the increased effective weight to be overcome and also the effective trajectory of the seat is encroached upon by the curvilinear path of the aircraft. It has been found (15) that these factors have little appreciable effect if the aircraft g forces do not exceed 5 g. Actually at small additional g loads the ejection velocity of the seat is increased owing to improved thermodynamic efficiency of the catapult.

Increased drag-over-weight ratios result in more rapid horizontal slowing of the seat relative to the aircraft and, hence, a need for greater vertical velocity to avoid impact with the tail. The lift-over-drag ratio of the seat is also of great importance because in some attitudes of the seat a negative lift results in a lowered trajectory and a greater

chance of colliding with the aircraft. A seat, on ejection, usually tumbles at high speeds because of unsymmetric aerodynamic loading. At low indicated speeds tumbling also occurs because the ejection force is tangential to the occupied-seat center of gravity. If the seat could be stabilized in an attitude giving a high positive lift-over-drag ratio this would obviously be of great advantage in clearing the aircraft and in gaining valuable altitude on low level ejections. A negative lift is advantageous in downward ejection.

BIODYNAMICS OF EJECTION. All factors are considered in deriving the requirements for the ejection seat trajectory. It is a simple matter to determine the amount of force required to attain the desired trajectory; however, the engineering problems are complicated because the maximum velocity must be imparted to the seat in a limited distance of travel along the rails and still remain within human tolerances to acceleration. From the standpoint of design criteria the g load tolerance limits have been determined to be approximately 20 g for upward and 12 g for downward acceleration in the seated position. As so well demonstrated in Stapp's work (16) the rate of onset of this acceleration, quite apart from its peak, must be limited if impact injury is to be avoided. A rate of onset of 250 g per second upward and 125 g downward are considered to be within tolerance limits. Present catapults are designed to operate well within these limits; for example; the most powerful U. S. Air Force upward ejection catapult produces an occupied seat (350 pounds) velocity of 81 feet per second with a rate of onset of 115 g per second and a peak g force of 17. Although these acceleration values may be designed into the equipment with great accuracy it is found that in practical application the g forces imparted to the seat occupant may greatly exceed the stated limits. This is because of the complex mechanical behavior of different parts of the body in relation to each other and of the body in relation to the seat when the body-seat system is subjected to ballistic forces. The body-seat system is mechanically a multiple mass system linked together with elastic elements. An externally applied force results in internal dynamic interactions within the system involving time lags of parts of the system and temporary energy absorption by elastic elements with later release of this energy causing overshoots in peaks of acceleration in parts of the system. This has a very practical application in the type and thickness of a cushion which might be used between the man and seat. It is obvious that when a thick, easily compressible, elastic cushion is used the seat will be well on its way toward its velocity goal before the man has moved at all; yet, when the final velocity is attained the man and seat will be moving at the same speed. This means that the rate of onset of acceleration (jolt) in the man will be greater than in the seat itself. This increase in jolt as a function of time lag in cushion compression may be of importance in spinal injury.

Peak acceleration values in parts of the body are also increased beyond the basic seat acceleration. If the time-force characteristics of the acceleration and the decay rate of acceleration are in harmonic resonance with the natural frequency of the man-seat system, severe overshoots in peak acceleration of the body can be produced. Therefore, particular rates of onset of acceleration in combination with certain durations may be especially dangerous. Latham (17), in his study in body ballistics, in which several types of cushions were used, found that accelerations of less than 0.2 second duration and of approximately 400 g per second rate of change are likely to produce a maximum acceleration overshoot in the man. If the duration of the change in acceleration can be prolonged beyond the period of natural frequency of the man-seat system, the acceleration overshoots caused by dynamic interaction or oscillation are minimized. Thus, a prolongation of the increasing acceleration period to a value as little as 0.23 second will result in a minimum overshoot of acceleration in the man. Latham also states that the maximum limit of acceleration tolerable by the seated human body along the vertical axis of the spine is in the range of 300 g per second rate of onset and 25 g maximum peak. In spite of lower design criteria these figures have probably been exceeded by present ejection seat equipment as a result of the internal dynamics of the man-seat system. There is evidence to support this assumption in that a number of back injuries on ejection have been related to the use of thick, elastic cushions and to the circumstance of ejecting while in an inverted position or during a negative g maneuver with slack shoulder straps permitting a considerable space between the seat and the man.

A study (18) of 633 nonfatal ejections revealed 14 cases (2.2 per cent) of back fractures caused by seat ejection forces. The most important factors appeared to be incorrect position and separation from the seat at the time of the ejection. The effect of the latter in increasing the jolt seems to be most important. The importance of factors other than primary acceleration values appears to be supported by incidents reported by Stapp (19) in which accidental exposures of human subjects to between 30 and 33 g at 500 g per second rate of onset were sustained without injury in upward ejection experiments under ideal laboratory conditions. Although most vertebral fractures occurring upon ejection have been attributed to unequal distribution of forces on the anterior portion of the vertebrae, as a function of incorrect position, it is quite possible that in many cases a combination of circumstances exists, not only position but perhaps individual susceptibility as an anatomical function and some of the known and unknown phenomena of body ballistics. Additional study is required in this area.

Although the foregoing discussion applies primarily to upward ejection it is also applicable to downward ejection. Any differences are a function of the manner and points of application of the acceleration forces to the body. If a considerable portion of the force in downward ejection is transmitted to the shoulder girdle by tight shoulder straps combined with a loose lap belt, the upper thoracic vertebrae are quite vulnerable; particularly so, inasmuch as the normal order of weight bearing is reversed and anatomically these structures are not as well designed for this role as the lower thoracic and lumbar vertebrae which are of concern in upward ejection. Further, the dynamic interaction resulting from the elasticity of both the man and the linkage is most severe when the shoulder straps act as the primary linkage.

When the special lap belt with the tie down strap, previously described, is the primary linkage there is less oscillatory intensification of the acceleration. Tests (20) of downward ejection systems have shown that with a loose shoulder harness and a tight lap belt and tie down strap the man and seat move as a single unit. With tightening of the shoulder harness there is evidence of dynamic interaction which becomes maximal when the shoulder harness and the lap belt are tight and the tie down strap was removed entirely. This demonstrates rather conclusively the important role played by the tie down strap in making the lap belt the primary man-seat linkage.

POSTEJECTION FORCES. When the seat is ejected, the phenomena associated solely with the catapulting forces are scarcely noticeable to the seat occupant. This is partly because of the extreme rapidity of the action; however, it is also in great part a result of the formidable nature of other factors in the escape environment at the instant of entry into the wind stream. These important factors are, (1) wind blast; (2) wind-drag deceleration; (3) thermal effects; and (4) tumbling and spinning. Each of these has its own lethal potential and the various combinations which occur magnify this potential. The limits of human tolerance to these conditions have been in some measure determined and engineering effort is bent toward the solution of problems related to keeping within these limits in any escape situation. A brief discussion of these factors will reveal some of the problems and the present status of actual or proposed solutions to these problems.

AERODYNAMIC FORCES. Wind blast effects result from the forces exerted by the dynamic air pressure of the slip stream to which the man and seat are suddenly exposed upon ejection. The magnitude of this ram pressure force is a function of speed and air density and is commonly expressed in pounds per square foot (p.s.f.) as the q force. The symbol q is an arbitrary one used by the aerodynamicist and may appear in three forms; q or q_i (incompressible) representing freestream dynamic pressure and q_c (compressible) representing dynamic pressure corrected for compressibility effects at very high speeds. Ordinarily the q (q_i) value is used, representing the ram pressure calculated on the basis of speed and air density. At supersonic speeds, where compressibility effects are significant, a correction must be applied to include the additional pressure effects of the compressed stagnated air at the ram interface. Thus, it will be noted that q_c will have a considerably higher value than q or q_i. It has been pointed out by Greer (21) that q_c is a more true measure of the dynamic pressure that is actually felt by an ejection seat-man combination than q_i. This is because the man and seat present a large stagnation frontal area rather than a leading edge as in the case of aerodynamically shaped objects, hence, a large amount of air is trapped and stagnates. This stagnating air compresses and exerts its own intrinsic pressure just as if it were in a pressurized container. This pressure is additive to the calculated ram pressure. In actual fact, inasmuch as not all of the air flow at the ram interface will reach stagnation values, the true dynamic pressure will be greater than q_i but slightly less than q_c on the frontal area of the seat-man combination.

It is this factor of high dynamic air pressures encountered at high speeds which is responsible for the most formidable problems in escape from high performance aircraft. In the U. S. Air Force, criteria for escape system requirements are stated in terms of dynamic pressure capability of the aircraft. The *Handbook of Instructions for Aircraft Designers* (Air Research and Development Command Manual (ARDCM) no. 80-1), which is the basic guide for aircraft design in the Air Force, states that dynamic pressure capability (q_i) of over 289 p.s.f. (260 knots equivalent airspeed) requires an ejection seat and over 1540 p.s.f. (600 knots EAS) capability requires an enclosed escape system (ejectable cockpit or capsule). Using these criteria which reflect human tolerances to aerodynamic stresses, Greer (21) has calculated and charted the bioaerodynamic limitations to escape from aircraft for various magnitudes of the two critical parameters of flight, speed and altitude. This information is presented in figure 120. This chart indicates the type of escape system required for various regions of speed and

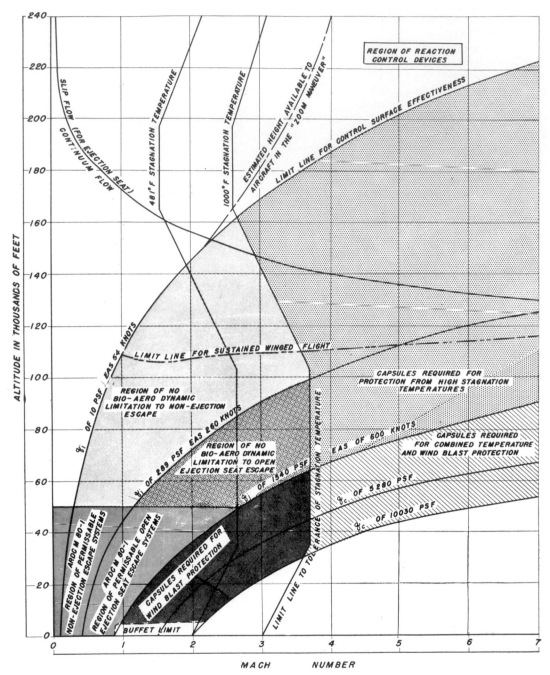

FIG. 120. Bioaerodynamic limitations to escape from aircraft. (From Greer (21).)

altitude and the conditions which the closed system protects against. Thermal protection is based on a temperature of 1000° F. which will be discussed in a later paragraph. It will be noted that two regions are marked "no bioaerodynamic limitation" and this has ref-

erence to the fact that ARDCM 80-1 imposes an altitude limitation of 50,000 feet beyond which a closed escape system is required. This limitation, therefore, has no relation to the problem of dynamic pressure. As a matter of fact, it is questionable if this altitude criterion is a valid one for closed escape systems in view of the fact that pressure suits are available which give full protection at any altitude.

Although the chart in figure 120 delineates the types of escape systems required for various Mach number altitude regions it does not presume to represent absolute requirements. Rather, it indicates regions which must be more thoroughly explored to find answers to the many unsolved problems of high speed, high altitude escape. The closed escape system will be discussed in a later section. At this point some of the effects produced by ram pressure will be discussed in order to amplify the chart and to bring into focus some practical aspects of the problems faced in open seat ejection.

The dynamic air pressure encountered by the body during escape is directly proportional to the speed and air density. Therefore, the higher the speed and the lower the altitude, the greater will be the ram pressure. A general conception of the tremendous air loads borne by the body in relation to speed and altitude can be gained from the data compiled by the NACA shown in table 62. It should be noted that these values are for subsonic speeds; at supersonic speeds the increase in dynamic pressure will be disproportionately larger because of the changes in aerodynamic flow characteristics. The effects on the escaping flyer resulting from these ram pressure forces may be divided into three categories. The first is the sudden direct wind blast force impinging on the man similar to that of a blast wave resulting from the detonation of a high explosive. The second type of effect is related to differential drag forces on various discrete areas of the man-seat mass resulting in loss of protective equipment, tearing of exposed skin and injury to the limbs and their attachments by flailing action. This is frequently termed wind blast erosion. The third category is the wind-drag linear deceleration, producing secondary dynamic inertial effects as the body is suddenly slowed down from a high velocity by the severe aerodynamic resistance. This category will be considered as a separate entity, distinct from wind blast.

BLAST EFFECTS. With regard to the first category, the possibility of classic blast injury from abrupt onset of wind blast pressure cannot be ignored. However, it is probable that the type of blast wave produced under the conditions which make escape feasible within limitations imposed by other parameters, such as wind-drag deceleration, will not result in injuries comparable to those of high explosive blast. Pressures will not be sufficiently high and also the onset of the dynamic pressure is several orders of magnitude slower than the onset of pressure resulting from explosions, thus minimizing shock phenomena. True blast injuries have not yet been produced in actual supersonic escape nor in experimental rocket sled studies (22) in which animals have been subjected to abrupt wind blast forces at velocities in excess of Mach 1.5 at sea level (q_c of approximately 5280 p.s.f.). These animals were protected with a windproof helmet, otherwise severe flutter and tear injury would have occurred. The hazards of facial injury were demonstrated by the German wind tunnel experiments during World War II with exposure of the bare face to wind blast in excess of 400 knots for several seconds which produced minor injuries of the eyelids, nostrils, lips and ears. Human experiments (23) in the United States, with the face protected, resulted in no injury attributable to wind blast *per se* at 562 knots. The uncovered face also presents the hazard of inflation of the stomach and conceivably excessive intrapulmonic pressure. Supersonic escape (24) without full face mask protection has resulted in stomach inflation of the

TABLE 62

Air Loads Borne by the Body in Relation to Speed * *and Altitude*

Altitude	Ram Pressure	Total Pressure to 4 Square Foot Drag Area of Man
feet	*p.s.f.*	*pounds*
50,000	158	632
40,000	288	1152
30,000	432	1728
20,000	692	2768
15,000	850	3400
10,000	1010	4040
5,000	1240	4960
Sea level	1440	5760

* Speed = Mach 0.9.

human and this has also been produced in animals on the rocket sled. No lung injury has been reported to have resulted from wind blast effects. Additional studies are required to determine if blast injury can be produced at technically feasible flight speeds. If such injury can occur this will establish an absolute requirement for protection of the body with a rigid shield such as the escape capsule or similar device. On the other hand, as indicated previously, it is highly probable that the factor of wind-drag deceleration in open ejection seats will limit the escape velocity to a level below the danger of blast injury. This of course may not be true if some methods such as streamlining, ballasting or use of the rocket catapult were successful in overcoming the wind-drag deceleration problem of open ejection seats. The probability of realization of such success in engineering design is discussed in later paragraphs.

WIND BLAST EROSION. There is no conjecture whatever regarding the hazards of the second group of ram pressure effects. Loss of vital protective equipment and flailing injuries have previously been mentioned. The upper extremity injuries which occurred in testing the downward ejection seat (14) at speeds below 400 knots (IAS) present adequate evidence of the dangers involved. British and French flyers have suffered lower extremity injuries, such as dislocation of the hips and fracture of the pelvis, from wind blast flailing. Premature deployment of parachutes by wind blast, with fatal outcome, has occurred. It is apparent that effective means of securing protective equipment and the extremities against the forces of supersonic wind blast will be difficult to attain without undue interference with aircrew performance. This is one of the many factors which may ultimately force abandonment of the open seat escape system in supersonic aircraft.

WIND DRAG DECELERATION. Of all factors to be dealt with in high speed escape perhaps the most formidable is wind-drag deceleration. The abrupt linear deceleration caused by the airloads imposed on the ejected occupied seat as it enters the air stream is in every sense a crash force. In fact, the lethal potentialities of wind-drag deceleration of a given magnitude are magnified beyond those of ordinary crash decelerations in that the duration of high g forces may be in the order of 10 to 20 times as long Further, the element of instability during deceleration, resulting in tumbling and spinning, produces a very complex pattern of mechanical forces acting upon the body.

If the complication of tumbling and spinning is ignored for the time being and a stable system is assumed, the rate of onset, magnitude and duration of deceleration forces are primarily dependent upon the following factors: speed at time of ejection (V), air density (ρ), exposed frontal area of the occupied seat (A), weight of the occupied seat (W) and its drag coefficient (C_D). A conception of the magnitude of g's produced by ejection at various speeds and altitudes is presented in figure 121; this chart, taken from Goodrich (25), also indicates the interrelations of Mach number, altitude and indicated air speed (calibrated). Calibrated air speed is actually indicated air speed corrected for installation and instrument errors. In common parlance the term indicated air speed (IAS) is preferable. It should be noted that the maximum linear deceleration g values indicated by the broken lines are practically constant for a given indicated air speed regardless of altitude. For example, in figure 121 it is apparent that the maximum linear deceleration experienced at Mach 1 at sea level is approximately the same as that experienced at Mach 2 at 39,000 feet. The progressive increase in g forces as a function of indicated air speed is very great. In fact, because of the variation of drag coefficient (C_D) with Mach number, calculations indicate (25) that g forces increase as the 2.47 power of the velocity. This means that a 15 per cent increase in indicated air speed results in a corresponding increase in g of almost 50 per cent. The g values in figure 121 were calculated as indicated in the accompanying formula using ejection seat drag coefficients from wind tunnel data. The 6.5 square foot frontal area and 325 pounds weight are representative of present ejection seats. These values vary considerably for different ejection seats and occupants and such variations will obviously affect the speed at which it is safe to eject. For exam-

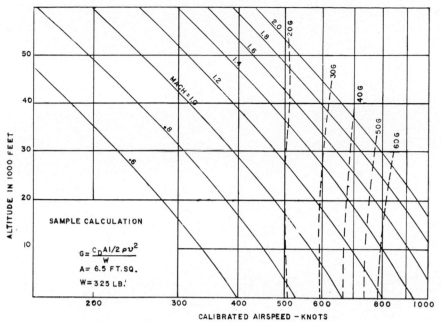

FIG. 121. Magnitude of g force as a function of calibrated airspeed, altitude and Mach number. (From Goodrich (25).)

ple, using a maximum peak of 35 g linear deceleration as a limiting value for safe escape, Goodrich (25) has calculated that this figure can be reached within a range of indicated air speeds from 575 to 725 knots, depending upon the variable ratios of area over weight possible in existing escape systems. This effect of just two variables upon the magnitude of wind-drag deceleration forces accounts in some degree for the marked differences in extent of injury sustained by individuals ejecting at the same speed. There are many other variables which affect the severity of deceleration injury including attitude of the body at time of ejection, effectiveness of body restraint, time of separation from the seat, spinning and tumbling and ejection altitude.

The last named factor is important from the standpoint of duration of deceleration which in itself imposes human tolerance limits. As the ejection altitude is increased the deceleration time is more prolonged. The increased altitude for any given indicated air speed results in a higher kinetic energy for the ejected occupied seat inasmuch as the kinetic energy is a function of the square of the true air speed (actual velocity). At 40,000 feet this kinetic energy is increased threefold

over that at sea level for a given indicated air speed. This increase in kinetic energy must be dissipated as a function of time in the less dense atmosphere at altitude. Figure 122 represents calculations (25) of deceleration decay times for the occupied ejection seat at different altitudes. It can be seen that it takes approximately twice as long for the deceleration g forces to decrease from 35 to 10 g at 40,000 feet as it would at sea level. The formula expresses the relationship that the duration of g forces at altitude (t_h) compared to that at sea level (t_{sl}) is proportional to the inverse of the square root of the density ratio of the air (altitude density over sea level density).

The importance of g force duration at relatively high levels has been emphasized by Stapp (23) in his experimental definition and evaluation of the time-force acceleration injury spectrum in the area between impact forces and centrifuge type hydrodynamic circulatory effects. It is in this area where tissue damage is produced very rapidly as a result of hydraulic displacement of body fluids. This high g hydraulic effect follows a latent period of 0.2 second and results in blood vessel rupture and pressure damage to cell membranes. The effects of acceleration

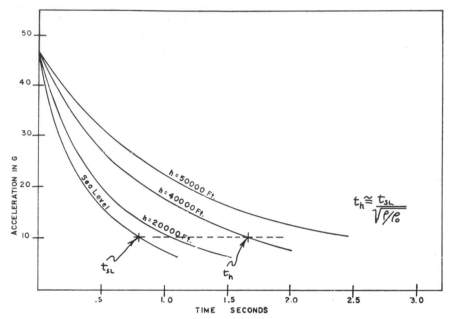

Fɪɢ. 122. Decay of deceleration as a function of altitude. (From Goodrich (25).)

forces are treated in detail in another chapter of the text; however, as a matter of convenience and emphasis, these parameters of human tolerance limits for acceleration forces as determined by Stapp (23), which are particularly applicable to wind-drag deceleration, are reiterated here: (1) for rate of change of deceleration the limit of tolerance is 1500 g per second at 40 g for 0.16 second duration or less; (2) for magnitude of force the limit is 50 g attained at 500 g per second rate of onset and duration of 0.2 second or less; and (3) the limit for duration is 1 second for forces averaging 25 g or more at 500 g per second rate of onset.

An apparent discrepancy may be noted between the above stated force magnitude tolerance limit and the previously mentioned 35 g limit. There are several reasons for this apparent discrepancy the most important of which is that the 35 g value has been proposed as an escape system design criterion limit which takes into consideration many important variables such as body attitude, effectiveness of restraints, seat stability and also the fact that following deceleration exposure, upon actual ejection, the individual must be physically and mentally capable of carrying out emergency survival procedures. The values as determined by Stapp were obtained under rather rigidly controlled conditions and represent tolerance limits for more or less pure decelerative force in the transverse axis applied to a forward facing seated subject. Further, the tolerance limit criterion used in Stapp's sled experiments was "reversible incapacitation"; this incapacitation, although reversible, could be rather prolonged and, therefore, not compatible with most survival situations following an emergency ejection.

An additional fact is that above the 35 g level small increments of force, as well as changes in direction of the acting force, very rapidly become more and more critical. The single value of 35 g maximum deceleration peak obviously expresses only part of the acceleration force parameter of escape system design. Figure 123, taken from Savely (26), presents other aspects of this parameter of design including rate of g onset and g duration as well as g peak, in the form of a time g curve. It is assumed that the force direction does not change, indicating that the system must be stabilized with the man in a forward facing seated position. It may be feasible with appropriate support and restraint, to use these same time g criteria for other body positions. This may be of importance in certain ejection seat designs which will be discussed later.

The above considerations make it obvious

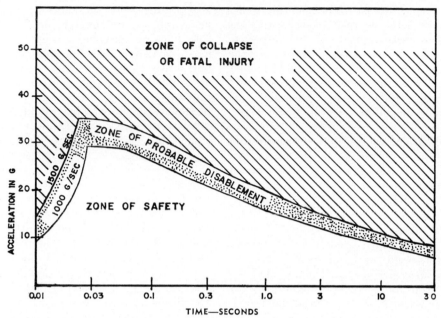

FIG. 123. Limits of human tolerance for escape systems. (From Savely (26).)

that critical problems are faced in the use of conventional ejection seats for escape in the upper range of speed and altitude capabilities of present day aircraft which are already well above 600 knots indicated air speed and 50,000 feet altitude, respectively, for all first line fighter aircraft. The seriousness of the wind-drag deceleration problem in ejection seat escape is re-emphasized with the advent of each ejection in the 600 knot speed range. A brief account of one of the early supersonic ejections will give a general picture of the type of hazard faced by the escaping flyer. The following information regarding this incident is abstracted from a report by Hegenwald and Blockley (24):

On the morning of 26 February 1955, George Smith, a civilian test pilot, ejected from an F-100A airplane over the Pacific Ocean. Ejection altitude was approximately 6000 feet. The aircraft was in a near vertical dive at Mach 1.05 or approximately 675 knots true air speed. The pilot was rescued from the water within 1 minute after landing. He was unconscious. Within 90 minutes he was receiving medical attention in a hospital. His condition upon arrival at the hospital was as follows: profound circulatory shock; head and face extremely congested; severe periocular edema; subconjunctival hemorrhages; superficial retinal hemorrhages; blood in both middle ears; bruises under arms and in groin; lacerations over eyebrow, on ankle and in groin; stomach distended; no broken bones; and no pulmonary or thoracic injury. He had intermittent loss of consciousness and later, amnesia, confusion and lethargy occurred. Subsequent examination revealed signs of intra-abdominal and retroperitoneal hemorrhage, concussion and dislocation or sprain of the hip joints. He developed jaundice indicating significant liver damage. Intestinal obstruction requiring surgery was a sequel to adhesions caused by traumatic perforation of the terminal ileum, which occurred during the ejection. Mr. Smith was in a critical condition for a prolonged period but had essentially complete recovery after several months' recuperation. He returned to test flying in high performance aircraft.

Almost all of George Smith's injuries were produced by wind-drag deceleration forces. Although it is true that some variations in modes of g force action were necessary to account for all of his injuries, the simple fact is that most of the serious injuries were produced by the crash impact effect of q forces. The q in this case was rather accurately determined to be 1280 p.s.f. at the instant of ejection. The time g curves resulting under conditions of the escape, together with the direction of force application with respect to body position, have been experimentally determined by Hegenwald and Blockley (24). This was done in high speed rocket sled ejection experiments using equipment, anthropomorphic dummies and dynamic performance modes based upon computations available from known data of the escape circumstances. These studies indicated that George Smith was exposed to the following forces at the head level: a peak acceleration of 64 g, a 700 g per second rate of onset of peak g, and duration of 0.12 second above 35 g and 0.29 second above 20 g. The direction of application varied because of bending of torso and tumbling but was predominantly "negative" which means that the body inertial forces were acting foot-toward-head. He was exposed to the following forces at the lower torso: a peak of 50 g, 1300 g per second rate of onset, 0.045 second duration above 35 g and 0.14 second above 20 g. The direction of decelerating force application was predominantly chest-to-back.

Very similar deceleration forces had already been experienced by Stapp (23) in February 1955, in his series of rocket sled deceleration experiments. Strikingly similar effects were produced, particularly with regard to shock and hydraulic effects, even though controlled conditions pertained in the sled run; most important of the controlled conditions being constant direction of force application (transverse) and absence of tumbling. The extreme negative g effects in the case of George Smith may be explained by forward bending of the body at the time of ejection permitted by loose shoulder straps. This set up a hydrostatic column from hips to head level and also severely compressed the lower abdomen with the lap belt. Deceleration in this position can be readily correlated with the concussion, eye damage and other negative acceleration effects. Violent abduction of the legs produced the hip injuries. Jolt impact transmitted by the lap belt could have been responsible for the traumatic perforation of the ileum. Tumbling in a high g force field could possibly have accounted for other visceral damage and hemorrhage. Some injury was also produced by parachute opening shock. Parachute panel damage indicated premature opening may have been produced by wind blast effect. The automatic lap belt and parachute release were set at 2 seconds delay each which should have permitted a minimum of 4 seconds decay in velocity before parachute opening. This would result in a velocity of approximately 140 m.p.h. which should have permitted safe parachute opening.

This case and many others which have followed, some fatal, indicate the seriousness of the wind-drag deceleration problem in present configuration open ejection systems. Proposed methods of attack on this problem include the following: (1) the use of drogue chutes to slow the aircraft down prior to ejection; (2) rocket thrust augmentation on the seat in the direction of flight to counter the deceleration g forces; (3) reduction of effective frontal area by streamlining or other method and increase in weight of the seat which together result in a more favorable drag over weight ratio (lower); and (4) stabilization of the seat in an acceptable attitude. Although each of these proposals has merit under certain circumstances, they also pose many technical difficulties. The use of aircraft drogue chutes, although technically feasible, would impose a serious weight penalty. Also, there is some question of practicability with respect to time and opportunity under emergency circumstances. Rocket thrust on the seat for both separation from the aircraft and counter g force augmentation is feasible and has many advantages, including a high trajectory which would be useful in low level escape. The blast of a rocket catapult is a serious hazard for multiple place aircraft and the wind blast problem may become of greater concern. Rocket ejection seats have been extensively tested and are now in operational use. Methods being applied to provide a lower drag over weight ratio have many practical limitations if the device is to stop short of an aerodynamically clean, ogive shaped capsule which is actually a step beyond the ejection seat. An important consideration which is encountered in the reduction of the magnitude of deceleration forces is the time factor. Increased deceleration time is required to make lower g force peaks possible. At low altitudes this time may not be available, particularly if the aircraft is in a diving attitude at the time of the escape. Some of the prototype systems now under development to solve these difficulties will be discussed in later paragraphs.

THERMAL STRESSES OF EJECTION. Thermal problems, so far encountered in escape from aircraft, have been limited to ambient temperature effects of high altitude which can result in serious frostbite unless all parts of the body are adequately covered with protective clothing. High temperature problems related to the aerodynamic heating of high speed have not yet been encountered under actual escape conditions. Structural limitations will, in all probability, preclude this as a significant escape problem at low altitude; however, at very high altitude where hypersonic speeds are possible the thermal barrier problem may become of importance from the standpoint of escape. With the advent of rocket aircraft and manned "boost-glide" vehicles, altitudes in excess of 300,000 feet will be traversed. If escape is initiated at such extreme altitude, free falling bodies build up velocities of very high Mach numbers in the extremely low density atmosphere. Aerodynamic heating is very great at high Mach numbers, a general rule of thumb being that the temperature rise in Farenheit will be approximately 75 times the square of the Mach number. Thus a speed of Mach 10 would yield a temperature of 7500° F. Heat transfer at extreme altitude is low, however, and considerable research will be required to evaluate this hazard.

At the present, information is available only for low altitude, high speed thermal exposure. High speed sled wind blast runs at Mach 1.7 have resulted in severe third degree burns on exposed areas of large animals. Exposure time at this speed was approximately 1 second with a total exposure time of less than 10 seconds at lesser velocities. Measured surface temperatures at Mach 1.7 vary between 300 and 320° F. Although it may seem incredible that severe third degree burns could be produced by such momentary exposure to relatively moderate temperatures it is apparent that the total heat

transfer must have been very great. No information is available regarding the heat flow rate in calories per unit area per unit time. Buettner (27) has shown that third degree burns can be produced in 10 seconds at skin temperatures of 60° C. (140° F.). It is, therefore, not surprising that under conditions of wind blast exposure involving a combination of pressure on the skin surface and a flow of heated dense air, unusual thermal injury may occur. The surface pressure effects may be of importance from the standpoint of collapsing blood vessels and increasing the density of the tissues; the former reducing the heat transfer effect of the circulation and the latter increasing the heat conduction to deeper tissue layers. A third factor of possible significance would be present in actual ejection; fluid stagnation effects of deceleration. High deceleration effects were not present in the sled wind blast studies.

It is quite evident that aerodynamic thermal stress may present a serious hazard, requiring an enclosed capsule for protection at extremely high speeds which may be attained at extreme altitude. Protective clothing has been developed which has successfully protected animals against the above described injuries produced at Mach 1.7 at sea level and it is possible that this can also be adapted to the flyer. However, consideration must be given to the increasing resistance which flyers have shown to acceptance of protective gear which must be worn on the body thereby compromising comfort and performance. The aerodynamic heat problem in the future could possibly be another factor which may ultimately tip the balance in favor of closed escape systems. Further evaluation of this problem is required.

ROTATIONAL STRESSES. The hazard of tumbling and spinning following ejection and during the free fall to opening of the parachute has not yet been fully evaluated. Although almost any type of gyration can occur after separation from the aircraft there are essentially two types of concern. One is head-over-heels tumbling about a bodily transverse axis, usually while still attached to the seat. The second is the so-called flat spin of the body during the free fall in which the body is stretched out in an essentially horizontal attitude and spins about an axis more or less parallel to line of fall. Sufficient incidents have been reported to indicate that both tumbling and spinning are potentially serious hazards, particularly at high altitudes. Combinations of tumbling and spinning in all degrees of freedom of rotation can occur.

Tumbling and spinning rates increase with altitude. For a given ejection seat system at a constant indicated air speed the rate of tumbling will increase as the altitude is increased because of the lower damping forces provided in the less dense atmosphere; the aerodynamic damping forces decrease whereas the force which produces the tumbling remains constant. The rate of tumbling for a given escape system at 40,000 feet approaches a value double that at sea level for the same indicated air speed (25). Extremely high rates of spin can develop during the free fall of the body from high altitude. Investigations (28) utilizing dummy drops from 83,000 feet and parachutist models in wind tunnels indicate that in a free fall from 83,000 feet the human body may spin at a rate of 465 r.p.m.

Tolerance limits for spinning and tumbling have been experimentally investigated with both animal and human subjects on the spin table (29). With the center of rotation at the heart, unconsciousness can be produced in humans in 3 to 10 seconds at 160 r.p.m. Under the same conditions a fatal outcome can be produced in animals in 2 minutes at 150 to 200 r.p.m. The more than 400 r.p.m. which can be expected in a free fall from altitudes readily attainable in present aircraft obviously exceeds the fatal rate for man. The effects of spinning and tumbling are a combination of "negative" and "positive" g and will vary with the location of the center of rotation. Cardiodynamic and general circulatory effects are maximal when the heart is at the center of rotation. In animals it has been shown that in this circumstance at 150 r.p.m. the A-V pressure difference and pulse pressure are reduced to less than 5 mm. of Hg and cardiac output can be considered to have virtually ceased. This, of course, results in tissue anoxia which may be fatal in itself or may result in fatal cerebral hemorrhage from damaged vascular

walls following the spinning when very high systolic blood pressure overshooting occurs. Circulatory impairment in the human is not serious at 125 r.p.m. The hydraulic effects and particularly the vascular damage of the "negative" g type at the head is increased when the center of rotation is in the lower part of the body. The longer the column of blood between the region concerned and the center of rotation, the greater the hydraulic effect. Conjunctival hemorrhage, periorbital edema and hemorrhage into the sinuses and middle ear are readily produced in this manner. Thresholds of petechial hemorrhage of the conjunctiva have been determined for man at various spin rate time values. With the center of rotation at the iliac crest the values vary from 3 seconds at 90 r.p.m. to 2 minutes at 50 r.p.m. When the center of rotation is at the heart, tolerances range from more than 10 minutes at 45 r.p.m. to 4 seconds at 120 r.p.m. Pain and diffuse headache are also produced and these symptoms have limited exposure of the human to 125 r.p.m. Vertigo and nausea are not commonly produced on the spin table except in prolonged slow down from the spinning and following repeated spinning with short intervals of rest.

Actual tumbling and spinning experience in the air includes reports of rotational speeds as high as 240 r.p.m. (28). This rate of tumbling produces a calculated radial accelerative force of approximately 37 negative g at the eye level which can obviously produce severe vascular damage. Spinning of drogue stabilized seats occurring in a free fall from 40,000 feet has produced severe disorientation, blurring of vision and nausea (30). Violent tumbling and spinning has occurred in downward ejections at an altitude of 45,000 feet (14) producing severe disorientation, nausea and vomiting. The predicted increased seriousness of the spin hazard at high altitude has recently been confirmed by the experience of 2 R.A.F. flyers who escaped from a Canberra aircraft which exploded at 54,000 feet altitude (31). Both flyers separated from their ejection seat approximately 2 seconds after ejection. One experienced violent spinning, the other did not. There is a probability of malfunction of the seat stabilizing drogue chute in the case of the former. Normally this chute should effect momentary stabilization after ejection and just prior to separation from the seat. It is apparent that with malfunction of the drogue chute the unstable seat imparted a spinning moment to the flyer and that his body configuration and the altitude perpetuated the spin and increased the rate during free fall. Spin injury sustained was severe with marked edema of the neck and face; severe subconjunctival hemorrhage; ecchymosis of the eyelids; nasal and middle ear hemorrhage; and petechiae of the soft palate, pharynx, fauces and dorsum of both feet. These injuries were owing entirely to spinning inasmuch as there would be no significant wind-drag deceleration at the observed ejection speed of 147 knots indicated. Although not fatal, the severity of the hydraulic vascular effects, a severe headache which lasted several days and a marked degree of incapacitation which occurred in this case indicate that spinning is a serious hazard. Had this escape been initiated at a higher altitude the outcome would probably have been fatal.

It is obvious that stabilization at the time of ejection is an absolute requirement for any ejection system for safe escape at extreme altitude. Available evidence at the present time indicates that stabilization at altitudes above 50,000 feet will be extremely difficult; existing methods have not yet been successful in accomplishing this objective. At lower altitudes various methods including the use of drogue chutes, aerodynamic surfaces and trailing booms have been successfully employed.

COMBINED STRESSES. Although the foregoing discussion has dealt separately with the several stresses of ejection into the wind stream it is fully recognized that exposure to all of them is almost simultaneous and they may combine with one another in a summating manner. Although combined effects have not yet been thoroughly evaluated some studies have made progress in this direction. The problem of combined acceleration, which occurs when the body rotates in a superimposed g field, has been studied on the epicyclic centrifuge (32). It is possible that certain rates of rotation in a g field may be beneficial; however, there are also rates of rotation which would produce additive effects. Although it may be useful to have a more complete definition of all possible variations in combined acceleration effects it is obviously more practical to stabilize the seat during wind-drag deceleration than attempt to effect a controlled rate of rotation. Investigations (33) have been made on the effects of simultaneous deceleration, tumbling and wind blast by ejecting chimpanzees from the Cherokee supersonic missile at a velocity of Mach 1.5. One ejection was done at 21,000 feet altitude using a standard B-47 downward ejection seat. The subject was killed when structural failure of the seat occurred during and following ejection. The maximum composite acceleration acting through the center of gravity was determined to be 34.4 g; obviously much higher peaks were produced at points away from the center of gravity. This test indicated that a stronger seat and a cleaner separation from the aircraft are essential for successful escape at Mach 1.5. A second test with a redesigned seat resulted in successful ejection and retention of structural integrity of the seat; however, premature deployment of the parachute by the wind blast resulted in destruction of the parachute and nonrecovery of the subject. This test indicated the need for a parachute pack which is wind-blastproof.

Studies of this type, including high speed sled ejections and evaluation of emergency ejections from operational aircraft, have served to emphasize the inadequacy of present open seat ejection systems for escape at supersonic speeds. This has resulted in a two pronged attack on the problem of supersonic escape. One direction has been toward modification and improvement of the open ejection seat and the other, a complete departure from the open system in favor of the closed or capsule system. Before discussing these efforts it will be useful at this point to briefly review the record with respect to the success and failure history of the open ejection seat. These statistics are useful in determining requirements for improved escape systems and in evaluating the potential returns to be expected from improved or new escape systems.

EJECTION SEAT EXPERIENCE. Data are available from U. S. Air Force (34) and U. S. Navy (35) operational experience. Although different types of ejection seat systems are used in the two services and certain differences exist in flying operations, the over-all data are very similar. U. S. Air Force statistics (table 63) cover the period August 1949 to July 1958 during which 1462 emergency uses of the ejection seat occurred. U. S. Navy statistics (table 64) cover the period August 1949 to July 1958. There were 463 emergency seat ejections during this period.

Although the ejection survival rate is less favorable than World War II over-the-side bailout survival rates, cognizance must be

TABLE 63
Injuries Received during Ejection Escape*

Injury	Number	Per Cent
None	679	47
Minor	264	18
Major	225	15
Fatal	294	20

* U. S. Air Force data from August 1949 to July 1958.

TABLE 64
Injuries Received during Ejection Escape*

Injury	Number	Per Cent
Minor or no injury	312	67.4
Serious injury	61	13.2
Fatal, lost or missing	90	19.4

* U. S. Navy data from August 1949 to July 1958.

TABLE 65
Per Cent of Successful to Total Ejections from U. S. Air Force Aircraft by Selected Periods

Period	Total Ejections	Successful Nonfatal	Unsuccessful (Fatal)	Per Cent Successful
1 August 1949 to 30 December 1953	347	266	81	77
1954	171	135	36	79
1955	241	183	58	76
1956	284	239	45	84
1957	304	257	47	85
1 January to 30, June 1958	115	88	27	77
Total	1462	1168	294	80

taken of the fact that in the majority of instances reflected in tables 63 and 64 conventional bailout would have been extremely difficult or impossible. The ejection seat must be recognized as an important lifesaving device. However, a continued high rate of major and fatal injury points to a need for improved efficiency of escape systems to match advances in aircraft performance. A more detailed analysis (table 65) of U. S. Air Force statistics (34) indicates the trend in success and failure rates over the 9 year period of ejection seat use.

It is noted that the success rate improved each year until an apparent reversal of this trend occurred in the first half of 1958. This reversal may be related to the increased percentage of low level escape attempts which, during this period, was doubled for altitudes below 1000 feet. Improvements in low level escape capability apparently resulted in undue optimism with regard to the margin of safety in this highly critical part of the escape profile. The fallibility of human reactions obviously makes it unwise to delay escape in an emergency until the absolute minimum ejection altitude is reached. Improved low altitude performance of automatic ejection seats evidently has encouraged such delays. This is reflected by the fact that an overwhelming number of fatal ejections result from insufficient time to separate from the seat or to deploy the parachute, as indicated in table 66 which shows the principal causes of ejection fatalities in the U. S. Air Force (34).

A review (34) of the causes of nonfatal major injuries indicates additional sources of difficulty in ejection seat escape. Table 67 indicates that fractures constitute the most common nonfatal injury. Almost all ejection force fractures were vertebral. Spinal cord injury was infrequent and complete recovery was the rule.

Three factors which have an important influence upon the success-failure rate of ejection are altitude, attitude and speed of the aircraft at the time of ejection. Analysis of Air Force experience (34) with regard to these factors and injury rate is shown in tables 68, 69 and 70.

The very high fatality rate (70 per cent) for ejections below 1000 feet altitude indi-

TABLE 66

Causes of Ejection Fatalities

Violent contact with ground or water		236
Still in seat	128	
Separated from seat but chute not deployed	99	
Fell out of chute or unfastened it too high	3	
Information in regard to release of seat, not reported	6	
Drowned		16
Struck by Empennage or fuselage		6
Exposure (cold water immersion)		3
Missing		13
Amputation of left lower extremity as a result of malposition at time of ejection; pilot expired 7 days later from pulmonary embolism		1
Pilot sustained severe injury at time of midair collision; death believed to be caused by exsanguination during parachute descent		1
Extreme opening shock of parachute at high speed while still in seat		1
Hypoxia		1
Exact cause undertermined		9
Probable fatal head injury sustained in escape (striking canopy, etc.)	6	
Probable hypoxia (ejection at 38,000 feet)	1	
Probably struck by flying debris (after midair collision)	2	
Unknown		7
Total		294

cates the critical importance of the low altitude escape problem. There is no indication that escape at very high altitude has yet become a serious problem in Air Force operations. The advantages which accrue from straight and level flight or a climbing attitude at the time of ejection, as opposed to ejection in a dive, are well illustrated in table 69. The experience relative to speed at the time of ejection indicates that this factor does not assume great importance until speeds in excess of 500 knots IAS are reached. Of the 38 cases reported in excess of this speed it is believed that only one fatal outcome resulted from incapacitation caused by wind-drag deceleration. Some of the fatalities were caused by contact with the aircraft structure and one was probably caused by parachute opening shock.

The available data clearly indicate that low altitude escape and escape at speeds in excess of 500 knots IAS pose serious problems with present equipment. These problems will become more serious as the performance of aircraft increases. The low level escape problem is a two headed monster in that low level, low speed escape requirements may be completely incompatible with those of low level, high speed escape. There is not yet sufficient operational data to indicate

TABLE 67

Causes of Primary Major Nonfatal Injuries during Seat Ejections

Injury Type	Total	Parachute Landing Accident	Ejection Force	Opening Shock of Chute	Cockpit Contact During Ejection	Struck by Canopy	Struck by Seat	Other and Unknown,
Fractures	119	45	36	11	12	1	2	12
Sprains, strains, dislocations	37	19	9	2	1	1	0	5
Surface wounds	37	4	1	4	13	2	2	11
Brain concussion	5	0	0	1	0	3	0	1
Amputation	1	0	0	0	0	0	0	1
Burns	14	0	0	0	0	0	0	14
Other	12	0	0	2	0	0	0	10
Total	225	68	46	20	26	7	4	54

the seriousness of very high altitude escape problems. It is probable that most of the important escape problems which will be encountered in future atmospheric as well as extra-atmospheric flight already have been defined by human factors groups of the services and industry who have been working jointly for several years in a concerted effort to make emergency escape possible under all

TABLE 68
Indicated Altitude Relative to Injury

Altitude	Total Bailouts	Fatal Injury		Major Injury	Minor Injury	No Injury
		Number	Per cent			
feet						
0 to 999	181	126	70	13	7	35
(0 to 499)*	(81)	(71)	(88)	(2)	(2)	(6)
(500 to 999)*	(67)	(23)	(34)	(11)	(5)	(28)
(0 to 999, unspecified)*	(33)	(32)	(97)	(0)	(0)	(1)
1000 to 1999	167	29	17	29	29	80
2000 to 2999	97	11	11	15	21	50
3000 to 4999	169	8	5	27	31	103
5000 to 9999	325	12	4	47	65	201
10,000 to 19,999	318	20	6	57	77	164
20,000 up	120	10	8	36	30	44
Unknown	85	78	92	1	4	2
Total	1462	294		225	264	679
Per cent of total		20		15	18	47

* The numbers in parentheses are a breakdown of the 0 to 999 feet altitude row.

TABLE 69
Attitude of Aircraft at Time of Ejection Relative to Injury

Attitude	Total Bailouts	Fatal Injury Number	Per cent	Major Injury	Minor Injury	No Injury
Climb	154	13	8	26	25	90
Level	571	45	8	73	99	354
Inverted	66	7	11	19	13	27
Spin	147	20	14	19	41	67
Bank	71	14	20	9	16	32
Spiral	53	11	21	16	10	16
Barrel or snap rolls	14	2	14	0	6	6
Dive	182	59	32	36	26	61
Unknown and/or other	204	123	60	27	28	26
Total	1462	294		225	264	679
Per cent of total		20		15	18	47

TABLE 70
Indicated Airspeed Relative to Injury

Speed	Total Bailouts	Fatal Injury Number	Per cent	Major Injury	Minor Injury	No Injury
knots						
100 to 199	443	43	9.7	66	76	258
200 to 249	342	29	8.4	42	66	205
250 to 299	157	5	3.2	35	37	80
300 to 349	126	9	7.1	29	31	57
350 to 399	64	7	10.9	8	19	30
400 to 449	45	7	15.6	12	13	13
450 to 499	26	6	23.1	8	6	6
500 up	38	11	28.9	15	5	7
Unknown	221	177	80.1	10	11	23
Total	1462	294		225	264	679
Per cent of total		20		15	18	47

flight conditions. The results of these efforts are indicated in the following paragraphs.

TECHNICAL ADVANCES IN EJECTION SEATS. Some of the improvements of the open ejection seat system have already been mentioned, as for example the adoption of the gas initiator system to eliminate mechanical linkages and to make reliable automation possible. The introduction of the automatic seat belt and automatic parachute opening device, now available in all first line aircraft, has been remarkably successful in reducing fatalities, particularly in low level escape. An indication of this progress is available in Air Force experience which indicates that the escape fatality rate fell from 24 per cent in 1955 to 15 per cent in 1957. During this period the percentage of automatic seats used in these ejections increased from 18 to 70 per cent. Data from Royal Air Force experience also reveal a remarkably high percentage of successful escapes with their automatic equipment when compared with the nonautomatic seat ejection fatality rate. Reduction of the time delays in the automatic belt and parachute release device to absolute minima has resulted in a very low altitude escape capability. A British system permits separation from the seat in less than a second with immediate opening of the parachute if sufficient decay of the deceleration rate has occurred. This is determined by an acceleration sensing device which is an integral part of the seat-parachute system. A three charge cartridge catapult assures a trajectory high enough to permit escape on the runway at moderate speeds. An aneroid control prevents activation of the rapid low level escape mechanism when ejection takes place above 10,000 feet. The present Air Force low level escape system has a 1 second delay in the lap belt separation and permits immediate activation of the parachute ripcord by means of a lanyard which bypasses the 1 second delay automatic parachute opening device. This system, unfortunately, has a manual feature in that the lanyard must be hooked and unhooked as required in order to avoid rapid deployment of the parachute at high altitudes or high speeds. A modification is underway to make this system fully automatic by the use of a speed sensing device to select either a 1 or 3 second delay for lap belt separation. An aneroid device prevents opening of the parachute above 14,000 feet; below this altitude the parachute opens immediately after separation from the seat. This system with the 80 feet per second catapult and a flat circular parachute canopy replacing the slow opening guide surface type will permit escape on the runway at speeds as low as 120 knots.

The development of a successful rocket catapult was a major contribution to the progress in emergency escape system development. It solves the problem of limited trajectory imposed by human acceleration tolerance limitations encountered in conventional cartridge catapults. With the longer force application (approximately 0.5 second) of the rocket catapult, a very high trajectory can be achieved without exceeding human tolerances. In the rocket seat the rocket propulsion device may either replace or supplement the cartridge in the catapult unit. A most important application of the rocket ejection seat is the replacement of downward ejection seats in very high performance fighter aircraft in which conventional cartridge catapults gave an inadequate upward trajectory for fin clearance at high speed. This will eliminate a highly unsatisfactory system which has caused many tragic low altitude ejection deaths. The rocket catapult will also improve low altitude, low speed escape capabilities inasmuch as at low speeds its trajectory is 44 per cent higher than that of the most powerful single cartridge catapult and the rocket thrust direction also imparts some forward velocity which assists quick parachute deployment. It is possible that zero velocity, "on-the-deck" escape capability can be realized with the rocket seat.

The rocket seat also ameliorates the wind-drag deceleration problem in that the forward thrust component counters the drag and thereby trades off deceleration force with time. At sonic speeds this effect reduces the magnitude of peak wind blast deceleration by as much as 15 g (36). The rocket seat, at the time of separation from the aircraft, has a minimum of eccentric loadings thus providing stability upon entry into the wind stream. The rocket thrust vector acts through the seat-man center of gravity thereby avoiding tumbling and permitting effective stabilization by fins, booms or drogue chute which must be activated just following separation from the aircraft.

There are some disadvantages. The deceleration time is prolonged although the peak is of lower magnitude; the wind blast overpressure and erosion effects are more severe and prolonged and separation of the man from the seat is retarded. The latter disadvantage may be critical at low altitude and may require correction by use of a separating device such as a bag inflated by a gas initiator cartridge. This can be done with little difficulty. However, the problem of protecting against abrupt compression and buffeting of the body walls as well as flailing of the extremities will become more and more difficult as higher speeds are realized. The closed ejection system may be the only solution to this problem. The rocket seat also introduces a new hazard in multiplace aircraft having seats in tandem under a single canopy. This is the hazard of incineration by rocket blast of an aircrew member in place behind an ejecting seat. This hazard can be controlled by shielding or by controlled sequence of seat firing. Rocket seats with fin and/or boom stabilization are now installed in operational jet aircraft and also in the X-15 rocket aircraft.

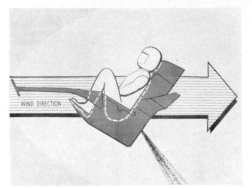

FIG. 124. "A" type seat with fins and skip-flow generator. (From Mohrlock (37).)

Improvements in existing ejection seat systems have not been the only developmental achievements in emergency escape. A large number of industrial organizations in the aircraft industry have pooled data and resources to solve the problems of supersonic emergency escape. They have operated through the Industry Crew Escape Systems Committee (ICESC) which has been responsible for remarkable progress in escape systems development. Many ideas have been explored and several new type seats have been proposed and are now undergoing development and testing. The problem has been made most difficult by the restriction that no radical changes can be made in existing cockpit and airframe configuration to accommodate any new escape system. Only two of many new systems now under development will be described. Both are open type escape systems and are called "A" and "B" type seats. Figures 124 and 125 taken from Mohrlock (37) depict these seats in schematic form.

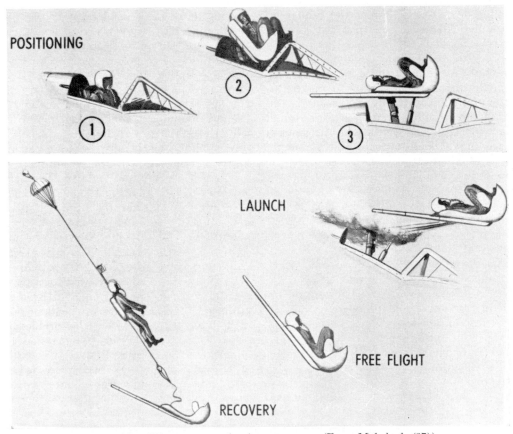

FIG. 125. "B" type seat; ejection sequence. (From Mohrlock (37))

The "A" type seat employs a unique device, the skip flow generator, which theoretically, at least, serves three functions; (1) presents a smaller effective surface to the wind blast and, therefore, reduces the magnitude of wind-drag deceleration, (2) forms a wind blast protective envelope for the seat occupant by wind deflection at high velocities and (3) provides stability by moving the center of gravity forward of the seat. Although the principle of the skip flow generator is appealing from the standpoint of functional simplicity, tests indicate that its range of effectiveness with respect to speed and altitude may be too limited.

The "B" type seat provides a means of protecting the aircrew member from overpressure and wind blast erosion effects by rotation of the seat and using its bottom as a wind blast deflecting surface. It is boom stabilized. Wind-drag deceleration is reduced by both the semistreamlining effect of the seat's attitude and the counter force of the rocket propulsion. Tests have shown this seat to be very stable and to have a very high trajectory which results from its aerodynamic characteristics and its dual rocket propelling unit. When ejected at a speed of 200 knots the "B" seat rises to an altitude in excess of 300 feet above the level of ejection. Ejection at an indicated airspeed of 735 knots produced g stresses which were well within human tolerances; the transverse g being 22 and the peak spinal acceleration being 9 g. The "B" seat configuration simplifies the problem of restraint and appears to meet the problems of wind blast, wind-drag deceleration and aerodynamic heating. Its high trajectory meets some of the requirements for low altitude escape although low forward velocity and diving attitudes may be severely limiting.

THE ESCAPE CAPSULE. There is little doubt but that future experience with emergency escape from supersonic aircraft will provide an absolute requirement for closed escape systems. There is already sufficient evidence to indicate that even the newer type open ejection seats do not provide an adequate escape system for existing high performance aircraft. It is recognized that the problem of wind-drag deceleration will not be solved by the closed system. Actually, it will be a more difficult problem in view of

the necessity of providing a harness to distribute the deceleration forces over as large an area of the body as possible which in the open system is transmitted to the entire frontal surface by the wind blast. Also, the low altitude escape problem may be more difficult. However, the solution of these aspects of capsular escape are technically feasible and the problems of wind blast pressure and erosion effects, as well as the thermal problem, are effectively solved in the closed escape system.

There are many other advantages offered by capsule escape systems including the use of the capsule as a survival unit for environmental protection on both land and sea. Designed for environmental protection both in flight and during emergency escape the closed system will permit the flyer to discard most of the protective and survival equipment now attached to his body and attain the much longed-for status of unencumbered "shirt sleeve flying." The closed system will obviously provide improved fire protection which would be extremely advantageous if a zero velocity ground level capsule ejection capability could be realized. Aside from offering a more vulnerable target for enemy action the primary difficulties presented by the closed escape system are the technical problems associated with design to meet the requirements of escape under conditions imposed by the many complex combinations of speed and altitude presented in the flight envelope of high performance aircraft. It is presumed that these technical problems will be solved.

Closed escape systems are basically of two types; one involving the separation of the entire cockpit area from the aircraft. This may be in the form of a jettisonable nose section containing the cockpit or an ejectable cockpit section encompassing the normal crew station and its integral boundary structure. The second type is simply an encapsulated seat which is ejected from the aircraft in a similar manner to the present ejection seat. The latter type appears to be technically more feasible unless the concept of aircraft design is radically changed to provide primarily for an escape cockpit around which the aircraft is secondarily constructed.

Experience with closed escape systems is

at present meager. The German DFS-228 aircraft had a detachable nose but was never used in an actual emergency. The U. S. Navy D-558 and the U. S. Air Force X-2, both rocket aircraft, had a jettisonable nose section. That of the X-2 was used unsuccessfully in an emergency when the pilot failed to free himself from the jettisoned nose section. The major disadvantage of these systems was the demand placed upon the pilot to bail out of the jettisoned nose by sheer muscular force. This was an unrealistic requirement under a situation loaded with an abundance of potentially overwhelming environmental stresses. Other closed systems which have reached various stages of developmental design are of lesser mass and employ a parachute which supports the cockpit capsule or seat capsule permitting the flyer to remain inside during descent and landing. Present trends indicate that the first operational closed system will be of the ejectable seat capsule type. This type is proposed for the B-58 supersonic bomber and some of its design features, as presently conceived, will be briefly described (38).

The general configuration and some of the ejection sequence features of the encapsulated seat are shown in figure 126. It will be noted that the capsule is closed by a series

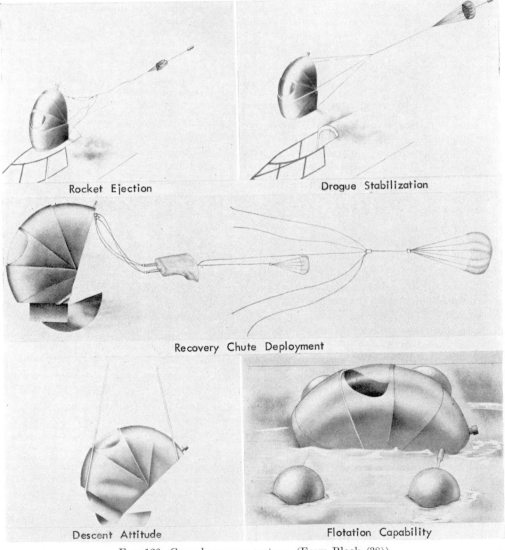

Rocket Ejection

Drogue Stabilization

Recovery Chute Deployment

Descent Attitude

Flotation Capability

FIG. 126. Capsule escape system. (From Bleck (38))

of overlapping doors which rotate down to the closed position from the top of the seat. Upon activation the system automatically withdraws the flyer's feet into escape position, activates body restraint devices, closes and pressurizes the capsule. The control stick is contained in the capsule and permits a "fly-down" capability, should immediate ejection following an emergency not be necessary. The pilot can see essential instruments through the window provided in one of the door sections. The capsule is ejected by rocket propulsion and has a ground level escape capability at 100 knots. It is stabilized by a drogue chute during deceleration and during free fall if above 15,000 feet, below which altitude the recovery parachute is automatically deployed, permitting the escapee to land inside the capsule on either land or water. A flotation system permits water survival in heavy seas. All essential survival gear for all types of environmental conditions are attached to or stored in the capsule. Protective and survival equipment attached to the individual will be reduced to a minimum. This system, which is now under development, is said to approach the ideal of "shirt sleeve flying" with adequate provisions for emergency escape and survival.

SEPARATION FROM THE EJECTION SEAT. At this point it is necessary to revert to the discussion of present conventional escape systems about which consideration has already been given to the problems of pre-ejection, ejection and immediate post-ejection. This final consideration is concerned with separation from the seat and descent in the parachute to the survival situation. The problems of separation from the seat are of two categories, high altitude and low altitude. At high altitudes it would appear to be advantageous for the flyer to remain in the seat until a safe level of approximately 15,000 feet is reached. This would permit attachment of emergency pressure suit oxygen supply and control equipment to the seat thus allowing greater space in the survival kit for surface survival equipment. Further, if the seat is stabilized there would be no concern for the hazard of the flat spin to which a free falling body is subject. If separation is immediate, then consideration must be given to stabilization of the man in addition to initial stabilization of the seat.

Present systems employ both immediate and delayed separation at high altitudes. The small number of very high altitude ejections has not permitted evaluation of the relative merits of the two. It is obvious that successful low level escape demands quick separation from the seat and immediate deployment of the parachute. Some systems employ a positive separation action whereas other systems depend upon differential air drag to separate the man from the seat. Although tests using anthropomorphic dummies have shown differential drag separation to be as rapid as that produced by a supplemental force, it has been pointed out that a human may unconsciously cling to the ejection activator sufficiently long to delay separation. At very low altitudes any delay is of great significance. Review of the problem has also pointed up the fact that new rigid type global survival kits, which must separate with the man, cause some delay in separation in the absence of a supplemental separating force. Further, it has now become apparent that the improved stability of rocket seats makes differential drag less effective as a man-seat separation force. Indications are that a positive separation device will be required on all ejection seats. Present methods include spring loaded ejectors, drogue activated slings and bags inflated by gas initiator cartridges. Following separation the escapee's problems become those of the parachutist which have been discussed in the first section of this chapter. During parachute descent and following landing the problems of survival and rescue become of primary concern. These will be discussed in succeeding sections.

SPECIAL ESCAPE PROBLEMS. In closing this section on escape, mention should be made of some special category escape problems which are of interest. These include escape from VTOL aircraft (vertical takeoff and landing), escape from submerged aircraft and escape from the so-called "flying platform."

Vertical takeoff aircraft have the unique problem of permitting escape of the pilot during conventional flight at high speeds and high altitude as well as in a vertical attitude with a zero horizontal velocity during takeoff and landing. Present developments include a seat which can be rapidly rotated to accommodate for change in attitude and provision for quick man-seat separation with immediate deployment of the parachute during vertical low level flight. It is probable that the rocket catapult can advantageously be adapted to VTOL aircraft to provide for escape in all attitudes and particularly in the vertical attitude at low level during zero horizontal velocity.

Escape from submerged aircraft by use of the ejection seat is especially applicable to naval operations. One instance has already been recorded in the U. S. Navy (39) in which the aircraft went over the side of the carrier landing in the sea inverted. The pilot was stunned but recovered and fired the ejection seat after submersion. During his underwater journey he passed through the turbulence of the ship's wake and emerged approximately 1000 feet astern, where he was promptly picked up by a helicopter. The pilot did not recall any excessive force of the ejection and was confident that his automatic lap belt release functioned normally. He was on 100 per cent oxygen at the time of the accident. A similar instance has been reported in the Royal Navy and experimental live underwater ejections were made in the United Kingdom (40) which confirmed the feasibility of using standard ejection seats for submerged escape. These investigations indicated that forces acting on the aircrew, when using either 60 or 80 foot per second ejection systems for escape from a submerged aircraft, are tolerable. It is recommended that manual escape with the help of the Mae West life vest be used if the canopy is open or off when submersion occurs. However, if submersion occurs before it is possible to remove the canopy then it is preferable to eject through the canopy rather than attempt to jettison the canopy before ejecting. Recommended procedure for escape includes breathing 100 per cent oxygen until ready for ejection, inhaling normally and blowing out slowly. After activating the ejection catapult the parachute harness is released and the Mae West inflated. After pushing free of the seat and as the Mae West carries the flyer to the surface, he should blow off excess lung gases to avoid aeroembolism. The oxygen mask is removed at the surface. If the flyer becomes entangled and cannot separate from the seat,

inflation of the dinghy will carry both him and the seat rapidly to the surface. Such escapes should be carried out before the aircraft sinks to 100 feet depth although it has been calculated that escape is possible down to depths of 300 feet.

Escape from the individual "flying platform" at altitudes below 100 feet and low or zero horizontal velocity poses the unique requirement for a parachute which will open instantaneously and give immediate support at the time of opening. An ultrafast opening parachute has been developed (41) for this purpose. This device is ballistically operated and will fully deploy in 0.8 second. It consists of a back style assembly using a standard Army troop type, reserve parachute canopy modified for use with a pyrotechnic deployment and opening device. The operational sequence consists of two stages. The first stage is initiated by pulling the emergency ripcord which fires the deployment charge, projecting the canopy pack upward with a force of approximately 1100 pounds. Within 0.4 second the pack reaches its peak, fully extending the risers and suspension lines. Snubber lines decelerate the canopy pack, thus, setting off an inertia activator which fires the canopy ejection charge. This charge fires 24 metal slugs radially from a 24 barrel cylinder. The slugs are permanently attached to the canopy skirt, one at each suspension line attachment point. Propulsion of the slugs outward deploys the canopy skirt within 0.4 second resulting in a completely opened and functioning parachute. This ultrafast opening parachute is effective at near zero airspeed from altitudes as low as 15 feet above the terrain. It can be used at an altitude of 30 feet at airspeeds up to 50 m.p.h. Higher airspeeds make its use unsafe and it is calculated that extremely high parachute opening shocks will be experienced at airspeeds higher than 80 m.p.h.

ADVANCED ESCAPE SYSTEMS. Manned satellite and space operations present requirements for escape systems of greater sophistication than those now available, even for rocket aircraft. The same principles of humanity relative to reasonable assurance of safe escape and survival of crews will hold in astronautics as now exists in atmospheric flight. Available data indicates that crew escape can be provided for most emergency conditions in manned rocket space operations. Present engineering designs of rocket vehicle escape systems provide for separation of the sealed cabin from the primary vehicle by rocket thrust and subsequent parachute recovery of the entire cabin. The liftoff phase and climb to rocket burnout are most critical from the standpoint of probability of emergency. In the event of malfunction or explosion, rocket separation and propulsion of the occupied cabin to a safe altitude for parachute recovery is feasible while the space vehicle is still on the launching pad. Similar escape can be effected during climb of the vehicle under maximum q conditions and at extreme altitude. Once the vehicle has entered orbit or similar phase of its space flight the escape mechanism will be esentially that of whatever means are provided for re-entry into the earth's atmosphere. This can be activated by the crew in the event of an emergency. Following re-entry the occupied part of the space vehicle will be supported by a recovery parachute and a safe landing can be made either on land or sea. Search and recovery of the survivors will be supported by the most advanced techniques of electronic monitoring and communication. Supplies for sustenance and necessary equipment will be available in the cabin for prolonged survival under environmental extremes in order to assure successful rescue from any accessible part of the earth.

SURVIVAL

The flyer who has abandoned a disabled aircraft, whether it be by conventional bailout, ejection, other in-flight means or through an emergency hatch after a crash landing or ditching, may immediately face a situation more formidable than the escape from the aircraft. Survival conditions are extremely variable, unpredictable and usually less well prepared for than escape. The global nature of air operations, whether civil or military, imposes almost unattainable requirements for survival equipment and techniques. Space and weight considerations severely limit the type and amount of survival equipment available to those who are forced to abandon a disabled airplane. Neverthe-

less, if appropriate equipment and techniques are not employed the outcome can be just as fatal as escape at high altitude without a parachute. A crew member may successfully eject and arrive at the surface of the earth in excellent condition only to die of exposure a few minutes later in icy northern latitude waters. In some survival situations certain equipment and techniques are absolutely mandatory. In other situations the outcome is more dependent upon the man; his background, training and physical and psychologic liabilities and assets. In the following paragraphs it will only be possible to briefly outline the hazards and stresses of general categories of survival situations and the means of countering these by survival techniques, equipment and man's ingenuity, resourcefulness, stamina and courage. Many volumes of factual accounts of survival experiences are available in the open press and detailed survival manuals can be obtained from the military services and national and international governmental sources.

Prelude to Survival

More often than not, when a survival situation is entered the outcome has already been determined by events prior to and during the emergency. Considerations prior to the emergency center upon how well the flyer is prepared for the emergency and subsequent survival. Essential equipment must be available when needed, its functional condition must have been assured by prior periodic inspection and the user must have had complete and thorough training and practice in its operation. During the emergency, decisions made by the flyer or aircraft commander, promptness in declaring an emergency, effective communication with rescue agencies and effectiveness of the technique of bailout, ejection, crash landing or ditching, are all critical. Preabandonment communication with rescue agencies is probably the single most important factor in isolated areas with severe environments such as the arctic or northern latitude seas.

The decision whether the airplane will be abandoned in flight or crash landed or ditched ordinarily rests with the airplane commander. In the case of civil air carrier and some military transport operations the decision has already been made by the policy that parachutes are not carried. Crew members of high performance military aircraft have little choice inasmuch as the forces involved in ditching or crash landing on unprepared surfaces almost always produce serious injuries and, frequently, fatal injury. Ejection is relatively safe, naval experience indicating that the chance of fatal outcome is increased from 1 in 40 for ejection to 1 in 4 for ditching of high performance aircraft. In low performance aircraft, if there is a choice, it is usually better to crash land in isolated arctic and desert areas and to ditch in open sea areas remote from land rather than to abandon the ship in flight. This procedure will usually provide more adequate survival equipment and supplies, mutual support of a number of survivors and improved chances of location by search and rescue operations.

If the aircraft is abandoned in flight the flyer must have attached to his person essential survival equipment and supplies. Aircrew who eject are usually well equipped with a global survival kit and flotation equipment if needed. This equipment is contained in the recesses of the back or bucket of the ejection seat and attached to the parachute harness. Those who must abandon an aircraft by conventional bailout are frequently not as fortunate inasmuch as survival kits must be manually attached before jumping and the emergency timing does not always permit this. Also, it is not always practical to clear available exits by manual bailout with bulky survival kits. In the case of multiple place aircraft different crew members may be responsible for different items of survival equipment as for example, the radio technician usually carries the communication equipment. Following abandonment the survivors, if possible, assemble to join forces in a coordinated survival effort.

Although the flyer who ejects from a modern high performance aircraft is most frequently alone, he is usually also well prepared for survival. He usually wears special survival clothing and his survival equipment is designed and selected for specific operations in which he is participating. After ejection, survival procedures may begin almost immediately. A cloud of radar sensitive "chaff" may be released from his ejection seat. This floats slowly to the surface and may be picked up by radar search aircraft for periods as long as 100 minutes, thus providing a good "fix" for localized search activities. During descent in the parachute the survival kit is deployed before reaching the surface. This provides an inflated raft a few feet below the man on a static line attached to the parachute harness, ready for immediate occupancy if over water. At the end of the static line below the inflated dinghy is the accessory kit containing essential survival supplies and equipment. If over land this arrangement reduces the landing force by lessening the load on the parachute just prior to impact of the man.

When crash landing or ditching is the selected or forced method of aircraft abandonment the technique of the pilot becomes of paramount importance. Procedures for each type of aircraft are contained in appropriate manuals. Each crew member has specific functions. Training and simulated drill in these activities are of utmost importance. Indoctrination of passengers is important but frequently inadequate. Of primary concern is the prevention of injury or incapacitation during the emergency landing. Appropriate use of restraint harness and specific positioning on some types of combat aircraft are important. Rearward facing seating with adequate g stressing would be of great advantage in passenger aircraft. Special positioning or restraint for some crew members is highly desirable to guarantee expert assistance to passenger survivors at a highly critical time of the emergency. Fire following the successful crash landing or ditching is the greatest hazard. Rapid evacuation may be delayed by inadequate supervision as well as physical injuries and psychic trauma. More serious problems are faced in such emergencies by the crews of aeromedical evacuation aircraft loaded with patients. In civil air operations, aged, young and those with limited physical capacity among the passengers create similar problems. Special aircraft design, equipment and procedures have been developed to insure rapid escape in emergency crashes. Subsequent survival is affected in great measure by the effective use of these by trained crew members and well indoctrinated passengers.

Land Survival

In most land survival situations there are certain fundamentals which are almost universally applicable and there are also principles and procedures which are only applicable to specific situations usually determined by geographic and climatic considerations. Following a brief discussion of some general principles of survival, the special problems faced in desert, tropic and arctic survival will be considered separately.

When a crash landing has occurred the primary consideration is removal of all survivors to a safe distance from the airplane until there is no danger of fire. If fire does not occur all supplies and useful equipment, particularly emergency radio equipment, should be immediately removed from the aircraft. The injured should be given first aid and shelter should be provided if possible. The parachute serves well for this, and many other purposes, when available. In cold climates a fire should be built as soon as possible. In situations with several survivors the survival effort must be organized. Leadership must be assumed and specific duties assigned. Immediate efforts should be directed toward the use of communications equipment. Many types of radio signalling and transceiver devices have been developed and have been used with variable success. When available and functioning the radio is the best rescue aid. It is conceivable that recent progress in electronics and semiconductor development may produce more reliable devices with greater range. Automatic transmitting devices, which are jettisoned from the aircraft and activated by the crash forces, have been developed and will soon be in service. The problem of communications is the most critical of all problems in the field of survival and rescue. Significant advances in communications will pay the greatest dividends and minimize the importance of many survival problems for which man's best efforts have so far been able to produce only compromise solutions.

As a general rule it is advisable to stay near the crashed aircraft. This will, in most cases, aid search and rescue operations.

Where possible, signal devices such as colored panels or paulins should be displayed. Recently developed parachutes use multicolored panels which provide for conspicuity, signalling and even camouflage. Other means of signalling, such as arrangement of foliage or rocks and turning of turf are useful in the absence of signalling equipment. When available, pyrotechnic signalling devices are effective when search aircraft are within appropriate range. Smoke grenades, flares, Very cartridges, flashlights and fires of any type are useful. One of the most effective devices in sea, arctic and desert survival is the heliograph signalling mirror. This is standard equipment in all survival gear and has been responsible for many rescues. In routine survival procedure the horizon is periodically scanned with the signal mirror inasmuch as search aircraft can detect a mirror flash long before the aircraft can be detected by the survivors.

The classic problems of survival are associated with food, water, clothing, shelter, fire building, survival weapons, geographic orientation, travel and health hazards. The approach to these problems will vary with geographic and climatic areas and will, therefore, be considered in context with the major types of survival conditions.

Desert Survival

The severe environment of deserts and the large number of desert areas in the world place this subject in a position of importance to the global air traveler. One survival publication (42) lists some 69 important deserts of the world, one of which is three million square miles in area. The most serious aspect of desert survival devolves upon the heat and the effects of the sun combined with a shortage or complete lack of water. An analysis (43) of 382 successful desert survival episodes of World War II provides an abundance of information which will be drawn upon in the following discussion.

Most recorded emergencies leading to survival in the desert were the result of enemy action although other conditions included navigational errors, fuel shortage and mechanical failure. Crash landings and bailouts occurred with equal frequency. All of the survivors were able to walk back to their own lines or enemy lines and surrender; however, with modern search and rescue methods it would probably now be preferable to remain in the vicinity of the crash or bailout. In the above study the men who survived were in the desert 1 to 29 days and traveled 10 to 350 miles across desert terrain (average: 5 days and 50 miles). Individuals who strayed from survival groups were never seen again. The primary environmental hazards were heat, sun and water shortage. Other factors included sun glare, cold nights, dust, sand and sandstorms. Water supplies were meager and obtained from wells, cisterns and oases. Water rationing was attempted but was probably unwise in the light of present concepts. Travel was best accomplished at night or in the cooler part of morning and evening. Most survivors found that day travel was too exhausting. Rest and shelter in the day was of great importance. All survivors learned that complete coverage of the body with clothing was essential. Only the sturdiest of shoes held up under desert travel. Considerable

difficulty was experienced with blisters and sore feet. Postwar trials have indicated that this may be prevented by wearing two pairs of socks, inner nylon and outer woolen. In general, the health of the survivors was good except for attacks of dysentery and desert sores from minor abrasions. Sunburn was distressing to the fair skinned. Food was not a serious problem and men short of water had little desire to eat solid food. Wild animals were used for food more frequently than plant life. Small insects, such as flies, sand flies and mosquitoes, were most distressing. Large animals and snakes were not involved as a hazard. Natives, made contact with, proved to be friendly and helpful. Signaling equipment was scanty and not very effective. Modern radio equipment should correct this defect and mirror signaling should be very effective in desert regions.

The problem of water is obviously of greatest significance in desert survival. The most important contribution to an understanding of this problem is the work of Adolph and associates (44) concerning human physiology in the desert environment. Their studies provide invaluable information relative to man's water requirements under various environmental conditions. The concept that men could be "trained to do without water" by a rationing procedure was thoroughly debunked by these investigators. There is no advantage in water restriction inasmuch as the requirement for water under desert conditions goes on whether it is taken in or not. Delay in drinking or spreading intake over long periods with small amounts only results in dehydration which must be "made up." Increasing the intake of water does not increase sweating and so long as a man desires water he will not be overhydrated. Water in the man will be utilized more economically than that in the canteen. Table 71, from Adolph and associates (44), shows the critical nature of water requirements under desert survival conditions. This table shows that survival time is not appreciably increased until the available water is about 4 quarts which is approximately the amount necessary to maintain water balance for 1 day at the high temperatures of the desert. The concept of "rationing the sweat" has replaced that of water rationing. In other

TABLE 71

Days of Expected Survival in the Desert under Two Conditions

Condition	Maximum Daily Shade Temperature	Available Water per Man in U. S. Quarts					
		0	1	2	4	10	20
	°F.						
No walking at all	120	2	2	2	2.5	3	4.5
	110	3	3	3.5	4	5	7
	100	5	5.5	6	7	9.5	13.5
	90	7	8	9	10.5	15	23
	80	9	10	11	13	19	29
	70	10	11	12	14	20.5	32
	60	10	11	12	14	21	32
	50	10	11	12	14.5	21	32
Walking at night until exhausted and resting thereafter	120	1	2	2	2.5	3	
	110	2	2	2.5	3	3.5	
	100	3	3.5	3.5	4.5	5.5	
	90	5	5.5	5.5	6.5	8	
	80	7	7.5	8	9.5	11.5	
	70	7.5	8	9	10.5	13.5	
	60	8	8.5	9	11	14	
	50	8	8.5	9	11	14	

words, the conservation of sweat by limited activity, protection from the sun by shade and clothing and conduct of necessary activities only during the low night temperatures will save water. Available water should be used to prevent dehydration which will markedly lower efficiency. Man does not acclimatize to dehydration and in this state there is no appreciable lessening in output of water for cooling, therefore, water can only be conserved in the desert by minimizing man's heat gains. Efficiency loss by dehydration is quickly restored by drinking water; even recovery from dehydration collapse can occur in a few minutes. Severe symptoms can result from a water deficit to the extent of 4 to 6 per cent of the body weight. There are no permanent ill effects which result from this level of dehydration. Deficits of 15 to 25 per cent are fatal at ambient temperatures above 85° F for the lower figure ranging to the higher, below 85° F. As a general rule it is considered that a man will survive if rescued before the deficit exceeds 20 per cent.

Heatstroke or sunstroke, involving hyperpyrexia and cessation of body sweating, has been mentioned as a hazard in desert survival. This results from prolonged excessive environmental heat with no surcease. It is apparent that under desert survival conditions this is rare if it occurs at all. Adolph's studies showed that men short of water suffered slow prostration instead of succumbing to a sudden stroke. If heatstroke should occur it is a medical emergency demanding immediate cooling by the fastest means if a fatal outcome is to be prevented.

Heat exhaustion and heat cramp can occur in unacclimatized individuals, usually resulting from a shortage of fluids and sodium chloride. Acclimatization to hot climates conserves salt by reducing the amount excreted in the sweat and occurs in a few days. Salt deficiency is uncommon in desert survival and in the presence of a shortage of water the use of salt tablets is contraindicated.

Many studies in survival ration development have attempted to determine the value of low protein diets in conserving water. Reduction of nitrogen urinary solutes requiring water for clearance can possibly be of some significance. A reduced food intake limited to carbohydrates will spare protein catabolism which would contribute more urea to the urine. However, in desert survival, if water is totally lacking, dehydration will be very rapid and food will play practically no role at all. Limited water in the desert results in dehydration which causes an aversion to food. This severe anorexia will naturally limit food intake. Under these circumstances a few packages of candy will suffice inasmuch as little else would be eaten even if it were available. It is probable that under sea survival conditions with slower dehydration the high carbohydrate diet may be of more significance in maintaining a favorable nutritional status and in slowing the rate of dehydration. It is the opinion of Adolph and his co-workers that "under no circumstances should a significant part of a load carried by a man stranded in the desert consist of food when water could be carried instead."

Tropic and Jungle Survival

It is probable that the least formidable of all survival environments are presented by the tropical regions. This is primarily because of the general abundance of food and water and the frequent presence of friendly natives. The survival situation may be limited to sea survival or jungle survival or may be a combination of both. The more important aspects of sea survival will be discussed in a later section. Most of the salient features of survival in tropical areas are available in an analysis of 1000 survival experiences in the southwest Pacific (45). This study is the major source of the information in the following paragraph.

The most frequent cause for in-flight emergencies leading to survival incidents in the southwest Pacific was a shortage of fuel. Other causes, in order of frequency, included enemy action, navigational errors and mechanical failure. Most survivors escaped by bailout, some ditched and a few crash landed. This is an expected variant from desert incidents. The duration of individual survival episodes was very short, averaging less than 48 hours before contact was made with natives or rescuers. The natives encountered were friendly and cooperative 90 per cent of the time. It was found that 90 per cent of survivors were injured before being rescued; 60 per cent during landing. This emphasizes the importance of training in first aid and the availability of survival medical kits. The most important health hazards were gastro-intestinal and insect borne diseases which required the use of water sterilization, insect repellents, protective clothing and malarial suppressive medication. The need for a variety of medical supplies is obviously greatest in tropical areas. Sunburn, as in the desert, was particularly a hazard in tropical ocean survival. Water and food were lesser problems than in other survival areas. Water purification tablets were usually available and besides fresh water lakes and streams additional sources of water included clear sap from plants (milky and colored plant juice avoided), coconut milk and rain water. The latter was the most important source in tropical sea survival. Foods were of both plant and animal origin; care being taken to avoid bitter plants and plants with a milky sap. Little or no difficulty was encountered with animals or reptiles. Leeches were quite troublesome, difficult to remove and sometimes caused infected sores. Travel in some areas was rather difficult; however, natives were usually encountered within relatively short distances. Signaling equipment and techniques were relatively unsatisfactory although mirror signaling was very effective in the open sea.

Arctic Survival

The most difficult problems of survival are presented by extremely cold environments. Arctic survival requires better physical and mental conditioning, more training, more equipment and more supplies than any other type of survival. It also requires considerable fortitude, courage and ingenuity on the part of the individual and oftentimes a good measure of luck is necessary for success. Because of the extreme difficulties presented by arctic survival problems, great efforts on a national and international scale have been expended in terms of accumulation of knowledge and experience, training and the development of survival techniques, clothing, equipment and supplies. The success of these efforts insofar as the flyer is

concerned has not been too encouraging. In the case of the military flyer adequate protective equipment and supplies to afford a reasonable chance of survival and rescue in all arctic areas almost completely negates his primary mission performance capability by severe encumberance of mobility. In the case of civil air carrier operations, space, weight and passenger equipment limitations make it all but impossible to provide arctic survival capabilities. In spite of this rather pessimistic picture there are available many items of survival equipment, survival techniques and useful knowledge which will provide for successful survival and rescue in many arctic survival situations. Volumes are available on the subject of arctic survival; only a very limited discussion will be presented here.

The success of a survival encounter in the arctic depends primarily upon how well prepared the individual is and how rapidly rescue is effected. If possible it is advisable to crash land or ditch rather than bail out in the arctic. Once at the surface, the survivor's activity during the first 15 minutes will probably determine whether he will come out alive or not. If he protects himself from the cold, particularly his hands, during this initial period and performs useful activities he will usually avoid becoming a casualty. During this critical period the "first-firsts" consist of securing all of the survival equipment and supplies, applying first aid to the injured, constructing an emergency shelter, building a fire and starting radio signaling. The struggle against the cold follows. Experience has shown that survivors should stay at the scene of the crash and not attempt to travel unless so instructed by rescue parties. Clothing and equipment available are seldom adequate. Some arctic experts still contend that the best of modern technology in the textile and tailoring industry have failed to provide arctic clothing equal to the skin and fur apparel of the Eskimo. The multiplicity of types of arctic protective clothing almost defies description; at least within the confines of a single volume. It can only be said here that the survivor must keep dry and preserve the insulative values of his clothing, whatever kind it may be. Wet clothing or footgear will result in serious cold injury in the winter arctic in a very short time. One most important item which is usually available to the military aircrew survivor is the arctic sleeping bag. Vacuum packing of this makes it available even in the smallest of arctic survival kits.

Survival publications (46, 47) are replete with various methods of providing shelter in the arctic including igloos, snow caves, "fighter" trenches, parateepees, "paraigloos" and others. Space does not permit description of these; however, they are mentioned to emphasize the importance of shelter in the arctic. Life rafts can be used as shelters and for insulation against snow and ice surfaces. Aircraft, particularly those which are insulated, may serve as effective and convenient shelters. In closed shelters with fires, adequate ventilation is a must to avoid the carbon monoxide hazard which has claimed many lives in the arctic. An understanding and avoidance of wind chill is of utmost importance if cold injury is to be avoided. Wind chill refers to the cooling effect of air movement on exposed skin. Charts are available which provide wind chill data on various combinations of air temperature and wind velocity. The importance of this factor can be gained from the fact that a temperature of 34° F. with a wind velocity of 20 m.p.h. has a cooling rate equivalence of −38° F. with no wind. In a 20 m.p.h. wind at −32° F. exposed flesh will freeze in 1 minute. Frostbite is the most frequent injury of arctic survivors and most cases among those who have been rescued could have been prevented had proper precautions been exercised. There is no substitute for good training in arctic survival. Without doubt, many who failed to survive could have been rescued had not local cold injury incapacitated them. In these cases the local injury resulted in an inability to accomplish necessary survival tasks with ultimate death from general hypothermia. Severe frostbite is best treated by rapid rewarming (water 107° F.); however, this is seldom practicable in a survival situation and other means of warming must be used. General hypothermia occurs after prolonged exposure in cold air or acutely after a few minutes exposure in icy arctic waters. Death usually results from ventricular fibrillation or cardiac asystole as the body temperature falls below 25° C. (77° F.).

In addition to clothing and shelter most arctic survivors have been able to have some type of fire. Hydrocarbon fuels from the aircraft, trees and bushes, driftwood and animal fats have been used. Small stoves and Sterno heaters are included in some survival kits. In some situations it is impossible to have a fire and the body is totally dependent upon metabolic heating. In this instance shelter, clothing and conservation of energy are of utmost importance because food in the arctic is a serious problem. Food supplies aboard aircraft are almost always inadequate and arctic survivors are rarely successful at foraging. In some areas, such as the north polar basin, there is absolutely no animal life available for food. Polar bear liver must not be eaten because of its extremely high vitamin A content which will produce the hypervitaminosis-A syndrome. The question of special rations for arctic survival has been investigated for many years and many types have been developed. It is generally considered that a very high caloric density food is required for arctic survival rations and "pemmican" (meat-fat bar) is an example of this type. Newer arctic survival rations are more palatable than "pemmican" and provide approximately 3500 calories. Starvation is a real danger because of the large energy requirements.

Water is usually obtained by melting snow or ice. If in the north polar basin, old sea ice which has lost its salt can be used. This is recognizable by its blue color and rounded edges. When fuel is not available for thawing ice, body heat may substitute by use of a plastic container under the clothing. It is advisable to avoid eating snow and ice because of the painful local cold injury of the mucous membranes of the mouth and pharynx.

Snow blindness is a moderately serious hazard and the eyes should be protected by arctic sun glasses available in survival kits or by improvised paper or fabric protectors with narrow slits opposite the pupils for vision. During the summer, mosquitoes and black flies are a plague and require protective measures. Ice fogs and arctic "whiteout" present a serious hazard when it is necessary to travel. Other serious handicaps to travel in the arctic include the great expenditure of energy required, constant darkness in the winter, bad weather, avalanches, crevasses and complete unreliability of the magnetic compass. Travel on sea ice is probably most treacherous of all, whether on floes where the ice is broken up or on pack ice where leads may open up at any time. The previously stated rule of remaining at the site of the crash appears to be a good one. Available records show that few arctic survivors have been able to "walk out" and many have died trying.

The need to solve the almost insuperable problems of arctic survival is being heightened day by day. The strategic importance of arctic routes for military operations is obvious. This necessitates constant and sustained air operations over the Arctic even during what is referred to as "peace time." Additionally, the polar routes from Europe to the western United States and to the Orient are now becoming well traveled by civil air carriers. Survival capability should be improved not only to assure the return of highly trained combat aircrew but also because of its impact on combat effectiveness. Flyers who have reasonable assurance of survival and rescue will pursue assigned objectives with a greater determination and confidence. Extensive research and modern technology have failed to provide all of the needed answers. Physiologic and metabolic studies of the Eskimo have failed to reveal any "secrets" of acclimatization to the arctic environment. As a matter of fact, there is probably no inborn factor or real physiologic acclimatization which explains the successful existence of the Eskimo in the north. It is more a matter of physical and mental adaptation to every aspect of the arctic environment; a matter of attitude and know-how combined with robust physical fitness. If this be true, then it is apparent that one of the most important keys to arctic survival is adequate training.

Sea Survival

The importance of sea survival is emphasized by two facts; open water represents four-fifths of the earth's surface and the unforgiving sea can deal swiftly and finally with human life, either through drowning or exposure. For the latter reason, immediate availability of life-saving procedures without delay upon entry into the sea is imperative. When ditching is the method of entry preditching procedures, ditching technique, emergency crew performance, passenger indoctrination and ready availability of flotation equipment both personal and general are factors which will determine the success of the initial phase of sea survival. The frequency of civil air carrier ditchings is not great; however, the survival rate leaves much to be desired. A CAA report lists 18 civil transport ditchings during the 10 years from 1946 to 1956 in which 53 per cent of the 484 passengers survived. If the escape to the sea is by bailout or ejection, essential lifesaving and survival equipment must be securely attached to the individual. Normally the parachutist actuates his water survival equipment prior to reaching the surface and his equipment and inflated raft are suspended below him. Usually one side of the life vest is inflated and the flyer is prepared to release the parachute by one of several methods as he enters the water. Failure to do this may result in being dragged under the water by surface winds. Excellent swimmers have been drowned in this manner. If drowning doesn't occur acute illness from swallowing water and exhaustion may compromise further survival efforts. Immediate occupancy of the life raft is essential for most sea survival situations.

In some northern latitude waters a protective exposure suit is essential for successful survival. Quick donning exposure suits, available in some transports, can be put on prior to ditching. Aircrew of operational aircraft must wear the immersion suit as part of the flying clothing if they are to be adequately prepared for emergencies over cold sea areas. In the absence of adequate protection from cold water the survivor will become helpless within a very few minutes with death from immersion hypothermia quickly following. In very cold sea water, death has occurred in less than 10 minutes and even when the water temperature is as high as 70° F. the time that a man immersed in it will remain alive is limited to about 40 hours. There is wide individual variability in fatal exposure times. Table 72 indicates the approximate periods a man immersed in sea water at various temperatures may be expected to survive without the protection of a water tight garment.

In warmer waters the hazard of sharks makes it advisable to get into a raft as quickly as possible and in heavy seas a raft is necessary to prevent exhaustion and drowning which frequently occur when only life jackets or vests are available.

Once aboard the raft, either following bail-out or ditching, the second phase of sea survival begins. This is concerned primarily with protection against exposure, sustenance with limited food and water and the use of all possible measures to communicate with rescuers. Most survivors who will be recovered will be rescued within 2 weeks. One analysis of 607 sea survival incidents showed that approximately 80 per cent of the rescues occurred in the first 48 hours and few recoveries were made after 14 days. The longest raft survival recorded was that of Poon Lin, a Chinese survivor of a torpedoed transport who drifted for 131 days on a ship's raft. The longest survival period in a flexible raft following escape from an aircraft is 47 days.

Immediate activities aboard the raft consist of securing all survival equipment and supplies, connecting rafts with lines when more than one, transmission of distress signals, erection of radar reflector and the readying for appropriate use of all other signaling devices including the heliograph mirror, pyrotechnics, sea marker dye, lights and the police whistle. Readiness and appropriate use of these devices are critical in sea rescue. Location and detection of small rafts by air search or sea search is extremely difficult. Use of a sea anchor delays movement away from the site of the ditching or bailout and also makes the raft more stable in heavy seas. All possible means of protection against the elements should be utilized; this includes the sun in warm oceans and the spray and cold in the north.

Drinking water represents the most critical need in sea survival. Calculated periods of survival at sea without water (44) vary from approximately 12 days in an air temperature of 40° F. to 4 to 5 days in an air temperature of 90° F. If 1 gallon of water per person is available in the emergency kit these times will be prolonged 1 or 2 days. Less water in emergency kits is of little practical importance and serves mainly to bolster morale. Besides "canned" water other sources in sea survival are the use of solar stills and desalting kits, collection of dew on paulins and rain catchment. The latter is most important and is feasible over most ocean areas. Charts are available (44) which indicate frequency and adequacy of rain water catchment over all ocean areas, for each season. Availability of plastic bags or other containers for rain water storage is important for survival on a raft. In addition to taking advantage of all possible sources of water, conservation is also important. This is possible through the use of paulin sun shelters and evaporative cooling of wet clothing. External garments should be dampened with sea water only during the day and when the temperature is above 80° F, otherwise the chilling effect will be uncomfortable as well as stressful. Elimination of unnecessary activity in warm ocean areas is also helpful. Sea sickness is also a source of dehydration and if available, sea sickness preventives should be taken. Under no circumstances should sea water be drunk, either undiluted or mixed with fresh water, to "stretch" the supply. The electrolyte intake with ingested sea water requires a greater volume of water to be eliminated from the body, which it must be, than the volume of sea water taken in. Any amount of sea water will, therefore, hasten dehydration.

Food is not as critical as water, but if

TABLE 72

Survival Time in Sea Water without Water Tight Garment

Water Temperature	Survival Time
°F.	hours
32	Less than 1
40	½ to 3
50	1 to 6
60	2 to 24
70	3 to 40
80	Indefinite

water is available food is necessary to maintain strength and endurance. It is agreed by many investigators that if the water supply is limited it is advisable to limit the calories and to use principally carbohydrate for its sparing action on protein catabolism. This is not universally accepted. In northern areas cold will increase the requirement for food. The sea is a good source of food, most fish in the open sea being edible. Raw fish or fish "juices" are not a source of water. Fishing kits are most always available in survival equipment and if not, can be improvised from many personal or incidental items. Many survivors at sea have also been able to catch birds. Plankton, frequently mentioned as survival food, has not proven to be a practical source of food and some species are very poisonous.

Some of the health hazards of sea survival include immersion foot, glare conjunctivitis, salt water sores, frostbite, sunburn and severe mental disturbance. Sharks can be a serious hazard and a chemical repellent has been used with doubtful success. Survival swimming techniques, raft seamanship and techniques to be used for going ashore under various circumstances are included in referenced survival manuals. Training in these aspects of sea survival is rarely adequate. The great hope of all sea survivors is an effective search and rescue system quickly brought into action by emergency communications.

Survival Equipment

In spite of some of the pessimism regarding present survival clothing and equipment there are many excellent items available and present developmental efforts give great promise for some important "break-throughs." The most difficult aspect of the survival equipment problem concerns integration of the many items necessary for both survival and air operation functions. The problems of space and weight are ever present and force compromises which often result in the abandonment of provisions for survival capability.

Some examples of outstanding progress in survival equipment development include "omnienvironmental" suits which protect against high altitude flight as well as against cold water immersion, combination dinghy-sleeping bags, reliable flotation equipment for infants, compressed air inflation devices for rafts to replace CO_2 which does not function in extreme cold, silicone impregnated garments, plastic foam arctic clothing and many others. Space does not permit discussion of the hundreds of items of survival equipment; however, extensive listings with complete descriptions are available (48–50).

Survival Nutrition

It has been noted in the discussion of each specialized survival category that consideration has been given the question of type-specific survival rations to match the requirements imposed by different environmental conditions. This concept has been accepted by many investigators and is supported by experimental evidence. However, the recent extensive and intensive studies of Sargent and others (51) has resulted in the concept of an all-purpose survival ration. This concept includes many aspects which are counter to some presently accepted tenets. For example, the experimental evidence of this group indicates that the use of a pure carbohydrate ration in a limited water supply situation for the purpose of retarding dehydration by sparing protein catabolism is in error. New evidence has shown that in limited water regimens too little osmotic intake (pure carbohydrate) will accentuate rather than retard dehydration. It is the conclusion of this group that a single all-purpose survival ration will suffice for all environments and all daily work loads. In their carefully designed ration they have found the best combination of carbohydrate, protein, and fat which will minimize deterioration in temperate, hot and cold conditions regardless of work load and water intake. Wide deviations toward more carbohydrate, more protein or more fat was found to invariably result in measurably enhanced deterioration of the subjects.

The recommended composition and characteristics of the all-purpose survival ration are as follows:

1. Two thousand calories per man per day with a calorie percentage of protein 15 per cent, carbohydrate 52 per cent and fat 33 per cent.

2. A water allowance goal of 3 quarts per

man per day for hot weather and no less than 1 quart per man per day under any circumstances.

3. Optimal osmotic intake, neither too large nor too small with a goal of 700 milliosmols per day, provided by the sum of protein and minerals.

4. Within the limits set by the recommended proportions of carbohydrate, protein and fat, minimal ketogenicity, minimal specific dynamic action and maximal water of oxidation.

The concept of an all-purpose survival ration will recieve further consideration in future survival ration development and testing. It is the belief of Sargent and his group that a castaway's survival potential can be protected by an appropriate ration whereas, under some circumstances, an unsound survival ration may actually produce deterioration faster than will starvation, particularly when water is limited. The meat-fat bar and pure carbohydrate survival rations are considered to be unsound and to have intrinsically undesirable effects on a castaway's organic functioning and total efficiency. Readers who desire more complete information concerning survival nutrition are referred to the extensive bibliography of the paper by Sargent and associates (51).

Stress Reactions and Survival

One aspect of survival which is now receiving more emphasis than heretofore is an understanding of man's combined physiologic and psychologic reactions to the stress of hostile or unusual environments. Many of the physiologic considerations have already been discussed; the physiologic and psychologic are always intermingled, one affecting the other. However, it is the psychologic reaction which is, more often than not, unpredictable and more difficult to understand. For this reason it is important that aircrew members, who may at any time be faced with survival, be as well trained as possible in the understanding of physiologic and psychologic mechanisms involved in survival stress reactions. Most of the preceding discussion on survival has emphasized the use of certain equipment, supplies and techniques in meeting specific survival problems. Not much has been said about the man and his reactions and how he manages them. The importance of this aspect of survival cannot be ignored and is aptly stated in the following quotation from a survival report: "Whether a man returns after being forced down in either jungle or enemy territory depends largely on the individual concerned. No amount of survival equipment will help some men while others, through sheer ingenuity and determination and under similar circumstances, will fare much better and return regardless of whether they possessed such equipment or not. It's largely a mental outlook—the will to survive is the deciding factor." The importance of this facet of survival has been recognized and service survival schools are giving a great deal of attention to the analysis of this "will to survive" and are providing realistic training which will activate and develop this most important element of survival success.

Some of the psychologic factors in the management of survival stress reactions have been studied in relation to survival training by Torrance (52) and are briefly summarized in the following paragraphs.

Fear and anxiety with all of the concomitant physiologic and psychologic repercussions, constitute survival reactions of critical importance. These, of course, are normal reactions but the manner in which they are handled may spell the difference between life and death. Fear may, on the one hand, destroy a man's chances of survival and, on the other hand, may improve them. An understanding of the mechanism and source of fear reactions such as fear of death, injury, the unknown, loss of prestige or support, is essential and will favor an adaptive response of increased alertness and stimulation to emergency action. The absence of understanding and insight will favor a disruptive response with fear in complete command, the individual reacting to his feelings and imagination rather than to the external activity in progress. Fear may be intensified by physical debilitation, contagion from others, helplessness and hopelessness. Automaticity of functioning which can result from training and practice is a potent force in the control of fear. Other antifear factors are leadership, discipline, activity, contagion and confidence in survival and rescue resources.

The subjective reactions to such stresses as pain, cold, heat, thirst, hunger, fatigue, sleep deprivation, isolation, boredom and loneliness can have serious additive and cumulative effects which may endanger the success of the survival effort or even guarantee its failure. The dangers from these stresses must be recognized and understood. The means of effectively combating these stresses are frequently not available in which event the individual must recognize the concessions that have to be made to his "normal" state of comfort. He can learn in survival training that these reactions may be suppressed from conscious awareness by strong motivation to do what is necessary to survive.

One helpful concept which is now emphasized in survival training is that of "set" for survival. "Set" represents a preparatory attitude or state of readiness for any emergency or survival situation which may be expected to occur. There are both positive and negative aspects of psychologic set relative to survival. On the positive side the full acceptance by an individual of survival training and conscientious recognition of its importance will result in a preparatory attitude which, under emergency conditions, should provide an appropriate response. A prime example of the negative aspect of "set" is seen, all too frequently, in the individual with the attitude of "it can't happen to me." This is the antithesis of "preparatory set" and will seriously endanger the chances of survival. The absence of any "set" at all can be the cause of panic even in individuals who ordinarily appear to be quite stable.

The psychologic problems and stress reactions are intensified and made more complex when complicated by enemy action. This is particularly true when the survivor is in a prisoner of war or evadee status. Under these circumstances the ramifications of psychologic reactions become very complex and constitute a subject beyond the scope of this discussion. The problems of group behavior under survival conditions also constitute a subject of some importance and in survival training must receive appropriate recognition. Those especially interested in the psychologic aspects of survival are referred to the listed reference of Torrance and his extensive bibliography on this subject.

RESCUE

The world-wide search and rescue operations which today are organized on an international level represent a response to a wartime requirement. Paradoxically, this is true of many humanitarian and lifesaving procedures and devices. At the opening of World War II the German Air Force had a well organized air-sea rescue service and soon after the beginning of the war British and American forces recognized the necessity of establishing an organized air-sea rescue effort for the purpose of rescuing aircrews in distress. As a consequence many thousands of airmen were saved who would have otherwise been lost. During the Korean War organized rescue units evacuated almost 10,000 wounded in Korea and successfully rescued more than 1000 United Nations personnel from behind enemy lines. The benefits of an effective search and rescue capability are concerned mainly with aircrew morale, return of highly trained personnel and humanitarian principles.

Organization

The International Civil Aviation Organization (ICAO) provides a common meeting ground for international standards and recommended practices for search and rescue. The Search and Rescue (SAR) Division of the ICAO publishes manuals and administrative directives which provide guidance for the participation of the Contracting States in International Search and Rescue Operations. The United States, as one of the Contracting States, is obligated to furnish certain SAR facilities. The U. S. Coast Guard provides these with the assistance of the Air Force Air Rescue Service when requested.

Although there is no primary rescue agency within the U. S. government, the President's Air Coordinating Committee has the responsibility for coordinating all United States SAR interests. There has also been formulated a National Search and Rescue Plan which establishes three regional coordinators with broad responsibilities as follows: (1) inland region, the Air Force; (2) maritime region, the Coast Guard, and (3) overseas region, the Overseas Unified Command. The purpose of this plan is to insure effective utilization of all available facilities in all types of search and rescue. Although each military service is responsible for search and rescue support of its own operations, almost all SAR activities involve many mutually supporting organizations both military and civil. These activities are coordinated by local agreements between military commanders and local agencies. Agencies concerned with SAR include the Army, Navy, Air Force, Coast Guard, Federal Aviation Agency, Civil Air Patrol and state, local and private organizations. The Air Rescue Service of the Air Force constitutes the most important world-wide primary air SAR organization. Units of the Air Rescue Service are globally employed to perform tactical and strategic air rescue missions.

Operations

Air rescue operations entail one or a combination of four mission phases: (1) notification, (2) search, (3) aid and (4) rescue. The notification phase is performed by anyone having knowledge of an aircraft incident. Most commonly this is an air traffic control agency. After notification the second phase involves communications or physical search to locate the aircraft in distress or scene of the crash. The third phase consists of providing survivors with immediate and continuing aid until the final phase of recovery and delivery of survivors to the proper receiving agency can be effected. Rescue operations are directed from a Rescue Center which collects and centralizes SAR information, integrates the capabilities of assisting agencies into an area SAR plan and coordinates the combined efforts of all facilities during SAR operations. There are a number of types of centers which have desigantions corresponding with the level of the operation. Communications is the most important element of the rescue center.

The time element is of utmost importance in rescue operations because the probability of finding survivors and their chances of survival diminish with each minute that passes after an incident occurs. Records have proven that the life expectancy of injured survivors decreases as much as 80 per cent in the first 24 hours following an accident whereas the chances of survival for uninjured survivors rapidly diminish after the first 3 days. These facts emphasize the need for an effective and reliable automatic crash locator device in every aircraft. The length of search operations varies with the circumstances of each incident and termination of activities is based upon the probability of finding survivors.

The search phase is the most difficult of the four mission phases of SAR activities. Aerial search methods include visual search, radar search and radio search. All types of aircraft may be used including alerted civil air carrier aircraft transient in the vicinity of a reported incident. Surface vessels may assist in search at sea. The most difficult search conditions are probably those of the north polar basin which is enveloped in darkness in the winter and covered by low clouds almost constantly through the other seasons. Additional difficulties are imposed by the lack of electronic navigational aids, difficulty of navigation by natural aids and severe interference with radio communications. Search over water is also very difficult and emphasizes the importance of timely assistance by the survivors with flares, heliograph mirror, marker dye or other means. The perfection of SOFAR (Sound Fixing and Ranging) techniques could possibly, in the future, solve the problem of accurate and rapid location of survivors at sea.

Once the survivors are located it may not be possible to immediately rescue them. In this event it will be necessary to supply them with essential survival gear, medical equipment and subsistence. Survivors in the arctic have been maintained for weeks by air supply before successful recovery could be accomplished. Delivery of airborne equipment is a routine procedure for air rescue units and special kits have been designed for use under varying situations for both land and sea survivor aid. An example is the free fall, sea rescue kit which consists of two pneumatic rescue raft containers and three sustenance containers. Each container is interconnected by 210 feet of buoyant line. The rafts which are at either end of the kit, inflate during descent and all the components string out to create 800 feet of floating life line. The entire assembly tends to encircle the survivor, minimizing the danger of his not being able to reach the rescue equipment.

At times it may be necessary to provide human aid to the survivor immediately following his location. This is accomplished by highly trained pararescue teams which can make jumps under almost any condition such as, open field, water, night, snow, trees and at altitude. When it is impossible to parachute to the survivors the rescue team must use surface means of reaching them.

Recovery of survivors is accomplished by various means depending upon the survival situation. At sea, recovery may be made by surface vessel, seaplane, amphibious aircraft or by helicopter operating from land or from ship. Land rescue may be by helicopter, conventional aircraft or aircraft fitted with skis, seaplanes or amphibious aircraft on inland waters, motor vehicles, dog teams, rescue teams on foot or other means. The helicopter has become one of the most important and versatile means of survivor rescue. In addition to its rescue capabilities in almost any type of terrain, either by hovering or landing, it may also be used effectively to combat or control fire at the site of the aircraft accident. This is done by directing the rotor wash into the flames to provide a path whereby rescuers can reach and remove survivors.

The amount and type of immediate medical aid given survivors varies with the situation and capabilities of the rescue team. Training of rescue and survival technicians in emergency medical procedures is as extensive and thorough as practicable. The practice of training physicians as pararescue personnel was discontinued when the requirement for this capability was markedly reduced by helicopter rescue operations. Medical kits are well designed to give maximum lifesaving capability although in many instances it is not possible to provide immediate essential treatment. For example, in severe immersion hypothermia, rapid rewarming in baths at 115 to 120° F. can be lifesaving; however, if rescue is by helicopter this procedure is manifestly impossible. Some surface craft can provide this facility and during World War II the Germans developed special rewarming devices for rescue vessels.

The development of an efficient electrically heated casualty bag may provide an answer to this problem. Many equally difficult problems still exist. Research and development in the field of rescue and survival is actively engaged in meeting the many requirements imposed by military as well as civil air operations. One example of a rather sophisticated endeavor is the development of a human pickup system, capable of rescuing survivors in areas not suitable for landing an aircraft. This system will provide for pickups of personnel with aircraft other than helicopters by the use of a capsule that is dropped to the survivors; rescue at speeds up to 180 knots will be possible. Existing procedures, equipment and techniques used in search and rescue operations represent tremendous advances since the establishment of this important specialized field in World War II. The interested reader will find details of rescue operations and accomplishments in this field in works already published (53, 54).

REFERENCES

(1) Scheubel, F. N.: Parachute opening shock. In German Aviation Medicine, World War II, Vol. I. Washington, D. C., Government Printing Office, 1950, chapter VI-D, p. 599.

(2) Determination of the Rates of Descent of a Falling Man and of a Parachute Test Weight. Air Corps Information Circular, Vol. 7, No. 628, Washington, D. C., 1928.

(3) Armstrong, H. G.: Principles and Practice of Aviation Medicine, Ed. 3. Baltimore, The Williams & Wilkins Co., 1952, p. 465.

(4) Oxygen Requirements in Parachute Descent from 30,000 Feet. Memorandum Report, Army Air Corps, Material Division, No. EXP-M-49-696-6, Wright-Patterson Air Force Base, Ohio. 1942.

(5) Bailing Out Above 30,000 Feet. Memorandum Report, Army Air Forces, Material Center, No. EXP-M-49-696-6A, 1942.

(6) Injuries Associated with Parachute Escapes. Medical Safety Division, Army Air Forces, Air Surgeon's Bulletin, Vol. I, No. 5, Washing, D. C., 1944.

(7) USAF Publication M-16-52, Medical Safety Division, Office of the Inspector General, USAF, Norton Air Force Base, California. 1952.

(8) Handbook for Survival Training and Personal Equipment Personnel. AF Manual 64-4. Washington, D. C., Department of the Air Force, 1954, p. 240.

(9) Dugan, P. D.: Problems in design of Navy escape system. In Proceedings of a Symposium on Escape From High Performance

Aircraft. Los Angeles, Institute of Transportation and Traffic Engineering, University of California, 1955, p. 50.

(10) ZELLER, A. F.: Psychological factors in escape. In Proceedings of a Symposium on Escape From High Performance Aircraft. Los Angeles, Institute of Transportation and Traffic Engineering, University of California, 1955, p. 43.

(11) MASON, J. K.: The Influence of Aviation Pathology on Flight Safety. Report from RAF Institute of Pathology and Tropical Medicine, Holton, England, 1957.

(12) SHAW, R. S.: Test Firing of T-7 Catapult for Downward Seat Ejection. Memorandum Report DMCREX-695-74 I, Wright-Patterson Air Force Base, Ohio, 1948.

(13) Pilots Ability to Simulate an Emergency Escape with Various Types of Ejection Seats While Subjected to Fluctuating Acceleration. Letter Report MA-4 No. 10467, TED ADC AE 6303. Johnsville, Pennsylvania, Naval Air Development and Material Center, 1953.

(14) SPERRY, E. G., NIELSON, H. P., AND BARASH, I. M.: Downward ejections at high speeds and high altitudes. J. Aviation Med., **26:** 356–372, 1955.

(15) HABER, F.: Notes on physics of escape from aircraft. In Proceedings of a Symposium on Escape from High Performance Aircraft, Los Angeles, Institute of Transportation and Traffic Engineering, University of California, 1955, p. 18.

(16) STAPP, J. P.: Crash protection in air transports, Aeronautical Engineering Revs., **12:** No. 4, 1953.

(17) LATHAM, F.: A study in body ballistics: seat ejection. Proc. Roy. Soc., London. ser. B, **147:** 121–139, 1957.

(18) The Problem of Back Fractures During Ejection from USAF Aircraft. Publication 2-57. Directorate of Flight Safety Research, USAF, Norton Air Force Base, California, 1957.

(19) STAPP, J. P.: Human factors of supersonic escape. Unpublished paper, 1958.

(20. ROTHWELL, W. S., AND SPERRY, E. G.: Escape from aircraft by downward ejection. J. Aviation Med., **24:** 322–327, 1953.

(21) GREER, R. L.: Operational Regions and Bioaerodynamic Limitations of Future Aircraft Escape Systems. WADC Technical Report 57-590. Wright-Patterson Air Force Base, Ohio, 1957.

(22) STAPP, J. P., AND HUGHES, C. D.: Effects of mechanical force on living tissues. II. Supersonic deceleration and windblast. J. Aviation Med., **27:** 407–413, 1956; and later unpublished data.

(23) STAPP, J. P.: Effects of mechanical force on living tissues. I. Abrupt deceleration and windblast. J. Aviation Med., **26:** 268–288, 1955.

(24) HEGENWALD, J. E., JR., AND BLOCKLEY, W. V.: Survivable Supersonic Ejection. A Case Study to Correlate Analytical, Experimental, and Medical Data by Reconstruction of an Incident. Report No. NA-56-452. Los Angeles, North American Aviation, Inc., 1956.

(25) GOODRICH, J. W.: Escape from High Performance Aircraft. WADC Technical Note 56-7. Wright-Patterson Air Force Base, Ohio, 1956.

(26) SAVELY, H. E.: The physiology of escape. In Proceedings of a Symposium on Escape from High Performance Aircraft. Los Angeles, Institute of Transportation and Traffic Engineering, University of California, 1955, p. 35.

(27) BÜETTNER, K.: Conflagration heat. In German Aviation Medicine, World War II, Vol. II. Washington, D. C., Government Printing Office 1950, chapter XIII-A, pp. 1167–1188.

(28) WALCHNER, O.: Parachutists' Spin Problem. Unpublished report presented at the AGARD Aeromedical Panel Meeting, Copenhagen, Denmark, 1958.

(29) WEISS, H. S., EDELBERG, R., CHARLAND, P. V., AND ROSENBAUM, J. I.: Animal and human reactions to rapid tumbling. J. Aviation Med., **25:** 5–22, 1954.

(30) MAZZA, V.: High altitude bailouts. J. Aviation Med., **22:** 403–407, 1951.

(31) ROXBURGH, H. L.: Biological Problems of Escape at High Altitudes. Unpublished paper presented at AGARD Aeromedical Panel Meeting, Copenhagen, Denmark, 1958.

(32) LOMBARD, C. F., AMES, S. W., ROSENFIELD, S., PAGRUND, R. S., AND BROOKS, P. M.: Studies with the Epicyclic Centrifuge on Animals and Humans. Project NR-161-014, Office of Naval Research, Department of the Navy, Biological Science Division, Washington, D. C., 1951.

(33) ENGSTROM, B. A.: The Effects of Simultaneous Deceleration, Tumbling and Windblast Encountered in Escape from Supersonic Aircraft. WADC Technical Note 54-18, Part II (ASTIA Document No. AD-118328). Wright-Patterson Air Force Base, Ohio, 1957.

(34) MOSELEY, H. G.: U. S. Air Force experience with ejection seat escape. J. Aviation Med., **28:** 69–73, 1957 (statistics revised to July 1958 by personal communication).

(35) WILBUR, C. E.: U. S. Navy operational experience with ejection seat escape. J. Aviation Med., **28:** 64–68, 1957 (statistics revised to July 1958 by personal communication).

(36) MOHRLOCK, H. F., JR.: The development of RESCU (rocket ejection seat catapult, upward) Mark 1. In Jet Propulsion. American Rocket Society, 1957.

(37) MOHRLOCK, H. F., JR.: Industry Crew Escape Systems Committee Report (I.C.E.S.C. upward "B" seat). Presented at the 37th AF-Industry Conference on Emergency Escape, Palm Springs, California, 1958.

(38) BLECK, M. E.: Capsule escape system specific

design approaches and problem areas (FZM-1253, Part II, B-58 Capsule Escape System). Presentation at the 37th AF-Industry Conference on Emergency Escape, Palm Springs, California, 1958.

(39) Over, under and out. In Approach. The Naval Aviation Safety Review, NAVER 00-75-510, Naval Air Station, Norfolk, Va., 1957, pp. 20–21.

(40) RAWLINS, J. S. P.: Escape from submerged aircraft. I. Unpublished report presented at the AGARD Aeromedical Panel meeting, Copenhagen, Denmark, 1958.

(41) Ultra-fast Opening Parachute. Progress Report XMP-2. Technical Memorandum WCLE-TM-58-34. Wright-Patterson Air Force Base, Ohio, Wright Air Development Center, 1958.

(42) POND, A. W.: Afoot in the Desert. ADTIC Publication No. D-100, Air University, Maxwell Air Force Base, Alabama, Arctic Desert Tropic Information Center, 1952.

(43) HOWARD, R. A.: Sun, Sand and Survival. ADTIC Publication No. D-102. Air University, Maxwell Air Force Base, Alabama, Arctic Desert Tropic Information Center, 1953.

(44) ADOLPH, E. F., AND ASSOCIATES: Physiology of Man in the Desert. New York, Interscience Publishers, Inc., 1947.

(45) HOWARD, R. A.: 999 survived. An analysis of survival experiences in the southwest pacific. ADTIC Publication No. T-100, Air University, Maxwell Air Force Base, Alabama, Arctic Desert Tropic Information Center, 1950.

(46) Survival. AF Manual 64-5. Washington, D. C., Department of the Air Force, 1952.

(47) HOWARD, R. A.: Down in the North. ADTIC Publication No. A-103, Air University, Maxwell Air Force Base, Alabama, Arctic Desert Tropic Information Center, 1953.

(48) Handbook for Survival Training and Personal Equipment Personnel. AF Manual 64-4. Washington, D. C., Department of the Air Force, 1954.

(49) Safety and Survival Equipment. U. S. Navy Manual NAVAER 00-80T-52, Washington, D.C., 1959.

(50) Air-Sea Rescue and Equipment Guide. Report NAVCG-117. Washington, D. C., U. S. Coast Guard, Air-Sea Rescue Agency, 1945.

(51) SARGENT, F., II, AND JOHNSON, R. E.: The Physiological Basis for Various Constituents in Survival Rations. Part IV. An Integrate Study of the All-Purpose Survival Ration for Temperate, Cold and Hot Weather. WADC Technical Report 53-484, (ASTIA Document No. AD 142233). Urbana, University of Illinois, 1957.

(52) TORRENCE, E. P.: Psychological Aspects of Survival. HFORL Report No. 35 (ASTIA Document No. AD-7860). Andrews Air Force Base, Maryland, Air Research and Development Command, 1953.

(53) Rescue Operations Manual. ARS Manual 55-1. Air Rescue Service, Military Air Transport Service, USAF, Scott Air Force Base, Illinois. 1957.

(54) ARNOLD, E.: Rescue. New York, Duell, Sloan, and Pearce, Inc., 1956.

21

AVIATION
OPHTHALMOLOGY

James L. Fuelling, M.D.

The eye is the most important of all of man's sensory organs which come into play when he is flying. A pilot needs excellent distant vision for locating his plane in space, for spotting enemy planes and targets and for proper identification of signal lights and flares. Faulty interpretation of a colored signal may be disastrous to him or to persons on the ground. Because of the great complexity of instruments in the modern aircraft, proper near vision has increased in importance. The pilot must always see well when watching instruments and indicators. Good depth perception is necessary for landing an airplane or for formation and precision flying. Ground personnel working near runways also must have good distant vision and color perception in order to avoid misinterpreting colored lights from the control tower used as signals for crossing these runways.

A knowledge of the fundamentals of ophthalmology is essential for proper selection and care of the aviator. Eye defects account for about half of the physical disqualifications among applicants for flight training and constitute the most common cause for disqualifications or limitations of the older pilot. Fortunately, the aviator is especially conscious of his eye and usually seeks advice from the flight surgeon when the slightest symptom presents itself. An expression commonly heard in the eye examining room is, "I don't want anything to happen to my eyes, Doc." This extreme concern about his eyes raises questions concerning pathologic conditions, exercises, glasses, etc. Should an ophthalmologic problem arise which is not clear to the flight surgeon, he should consult a qualified ophthalmologist.

ANATOMY AND PHYSIOLOGY

The human eye is a wonderful camera. The cornea and lens refract the light as does the lens of a camera. The iris acts as a shutter, permitting the correct amount of light for a clear picture and eliminates the peripheral light rays of the cornea and lens, thereby minimizing spherical and chromatic aberrations. The cornea has about 40 diopters of refracting power while the lens has about 20 diopters which gives a total of about 60 diopters of refracting power for a normal eye. This corresponds to a very strong convex lens, being five or six times stronger than the usual magnifying glass.

Retina

The retina of the eye corresponds to the film of the camera. Parallel rays of light entering a normal eye are brought to a sharp focus on the retina which has a depth of focus of about 0.50 diopter. As long as the point focus is on the retina or within 0.25 diopter on either side, a normal eye can see 20/20 or better.

In a myopic eye (near sighted) the sharp

focus is in front of the retina, resulting in a blurred image; accommodation in this case must be completely relaxed for best distant vision. In a hyperopic eye (far sighted) the sharp focus is behind the retina unless the eye can accommodate sufficiently to bring the focus forward to the retina. An astigmatic eye does not have a sharp focus but has an elongated, blurred one which is called a conoid. If the conoid is in front of the retina, it is myopic astigmatism; if behind, it is hyperopic astigmatism. Mixed astigmatism results when one end of the conoid is in front of the retina and the other end is behind it. The condition of astigmatism is caused usually by a difference in power of the various meridians of the refracting surfaces and is usually greater in the cornea than in the lens. An eye with an astigmatic focus of not more than 0.50 diopter can see 20/20 if the center of the focus is on the retina. Many astigmatic eyes can see 20/20 with a blurred focus of 0.75 diopter; such eyes usually see better than 20/20 when the astigmatism is corrected by lenses.

Best vision is obtained if the eye can adjust the accommodative mechanism so that the midpoint of the conoid is on the retina. This is possible in hyperopic or mixed astigmatism but not in myopic astigmatism except on viewing close objects. Thus, a normal eye relaxes accommodation when looking at distant objects but accommodates for near objects, a myopic eye relaxes for distant objects and accommodates only slightly or not at all for near objects and a hyperopic eye must accommodate somewhat for distant objects but considerably more for near ones. Myopes are relaxers whereas hyperopes are accommodaters. Myopes have blurred images of distant targets; hyperopes have clear images except they must work to see.

When light falls on the retina it starts a nerve impulse in the rods and cones which is transmitted through one or more neurones to the ganglion cells of the retina. This impulse then travels along the axon of a ganglion cell, through the optic disk, back through the optic nerve to the chiasma. Those axons from each nasal retina cross over in the chiasma to join the axons from the temporal retina from the opposite eye and then go back to the lateral geniculate body. The axons concerned with the pupil reflex and accommodation terminate in the midbrain. New axons originating in the lateral geniculate body pass backward to terminate in the occipital cortex. When the impulse finally reaches the cortex there is conscious vision. Even though extremely rapid in action all of this transmission of nerve impulses takes a considerable amount of time.

Rods and Cones

The cones and rods are the photosensitive cells of vision. Under normal conditions they are stimulated by light and cause the sensation of light in the cortex. When stimulated by some other means, such as electricity, they still cause the sensation of light. The cones are densely packed at the fovea and diminish in number toward the periphery; rods are absent at the fovea but are present everywhere else. Most cones are connected individually to a separate bipolar cell, whereas several rods are connected together to a single bipolar cell. Inasmuch as the cones have this direct connection, they have a greater degree of discrimination, and so a greater degree of visual acuity is possible at the macula. Normal 20/20 vision is macular vision. Only a few degrees peripheral to the macula the vision is only 20/200.

Cones and rods are both sensitive to light but they differ in that the cones work better in daylight whereas the rods work only in dim light. Cone vision is best at the fovea but, inasmuch as no rods are present here, this region is blind for night vision. The eye must look directly at an object for best cone vision but a few degrees to the side of the object for best night vision. Rod vision is nighttime vision whereas cone vision is daytime vision. Cones work best in bright light as long as there is no glare, and cease to function in twilight. They not only have excellent discrimination for fine details, but they also have excellent color perception. Rods have rather poor discrimination for details but excel in detecting movement of objects. They see only shades of black and white and have no color perception. They start functioning when illumination is about equal to that of a full moonlight night and are the only part of the retina that can see an object in starlight.

Good Vision

Vision is the act or faculty of seeing. It is more than being able to read the 20/20 line on the Snellen chart. It is more than being able to read Jaeger 1 size letters on the near vision card. It depends on the proper development of the function of the eyes, their proper utilization and then the proper interpretation by the brain.

Development

At birth an infant has very little vision but he soon learns to see large and bright objects, and in a short time his eyes are held in good alignment so that each eye sees the same object. Fusion develops so that the pictures from each eye are blended into one single picture, and accommodation develops so that this picture is seen more clearly. The brain learns to adjust the eyes so that they always point toward the object of regard. Usually, each eye moves in the same direction but upon looking at a near object each eye turns inward. The midbrain makes these adjustments automatically.

As he develops, certain areas, such as the macular areas in each eye, normally work together and he learns that a point in the nasal retina of one eye usually sees the same object as a point in the temporal retina of the other eye. Such areas in each eye which normally see the same object are called corresponding retinal points and from these points he learns to interpret location as well as distance. If corresponding points are stimulated in each eye, the brain thinks the object is the same distance away as an object being viewed by the maculae. Those objects which stimulate corresponding points lie on a line called the horopter. Objects located off the horopter stimulate noncorresponding points and are seen as two objects (physiologic diplopia). If the diplopia is crossed, the object is nearer than the point of fixation; if the diplopia is homonymous or uncrossed, the object is farther than the point of fixation. An object that is very near the horoptor is not seen as two objects, even though there is a slight noncorrespondence but the sense of depth is still obtained.

This ability to detect depth because of a noncorrespondence, but not sufficient noncorrespondence for diplopia, is called stereopsis. Proper stereopsis depends on proper alignment and may be handicapped by a high phoria, especially with fatigue or hypoxia. Some people have a highly developed stereopsis, whereas others have considerably less or none at all. Development of vision is completed at about age 5 or 6 years, when it normally reaches 20/20. Eyes are held in good alignment and stereopsis has developed. Psychologically, however, there is still much to be developed.

Even if it has developed to 20/20 or better and alignment is good, vision still depends on many factors. Together, both eyes see a visual field of about 185 degrees. Nearly all the vision in this area is 20/200 or less except the portions seen by each macula where it approaches 20/20. In order to see a small object or a large object far away one must look with the fovea. A quick glance does not tell much. One must look directly at the object for a second or two to really see it. When trying to see another plane in the sky, one must systematically cover every 5 to 10 degree area with a 1 second look. Scanning without hesitation every few degrees is not good and scanning too rapidly means loss of details but systematic scanning by hesitating every few degrees is excellent. Many times the peripheral vision detects slight movement, attracting attention for a proper look.

Among the many factors upon which vision is dependent the following may be mentioned briefly. Clearness of atmosphere aids vision as one cannot see well through a haze or fog. Proper contrast helps; more light is needed to see dark thread on dark cloth than for white thread on dark cloth. Camouflage attempts to destroy this contrast. Glare as well as a dirty windshield or canopy reduces vision. The spots of dirt may even be mistaken for distant objects. Familiarity aids in locating an object in the visual field as a mental picture helps in attracting the mind's eye. Accommodative mechanism comes into play when adjusting the focus for near in order to look at charts or instruments and relaxes in order to see distant objects clearly. Complete relaxation takes a few minutes and is aided by viewing a definite distant object, such as the wing tip of large planes or an accompanying plane. During World War II pilots benefited from psychologic training in recognition which was carried out by having them glance very quickly at models or pictures of planes and ships.

As an aid to vision orthoptic exercises have undoubtedly increased the vergences and have been beneficial in some cases in helping to overcome certain heterophorias. Their permanent beneficial effect, without continuation of such exercises, is often questioned in the adult age group. Exercises for changing the refractive state of the eye have been attempted but usually proved unsatisfactory. So often such patients only improved their interpretation of blurs, enabling them to read another line on the eye chart but not really improving their ability to see a smaller object farther away. Correct examination and application of current physical standards on the original flight examination usually eliminates these problems.

Good vision, therefore, depends on a normal optical system, an unobstructed view, correct accommodative adjustment, proper alignment of the eyes, familiarity of objects to be observed and a properly planned scanning procedure consisting of momentary stops for about 1 second every 5 to 10 degrees.

NIGHT VISION

There are two facts about night vision that are important to remember. The first concerns foveal, or central vision. The daylight vision in this area is 20/20 but there is practically no night vision. When an eye attempts to see an unlighted object at night, it will not see that object unless the gaze is directed 5 to 10 degrees to one side. This night blindness of the foveal region is owing to the absence of rods at the fovea. The other important fact to remember is that bright light breaks down the photochemical substances of the rods. It takes time to re-

build these substances before maximum sensitivity is regained.

Adaptation

Cones and rods must have a period of adaption for best vision. Cones light adapt in a matter of a few minutes, but rods do not function at this maximum except in dim light and must go through a longer period of adaptation before they reach this peak. Any sudden exposure to bright light will nullify previous adaptation. About 30 minutes of dark adapting will enable the rods to detect a light about 10,000 times dimmer than when the eye is light adapted. During this time the rhodopsin, or visual purple, builds up in the rods and the iodopsin, or visual violet, builds up in the cones. Excessive light breaks down these substances; even ordinary daylight breaks down the rod substance. The cones reach maximum sensitivity after exposure to bright light in about 8 minutes; rods require about 30 minutes of absolute darkness to reach maximum sensitivity. Light with a wave length greater than 600 mμ is not absorbed by visual purple. The red color of the visual spectrum has this wave length. If such a light is used, the eye is able to see by cone vision and at the same time protect the dark adaptation of the rods. This is the reason for wearing red goggles when becoming dark adapted. Rods, having no color perception, see only by contrast, objects being only lighter or darker than the background. This contrast difference is slight; thus, any obstruction such as a dirty canopy, dirty goggles or a haze is a great handicap. Military pilots are taught to fly low over dark terrain to be below enemy planes and to fly higher over snow, desert and white clouds so that they are above enemy planes if they are to avoid detection at night.

Pilots should be thoroughly dark adapted prior to takeoff at night. They may accomplish this by remaining in total darkness for 30 minutes or by wearing red goggles in a semilighted room. The latter permits them to read maps and see sufficiently to move about. Red goggles are also extremely useful for pilots who need to remain dark adapted for long periods. Although a period of 30 minutes is necessary for dark adaptation, the effect can be lost in a second if a person is

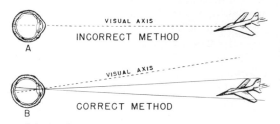

FIG. 127. The correct and incorrect methods of looking at an object in dim illumination.

exposed to a bright light. The eyes work independently so far as adaptation is concerned. Adaptation can be lost in one eye without the other being affected; therefore, if it is necessary to look at a light, such as a search light, gun flash or lighted match one eye should be covered to preserve the adaptation in that eye.

Flashes of lightning occurring during thunderstorms can destroy dark adaptation but this loss is not particularly detrimental because there is scarcely any visibility outside the cockpit. During such flying close observation of instruments is most important and for this, cone vision should be used with about 10 foot candles of white light. Military pilots receive frequent night vision training demonstrations. The present trainer is a projector which pictures typical night outdoor activities projected on a screen at levels of illumination found at night.

Hypoxia and Night Vision

Night vision is decreased by lack of oxygen; at 4000 feet there is a 5 per cent loss which gradually increases to 40 per cent loss at 16,000 feet. In order to avoid even a slight hypoxia, night pilots should use 100 per cent oxygen from the ground up. Excessive smoking may cause an accumulation of carbon monoxide which decreases available oxygen and, in turn, night vision. Accumulation of carbon monoxide from smoking three cigarettes in a row may reduce night vision as much as 25 per cent.

Autokinetic Movements

Eyes may play tricks at night. When staring at a stationary light, autokinetic movements of the eyes may occur, giving the illusion that the light is moving or swinging in wide arcs. If it is a moving light, it may seem to move from side to side. This illusion could be a hazard in formation flying. Sometimes there is an apparent contraction or expansion of light when actually it is approaching or going away. These illusions can be avoided by shifting the gaze to eliminate staring.

Night Myopia

An individual with normal eyes may be somewhat myopic at night. This night myopia may range from 0.25 to 0.75 diopter.

It is thought to be caused by an involuntary accommodation and to spherical aberration from the widely dilated pupil.

Cockpit Illumination

Instrument lighting must be sufficient to enable the pilots to see instruments clearly, but must not be visible to the enemy, nor should it be so bright as to cause loss of dark adaptation. Inasmuch as it is impossible to have optimum light for all purposes, compromises must be made. Over the years there have been three general types of lighting systems in use: (1) ultraviolet flood lighting of fluorescent instrument markings, (2) red flood lighting and (3) red indirect lighting. In the first type which was in use for a long time, a bluish-green fluorescent paint was used on the instruments. That proved to be a poor light for preserving dark adaptation; therefore, an orange fluorescent paint was substituted which provided good contrast. It was satisfactory for reading instruments, but without background lighting there was some trouble with autokinetic movements, fogging of vision by ultrafluorescence of the crystalline lens and loss of dark adaptation. The disadvantages almost outweighed the advantages.

Red flood lighting has been accomplished by lighting the entire instrument panel. In this type of system the total amount of light must be high. There is often difficulty in locating the light source so that all instruments can be seen and still have reflections directed downward away from the pilot's eyes. Red light is most desirable for preserving dark adaptation but it disturbs color relationships on the instruments, maps and charts. Because red objects or lines appear very light while green or blue objects appear very dark and small printed information on aeronautical maps is often unreadable, such markings often become useless to the night flyer. When it becomes necessary for a pilot to read such charts, he may have to use a flash light, preserving dark adaptation at all times by keeping one eye closed. Larger aircraft have compartments where use of white light may be permitted.

Most modern military aircraft use red indirect lighting. Each instrument or group of instruments has a small bulb concealed under the rim or under a small shield which reflects the light onto the face of the instruments. Several rheostats permit control of brightness of various groups of instruments so that illumination with red light having a wave length greater than 600 mμ is provided. This system has several advantages: it is confined to the instrument face and does not flood the cockpit, glare is controlled by rheostats and proper location of the shields, it is not visible to an enemy, and it is excellent for maintaining dark adaptation. However, there are also disadvantages: some markings, knobs and switches are not a part of an instrument and are, therefore, poorly lighted. Attempts have been made to correct this in some planes by having a red light above and behind the pilot for illuminating these unlighted areas. A few instruments are partially obstructed by the lighting shields, especially when viewed at an extreme angle. Red indirect lighting is not the final answer to cockpit lighting but at the present time it is the most satisfactory of all the methods.

Vitamin A

Vitamin A deficiency decreases night vision but an excess does not increase it. Vitamins A, B and C are indicated when the diet is inadequate. Several weeks or months of treatment may be necesary after a starvation diet. In spite of sufficient Vitamin A night vision often decreases with age, especially after 40.

VISUAL PROBLEMS OF HIGH ALTITUDE

Modern aviation has presented many new problems. In the early days of flying the problems were chiefly mechanical, the planes were crude and slow, engines had only low horsepower and altitudes over 10,000 feet were unusual. Fatigue presented somewhat of a problem but most planes could not remain aloft long enough for this to be important. Then the designs improved, horsepower was increased and a host of new problems presented themselves.

High Altitude Hypoxia

From the standpoint of the eye, low oxygen tension was one of the first problems encountered. Ordinary daytime vision begins to be affected by hypoxia at 10,000 feet; from 10,000 to 16,000 feet the pilot is able to overcome most visual difficulties unless he remains at this altitude for several hours. The effects of decreased oxygen tension in this altitude zone gradually increase as the altitude increases. The retinal vessels become dark and cyanotic; retinal arterioles increase 10 to 20 per cent in diameter; retinal blood volume increases up to four times; retinal arteriolar pressure increases along with the systemic blood pressure; intraocular tension shows a slight increase; the pupil constricts; and accommodation and convergence powers are decreased (1, 2). There is a decreased urge to hold fusion and so less ability to overcome heterophoria. There is even an increased tendency toward esophoria with less fusion ability to overcome it. Night vision at altitude is affected as low as 4000 feet where there is about a 5 per cent loss. At 6000 feet there is a 10 per cent loss, at 10,000, a 20 per cent and at 16,000, a 40 per cent loss. To avoid visual difficulties owing to hypoxia it is necessary to use oxygen above 10,000 feet in daytime flying and above 5000 feet in night flying.

From 16,000 to 25,000 feet only a few minutes without oxygen slows the visual reaction time. The fusion mechanism can no longer control heterophorias and they become heterotropias with double vision. Depth perception by stereopsis is lost, accommodation is weakened and instruments appear to be blurred and double. All these difficulties are eliminated by breathing oxygen. Above 25,000 feet, even when breathing 100 per cent oxygen, symptoms of hypoxia begin to appear which are similar to those encountered at lower levels without oxygen and at 42,000 feet oxygen tension equals that experienced at 18,000 feet while breathing air.

Decompression Sickness

Symptoms of decompression may occur even with the use of 100 per cent oxygen at 25,000 feet or above. Cerebral air emboli can produce migrainelike symptoms with scintillating scotomata which are often hemianopic in type and vision is reduced. Decompression sickness is usually prevented by denitrogenation prior to flying and by pressurization equal to 25,000 feet or below when flying.

Acceleration

Changes in acceleration affect vision regardless of the attitude. When centrifugal force is increased in the head-to-seat direction (positive g), there is less blood flowing to the brain and retina. If the retinal arterial pressure falls below the intraocular pressure (usually 20 mm. of Hg), visual function is impaired. In general, a force of 3.5 to 4.0 g causes loss of peripheral vision with a greying of central vision, called a grey out. A force of 4.0 to 4.5 g or more produces a total loss of vision, with the sensation of blackout. The g tolerance may be increased by placing the pilot in a dorsal or prone position, but inasmuch as this is usually impractical, tolerance is increased by pressure breathing or by enclosing the lower part of the body in a g suit. Forces in the seat-to-head direction (negative g) cause a congestion of the upper part of the body from which hemorrhages of the retina and anterior chamber might be expected but have not occurred experimentally. A sensation of red out has been described and is also difficult to produce experimentally. It is thought to be caused by the movement of the lower lid up over the eye, obstructing the vision, but this explanation has often been questioned.

Glare

Whiteside (3) has referred to a reversed light distribution present at high altitudes and first noticed at about 30,000 feet where the greater part of the atmosphere is underneath. At lower altitudes the bright sky usually seen is the result of light reflected from particles in the atmosphere but at high altitude most of the atmosphere is below and so the brightness is from below. Above, it is relatively darker except in the direct sunlight which appears brighter because of the absence of air. The brow and upper lid will protect the eye from the glare at lower altitudes but not at higher ones where there is an increased brightness in the lower lateral parts of the visual fields. This brightness causes a scattering of light within the eye which results in haziness of vision. Such glare is best controlled by sun glasses or visors. Reversed light distribution also accounts for less light on the instruments as the light from the atmosphere below cannot reach them. This resulting poor contrast can be aided by increased lighting of instruments. Windows on the side walls of the cockpit would help

provided there was no direct glare to the pilot.

Space Myopia

At lower altitudes the eyes nearly always have some object in view; it may be an object on the ground or a cloud in the sky. When looking for distant objects such as approaching aircraft, it is easy for the accommodative mechanism to adjust for distance. When a picture is formed on the retina, the accommodative mechanism attempts to adjust itself for the clearest possible picture. When there is nothing to see, there is no incentive for this adjustment to occur so that instead of the complete relaxation needed for viewing a distant object, there may be an accommodation of 0.50 to 1.50 diopters. This would be excellent for a hyperopic eye but is bad for a normal or myopic eye. In the latter, objects must be larger or closer before they can be detected. This tonic state of accommodation may be increased by nervous tension, or by frequent viewing of near objects, such as instruments or particles of dirt on the canopy.

A satisfactory answer to the empty visual field problems is difficult. Selection of pilots who are about 1.00 diopter hyperopic might be considered because when such eyes are accommodated 1.00 diopter, the eye would be adjusted to distant objects. Pilots with normal or slightly myopic eyes frequently interrupt the distant scanning procedures by looking at a definite object, such as the tip of the wing, provided it is at least 20 feet away. Inasmuch as modern planes have wings shorter than 20 feet, the pilot should look at an accompanying plane at frequent intervals, probably every 3 or 4 seconds. Perhaps a better solution lies in an electronic device which will do the seeing for him.

VISUAL PROBLEMS OF HIGH SPEED FLYING

Speeds in excess of 1200 miles per hour have been reported. Recent advances in technical skill and materials make the speed of the future not only unpredictable but almost unbelievable. The mechanism of seeing, which takes a certain amount of time, provides insufficient vision at these speeds.

Byrnes (4) has discussed this problem in an excellent manner and has made calculations of this time and speed. It takes 0.4 second after an object is detected in the periphery before it is seen by the fovea and 1.0 second elapses before the object is recognized. A plane going 1800 miles per hour covers about 1 mile every 2 seconds and would, therefore, travel 3683 feet from the time of appearance of an object to the time of its recognition. Byrnes further stated that if two planes emerged from clouds on collision courses 3000 feet apart, they would collide before the pilots could do anything to avoid it. If the planes were only 500 feet apart, they would collide without either pilot seeing the other. Byrnes stated that it takes 2.39 seconds to turn the eye from clear distance vision to an instrument, accommodate properly, read the dial with recognition, turn the eyes back to the distant object and relax the accommodation properly for clear distant vision. A plane could travel 6336 feet while this cycle was being completed. In older pilots accommodation time as well as relaxation time when changing from near to distant vision is even longer.

Concerning acceleration effects which have also increased with the speed of planes, Byrnes pointed out that at 2000 miles per hour a pilot could not turn in a circle less than 18 miles in diameter without blacking out because of a centrifugal force of 6 g.

Other problems of high speed flying are those of depth perception and vibration. Depth perception may be erroneous because of displacement of an object by the optical effect of shock waves as well as of heat waves. Vibration may account for a transient blurring seen often when passing the sonic barrier. Increased temperatures of aircraft at supersonic speeds has been suggested as a possible hazard to vision, but the eyes can actually withstand an air temperature higher than the lungs can tolerate, somewhere around 240° F. Eyes can also probably withstand greater air blasts than the surrounding facial tissues if ejection at extremely high speeds becomes necessary.

All these figures and facts serve to point up the necessity for installing electronic devices in supersonic aircraft. Such devices which react much faster than any human are currently being developed.

VISUAL PROTECTIVE DEVICES

In the earlier days of aviation when planes had open cockpits, goggles were worn to protect the eyes from wind and dirt. The modern plane has a closed cockpit, but eyes still need protection from harmful rays of the sun, glare, fire, extreme cold, wind, enemy flak and loose objects in the aircraft. Recent high altitude flying has emphasized the importance of protection from glare and invisible rays.

Visible light includes electromagnetic wave lengths from 400 to 750 mμ (5), and most people are comfortable as long as the light intensity is not over 10,000 foot candles which is the usual intensity at sea level on a clear day. At 10,000 feet the intensity of light is 12,000 foot candles and about 13,600 foot candles in extraterrestial space. At these levels light is too intense for comfort. Eyes are also uncomfortable when there is too much reflected light or glare as from snow, white sand and clouds. Snow sometimes reflects back 85 to 90 per cent of the light which strikes it resulting in not only an uncomfortable glare but also in diminished vision by interference with cone adaptation.

Excessive light and glare contain other wave lengths which are not visible. Below 400 mμ are the ultraviolet rays which can produce a slight haziness in vision by their scattering effect in the lens and also can cause an actinic conjunctivitis by their absorption in the cornea and conjunctiva. This condition resembles the familiar flash burn of the welder. At high altitudes there is not only a greater intensity of light but also more ultraviolet rays. These rays, which are partially absorbed by dissociated oxygen, are more numerous above 100,000 feet and may become more of a hazard at extremely high altitudes. Infrared rays range from 750 to 2100 mμ wave length. These rays penetrate deeper into the eye and can cause retinal burns with permanent damage to the macular area. Cataracts have developed after repeated long exposures to infrared rays in certain occupations, such as in glass blowers.

Sun Glasses and Visors

Various filters which serve to eliminate or filter out a portion of the light are used to protect the eyes. Inasmuch as these filters have the same effect on normal light as they do on glaring light, sometimes vision is handicapped in the reduction of normal light in the effort to reduce or get rid of the glare.

Crown glass, the glass usually used in spectacles, eliminates most of the ultraviolet light and transmits all but about 8 per cent of visible and infrared light; with the addition of a coating of magnesium fluorite it will transmit all but 4 per cent. Ordinary clear plastic lenses transmit ultraviolet light, as does the plastic currently used in aircraft canopies, whereas most dark tinted plastics transmit infrared but not ultraviolet.

COLORED FILTERS. These filters absorb more light of certain wave lengths. Generally, a green glass permits more of the color green to come through but eliminates a higher percentage of the other colors whereas yellow eliminates more blue and dark green and permits more red, orange, yellow and light green to be transmitted. The major criticism concerning the use of colored filters centers around the slight distortion of colors which they cause. The green sunglass in common use, such as the "Calobar D" or the "Ray-Ban 3," transmits about 25 per cent of visible light, less than 5 per cent of ultraviolet and less than 10 per cent of infrared. Except for the slight color distortion they are quite satisfactory. The use of yellow filters has been advocated in fog or haze. Blue and blue-green light is scattered more under these conditions and not transmitted by yellow. There is a sensation of increased brightness, but carefully controlled experiments have failed to show any increase in vision through the use of yellow or amber lenses in a fog or haze.

NEUTRAL FILTERS. Neutral filter sun glasses and visors are currently being used by the aviation branch of the armed forces. These absorb equal amounts of all wave lengths of light, always appear to be grey in color and serve to reduce light without changing or distorting the colors. These sun glasses have a lens similar to the "Ray-Ban G-15," and light transmission is like that of green sun glasses but may even eliminate a little more of the infrared. The main advantage of the neutral grey sun glasses is in the lack of distortion of colors.

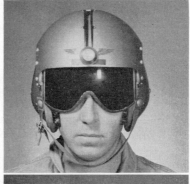
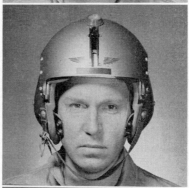
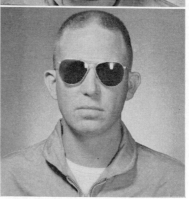

FIG. 128. Photographs showing, from top to bottom, helmet with sun visor down, sun visor up and aviation sun glasses.

Sun visors now used by the armed forces are also neutral grey. Some of them are lighter in the lower part to facilitate reading of the instrument panel. In order to satisfy individual preferences of the pilots there are four different shades. The very dark shade transmits 5 to 6 per cent light; dark transmits 6 to 8 per cent, medium dark 8 to 10 per cent, and the lightest shade transmits 10 to 20 per cent.

REFLECTING FILTERS. A portion of light is

transmitted and the remainder is reflected back through the use of reflecting filters. They act like silvered mirrors and have the appearance of a small mirror. The reflecting coating usually is a mixture of chrome and nickel. Most neutral reflecting lenses transmit more infrared than the neutral absorbing lenses. Another disadvantage is that the coating is easily damaged when the glass is cleaned. Colored sun glasses often have a reflecting filter added to the upper one third or to both the upper and lower thirds of the lenses. Such glasses are commonly called "graded density lenses." Use of these is advantageous when intense light and glare from above and below is present, as when boating or when travelling over snow.

POLARIZING FILTERS. This type of filter transmits only light vibrating in a certain direction and absorbs light vibrating in other directions. They transmit usually about 30 per cent of the light unless they are polarized in one particular plane and are ordinarily combined with a color filter when used as sun glasses. Polarizing filters are not neutral ones and transmit more of some wave lengths than others. They are laminated lenses which are difficult and expensive to make especially when curved ones are necessary. The use of polarizing lenses has been advocated for seeing submerged objects, such as submarines, because of absorption of polarized light from the surface of the water. However, they not only absorb this polarized light but also light from the surface of the submerged object and thus offer no advantage. Experimental tests have failed to show any superiority of polarizing lenses for seeing submerged objects. They are useful only in reducing over-all brightness and glare especially when the sun is glaring off a pavement or off water directly into the eyes. In this instance they have a specific effect of eliminating the bright glare more than the surrounding light. Only a polarizing glass can do this.

In general, sun glasses and visors reduce over-all brightness to a level comfortable for the eyes. Lenses with 10 to 15 per cent light transmission are probably best for sun glasses. Neutral grey is probably the best filter. It is preferable to have visors somewhat darker, about 8 to 10 per cent light transmission for high altitude flying. There it is excellent for glare but does not permit sufficient light for landing, especially on a cloudy day. If visors darker than 10 per cent transmission are used, they should be removed prior to landing. Visors are worn at high altitudes to protect eyes against glare and they act as protection against wind blast as well as help to hold the oxygen mask in place in case of bailout at high speed. Sun visors, now used, give little or no protection against infrared; even if they are very dark, they give a false sense of security against infrared. Aviators should be cautioned against looking directly into the sun.

GOGGLES. Goggles are still used in low flying planes which are open. They are useful in protecting eyes from wind, flash flames, prolonged fire and from flying missiles from gunfire. Goggles usually are made of plastics and require especial care in cleaning to avoid scratching. In high altitude flying they have almost been completely replaced by the visor which is attached to the helmet.

Red goggles are used for dark adaptation prior to night flying. For best night vision they should be worn 15 minutes in light followed by 15 minutes in absolute darkness. They are usually contained in a leather frame so they may be folded for easy storage in a pocket and, thus, be available if lights are turned on in the aircraft.

COMPARISON OF VISUAL STANDARDS OF TRAINED AND STUDENT AVIATORS

Especially in the military services, visual standards vary with training and experience of the aviator. Once a man is a trained pilot, it is a matter of deciding if he is safe to continue flying. When examining an applicant for flight training, however, the flight surgeon must decide not only whether the candidate is safe to fly but also whether he will be a safe flyer for a period which may vary from 5 to 20 years, depending upon the needs of the services.

Trained Aviator

To be safe to continue flying the trained pilot must have normal distant vision, normal depth perception and normal near vision.

Normal distant vision is considered to be 20/20 on a Snellen chart. Eyes with small refractive errors can usually attain that score through the process of squinting which involves a contraction of the orbicularis oculi, partially closing the lids and exerting a slight pressure on the eyeball. If an eye of 20/30 or better is correctable by lenses, it is ordinarily safe to assume that it can see 20/20 by squinting. Eyes of worse than 20/30 visual acuity cannot see 20/20 by squinting and have enough refractive error to usually justify corrective lenses. Experience has shown that whereas most people with 20/40 vision can do most jobs without glasses, a pilot, however, must be able to produce 20/20 vision without lenses when necessary; therefore, he must have at least 20/30 vision without squinting in each eye. Usually, eyes which cannot be corrected to 20/20 by squinting have had some pathology or did not develop to 20/20. Pilots who fly the high altitude, high speed planes of today have enough difficulties with helmets, visors, oxygen masks, pressure suits, bailout equipment, etc., so that the wearing of corrective lenses, although perhaps not impossible, is certainly impracticable and is not recommended. A trained aviator, therefore, should have an uncorrected visual acuity of 20/30 or better to fly unrestricted. Perhaps future flying will emphasize the importance of near vision over distant vision, but airplanes still must land; distant vision is then a necessity.

Normal depth perception, also a must for unrestricted pilots, is present when visual acuity is not worse than 20/30, but squinting to attain this may be necessary. Current tests of depth perception are mostly tests for stereopsis and include the Verhoeff Stereopter test for stereopsis at 1 meter and the Howard-Dolman apparatus test for stereopsis at 20 feet. The latter is not an apparatus for testing pure stereopsis unless the test is given properly and even then parallax and familiarity of sizes may aid the subject in obtaining a score sufficient to pass. Older aviators, especially those who are hyperopic, may have lost some of their accommodative ability. They may have normal stereopsis by the Howard-Dolman test at 20 feet, but may not have sufficient stereopsis at 1 meter to pass the Verhoeff test. Accurate depth perception is required more when landing a plane and when estimating the position of distant objects. All pilots should have sufficient depth perception to pass the Howard-

Dolman test but it is not considered necessary for older pilots to pass the Verhoeff test at 1 meter, assuming their previous flying has demonstrated good depth perception by their having had no difficulty with landings or formation flying.

The ability to read maps, radio dial settings, and instruments quickly and accurately is an essential for the unrestricted pilot. Near vision, which is usually measured by Jaeger test types, should be such that he is able to see Jaeger no. 1, and he should have enough accommodative ability to see it as close as 40 cm., or about 16 inches. This indicates an accommodation of about 2.5 diopters. If a pilot is unable to read the small print within 16 inches, corrective lenses for near are probably indicated; thus, he should not be permitted to fly unrestricted.

Private flying in small cabin planes, ordinary commercial flying and certain military flying can be carried out without the use of helmets, visors and oxygen masks. In such flying pilots may be permitted to wear corrective lenses, but their uncorrected vision should not be so poor that a safe landing in case of emergency could not be accomplished without glasses. Visual acuity then should not be worse than 20/50, correctable to 20/20 by lenses, because when worse than that or when accommodation is less than 2 diopters, pilots flying without wearing corrective lenses are not considered safe. Even when wearing them they may not be safe in certain emergencies. Some military pilots whose vision becomes worse than 20/50 are permitted to fly military aircraft only if they are accompanied by an unrestricted pilot as a co-pilot. If their vision becomes worse than 20/100, they are no longer permitted to fly a military plane.

Student Aviator

When a candidate student aviator is examined for private flying, the standards of the trained aviator may often be applied but when he is examined for training as a military pilot, the standards must be more stringent. He should have 20/20 vision in each eye without correction. Refraction should be done and should show no myopia or, at most, not more than 0.25 diopter. Young men near 20 years of age sometimes become more myopic. If they are myopic at that age, they may progress so much they will be unable to see 20/30 before they have done any useful flying as unrestricted pilots. There should not be more than 0.75 diopter astigmatism. More than this gives a focus too blurred for normal vision and, in addition, these astigmatics often suffer from eye strain when reading or flying by instruments. There should not be more than 2.00 diopters of hyperopia if the selection is for 15 or 20 years unrestricted flying. Those pilots with more hyperopia than this will probably have eye strain symptoms in their late thirties and may need correcting lenses for near, placing them in a restricted status. If selection is for only 5 or 10 years of unrestricted flying, a hyperopia of 2.50 diopters would be permissible.

Anisometropia (each eye having a different refractive error) should not be greater than 0.75 diopter. A difference of refraction of only 0.75 to 1.00 diopter has been the cause of eye strain symptoms. An anisometropia of 2.50 to 3.00 diopters usually makes good central fusion impossible or extremely difficult. Students with such eyes may have some stereopsis but usually not sufficient to pass the Verhoeff test. A student should have sufficient stereopsis to pass this test.

Accommodation should not be less than 3.00 diopters below the normal for his age. If less than this, he may tire too easily when reading or doing instrument flying, needing corrective lenses for near vision sooner than normally expected. If accommodation is greater than normal, he may have extremely good accommodative power or it may be indicative of a myopia, in which case his distant vision would not be normal.

Indications for Corrective Lenses

Corrective lenses for an adult have two main indications. They either help the patient to see better or they help him to feel better. They often do both. In aviation greater emphasis is placed on helping the pilot to see better, although sometimes the purpose is for comfort alone.

When distant visual acuity is worse than 20/30 in either eye because of a refractive error, lenses should be prescribed for distant vision. If there is such anisometropia that it interferes with proper stereopsis, then lenses may be prescribed for this reason. When accommodation is less than 2.50 diopters, lenses should be prescribed for near vision. If lenses are needed for distant vision, accommodation should be measured with the correction in place to be certain near vision is adequate. A pilot must always have clear distant vision and clear near vision available at all times. If the distant correction does not permit adequate near vision or if the near correction does not permit adequate distant vision, then a bifocal should be worn. If lenses are considered necessary for distant vision, they should be worn most of the time so that the pilot becomes accustomed to them. Depth perception is often different with a correction. It is usually improved when the eyes become accustomed to the lenses but, at first, it may be erroneous. It is often advisable for a pilot, making his first flight with corrective lenses, to be accompanied by another pilot in order to be certain his depth perception is not erroneous.

Pilots with a slight refractive error, such as a myopia of 0.25 to 0.50 diopter, but who can still see 20/30 or better without lenses, often desire a correction for this error. If the type of flying they are doing allows the use of spectacles it is permissible and often wise to wear a correction. In order to ensure proper depth perception such lenses should be worn most of the time for distant vision. If the lenses are worn only occasionally, then they should not be worn when flying. If the type of flying prohibits the use of spectacles, the lenses should not be worn more than occasionally.

When prescription lenses are needed for any reason while flying, both clear glasses and sun glasses should be prescribed. Prescription lenses should be free from defects. They should be properly placed so that the optical center is directly in front of the pupils to avoid prismatic effect. The line of sight should strike the lens at a perpendicular when a person is looking straight ahead or slightly downward to avoid undesirable cylindric effect. Frames should fit snugly but should not be uncomfortably tight.

Contact lenses have been suggested for aviators. They have an advantage over spectacles in that they could be worn with the usual oxygen masks, helmets and visors.

They also have some disadvantages. Many people cannot tolerate them. The small corneal type contact lens, which seems to be tolerated best, sometimes becomes displaced under the lid or is dropped. Removal and replacement of the lens for relief of irritation or for changing from a tinted to a clear lens would be difficult to accomplish while piloting the modern high speed aircraft. In general, the disadvantages outweigh the advantages and the use of contact lenses is not recommended for aviators at the present time.

The Prescription

In order to prescribe lenses correctly the true total refractive error of the eyes must be known. This is probably best determined in patients under 30 years of age by a cycloplegic refraction. For patients over 30 years the fogging type of refraction is usually satisfactory if done properly. Once the refractive error is known, one must decide if corrective lenses are indicated. An aviator who has normal distant vision, near vision and depth perception, and who has no symptoms indicating eye strain, does not need corrective lenses and none should be prescribed. If there are symptoms of blurred vision or eye strain, then the following suggestions may be used as a guide. Glasses may be indicated for aviators with:

1. Myopia of 0.75 or more diopters to improve distant vision.
2. Astigmatism of 1.00 or more diopters to improve vision and eliminate eye strain.
3. Anisometropia of 1.00 or more diopters to eliminate eye strain and improve stereopsis.
4. Hyperopia of 3.00 or more diopters to eliminate eye strain and improve near vision.
5. Hyperopia greater than half of the amount of normal accommodation for his age to eliminate eye strain and improve near vision.
6. Emmetropia with inadequate accommodation, to improve near vision.

When glasses are indicated, the proper prescription must be determined. To do this, it is well to know the spheric equivalent of the refractive error of each eye. Spheric equivalent is the total of the spheric correction added to half of the cylindric correction.

For example, a refractive error of +2.50 sphere combined with a −1.00 cylinder at axis 180 degrees has a spheric equivalent of +2.00 diopters. The direction of the axis is not used in this determination. If the spheric equivalent of the correcting lens is positive, the eye is hyperopic or has hyperopic astigmatism. Hyperopic eyes accommodate to see well and are accustomed to accommodating. If the spheric equivalent is negative, the eye is myopic or has myopic astigmatism. Such eyes must relax to see well at distance and are accustomed to relaxing accommodation. In general, an eye with a negative spheric equivalent will like the full basic correction, and this should be prescribed if it is comfortable. Never prescribe more negative than the full error. An eye with a positive spheric equivalent is accustomed to accommodating and will usually not be comfortable with the full basic prescription after the effects of the cycloplegic are gone. For purposes of comfort and to avoid blurred vision in the distance, the spheric component of the correction should be reduced. For example, an older aviator with an error of +2.50 sphere combined with −0.50 cylinder at axis 180 degrees may see only 20/40 with this correction, but will be comfortable and see 20/20 with a reduction of +0.75 sphere, the resulting prescription then being +1.75 sphere combined with −0.50 cylinder at axis 180 degrees. Usually the power of the cylinder should not be changed. Inasmuch as accommodation is usually equal in each eye, if the spheric value is reduced in one eye, it should be reduced the same amount in the other. The amount of reduction is determined by reducing the spheric component of the correction of both eyes at the same time until good comfortable distant vision is obtained. It should never be reduced an amount equal to or greater than the spheric equivalent. For example, if the error of +2.50 sphere combined with −0.50 cylinder at axis 180° degrees, having a spheric equivalent of +2.00, were reduced 2.25 diopters giving a +0.25 sphere combined with −0.50 cylinder at axis 180 degrees, a person would be wearing a spheric equivalent of plane glass, and his symptoms would probably not be relieved. He actually must accommodate more wearing this correction than he did without any correction.

He would have only the benefit of a sharp focus instead of an astigmatic focus.

After the prescription is determined for distance, near vision should be checked. If he can read Jaeger no. 1 print comfortably at about 33 cm. or 13 inches, the prescription is also adequate for near vision. In older aviators who are presbyopic, more positive sphere may have to be added for near vision. In such cases bifocal lenses should be prescribed. An addition of at least +1.00 diopter is usually necessary before bifocals are indicated. They are seldom necessary prior to age 40 and often not until ages 46 to 48.

Functional Visual Difficulties

Recent advances in speed and altitude have increased the responsibilities and the work load of the pilot. He has more things to see and do and less time in which to do them. Sometimes the problems become too great for him, but his pride will not permit him to quit. Such pilots may develop defective visual acuity for distance or for near and accommodation may be less. They may complain of blurred vision or a defect in the field of vision. Visual fields are often constricted or the size of the field may be the same for several distances from the screen. Pilots may complain of photophobia, headaches, weaknesses and maybe even diplopia. These symptoms are more prevalent among student aviators, especially those who are nearing completion of their training. A careful thorough ophthalmic examination is always indicated. Usually, the findings are variable and inconsistent and, along with the absence of pathologic findings, are indicative of the functional nature of these conditions. Such cases deserve a thorough psychiatric evaluation and often are not considered safe for continued flying.

REFERENCES

(1) Department of the Air Force: Flight Surgeon's Manual. AF Manual 160-5. Washington, D. C., United States Air Force, 1954.
(2) Department of the Navy, Bureau of Medicine and Surgery: Aviation Medicine Practice. NAVPERS 10839-A. Washington, D. C., Government Printing Office, 1955.
(3) Whiteside, T. C. D.: The Problems of Vision in Flight at High Altitude. NATO AGARDograph 13. London, Butterworth Scientific Publications, 1957.
(4) Byrnes, V. A.: Visual Problems of Supersonic Speed. Am. J. Ophth., 34: 169–177, 1951.
(5) Adler, F. H.: Physiology of the Eye: Clinical Application. St. Louis, C. V. Mosby Co., 1950.

22

CARDIOVASCULAR CONSIDERATIONS

Lawrence E. Lamb, M.D.

The circulatory system provides a means of internal respiration and metabolism at a cellular level. It is one of the vital functions of the body. Transitory changes in circulatory dynamics may drastically impair body function or result in loss of life itself. Aviation presents many unaccustomed stresses to body function. In order to cope successfully with these environmental changes adaptations must be made. Not infrequently, successful adaptation to flying stresses is dependent upon the response of the cardiovascular system. As such, the cardiovascular dynamics associated with the stresses of modern aviation provide a major and interesting segment of aviation medicine. A very high percentage of medical problems related to flying which confront the flight surgeon are cardiovascular in nature. The importance of the circulatory system as a limiting factor in man's adaptation to the flying environment has increased as the biologic stresses attendant to modern aviation have increased. At the threshold of man's conquest of space, cardiovascular dynamics may prove to be man's greatest obstacle to success.

Mechanics of Circulation

In carrying out its vital function of delivering oxygen to the body cells and transporting carbon dioxide to the lungs for dis-posal, the circulatory system is the transport mechanism between the source of supply and the point of demand. Alterations in the supply of oxygen to the circulating blood or changes in oxygen demand (metabolic requirements) necessitate circulatory adaptations and may alter circulatory dynamics. With increased metabolic states, more oxygen must be delivered by the circulatory system to the tissue cell in order that its increased metabolic function may be carried out. In hypometabolic states the requirement for oxygen delivery is diminished and the circulatory system need not deliver so much oxygen to the cell.

The characteristics of the circulatory system as a transport mechanism are commonly defined in terms of content, capacity, saturation and tension. Relative to oxygen, the following terms can be defined:

Oxygen content is the amount of oxygen which is being carried in the circulating blood volume (19 cc. per 100 cc.). The amount of oxygen within the blood stream is the amount of oxygen being carried by the red blood cells as well as the plasma.

Oxygen capacity is the amount of oxygen that the blood is capable of containing. Thus, if the blood were to be completely saturated with as much oxygen as it could possibly contain, this is spoken of as its oxygen capacity. In common usage, oxygen capacity

415

is ordinarily given in values which are obtained at ground level; however, it may be expressed in reference to other environmental circumstances.

Oxygen saturation is the ratio of the amount of oxygen contained within the blood (content) to the capacity of the blood stream to carry oxygen. Thus, if 100 cc. of blood contains 15 cc. of oxygen (oxygen content equals 15 cc.) and, on exposure to room air,

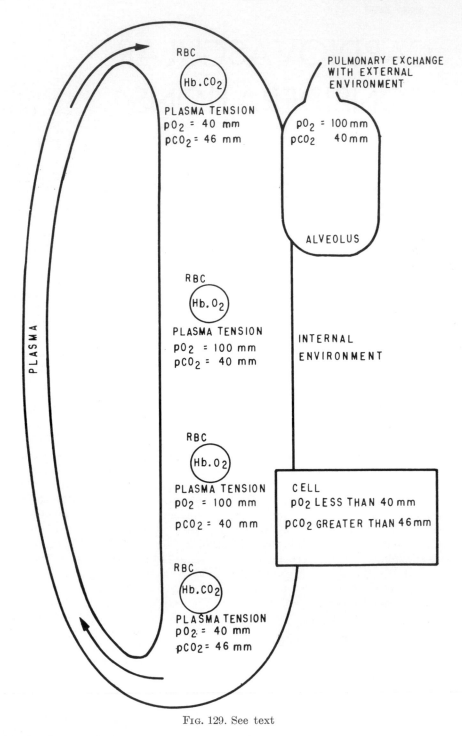

Fig. 129. See text

it absorbed 20 cc. of oxygen (oxygen capacity equals 20 cc.), the oxygen saturation is 75 per cent.

Oxygen tension is the pressure in millimeters of mercury exerted by oxygen within the plasma. Assuming no other complicating factors are present, the exchange of gases into and out of the circulating blood is entirely dependent upon the pressure exerted by the gas within the circulating blood volume and the pressure of the gases in the surrounding medium (fig. 129). To indicate oxygen tension the symbol pO_2 is used.

The relationship between the supply, demand and transport mechanisms can best be illustrated by a practical problem (fig. 130). If the body utilizes (demands) 200 cc. of oxygen per minute, the ventilatory mechanisms must supply 200 cc. of oxygen to the circulating blood. Let it be assumed that when the circulating blood leaves the point of supply at the alveolus it contains 19 cc. of oxygen for each 100 cc. unit of blood. As the cellular tissues are bathed with the cir-

culating blood, oxygen is removed to supply the metabolic demands. If 5 cc. of oxygen are removed from each 100 cc. units of blood which perfuses the body tissues, the oxygen content of the circulating blood when it returns to the right heart will be 14 cc. of oxygen per 100 cc. of blood. Therefore, 5 cc. of oxygen were extracted for each of the 100 cc. units of circulating blood (19 cc. minus 14 cc.). In order to deliver 200 cc. of oxygen demanded by the body, 40 units of blood, each amounting to 100 cc., must perfuse the body tissues (40 times 100 cc., making a total of 4000 cc.), or the cardiac output required to deliver 200 cc. of oxygen from the point of supply to the point of demand is 4 liters.

Alterations in the metabolic demands of the body necessarily affect both the supply and transport mechanisms. As a simple illustration, during physical activity the metabolic demands are increased. If the metabolic demands require 400 cc. of oxygen per minute, the ventilatory system must

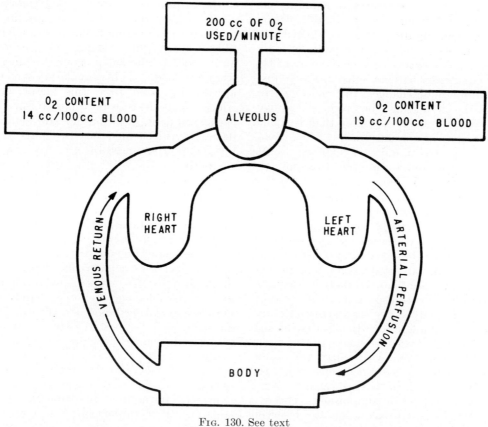

Fig. 130. See text

adjust in order to provide a constant supply of oxygen to efficiently saturate the circulating blood volume. The circulatory system in this instance could double its cardiac output to 8 liters per minute in order to deliver the 400 cc. of oxygen. Another mechanism of adjustment by the circulatory system is increased extraction of oxygen from the circulating blood as it perfuses the body tissues. Both increased cardiac output and increased oxygen extraction are commonly employed compensatory mechanisms.

Metabolic demands may be increased by physical activity, digestion or excitement, and must be considered in the total picture of circulatory dynamics during flight. Alteration in oxygen supply is commonly encountered in aviation and affects the circulatory dynamics. Under usual circumstances in aviation, these are associated with increasing altitude. The ventilatory system makes the early adjustment for these changes. In so doing, it maintains a normal oxygen tension within the alveolus of approximately 100 mm. of Hg. Simple diffusion across the pulmonary membrane creates an equal oxygen tension of 100 mm. of Hg in the plasma. When compensations by the ventilatory mechanisms are no longer capable of maintaining an oxygen tension of 100 mm. of Hg, the circulatory system must make adjustments for these changes. In essence, at this point the circulating blood receives less oxygen from the point of supply than it should under normal circumstances. This means that more blood must be exposed to the lower oxygen tension in order to supply the cellular demand. Thus, as the oxygen tension decreases within the alveolus, circulation must increase.

The mechanics of the circulation are markedly affected by changes in the transport mechanism or the circulating blood volume. When the metabolic demands remain constant and the ventilatory supply is adequate, changes in the transport mechanism alone can profoundly alter cardiovascular dynamics. A simple illustration is that of anemia. Normal oxygen tension may be present in the alveolus but when there are insufficient numbers of red blood cells within the circulating blood, the oxygen capacity of the circulating blood is diminished. The red blood cell is best looked upon as a reservoir

for the transport of gases. Oxygen combines with hemoglobin within the red blood cell molecule at a ratio of 1.34 cc. per gram of hemoglobin. When the hemoglobin content within the cell is diminished, or if hemoglobin in the circulating blood is diminished by virtue of absence of red blood cells, it is obvious that less oxygen can be transported per unit of blood. This requires that many more units of blood must be circulated to supply the same amount of oxygen demanded by the tissues. This same mechanism may be precipitated by a variety of circumstances which cause the hemoglobin to become ineffective, including the hemoglobinopathies such as sickle cell anemia, and chemical alterations in hemoglobin resulting from toxic influences such as carbon monoxide.

It is clear that the approach to the circulatory dynamics in any one individual during exposure to flying stresses must involve consideration of all three principles—supply, demand and transport. Although an individual may sustain a minor variation in one of these areas, compounding the stress with changes in all three areas can cause an individual to be unable to make the adaptations necessary during flight. Let us consider an individual who has a significant anemia. The work load upon his circulatory system is already increased from this factor alone, which affects the transport mechanism. If he is engaged in physical activity, the metabolic demands will be increased by muscular effort. This, too, increases the load on the circulatory system. If, in addition to these two problems, we expose such an individual to sufficient altitude as to diminish the supply of oxygen to circulating blood, we introduce still a third reason to increase the work load on the circulatory system. When all three are significant factors (severe anemia, marked increase in metabolic demand and diminished oxygen supply), life itself may not be possible. On the other hand, with normal circulating blood for the transport mechanism and lungs able to compensate for altitude changes in maintaining an adequate oxygen supply to the circulating blood volume, the increased metabolic demands occasioned by exercise could have no significance. Without a fundamental understanding of the interrelationship of these three fundamental mechanisms—supply, demand and transport—one cannot possibly evaluate the stresses imposed upon the circulatory system in any individual case.

CAPILLARY CIRCULATION

Exchange of fluid between the circulating plasma and the extracellular compartment is a function of the capillary circulation. The plasma proteins exert a hydrostatic pressure which tends to draw fluid into the circulating blood volume. Normally the pressure within the vessel at the precapillary level is greater than the hydrostatic pressure of the plasma proteins. Fluid is driven out of the capillary and bathes the tissues. Extravascular tissue pressure and other local environmental influences affect the amount of fluid migration.

The intravascular pressure created by the blood normally diminishes at the venous end of the capillary. The hydrostatic pressure of the plasma proteins is greater than the intravascular pressure and fluid returns to the circulating blood volume. The simple balance of exchange of fluid across the capillary maintains adequate circulating plasma volume and prevents localized edema.

Increased *g* forces accelerate the outward migration of fluid at the precapillary level. This is particularly apt to happen in areas where supporting tissue pressure is reduced. Under increased *g* forces, the weight of the circulating blood is increased and this may cause the intravascular pressure to exceed the hydrostatic pressure of the plasma proteins. When this occurs, fluid is not returned to the capillary at the venous end. Edema and loss of circulating blood volume ensue. The *g* suit affords some protection in this regard by increasing the extravascular tissue pressure.

REGULATION OF CIRCULATION

Cardiovascular dynamics are profoundly influenced by reflex mechanisms. Many of the major alterations in dynamics induced in flying environment are direct results of complex reflex action. Cardiovascular reflexes may cause circulatory collapse with all its hazards. The major role of cardiovascular reflexes in the maintenance of normal circulation makes an understanding of them by the flight surgeon mandatory. Hypoxia, *g* forces, respiratory changes and complications attendant to cardiovascular pathology are directly related to reflex action.

Cardiovascular reflexes are extremely complicated and many facets of them are still not completely understood. Essentially there are three types of reflexes which influence the heart and vascular system. There is the simple reflex arc which has receptors within the heart itself and may affect cardiac function without involving the higher centers. A second type of reflex includes those which have receptors within the heart itself which transmit impulses to the cardiovascular centers of the brain initiating impulses to be sent back to the heart. An example of such a reflex is the Bezold phenomenon which receives impulses from the heart and stimulates the cardiovascular centers to induce cardioinhibitory responses. A third type of reflex affecting cardiovascular dynamics includes those which have receptors outside the heart. Such receptors are distributed throughout the body and act upon the cardiovascular centers. In turn, the cardiovascular centers carry out the appropriate action on the cardiovascular system. A simple illustration of the latter is stimulation of afferent fibers in the vein during venipuncture. This results in stimulation of cardioinhibitory centers inducing marked bradycardia and, in some instances, fainting.

The cardiovascular centers may be identified as cardioinhibitory to decrease cardiac rate, cardioaccelerator to increase cardiac rate, vasopressor to increase peripheral resistance or elevation of blood pressure, and vasodepressor to decrease peripheral resistance or lower blood pressure. The centers regulating these dynamics are profoundly influenced by the action of each other and their various actions require intercoordination.

Despite the complexity of the individual reflexes which may be encountered in control of cardiovascular dynamics, their effects may be greatly simplified. Reflex action may induce tachycardia. The principal reflex associated with this phenomenon is the Bainbridge reflex. Increased velocity of flow of venous blood into the right atrium stimulates the heart to increased activity. The increased rate of the heart through the Bainbridge reflex is mediated to vagal afferent nerves which apparently diminish vagal efferent inhibition of the heart. It has also been recognized that the Bainbridge reflex may act as a simple reflex arc in certain circumstances and, although it may be initiated by vagal afferent fibers, it may also act in the absence of vagal impulses. The Bainbridge reflex secondarily influences respiration and hyperventilation also.

Closely related to the mechanisms of tachycardia is the second mechanism induced by reflex action, that of vasopressor reaction. Vasopressor reaction, for the most part, is accomplished through the sympathetic nervous system and is induced by the constriction of peripheral vessels. The vasopressor phenomenon from reflex action is further complicated by humoral influences. The sympathetic nervous system is directly related to the secretion of adrenaline and noradrenaline. In recent years it has become apparent that peripheral constriction is largely influenced by noradrenaline, whereas adrenaline itself may induce peripheral dilation. Thus, the humoral consideration of noradrenaline and adrenaline further complicates the vasopressor response in the individual subject. This may, in fact, account for a great deal of the individual variation noted in cardiovascular dynamics under stress.

The third type of response which may be induced by reflex action is bradycardia or slowing of the heart. This is largely effected through vagal influences on the cardiac mechanisms. The afferent receptor fibers may be widespread.

The bradycardia influence induced by vagal influences is often accompanied by the fourth reflex mechanism, the vasodepressor response, with fall in blood pressure. The combination of bradycardia with vasodepressor reaction has given rise to the term of bradycardia collapse, commonly utilized by German investigators. The cardioinhibitory-vasodepressor reflexes are of major importance in aviation. They include the Bezold type phenomenon, which has afferent fibers within the heart and perhaps within the pulmonary vascular tree. By their reflex action they cause marked cardioinhibition responses with bradycardia and marked decrease in peripheral resistance. Under normal circumstances this reflex is quiescent. It may be stimulated by administration of

drugs; however, it may be induced to activity by numerous stimuli. The Bezold reflex may well be regarded as an antagonistic reflex action to the Bainbridge response.

The best known reflexes which induce bradycardia and vasodepression are those which have afferent fibers in the carotid sinus and aortic body. Stimulation of the carotid sinus normally induces cardiac slowing and may induce significant bradycardia or cardiac arrest. Elevation of blood pressure within the aorta and carotid artery stimulates afferent receptors of this reflex which, in turn, induces bradycardia with vasodepression. It should be clearly understood that a very high percentage of normal subjects will have bradycardia and circulatory collapse with continued massage of the carotid sinus. The individual with a hypersensitive reflex of this type is the one who has an immediate reflex action on very minor stimulation of the carotid sinus.

One of the more important vagal reflexes which is capable of inducing bradycardia and vasodepression arises from the lung itself. Inasmuch as aviation constantly stimulates the pulmonary tree by changes in breathing mechanics and the introduction of artificial breathing mechanics, for example pressure breathing, this reflex is commonly stimulated. It is called the pulmonary stretch reflex (fig. 131). Afferent vagal fibers are stimulated upon stretching of the lung and pleura. Efferent vagal action is the same as that for other cardiovascular, vago-vagal, depressor phenomenon. Vagal afferent fibers in the pulmonary vessels may be stimulated by distention of the pulmonary vascular bed. These too may induce bradycardia and vasodepression and vasodepressor reaction.

Exposure of an extremity to cold (in a classic example, the cold pressor test) may likewise stimulate vagal afferent fibers with reflex bradycardia and vasodepression. Pain from any source within the body is apt to stimulate afferent fibers culminating in this end result. Even the skin of the face has afferent fibers which may be stimulated by wind blast during flight and, thus, induce a vagal response. It is clear that there are multiple sources of stimulation from all points of the body which are capable of inducing vagal inhibition of heart rate and vasodepression. Their multiplicity makes the

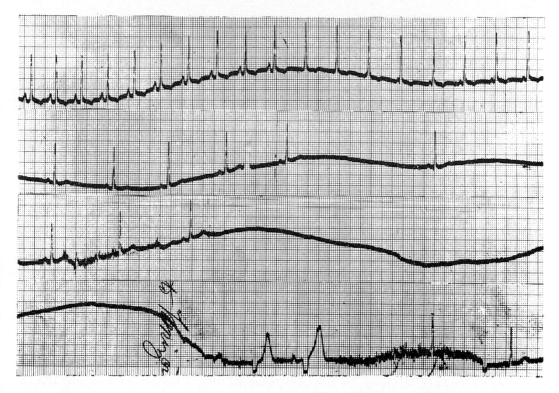

Fig. 131. Progressive bradycardia and cardiac arrest induced by breath holding and terminated by escape beats.

problem of identifying the precipitating factor to such a reaction extremely difficult.

All four mechanisms, tachycardia, vasopressor, bradycardia and vasodepressor, are closely interrelated. The action of the organism as a whole during the reflex stimulation is largely dependent upon the balance between sympathetic and parasympathetic stimulation. In those circumstances in which bradycardia is associated with elevated blood pressure one might assume that the parasympathetic nerves are largely effective on the heart, producing cardiac inhibition, whereas the sympathetic fibers have a greater degree of control over the vascular bed and induce vasoconstriction. When, for any reason, the relationship is changed or the sympathetic influences are no longer capable of coping with the parasympathetic influences at the vascular level, bradycardia with vasodepression ensues. It is pertinent to point out that many drugs which have been used to investigate reflexes of this nature have relatively selective action; notably, atropine inhibits the cardioinhibitory

action of the vagus nerve but has relatively little, if any, effect on the vasodepressor action of the parasympathetic system.

The mode of response to vagal action may actually be categorized into two distinct groups. One of these groups may be called the acute vagal responses. In this group is the individual who has a hypersensitive carotid sinus reflex which, upon stimulation, develops immediate acute vagal response. He is a person who collapses immediately at the onset of venipuncture or immediately at the height of inspiration with stimulation of the pulmonary stretch reflex. These early or immediate responses to vagal stimulation are quite distinct in their mechanism from other types of vagotonic reaction. They are also much less common. A second mode of vagal action may be called the vagotonic storm. When the cardiovascular system is put under stress, inducing a sympathetic or accelerated phase, a form of rebound phenomenon may follow during the recovery period. During the sympathetic phase, the cardiac rate for example may reach 160 or more per minute and following this period of recovery after the stress has been removed, marked vagotonia may occur with bradycardia or even cardiac arrest. At this time the patient presents all of the findings of excessive vagal reaction including appearances of nausea, pallor, bradycardia and vasodepressor responses. The blood sugar may be lowered secondarily by vagal stimulation of insulin secretion. The susceptibility of an individual to a vagotonic storm of this nature is an individual matter. Its occurrence, however, is by no means infrequent.

HYPOXIA

The normal cardiac muscle is relatively resistant to hypoxia. It is unique in utilizing lactic acid in its metabolic pattern. This prevents acidification of the cardiac muscle. Oxygen saturation of the coronary blood below 25 per cent still permits absorption of lactic acid from the blood stream by cardiac muscle. The muscle function can continue for hours at extreme altitudes of 32,000 to 42,000 feet. Function ceases by exhaustion of myocardial reserve. Hypoxia should not be confused with asphyxia. The former implies simply diminished amount of oxygen supply whereas the latter also implies retention of carbon dioxide. Cardiac muscle tolerates asphyxia poorly as compared to hypoxia. An example of localized asphyxia may be assumed in the presence of acute coronary occlusion with absent blood flow to a specific segment of muscle. Under such circumstances, relatively large amounts of lactic acid accumulate and myocardial failure of the tissue involved may ensue. Asphyxia may cause sudden changes in the heart and extra systoles are said to occur within 3 minutes after the onset of asphyxia.

The response of the heart and circulation to hypoxia which may be encountered in aviation problems is primarily caused by complicated cardiovascular reflex mechanisms. The effects of prolonged gradual hypoxia may be generalized into three stages. In stage one there is an increase in circulation. In part, this is brought about by the decreased alveolar pO_2 requiring a greater circulation to deliver the usually required amount of oxygen to the tissues. With the exception of the cardiac muscle, the peripheral tissues do not utilize lactic

acid efficiently and acidification owing to accumulated metabolites occurs. This results in the opening of numerous, functionally closed arteriole venous channels. The over-all effects of peripheral vascular dilation owing to accumulated metabolites and decreased alveolar pO_2 result in a marked increase in circulation rate and a decrease in peripheral resistance.

The increased velocity of venous return invokes reflexes responsible for acceleration of cardiac rate. The best known of these is the Bainbridge reflex. Stage two occurs during the hypoxic stimulation of the cardiovascular centers. In reality, hypoxia tends to stimulate all cardiac receptors. Variation in individual responses must be expected based upon the relative contribution of reflex components to cardiovascular dynamics in the individual concerned. The most commonly recognized response is bradycardia with increased blood pressure. Presumably this occurs because the vagal centers predominate in control of the heart and their stimulation results in cardiac slowing, whereas the sympathetic nervous system dominates vascular control and sympathetic stimulation results in vascular constriction. Individual response in regard to blood pressure may be influenced by the ratio of norepinephrine to epinephrine in any individual subject. The central sympathetic tone is sufficiently effective in this stage to counterbalance the vasodilating effects of accumulated metabolites. Stage three occurs when the metabolites accumulate in sufficient amount to negate the central vasoconstrictor influence of the sympathetic system. At this point, bradycardia and precipitous fall in blood pressure occur, resulting in collapse. In the light of recent observations, one may assume that a relatively high adrenaline to noradrenaline ratio could induce early peripheral vascular collapse. Adrenaline is chiefly a vasodilator whereas noradrenaline is a vasoconstrictor.

That hypoxia results in central reflex stimulation is generally accepted on the basis of classic experiments. Section of the vagus nerve abolishes a bradycardia response and complete denervation of the heart permits it to function at a rapid rate, deteriorating only after prolonged periods of hypoxia with exhaustion of myocardial reserve.

The response to sudden hypoxia is somewhat different from gradual hypoxia. It causes central stimulation of bradycardia influences and results in sudden cardiovascular collapse.

INFLUENCE OF *g* FORCES

The weight of a subject or an object is dependent upon the gravitational forces acting upon its mass. Gravity is a force which creates acceleration under proper circumstances; therefore, forces created by the earth's gravitational field as well as forces created by acceleration may be considered in a similar manner. Primarily their effect on the human organism depends upon the inertia of mass. The resistance of mass to change in its position or state of action accounts for the sensations associated with acceleration forces. The effects of *g* forces are initiated primarily through changes in the circulatory system. For the most part, failure in function of an organ on exposure to *g* forces is brought about by changes in its circulation. Changes in the visual field are secondary to changes in blood supply to the eye. Loss of consciousness may occur secondary to inadequate blood supply to the brain.

It is convenient to discuss the influences of *g* forces on the human organism in terms of longitudinal positive *g* forces, longitudinal negative *g* forces and transverse *g* forces. When acceleration forces or *g* forces are acting in a direction parallel to the long axis of the body, the weight of the column of blood depends upon the magnitude of the *g* force. In the upright position the weight of the column of blood from the heart to the brain increases as the height of the column increases. Under influence of acceleration forces the top of the column of blood may achieve sufficient weight to stop circulation to the head. These are strictly mechanical effects on circulation. The initial effects of significant *g* forces in the longitudinal direction with the person in the upright position then are mediated through decreased blood flow to the head and upper body. Diminished blood flow to the head results early in visual disturbances. Visual disturbances occur early because of intraocular pressure which counterbalances the perfusion pressure of the circulatory system. Normally, visual changes will begin between 4 and 5 *g*. With increase in *g* forces to 5 and 6 *g*, unconsciousness may occur. The inability of the circulatory system to perfuse the head and upper portion of the trunk is probably the greatest effect of longitudinal *g* forces. Obviously the heart must work very hard against the increased weight of the column of blood even before the organism becomes incapacitated.

It might be assumed that the increased weight of the blood column would tend to create pooling of blood in the lower regions of the body. This would prevent the return of blood to the heart or diminish cardiac return, resulting in circulatory collapse. In experimental observations, this aspect of the influences of *g* forces upon the circulation has not proved to be so critical. Dye dilution studies have demonstrated that the stroke volume of the heart is reasonably maintained in the presence of *g* forces or acceleration forces as great as 4 *g*. The blood pressure at the cardiac level is reasonably maintained. This is probably effected in part by the support mechanisms of the tissues surrounding the vascular bed and secondly because the circulating blood volume to the lower part of the body is augmented by the addition of blood from the head and the upper part of the thorax into the effective circulation. The upper part of the lungs has a marked decrease in pulmonary blood volume as visualized by x-ray. Redistribution of blood volume and tissue support undoubtedly contribute to maintenance of cardiac stroke volume. Nevertheless, with the increasing *g* forces the factor of diminished cardiac return becomes increasingly important. Stroke volume is maintained up to 5 *g*.

In the presence of longitudinal acceleration the carotid artery blood pressure begins to drop within 1 to 2 seconds after its onset. At 9 to 20 seconds, pressure reflexes are induced which help to compensate for the effect of the *g* forces on circulatory dynamics. One of the reflexes which deserve special mention in this regard is the carotid sinus reflex. Diminished pressure in the carotid artery stimulates an increase in blood pressure. Another effect of *g* forces is to increase the weight of the organs of the body. This may lead to stimulation of the pain receptors with adverse reflex responses.

The tolerance of a man to g forces depends upon the magnitude of the force, the duration of its action, its direction and time of onset. All individuals at ground level are constantly subjected to 1 g force without difficulty, although it should be pointed out that when the g forces are totally unopposed by common body mechanisms, as occurs by standing motionless in the upright position, even 1 g is capable of influencing the circulation to such an extent as to induce unconsciousness. Man may tolerate increases of g forces for a matter of several minutes at a level of approximately $3\frac{1}{2}$ g. Beyond this point the degree of tolerance to g forces over a period of time sharply diminishes. Five g can be tolerated for approximately 50 seconds and $7\frac{1}{2}$ g for only 5 seconds. Very large g forces may be tolerated for a very minute duration of time; for example, 20 g may be tolerated for 1 to 2 seconds. An individual's tolerance to g forces may vary from day to day. They are markedly influenced by fatigue, nicotine, alcoholic intake and febrile illnesses.

Almost all types of g forces of any magnitude for any duration of time are associated with marked increases in cardiac rate. It is exceedingly important to recognize that this is in essence a sympathetic phase of cardiac acceleration. During this period of time, sympathetic nerve stimulation is at its maximum, in part to induce vasopressor responses and counteract g forces. The total effect of acceleration on the circulatory system cannot be estimated by mere evaluation during the time the individual subject is exposed to g forces. Some individuals may be subject to the so-called vagotonic storms during the coasting period or recovery period following acceleration forces. These in essence are marked cardiac slowing with bradycardia and the development of significant cardiac arrhythmias. Great individual susceptibility to cardiovascular collapse following exposure to g forces is undoubtedly related to individual variations in vagotonic and sympathetic influences.

The g suit which is designed in part to protect against gravitational influences has special implications in circulation which require emphasis. Not only does it produce compression upon the external body to counteract diminution in atmospheric pressure or increases in g forces, but it has the property of displacing the volume of circulating blood from the external compartments into the pulmonary vascular bed. Distention of the pulmonary vascular bed by such mechanisms has been demonstrated by decreases in the pulmonary elasticity measured experimentally. Distention of the pulmonary vascular bed augments stimulation of the vagal afferent receptors which are capable of inducing cardioinhibitory and vasodepressor responses. It must be considered as one of the over-all factors influencing the possibility of occurrence of significant cardiac arrhythmias.

If acceleration is so directed that the forces of inertia of the blood column are directed in a headward manner and parallel to the longitudinal axis of the body, it may be spoken of as negative g. This results in distention of the carotid sinus and cerebral circulation. Human subjects do not tolerate this form of acceleration or g force well. Significant cardiac arrhythmias with vasodepression and cardiac arrest may be stimulated with less than 3 g in this direction.

The third group of acceleration of forces which has profound influence on the circulatory dynamics which require consideration are those of the transverse group. The g forces directed in the anteroposterior direction against the body are definitely better tolerated than those along the longitudinal axis. However, when these forces reach sufficiently large magnitudes (7 to 9 g), they may markedly inhibit the person's ability to breathe. A force of 10 g for a period of 1 minute largely arrests respiration for this period of time. It is cogent to point out that this is a sufficiently long period of time in many individuals to induce severe sympathetic discharge with tachycardia, and following the release of this stimulation, the vagotonic storm may ensue with cardiac arrest and loss of consciousness. The author has adequately demonstrated on numerous occasions that breath holding for periods of 45 seconds is sufficient to induce cardiac arrest in the recovery period following breath holding in many normal subjects. For this reason the transverse gravitational forces must not be considered totally innocuous.

Transverse g forces in the anteroposterior diameter and also in the lateral diameter are perfectly capable of twisting or distorting the position of various organs in the body, including the heart and mediastinum. Such displacements may produce mechanical obstructions or induce pain and other reflex reactions. In summary, it may be seen that gravitational forces affect the circulatory dynamics by their mechanical influences and by their initiation of reflex phenomenon. The latter may create arrhythmias as an immediate adaptive mechanism or during the recovery phase may result in a vagotonic storm.

SYNCOPE

Syncope or fainting is a frequent occurrence. The lay public and medical profession tend to regard it lightly because of its usual lack of complication and sequelae. However, syncope in aviation or transitory loss of consciousness may result in serious accidents and death. Aviation involves a man-machine effort and is a good example wherein split second failure of the man can have disastrous results. Particularly in the presence of high performance aircraft, the disastrous consequence of momentary loss of consciousness which might be expected has led to major efforts to prevent such an occurrence. Many questions concerning syncope remain unanswered. It seems relatively clear, however, that syncope may be induced in any subject when sufficient number of biologic stress phenomena are induced. Recent studies have indicated that even in a selected group of people who have already begun flying training, between 18 and 42 per cent have already experienced syncopal episodes prior to the beginning of their training.

Owing to the diversity of precipitating mechanisms which can induce syncope, it is wise to approach this problem on mechanisms or pathogenic factors rather than etiologies or precipitating causes. The author has found it convenient to classify mechanisms of syncope under six general categories: (1) venous, inadequate return of blood to the left heart; (2) cardiac, ineffective pumping action of the heart; (3) arteriole, change in routing of blood flow; (4) blood qualitative changes (abnormalities in the constituents of the circulating blood);

(5) blood quantitative changes (inadequate circulating volume); and (6) central nervous system, local disorders.

Although varicosities are frequently cited as factors contributing to syncope, clinically they are not found to be frequently associated with fainting. However, this is one of the causes why individuals with large varicose veins or other areas of loss of venous tone are not good candidates for flying activity. Under the influence of g forces, such areas of loss of venous tone can permit the entrapping of large volumes of circulating blood. Diminishing the volume of blood within the pulmonary vascular bed automatically diminishes the venous return to the left heart. The most commonly encountered mechanism of doing this in aviation personnel is pressure breathing. Breathing against pressure will diminish the pulmonary vascular bed and may contribute to inadequate circulation with syncope as the result.

The heart itself may be the major cause of syncope in a large number of individuals. It may be regarded as a pump and anything which interferes with this effective pumping action may contribute to inadequate circulation. If the heart beats too fast as noted in tachycardias, insufficient period of time may be permitted for diastolic filling and cardiac output diminishes. Clinical examples of these are paroxysmal atrial tachycardias, rapid auricular fibrillation and other mechanisms inducing rapid heart action. In order to maintain any degree of effective pumping action in the normal individual, the cardiac rate should remain, for the most part, below 180 per minute.

Cardioinhibitory responses or marked slowing of the heart is one of the more common mechanisms of pump failure. These may be induced by the reflexes as mentioned above, including carotid sinus massage, venipuncture, and many others. The pulmonary stretch reflex may be stimulated by merely taking a deep breath and holding it at the height of inspiration. At this exact point at the onset of breath holding, a certain number of individuals demonstrate transitory cardiac arrest with syncopal episodes. In recent evaluation of subjects having experienced syncope in flying population, and with subjects not having clinical syncope for controls, the author was impressed by the significance of cardiac arrhythmias as a mechanism of inducing syncope. It should be pointed out that in many instances these were not merely minor cardiac arrhythmias but were of the magnitude of cardiac arrests in some instances for as long as 12 seconds. Cardiac arrest induced by such simple maneuvers as the rigid upright posture was observed. Cardiac arrest in the recovery period following prolonged breath holding was observed. In addition to acute loss of consciousness, had these events not been terminated by clinical means, death would have resulted.

Breath holding, postural influences and other stress mechanisms were noted to induce less important cardiac arrhythmias even in additional subjects who did not experience syncope. These findings strongly suggest that even the common everyday syncope experienced by the lay population is profoundly influenced and often initiated in certain instances by cardiac arrhythmias induced through reflex mechanisms. Marked bradycardia response, arrhythmias, A-V dissociation and cardiac arrest can be abolished by the intravenous injection of atropine. This is in accordance with atropine's vagolytic action abolishing cardioinhibitory responses.

Changes in arteriolar tone can result in inadequate perfusion of the brain in the upright position. The subject who reclines in the horizontal position and then suddenly assumes the erect position must have contraction of the small arterioles in the peripheral vascular bed in order to prevent the arteriolar blood from gravitating to the lower regions of the body. Peripheral constriction at the point of the arteriole is accomplished by reflex means and results in maintaining a normal distribution of blood to the brain. If this reflex mechanism functions poorly, or not at all, syncope occurs on assuming the upright posture. Destruction of the nerves which are responsible for maintaining this reflex may induce such reactions. Sympathectomy is such an example. Neurologic diseases may also be responsible for loss of the arteriolar reflex.

The most common cause of loss of arteriolar tone is prolonged bed rest. A subject who remains at bed rest for a few days with or without an acute febrile illness will lose the normal active response of the arteriolar reflex. When he first begins ambulation, he will note that on arising he is particularly prone to orthostatic collapse. Any member of flying personnel who has been ill for any reason or retained or restricted to bed rest for any reason should be carefully evaluated with regard to his orthostatic tolerance (tolerance to assuming the upright position) prior to the time he returns to flying. This means that he should adequately demonstrate that he can assume the erect posture in a relatively motionless position for a period of at least 3 minutes without some significant change in circulatory dynamics, such as bradycardial collapse or excessive tachycardia with fall in blood pressure.

Arteriolar tone may be diminished by reflex actions such as the Bezold type or to vasodepressor responses initiated by extra cardiac afferent stimulus. Arteriolar tone, of course, is markedly influenced by heat and by drugs, for example, alcohol.

Changes in the circulating blood may cause a person to be more susceptible to loss of consciousness. Anemia results in opening up of arteriovenous channels and diminishes the ability of the circulatory system to adequately oxygenate the central nervous system. Every person engaged in flying should be evaluated relative to the presence or absence of anemia. Other blood qualitative changes which influence syncope may occur. These include hypoglycemia, carbon monoxide or other toxins. Hypoglycemia may be an associated finding in response to vagal discharge stimulating the secretion of insulin rather than being a primary cause of syncope. Lowered blood sugar, like fatigue, may lower one's tolerance of the circulatory system to withstand g forces or biologic stresses. Clinical cases of hypoglycemia which induce syncope are usually identified by recurring symptomatology and have already been detected. They concern patients who usually are under treatment and are not likely to be found in a flying population.

Changes in the amount of the circulating blood volume obviously may induce loss of consciousness. The most obvious example of this is acute blood loss. Dehydration from any cause, for example, gastroenteritis, may also contribute to or cause syncope.

There are a number of disturbances which

may affect the central nervous system locally and induce unconsciousness. These include abnormalities in the nerve cells as well as changes in the vascular supply to the brain. Small strokes, cerebral hemorrhages or hypertensive encephalopathy may induce syncopal reactions. In a young population the rare possibility of a congenital berry aneurysm of the brain must be kept in mind. Apparently because syncope results in loss of consciousness, much attention has been directed toward a possible underlying brain disorder or epileptic type behavior. Any normal brain cannot be expected to function without adequate blood supply. Lennox's figure of 0.5 per cent of epilepsy in the general population is in sharp contrast with the 20 to 45 per cent of the general population that has experienced syncope. The objective evidence of circulatory collapse inducing syncope makes it unnecessary to postulate that nearly half of the general population has a brain disorder.

A clear-cut understanding of the basic mechanisms which may create a syncopal episode are very valuable to the approach of any problem related to syncope. Inasmuch as the multitude of factors which may induce syncope are relatively common and part of everyday living, adequate protection against development of one of the mechanisms which might induce syncope has practical value. The M-1 maneuver, which is a modified valsalva, is a protective maneuver. The abdominal contents are compressed by contraction of the abdominal musculature. After taking in a very deep breath, rather than expiring against a closed glottis, the individual screams or exhales noisily immediately after the height of inspiration has been attained. Exhaling at this particular time helps to compress blood into the left heart and also it breaks continued stimulation of the stretch receptors which are capable of initiating significant cardiac arrhythmias.

Although it would be desirable to be able to eliminate those persons who are going to have a subsequent syncopal episode, there are no clinical tests at the present time which are adequate for such a prediction. A few individuals are frequent repeaters and can be detected by history. An individual who is susceptible to syncope today may not be tomorrow. The vast majority of individual subjects, therefore, are not necessarily constantly syncope prone nor is any individual subject constantly immune to the development of syncope. More often a combination of stresses are noted in people who have experienced clinical syncope. Among these are included recent rapid weight loss, acute infectious illnesses, fatigue, ingestion of alcohol and lack of sleep. Most of these are associated with something less than top hygienic conditions. Perhaps the most practical approach to preclude, insofar as possible, the occurrence of syncope during flight would be a closer examination of the general hygienic condition of the flyer before he begins his daily missions. Obviously the pilot who has recently been ingesting excessive quantities of alcohol or has permitted himself to get out of physical condition or is under excessive nervous strain or fatigue from other causes may well be inviting the chain of circumstances which culminates in a syncopal episode.

Caution should be utilized in evaluating experimental tests which are commonly used in laboratories for study of syncopal subjects. In a controlled series of normal subjects who had apparently never experienced syncope, it was interesting to note that many developed syncope with such procedures as utilization of the tilt table, carotid sinus massage, prolonged breath holding and even from orthostatic influences. These relatively standard procedures in no way separated those individuals who had known clinical episodes of syncope from those who had not. On the other hand, many individuals who had previously experienced known clinical episodes of syncope went through such a battery of tests without experiencing any syncopal attacks. This serves to point up the failure of such testing procedures in discriminating the individual who is syncope prone from the one who is not.

ARTERIOSCLEROTIC HEART DISEASE

Arteriosclerotic heart disease is not necessarily a disease of middle age or older. It has been well established that gross atherosclerosis of the coronary arteries is seen in as high as 70 per cent of young men with an average age of 22 years. Ten per cent of such a population exhibits significant coronary artery disease to the point of 70 per cent occlusion of one major vessel. No pilot should be considered free of atherosclerosis merely because of his age. There are now a number of well documented incidents of myocardial infarction associated with aircraft accidents. Benson reported the first episode of myocardial infarction occurring in flight. There are also well documented incidents of myocardial infarction in young people. Infarction has been noted in a 21-year-old aviation cadet. A routine survey of electrocardiograms in flying population has identified a number of young flyers below the age of 30 years who have already sustained myocardial infarction. As the age of the flying population is increased the incidence of atherosclerotic complications also increases.

Even though hypoxia normally causes dilation of the coronary arteries it is not likely that hypoxia can dilate an atherosclerotic vessel. Hypoxia of the normal heart is not to be confused with hypoxia in the presence of atherosclerotic heart disease. Significant atherosclerosis can sufficiently impair circulation to the region of the myocardium to induce asphyxia rather than hypoxia. With the accumulation of CO_2 within the tissue as well as oxygen want, significant disturbances in the metabolism in the area of muscle involved occur. Such changes in metabolism are capable of inducing serious cardiac arrhythmias.

One of the major unsolved questions in relation to unexplained aircraft accidents concerns the role of subclinical coronary artery disease in inducing cardiac arrhythmias with cardiovascular collapse. That differences in oxygen tension and carbon dioxide retention at specific regions within the heart muscle cause cardiac arrhythmia is an established fact. The frequency of occurrence in flying personnel remains an open question. Premature conclusion that any individual aircraft accident is the result of arteriosclerotic heart disease because of the postmortem finding of some degree of atherosclerosis is not warranted. With the high incidence of atherosclerosis it is to be expected that a number of aircraft accidents would involve individuals who present evidence of cardiac pathology at postmortem examination, irrespective of whether such pathology

had any influence upon the performance of the pilot. It is well known that a number of individuals with significant coronary artery disease and actual myocardial infarction have continued to fly without apparent difficulty. Like many other features of this disease, the problem of flying in relation to atherosclerosis has many variable facets and leaves relatively little room for dogmatic assumptions. Nevertheless, with the well documented evidence that arrhythmias and other unpredictable complications may occur as a result of significant atherosclerotic heart disease, particularly with previous myocardial infarction, a person presenting these findings should not be permitted to be the sole pilot in primary control of aircraft nor, from the individual's point of view, should he be exposed to the extreme stresses encountered in high performance aircraft. On the other hand, many such individuals are able to function adequately under controlled circumstances with a copilot in more conventional aircraft.

Inasmuch as it is obviously desirable to remove those individuals from flying occupations who are likely to have a repeated episode of coronary insufficiency with arrhythmia or actual myocardial infarction during flight, numerous methods have been advocated for screening. It cannot be overemphasized that in many instances the best clue to the presence of significant underlying coronary artery disease is the history itself. A typical history of chest pain and radiation into the left arm or neck, even in a young individual, should alert the clinician to the possibility of myocardial infarction. Such history has the value of being specific and individualized rather than being a probability factor.

In addition to the history, the other specific examination which may be applied to the individual case in detection of coronary artery disease is the electrocardiogram. There are a number of electrocardiographic findings which are specific for myocardial infarction. In this category one may include the localized QS deflections over the anterior precordial leads. When definite electrocardiographic findings are found which permit the diagnosis of myocardial infarction, this may be expressed as an individual matter for the individual being considered for selection.

One must be cautious in overinterpreting electrocardiograms in reference to myocardial infarction. There are other less clearcut findings such as nonspecific T wave changes, minor variations in the QRS complex and intraventricular conduction defects which are not produced only by atherosclerotic heart disease and may have questionable significance. Thus, the electrocardiogram provides a definite diagnosis in certain instances of atherosclerotic heart disease and may suggest the possibility of its presence on other occasions.

Certain laboratory studies have been recommended for the detection of probable atherosclerosis. It is extremely important to recognize that these are purely problematic factors. No blood tests have been devised to date which permit predicting, in a specific instance, that an individual is going to have a subsequent myocardial infarction or significant coronary artery disease. The presence of an elevated blood cholesterol or so-called abnormal ratios of S_f lipoproteins or even changes in the cholesterol or phospholipid ratio provide only an index of suspicion. There are many normal subjects who apparently never experience significant coronary artery disease who present so-called abnormal lipid profiles or elevations of their cholesterol levels. The chief drawback in utilizing such tests to detect individuals with coronary artery disease is the large amount of iatrogenic heart disease created by using such a nonspecific measurement. It is not good from the patient's point of view to frighten him with the prospects of subsequent coronary artery disease unless you can be rather specific for his individual case. If a number of the tests of this nature which have been advocated were employed for screening or diagnosis in large flying populations, there would be a large number of individuals removed from flying careers who would never experience subsequent coronary artery disease. They would remain emotional cripples as a result of overzealous attempts to apply such measurements to clinical disease.

With the widespread incidence of atherosclerosis, even in younger individuals, prevention of disease is a logical consideration. At the present state of our knowledge concerning atherosclerosis, a sensible, sane and moderate approach to a preventive program is about all that is indicated. This includes relatively general hygienic measures such as restricting the body weight or avoiding obesity, a well instituted program for maintaining adequate physical fitness and sufficient periods of relaxation or removal from the usual stresses of modern living. Fad diets of drastic fat restriction or low cholesterol diets are hardly indicated for the population at large. When more scientific information is available and the disease is more clearly understood, perhaps other factors can be instituted.

In the management of the patient who has already demonstrated the presence of clinical atherosclerosis one can be somewhat more strict. If for any reason such an individual is to continue a flying career certain precautions must be observed. Rapid weight reduction may well cause a person to be more susceptible to syncope and loss of g tolerance. Treatment with anticoagulant therapy is not recommended in flying personnel because of the complications which it may impose during accidents, exposure to g forces, with localized hemorrhages and other unpredictable events. The best approach to the management of the person who has demonstrated atherosclerosis is simple weight reduction; and if he should have grossly abnormal lipid profiles some value may be gained by restricting his diet in whatever fashion accomplishes the result for the individual concerned. The physician should always be alert to the possibility of hypoglycemia or other adverse circumstances which can accompany such dietary restrictions.

HYPERTENSION

There is considerable variation in opinion concerning what constitutes hypertension. A number of normal individuals present infrequent elevations of blood pressure, others present relatively fixed blood pressure and still others present complications commonly encountered in the presence of elevated blood pressure. For convenience it is easy to differentiate these people into three groups: (1) the vascular hyper-reactor; (2) essential hypertension; and (3) hypertensive cardiovascular disease. In the first group, one finds the individual with the labile blood pressure.

On being examined by the physician or during blood pressure determination for any cause, elevated readings may be obtained. Elevation may affect both the systolic and diastolic pressure. For the most part, elevations of the diastolic pressure are considered more significant clinically and are considered abnormal when they are 90 mm. of Hg or over. All individuals present some degree of vascular reactivity and on this basis vascular reactivity has been divided into the vascular hyper-reactor, the normal reactor and the hyporeactor. The vascular hyper-reactor has been defined as a person who presents with a diastolic pressure below 100 and after stress the diastolic pressure rises more than 20 mm. of Hg. Normal reactors are ones who present with a diastolic pressure below 100 mm. of Hg and after stress the pressure rises between 10 and 20 mm. of Hg. Hyporeactors are those individuals with an elevation if any of the diastolic pressure, after stress of less than 10 mm. of Hg. It is important to recognize that many normal individuals will have fluctuations in blood pressure. Certainly not all of these people should be classified as diseased. Many times elevated blood pressure is purely a manifestation of apprehension associated with physical examination. Frequently, normal pressures may be obtained in such individuals by reassurance or a short rest period.

In trying to decide whether a person truly has hypertension or is purely a vascular hyper-reactor, the best guide is to obtain some index of the over-all picture of the individual's blood pressure through long periods of time. For this reason it is common practice to do blood pressures twice or three times a day over a 3 day period. Sleeping blood pressures are also of help as they indicate the basal pressure when the individual is in a relaxed state. If there are no other evidences of complications seen in the presence of hypertension and the individual's pressure falls to normal limits with rest or subsequent determination, such individuals can be classified as vascular hyper-reactors and such a finding should in no way interfere with the ability to carry out flying operations. In the individual who presents more persistent elevations of his blood pressure and only occasional lower levels, it is advisable to carry out rather complete baseline evaluations.

The second group which may be encountered with relation to the problem of hypertension are those with true essential hypertension. In this category one includes those individuals who present persistent elevations of diastolic blood pressure above 90 mm. of Hg and who present no evidence of complications or cardiovascular disease. It is well to remember that the majority of the complications that occur as a result of hypertension are, in fact, atherosclerotic. A large number of individuals with hypertension develop coronary artery disease. Still others develop cerebral vascular disease as a result of changes in the vessels to the brain. Another group develops renal insufficiency associated with changes in the renal vessels. Some develop congestive heart failure which may, in part, be attributed to mechanics, but more often it is associated with accompanying coronary artery disease. Thus, the finding of essential hypertension in itself without complications is not always an incapacitating finding.

The prognosis of the individual with hypertension is dependent upon the development of complications. Early in the course of suspected hypertension as may be encountered in some of the more advanced vascular hyper-reactors or in the presence of definitely established essential hypertension, it is imperative that baseline studies be obtained. This includes x-ray of the chest demonstrating cardiac size, an electrocardiogram demonstrating the electrical characteristics of the heart insofar as hypertrophy or coronary insufficiency may be concerned and renal function studies. The latter includes the ability of the kidney to dilute and concentrate urine as well as to excrete foreign substances or dyes. No hypertensive evaluation is complete without adequate pyelography to demonstrate the absence of urinary tract disease, particularly structural or mechanical defects of the kidneys and lower urinary tract. There are occasional instances of young individuals with mechanical or structural defects which can be repaired to arrest the early onset of events which lead to fixed and irreversible hypertension. At yearly intervals, individuals presenting hypertension should have re-evaluation of their baseline studies in reference to their electrocardiogram, x-ray and renal functions. These provide an index to the rate of progression of disease or complications which might be expected. As a rule, the more rapid the development of complications (*e.g.*, progressive impairment of renal function or progressive enlargement of the heart), the more unfavorable will be the prognosis. In the absence of rapid progression, hypertension may be a long term finding and may even be compatible with a relatively normal life span.

Unless significant complications are present, a simple presence of hypertension should not limit the person's activity. Essential hypertension in a well trained pilot without evidence of complications need not terminate a flying career in all instances. A high degree of individuality is warranted in evaluation of the hypertensive.

The individual who is classified as having hypertensive cardiovascular disease not only presents hypertension but also clear-cut evidence of complications. These include evidence of coronary insufficiency or coronary artery disease, cardiac enlargement, significant renal insufficiency or cerebral vascular manifestations. The presence of any of these is adequate cause to remove such an individual from the stresses and strains attendant to modern aviation.

With the advent of drugs which may be utilized to control hypertension, much consideration has been given to their use in hypertensive individuals who wish to continue flying. For the most part, the individual who requires medication for hypertension should not be permitted to continue operational control of aircraft. All those medications which induce blocking or medical sympathectomy in effect reduce an individual's tolerance to *g* forces. Clinically we see such individuals develop syncope by merely assuming the upright posture. Obviously a person who is flying and being subjected to *g* forces cannot be medically sympathectomized prior to exposure to flight. Another group of medications include those with a sedative type reaction. All sedative type reaction drugs for control of hypertension slow down the reaction performance of the individual concerned. Their administration is not conducive to top-notch physical performance. In this conjunction, tranquilizers and Ranoffia preparations such as Serpasil are definite hazards to flying safety when administered to flying personnel. They also exert influences on the individual's ability to maintain adequate cardiovascular dynamics in the presence of biologic stress.

Medications which influence the electrolyte balance may have other side effects and if they are, in reality, successfully accomplishing their purpose may compromise the general ability to perform. Rice diets and other forms of severe caloric restrictions may reduce the individual's tolerance to *g* forces and may, in some instances, induce hypoglycemia or other adverse conditions.

Certain common misconceptions concerning the diagnosis of hypertension need to be pointed out. The amytal test is useful in determining the reactivity of the peripheral vascular bed but normal blood pressures induced by sedation or anesthetics do not exclude the presence of hypertension as a disease. Many hypertensive blood pressures can be significantly lowered by anesthetic measures. Perhaps the most valuable addition to specialized study of the hypertensive is the automatic recording of blood pressures over a long period of time. By recording the systolic and diastolic pressure automatically with a machine at frequent intervals over a prolonged period of time it is possible to obtain an objective measurement, over a matter of hours, of an individual's blood pressure. Such an objective measurement also avoids the pitfall of a technician becoming overly sympathetic to the flying applicant and recording biased readings.

Care should be exercised to avoid labeling the individual who presents acute glomerulonephritis as having bona fide hypertension. Some of these individuals who present advanced findings with eyeground changes and urinary tract findings may subsequently present little or no evidence of previous disorder. A portion of these individuals who demonstrate adequate recovery without complication and without the necessity of medication may adequately perform in the flying environment.

CONGENITAL HEART DISEASE

The presence of congenital defects frequently impose certain abnormalities in cardiovascular dynamics. Atrial septal defects have acquired some special significance in aviation medicine because of the possibility of transmitting emboli across such a defect. Normally, with small atrial septal defects, the shunt is from the left atrium to the right atrium and no cyanosis is observed, nor is there any tendency for embolic phenomenon in the peripheral vascular tree to pass into the systemic circulation and the brain. Insofar as decompression sickness is concerned, or possibility of fat emboli, or the release of nitrogen bubbles from fatty tissue, it is not necessary to postulate the presence of an atrial septal defect for their occurrence. There are abundant quantities of fatty tissue within the central nervous system itself and such tissue is heavily saturated with nitrogen. Direct release of nitrogen substances from the fatty tissue within the central nervous system is capable of causing neurologic disturbances without an embolus having to be transmitted across the septal defect.

The principal problem created by an atrial septal defect is the creation of an overload on the right heart and on the pulmonary circulation. Individuals with shunts from left to right which increase the load on the right heart and pulmonary circulation are frequently prone to syncopal attacks. Another complication which may be encountered is that with sudden increases in the pulmonary hypertension, the shunt may, in fact, be reversed. One of the first effects of hypoxia is to increase pulmonary hypertension. Either moderate hypoxia or pressure breathing may result in a reversed shunt from right to left. When such reversal occurs, cyanotic blood is being shunted directly into the systemic circulation and cyanosis may occur.

The principal congenital defects which one might encounter, presenting as a right to left shunt, are the atrial septal defect, patent ductus arteriosus, and ventricular septal defect. Almost all of the right to left shunts are associated with clinically detectable cyanosis and the elimination of such individuals from exposure to flying stresses does not present much of a problem. Insofar as air transportation is concerned, it should be constantly borne in mind, when dealing with defects which are associated with increased pulmonary vascularity or any compromise of the pulmonary circulation or pulmonary ventilation, that small degrees of hypoxia are capable of precipitating acute pulmonary

hypertension and this in turn can precipitate acute right heart failure.

Coarctation of the aorta is sometimes noted in individuals applying for training in a flying career. This particular abnormality is usually detected by the elevation of blood pressure in the arms and the clinical observation of diminished blood pressure in the legs. The systolic murmur is clearly heard over the base of the heart and a chest x-ray will frequently demonstrate rib notching caused by increased circulation through the intercostal arteries. Coarctation has some interesting theoretic speculations concerning flight. Inasmuch as the problem on exposure to longitudinal g forces in the head-to-seat direction is initiated by diminished flow to the head, one might assume that coarctation of aorta protects an individual against g force intolerance. The constriction of the aorta increases the pressure of the flow to the head and diminishes the flow to the lower extremities. A number of cases of coarctation of the aorta are associated with significant cardiac hypertrophy, aortic valvular disease or functional aortic insufficiency, and some are associated with medial necrosis of the aorta. Medial necrosis of the aorta is sometimes seen as an isolated finding or may occur in conjunction with other congenital abnormalities. Unfortunately it usually cannot be detected until actual dissection of the aorta has commenced. The stresses and strains associated with changes in g forces associated with flying can and do present a serious hazard in the presence of such a finding.

RHEUMATIC HEART DISEASE

A previous history of rheumatic fever and rheumatic heart disease has special significance in military populations and, in particular, for those individuals engaged in aviation. Not only must one be concerned about the damage which has already been incurred from previous episodes of rheumatic heart disease, but the use of prophylaxis to prevent recurrent attacks must be considered. It is now rather generally agreed that rheumatic fever is a response to streptococcal infections and that repeated attacks of rheumatic fever or reinfection with streptococcal organisms may lead to progression or development of serious heart disease.

In the care of the flying population, it is of importance to identify those individuals who have had rheumatic fever and those individuals who have underlying rheumatic heart disease. It is now an official recommendation of the American Heart Association that any such individual, regardless of whether he is engaged in aviation or whether he be military or civilian, should continue for life on a program of prophylactic antibiotics. Such a regimen is designed to eliminate the possibility of recurrent streptococcal infection and further progression of rheumatic heart disease. Military populations have recurrent exposure to multiple types of streptococcal organisms. The flying population has the added hazard of rapid changes of environments and rapid change in exposure to a large variety of different populations which may induce respiratory infections. A pilot may be in the desert in summer heat in the morning and spend the evening in a snowstorm; such rapid changes in environment are conducive to respiratory infections.

Respiratory infections lay the groundwork for streptococcal infection. For this reason all active flying personnel with previous rheumatic fever or detectable rheumatic heart disease should definitely be on a prophylactic program for the prevention of streptococcal infections. The American Heart Association has recommended, as prophylactic therapy, Benzathine penicillin G, intramuscularly, 1,200,000 units once a month, or an oral dose of penicillin consisting of 200,000 or 250,000 units twice a day. In those individuals who cannot tolerate penicillin, 1 gram of sulfadiazine may be administered orally once a day for adults.

An individual having rheumatic heart disease should receive additional prophylaxis during dental extractions or oral surgery which might precipitate bacterial endocarditis. For 2 days prior to surgery, 250,000 units of penicillin by mouth is given four times a day. On the day of surgery 250,000 units by mouth four times a day is continued plus 600,000 units of aqueous penicillin and 600,000 units of procaine penicillin injected shortly before surgery. For two days following surgery, 250,000 units is given orally four times a day.

Once an individual has developed rheumatic fever, he is treated in the customary fashion. Before return to flying status, however, it should be clearly demonstrated that he has made a complete recovery without any residual evidence of infection and with adequate physical tolerance. Rheumatic fever is a debilitating disease and leaves the individual with diminished physical reserves. It is important to demonstrate that the sedimentation rate has returned to normal and remains so despite physical activity and that the individual presents no evidence of excessive fatigue, circulatory instability, or significant damage to the cardiac valves which may adversely affect cardiovascular dynamics. Thus, resumption of flying activities becomes chiefly an individual matter requiring the proper clinical appraisal.

Valvular Heart Disease

Many young people presenting themselves for flying careers have cardiac murmurs. Not all of these are the result of underlying organic heart disease. A relatively high incidence of systolic murmurs heard at the apical region and over the pulmonary region are to be normally expected. Many of these murmurs may be brought out during the excitement of the examination or moderate exercise. As a general rule, any systolic murmur which is difficult to detect or can be detected only in the left lateral position or over the base of the heart of relatively low intensity and are not associated with any other evidence of organic heart disease may be considered as physiologic or unimportant. Exercise frequently brings out systolic murmurs. When exercise is necessary to produce systolic murmur, it is of questionable significance.

One of the characteristics of physiologic murmurs produced by exercise, excitement or other means which increase rapidity of blood flow, is their variability and tendency to disappear from one examination to the other. Exercise should be used to bring out diastolic murmurs and not systolic murmurs.

Another point of confusion frequently encountered in healthy individuals is the presence of split cardiac sounds. Split heart sounds are frequently confused with cardiac murmurs or evidence of heart disease. They are usually physiologic and do not represent any form of underlying cardiac disease. There are occasional clinical incidents in which split sounds are important. For the most part, these are right and left bundle branch block. Caution should be exercised in the evaluation of a split sound in the presence of apical systolic murmurs to avoid making the error of missing an opening mitral snap. The latter is indicative of underlying mitral stenosis.

Perhaps the most difficult murmur to evaluate from a clinical point of view in regard to its significance is the apical systolic murmur. An apical systolic murmur of moderate intensity (grade II by Levin's classification) is frequently seen as a physiologic finding; however, it may be evidence for underlying mitral insufficiency secondary to rheumatic fever. The usual approach to this problem is that if the individual presents a history of scarlet fever, family history of rheumatic fever or other evidence suggestive of rheumatic fever, the significance of the apical systolic murmur is given added weight. In the absence of such history it may be considered as insignificant. The diagnosis of mitral insufficiency of more marked degrees, of course, may be supported by the finding of other clinical phenomenon such as electrocardiographic abnormalities or radiographic demonstration of change in cardiac size or enlargement of the left atrium. Highly specialized diagnostic techniques may be employed in some such instances.

Significant mitral stenosis should preclude exposure to more severe stresses of flying. Mitral stenosis results in a small pulse pressure and greatly compromises the ability of the left heart to increase cardiac output under stress. Obviously, an individual with mitral stenosis who must increase his cardiac output to compensate for hypoxia or increased metabolic demands or the increased work against g forces would find it indeed difficult. Mitral stenosis is detected by the presence of a characteristic apical diastolic murmur and is easily diagnosed with careful auscultation.

Aortic stenosis results in a small pulse pressure and an increased load upon the left ventricle. The left ventricle is already subjected to an increased load in order to eject blood beyond the stenotic valve. When the weight of the column of blood in the great vessels is increased by g forces, the amount of pressure which the left ventricle is capable of exerting against these increased forces is minimal. In other words, the ability of such an individual to withstand g forces and prevent diminished cerebral insufficiency is markedly decreased. Aortic stenosis adds the problem of increasing the amount of cardiac muscle which must be supplied by coronary flow while at the same time diminishing the pressure head to perfuse the coronary vessels originating from the base of the aorta.

Aortic insufficiency permits diastolic regurgitation. To mention merely one hazard imposed by the stresses of flying in a person with aortic insufficiency, one need only to direct his attention again to the g forces and the weight of the column of blood in the vessels extending from the heart to the head. Marked diastolic collapse of the carotid arteries under the influence of g forces is to be expected in the presence of any degree of aortic insufficiency.

In summary, for the most part significant valvular lesions markedly compromise the circulatory dynamics at ground level and diminish the cardiac reserves which might be called upon during the particular circulatory stresses imposed by flying. In order for the heart to function effectively as a pumping mechanism, its valves must be expected to open normally and close completely thus preventing inefficient pumping action and undesirable cardiovascular reactions.

ELECTROCARDIOGRAPHIC FINDINGS

Inasmuch as the status of the cardiovascular system is of such vital importance in flying personnel, proved parameters of diagnostic evaluation are in demand. The electrocardiogram is a proved clinical tool in the diagnosis of cardiac disease. No cardiovascular evaluation is adequate without an electrocardiogram. The electrocardiogram has the advantage of being specific for the individual. Definite evidence of myocardial infarction is applicable to the individual and is not a probability factor. This frequently enables a specific diagnosis of heart disease in the individual concerned. Cardiac arrhythmias may be documented by objective evidence. Findings related to cardiac pathology, for example, left bundle branch block, may be detected only with the electrocardiogram and cannot be diagnosed by history, physical examination or other ordinary clinical means.

It must be recognized that there are many electrocardiographic findings which are not diagnostic and may be classified as nonspecific findings or equivocal findings which may run the gamut of a variation of normality to evidence of serious disease. This type of electrocardiographic finding requires expert clinical correlation. The electrocardiogram is subject to a number of variations from one examination to another. Changes may be caused by recording tracings at different times in relation to meals or during times when the individual is under stress with tachycardia or in different phases of respiration. Minor variations in technique or circumstances under which the recordings are made greatly influence a lot of the nonspecific findings. Minor variations are not frequently of any major significance in the more specific diagnostic findings of the electrocardiogram itself.

The electrocardiogram may be entirely normal in the presence of cardiac disease. This does not obviate its usefulness, however, in detecting those individuals with heart disease who do demonstrate electrocardiographic manifestations. At its present state of development and with limited normal values available, it cannot be used to predict the occurrence of cardiac disease. The electrocardiographic techniques are far short of their ultimate usefulness. New measuring techniques, refinement of method and serial analysis can be expected to greatly increase the clinical usefulness of this important diagnostic parameter. Because of the relatively large number of normal variations which may be encountered in electrocardiograms and the nonspecific changes which may be found subsequent to cardiac disease, a baseline electrocardiogram is very important. The use of comparative electrocardiograms is sometimes the sole means of establishing a clinical diagnosis or excluding it. Inasmuch as most of the electrocardiographic data has been collected from hospital and clinic facilities, there is relatively little information concerning the number of abnormalities which may be encountered in a relatively asymptomatic population.

The United States Air Force is currently conducting a survey of electrocardiograms in all its flying people. A significant number of electrocardiographic abnormalities have been detected in this flying population. This study is of particular importance because none of these people had been excluded from flying activities as a result of a screening electrocardiogram at the onset of their career. A sample of 5900 electrocardiograms recorded in individuals below the age of 40 and over the age of 25 years demonstrated 306 electrocardiographic abnormalities (5.23 per cent). The distribution of these abnormalities are presented in table 73.

Considering the relatively high frequency of electrocardiographic abnormalities, it is important to have some concept of the significance of such findings in individual cases. It is beyond the scope of this section to explain the details of the interpretation of such electrocardiographic abnormalities; however, their significance in flying personnel will be discussed.

Cardiac arrhythmias are frequently the result of hypoxia and g forces and many of them may initiate syncopal episodes. Thus, they constitute a major segment of cardiac problems in flying populations. It is pertinent to point out that cardiac arrhythmias are actually changes in the electrical mechanism of the heart and changes in cardiac rhythm which affect cardiac dynamics. They are not simply electrocardiographic findings. The electrocardiogram merely enables one to detect the changes in the dynamics which are occurring within the heart itself.

The normal cardiac rhythm is sinus in origin. Simple sinus tachycardia with cardiac rates of less than 180 per minute or sinus bradycardia with rates of 50 per minute and sinus arrhythmia present no known problems. The significance of marked sinus bradycardia or sinus arrhythmia may have to be re-evaluated in the light of more exacting requirements of future air flight.

Sinus arrest means failure of the sinus node to discharge or fire the heart. When this occurs, some lower center within the heart must assume the responsibility of initiating cardiac impulses. If this does not occur, cardiac arrest leads to loss of consciousness and death. An individual presenting episodes of sinus arrest under normal circumstances is not a likely candidate to withstand all the rigors of modern aviation. He is, in short, more susceptible to developing serious cardiac arrhythmia or cardiac arrest during

TABLE 73
*Abnormalities in 5900 Routine Electrocardiograms**

Abnormality	Number of Cases	Per Cent
Sinus arrest	1	
Atrial rhythm	16	0.27
Atrial premature contractions	14	0.24
Atrial fibrillation	1	
Nodal rhythm	5	0.08
Nodal premature contractions	15	0.25
Ventricular premature contractions	62	1.05
Ventricular extra systoles	3	
First degree A-V block	31	0.52
Second degree A-V block	1	
Complete A-V block	2	
A-V dissociation	6	0.10
Wolff Parkinson-White syndrome	11	0.18
Right bundle branch block	20	0.34
Left bundle branch block	4	0.06
Wandering pacemaker	10	0.17
Ventricular parasystolic focus	3	
Unclassified arrhythmia	3	
Nonspecific T wave changes	64	1.08
Nonspecific ST segment changes	3	
Left ventricular hypertrophy	1	
Atrial enlargement	2	
Total infarction problems	28	0.47
Other manifestations suggestive of infarctions	9	0.15
Total infarcts	19	0.32
Myocardial infarction, inferior wall	10	0.17
Myocardial infarction, lateral wall	1	
Myocardial infarction, anterior wall	8	0.13
Total abnormalities	306	5.23

* The actual number of abnormalities in this age group (20 to 40 years) is probably higher owing to sampling factors. Infarction of the inferior wall means a Q_3 of 0.04 second or over with Q waves in aVF and II. Other manifestations of infarction include Q_3T_3 of a more equivocal nature.

times of pressure breathing, the onset of hypoxia or recovery phases after extreme sympathetic cardiac action. Sinus arrest may initiate passive rhythms. Passive rhythm refers to the failure of the main pacemaker (the sinus node) with some other portion of the heart assuming the function of initiating cardiac impulses. Should the new focus for initiating cardiac activity fail, still another center must assume this function. Thus, passive cardiac rhythms develop as a result of failure by one of the higher centers.

Passive rhythms are in contrast to those rhythms which originate from an irritable focus (ectopic focus) or interrupt the normal mechanism of cardiac action. The latter are referred to as ectopic rhythms. A slow passive rhythm may be below the frequency discharge of an ectopic pacemaker. This permits an ectopic rhythm to assume control in the presence of a passive rhythm. An example of such is an individual with slow passive nodal rhythm suddenly developing nodal tachycardia (fig. 132).

An impulse within the atria is capable of assuming the role of the cardiac pacemaker. When an irritable or ectopic focus fires a premature discharge atrial contraction occurs. Atrial prematurities in themselves have no pathologic significance. Occasionally they are noted in the presence of underlying rheumatic heart disease or congenital disease with enlargement of the atria. Clinically, they may precede the subsequent development of more serious atrial rhythms such as atrial fibrillation. An individual presenting with atrial prematurity beats should be carefully evaluated clinically to exclude the possibility of underlying mitral stenosis or cardiac disease; and in the event that they are not so frequent as to be disabling and there is no evidence of underlying heart disease, they may be ignored. Reassurance of the patient who recognizes them by the symptoms they produce is oftentimes required. The elimination of poor hygiene, for example, desisting from smoking, excessive drinking of coffee and alcohol, and avoiding fatigue, are sometimes of benefit.

The irritable focus within the atria is capable of inducing paroxysmal rapid heart action, either atrial tachycardia, atrial flutter or atrial fibrillation. These mechanisms present the possibility of causing the heart to beat so rapidly that it does not have sufficient time for diastolic filling. When this occurs, the heart is no longer an efficient pumping organ. This may lead to serious impairment of cardiovascular dynamics. This possibility has led to the more or less accepted concept that individuals with episodes of rapid heart action are not suitable to be in primary control of aircraft. This approach may be re-

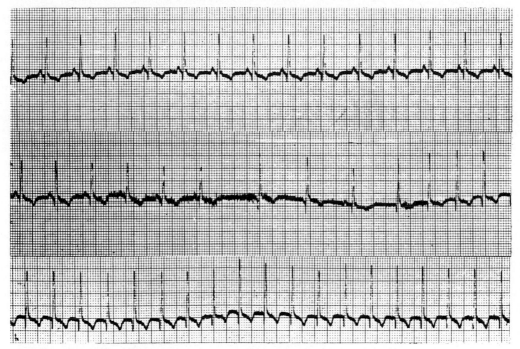

FIG. 132.In the middle strip passive nodal rhythm develops and is replaced by the onset of nodal tachycardia.

laxed somewhat in commercial aviation when one is dealing with passengers, or individuals involved in the flight operations, but never in primary control of the aircraft.

A focus within the atria may function as the pacemaker in a passive manner; that is, when the sinus node quits functioning, an atrial focus may act as pacemaker. In such instances, the cardiac rate is usually perfectly regular and slightly slower than that noted with the particular individual's sinus rhythm. The atrial focus may be located anywhere within the atrial chambers and affect the electrocardiographic configuration. Atrial rhythm may cause retrograde activation of the atria and can be confused with upper nodal rhythm. The location for the atrial pacemaker may change between the sinus node to numerous different locations within the atria. Such change in location from one cycle to the next is referred to as a wandering pacemaker. All individuals who present with atrial rhythm should be carefully evaluated with stresses of the type they might encounter in flying to be certain that no more significant arrhythmias occur under such conditions. There are still a sufficient number of pacemakers within the rest of the heart which can assume this function if the atrial focus fails to provide adequate safety factors. This point is essential in evaluating a passive rhythm and trying to exclude the possibility of cardiac arrest. As with other passive rhythms, however, at any time that the new pacemaker becomes overactive, an episode of tachycardia may ensue. The isolated finding of atrial rhythm without the demonstration of more significant arrhythmias should pose no major compromise to flying safety.

Nodal rhythms include premature contractions originating from a nodal focus, passive nodal rhythm and nodal tachycardia. An irritable focus within the node may produce a premature contraction and when these occur without the presence of cardiac disease, drug intoxication or other abnormal findings, they present no major compromise to cardiovascular dynamics. Nodal tachycardia with cardiac rates of 100 or more may be considered as another example of paroxysmal rapid heart action and as such may induce adverse cardiovascular hemodynamics.

Passive nodal rhythm implies that the cardiac pacemakers above the node failed to initiate cardiac impulses and the node itself must assume this responsibility. Beyond the node and its specialized conducting tissue, there remains only the ventricle as a possibility of running the heart in the case of a cardioinhibitory response. For this reason, individuals presenting passive nodal rhythm are not desirable candidates to be in primary control of aircraft. The author has had the experience of seeing pilots present the electrocardiographic finding of nodal rhythm and subsequently admit, during interrogation, to syncopal episodes. With the decreased cardiac rate attendant to slow nodal rhythms, the individual is somewhat more susceptible to syncope. Other than its effects upon the hemodynamics of the circulatory system so crucial to the flying population, nodal rhythm may have no significance insofar as the heart is concerned. It is seen on occasion in normal subjects.

Ventricular premature contractions are a frequent finding in normal populations. In their simplest form as isolated prematurities without evidence of underlying heart disease, they may be ignored. Not all ventricular premature contractions, however, are innocuous. A few, particularly the parasystolic type originating from a definite pacemaker within the ventricle, are capable of initiating ventricular tachycardia. All ventricular prematurities actually have this capability but it occurs infrequently in the majority of instances. Because of the high incidence of cardiovascular disease in the presence of multifocal ventricular premature contractions such a finding must be regarded with suspicion. A simple rule of thumb to follow is that the ordinary unifocal ventricular premature contraction which has a constant relationship to the preceding normal beat in the otherwise normal individual can be disregarded. If the ventricular premature contraction appears to arise from a parasystolic focus with inconstant coupling with respect to the preceding beat or if they are multifocal in origin, such an individual should be excluded from the greater stresses of flying occupations.

In the presence of simple uncomplicated ventricular premature contractions, individuals may experience clinical symptoms. This is particularly true in a somewhat introspective individual. Such individuals do

well with reassurance of the absence of clinical heart disease and instituting general hygienic measures of avoiding excessive fatigue, tobacco, alcohol and coffee. Simple ventricular premature contractions can result from underlying myocardial disease but unless other supporting findings warrant such a diagnosis, it is seldom justified. It is pertinent to point out that one of the earliest manifestations of asphyxia is the occurrence of ventricular premature contractions.

Conduction disturbances in the heart manifested by delay in transmission of the electrical impulse from the atria to the ventricle (A-V block) are a relatively frequent finding. First degree A-V block with simple prolongation of transmission of the impulse is frequently seen in an individual without any evidence of heart disease. It may also be due to atherosclerotic changes and carditis. Every individual presenting such a finding should be carefully evaluated to exclude unrecognized active carditis by using sedimentation rates, C-reactive proteins, antistreptolysin titers, and other well known clinical tools. If no evidence of active carditis can be demonstrated and there is no significant supporting evidence for atherosclerosis, this finding can be ignored.

Second degree A-V block presents the added complication of complete failure in transmitting some of the impulses to the ventricle. This is a somewhat greater degree of the abnormality and it is unlikely that an individual presenting second degree A-V block is free from underlying heart disease or significant change in their conducting mechanisms.

Complete A-V block, meaning that no impulses are transmitted from the atria to the ventricle, represents a manifestation of underlying heart disease. The slow ventricular rate encountered in this condition compromises the cardiovascular dynamics. The presence of underlying heart disease and the compromise in cardiovascular dynamics eliminates individuals with this finding as suitable candidates for primary control of aircraft.

A-V dissociation is not the same as A-V block, even though it is frequently confused with it. A-V dissociation means that an impulse below the atria is running the ventricles at nearly the same rate or slightly more rapid than the atria. This results in complete independence in the activation of the atria and ventricles. It is commonly produced by increase in the rate of the ventricle, usually through a nodal focus or, on other occasions, by suppression of the sinoatrial node. It may be seen in some normal subjects and is not necessarily a manifestation of underlying heart disease. It can result from myocarditis and drug intoxication. In order to have A-V dissociation one must assume that nodal rhythm or ventricular rhythm is present. At the present, our knowledge of the ability of individuals with this finding to withstand the flying stresses, which are prone to induce cardiac arrhythmias anyway, do not represent the most desirable candidates to be in primary control of high performance aircraft.

Aside from the usual arrhythmias encountered and discussed above there are others which have special significance in aviation. The Wolff-Parkinson-White syndrome or the short P-R interval with prolonged QRS complex has long fascinated people concerned with aviation medicine. Reportedly this finding is associated with a very high incidence of paroxysmal tachycardia, usually atrial tachycardia or atrial fibrillation. It is a congenital defect and can be readily diagnosed by electrocardiographic means. Because of the reported high incidence of arrhythmias in these individuals such a finding at the beginning of flying careers is probably adequate cause to recommend that the individual not pursue this occupation. For any individual who has already been trained and has begun his career the size of the investment may warrant a second thought before advising termination of a flying career.

In electrocardiographic surveys, it is now apparent that a relatively large number of individuals with this finding are flying and have apparently never experienced cardiovascular symptoms or symptoms of cardiac arrhythmia. This is probably caused by the difference in the type of population being discussed. The clinician who sees patients in his office with Wolff-Parkinson-White syndrome sees patients who seek him because of symptomatic findings; thus, reported instances of paroxysmal tachycardias in such individuals by the clinician is grossly colored by his clinical experience. In all likelihood, the incidence of paroxysmal tachycardia in this entity is nowhere near the usual reported incidence. For this reason it is perfectly sound to believe that an individual who presents no evidence of arrhythmia or history of paroxysmal tachycardia should continue an established flying career.

Right bundle branch block has long posed a problem in selection and maintenance of flying personnel. Not too long ago, right bundle branch block was considered as significant evidence of underlying heart disease. It is now well established that complete right bundle branch block may be seen relatively often in young people without evidence of underlying heart disease. In the younger age group, it is much more common than left bundle branch block and apparently can be of congenital origin without any other change in cardiovascular status. Right bundle branch block may be considered as caused by one of five general groups of causes: (1) congenital; (2) inflammatory (myocarditis); (3) degenerative (atherosclerotic); (4) right ventricular hypertrophy and dilation; and (5) influences of critical heart rate. In young individuals who present no evidence of any other underlying cardiac defect right bundle branch block should be considered as an innocuous finding. Inasmuch as right bundle branch block may be caused by significant atherosclerotic heart disease and a relatively high incidence of the older age group with right bundle branch block do have atherosclerosis, an early baseline electrocardiogram is very helpful in differentiating the possible causes of right bundle branch block in an older individual. Whereas one may be optimistic regarding the probable absence of cardiovascular disease in the young, asymptomatic individual with complete right bundle branch block, more caution must be exercised in the older age group.

Left bundle branch block is an infrequent finding. There is no reason to suppose that left bundle branch block occurs as an isolated congenital defect. Much confusion concerning the significance of left bundle branch block in comparison to right bundle branch block has been precipitated, as a matter of nomenclature. The prognosis for an individual subject with left bundle branch block or right bundle branch block may indeed be relatively the same if both individuals have underlying atherosclerotic heart disease.

However, the prognosis in the group of patients with left bundle branch block as a
whole as compared to a young group of individuals with right bundle branch block is
entirely a different matter. There are only
occasional instances of left bundle branch
block in young individuals and these are not
necessarily free of disease as myocarditis is a
common cause of left bundle branch block.

Reported incidents of so-called benign left
bundle branch block require close scrutiny.
The mere evaluation of a subject for a matter
of years following the finding of an electrocardiographic abnormality does not exclude
the possibility of underlying significant heart
disease. It is well known that individuals
who have sustained documented clinical myocardial infarction may survive for years after its occurrence; thus, simply observing a
case of left bundle branch block that survived for a period of 10 years does not imply that left bundle branch block is innocuous or is present without underlying heart
disease. Until such time as left bundle branch
block has definitely been demonstrated to
occur with sufficient frequency in individuals
without heart disease it is probably best to
regard all individuals who present with left
bundle branch block as having some underlying cardiovascular abnormality. This
should be considered strongly before recommending that such an individual be retained
in a flying career.

The term "incomplete right bundle branch
block" deserves special comment. For the
most part, unless serial electrocardiograms
show significant changes, intraventricular
conduction defects and incomplete right bundle branch block should be ignored. After a
review of thousands of electrocardiograms
obtained from a relatively normal flying population, recorded by numerous technicians
and read by doctors trained at all the different medical universities within the country,
it is quite obvious that the most frequent
cause of incomplete right bundle branch
block is an improperly recorded electrocardiogram. The error which commonly produces this is misplacement of the precordial
electrodes beginning in the third intercostal
space rather than the fourth; thus, such electrocardiographic patterns which have a terminal force directed upward and toward the
right shoulder may present with R' waves

over the precordial leads and be labelled as
incomplete right bundle branch block. Such
records when repeated with proper techniques no longer demonstrate the findings
which led to such a diagnosis. Even when
so-called incomplete right bundle branch
block is demonstrated it has rarely proved to
have clinical significance.

One of the most frequent electrocardiographic findings in the flying population are
ST segment and T wave changes. It should
be remembered that these are nonspecific
findings. They do not constitute sufficient
evidence to diagnose coronary artery disease
or hypoxia. The factors which will induce
such changes in the electrocardiogram are
multiple. It is true that such findings may be
the only manifestations of previous myocardial infarctions. On the other hand, they
may represent merely ingestion of a high
carbohydrate meal, minor variation in the
order of intraventricular conduction or other
innocuous events. Often the origin of such
electrocardiographic findings cannot be ascertained. Such findings should merely guide
the physician to interrogate more diligently
and pursue other diagnostic techniques to
exclude the possibility of underlying heart
disease. Among the things which may cause
ST segment and T wave changes in a young
flying population, it is well to keep in mind
that some of these may be associated with
vagotonic and sympathetic influences on cardiac rate, anxiety states and sometimes are
merely a manifestation of juvenile patterns.
Elevated ST segments are frequently encountered in normal healthy young people
and when associated with normal T waves,
should not be incriminated as evidence of
underlying heart disease.

The electrocardiogram has already demonstrated its usefulness in detecting a certain
number of subjects who have had asymptomatic myocardial infarctions. Obviously it
cannot and will not detect all such cases but
there are a significant number of these which
can be found by this diagnostic technique.
Caution should be exercised in over-reading
manifestations of myocardial infarction. Simple isolated findings of Q waves in lead III
is perhaps the greatest source of misinterpre-
tation. Many of these may be associated
with differences in body build which affects
the lead's length in respect to its geometric

and electrical characteristics. Individuals presenting equivocal findings of myocardial infarction should be carefully evaluated clinically, electrocardiograms should be recorded in different positions (inspiration and expiration) and other electrocardiographic lead techniques from the body should be utilized. These methods often serve to clarify the presence or absence of myocardial infarction.

Other manifestations of myocardial infarctions in the electrocardiogram do not permit much room for equivocation. Large negative QS deflections localized over the anterior precordium in a properly recorded electrocardiogram are rather conclusive evidence of myocardial infarction.

A frequent problem posed to the physician during a cardiovascular evaluation in flying personnel is the use of the exercise tolerance test. It should be emphatically pointed out that the exercise tolerance tests that are available at this time have no diagnostic value in the presence of a resting abnormal electrocardiogram. They are used solely to induce an abnormal electrocardiographic tracing in the presence of a normal resting electrocardiogram. They are not to be used in individuals who are known to have had previous myocardial infarctions. They are of no value in the presence of abnormal ST segment and T wave changes of undetermined etiology. Young, normal, healthy individuals with elevated ST segment changes and other nonspecific findings frequently present marked electrocardiographic changes after exercise without underlying heart disease. Interpretation and evaluation of electrocardiographic exercise tolerance tests should be handled by the expert and extreme care to avoid over-reading such tracings should be exercised.

Air Transportation of Cardiac Cases

The question frequently arises as to the advisability of transport of cardiac cases. In commercial or pressurized air-craft, this is often not a major problem; however, it must be recognized that even in a pressurized cabin the pressure is not comparable to sea level values during flight. Every individual case must be considered on its own merits. Most individuals with myocardial infarction can travel safely in commercial aircraft after they have recovered. Before any final answer is given to a patient, one should know the pulmonary status and the presence or absence of anemia. Minor degrees of congestive heart failure may result in massive right heart failure on exposure to moderate hypoxia. The presence of anemia may already have overtaxed the individual's cardiovascular dynamics and even moderate degrees of hypoxia may be sufficient to create a serious change in cardiovascular function. The presence of pulmonary disease of marked degree is relatively the same as living at altitude. Further exposure to even moderate amounts of altitude may present a crucial problem. In the event that it becomes necessary to transport even a seriously ill cardiac patient by aircraft, this can be accomplished in the pressurized cabin with the administration of oxygen. During inhalation of oxygen in the ordinary commercial aircraft, environmental circumstances comparable to sea level can be approached without difficulty. Air transportation routes are important considerations as lower altitude levels are being obtained in certain flight paths which do not necessitate flying over extremely high altitudes. One should keep in mind that travel by air in a pressurized cabin is less stressful than a journey over the mountains by auto, which takes the patient to altitude levels higher than that within the pressurized cabin. The individual's response to anxiety and apprehension are important considerations, particularly in the individual who may develop angina or coronary insufficiency precipitated by emotional factors.

The Threshold of Space

The possibility of man's journey into space presents even a greater degree of biologic stress than man has coped with in the past. A major consideration in man's ability to cope with these changing environmental circumstances will be his ability to adapt his cardiovascular dynamics. The first problem will begin with the launching of a manned satellite. If excessive g forces are utilized, one may expect a greater likelihood of cardiac arrhythmias to occur. It has already been demonstrated by animal experimentation that the launching is associated with a relatively marked tachycardia. This is entirely comparable to centrifuge experiments.

During the coasting or recovery period one might well expect that a bradycardia response would occur. Just as individual variations in animals have been noted individual variations in human subjects can be anticipated. One of the major problems associated with such a project is selecting the proper individual who will not have adverse cardiovascular responses secondary to g force problems. In the event that g forces are used in a transverse manner, respiration may be impeded for short periods of time. This is not wholly innocuous, as was mentioned in reference to breath holding during the recovery period. Following relatively short periods of breath holding, significant cardiac arrhythmias can and frequently do occur.

After successful launching has occurred one must then consider that the organism is exposed to a weightless state. Under such circumstances, the relative distribution of blood to the head and upper portions may be increased. These further stimulate vagal receptor fibers which are prone to create bradycardia responses. The individual who is prone to developing bradycardia collapse, who first experiences the sympathetic phase during launching and then is exposed to the weightless state, may well find it difficult to cope with this type of sequential environmental changes.

A relative degree of hypoxia for long periods of time which may be encountered in the gondola during the time that it is in orbit is capable of stimulating adverse cardiovascular reflexes, particularly of the bradycardia type, in susceptible individuals.

On re-entry, the possibility of even the small negative g forces must be regarded with caution. Negative g forces stimulate the carotid sinus and other vagal receptor fibers which can produce cardiac arrest and bradycardia collapse. Thus all three phases, the launching, orbiting with prolonged periods of hypoxia and re-entry, present major problems in adaptation to the cardiovascular system. These will require very careful selection in evaluation of the cardiovascular system. It is to be anticipated that a high proportion of relatively healthy subjects will not be suitable candidates for such a venture.

Once again as aviation frontiers move forward and multiply the intensity of biologic stresses, careful attention must be directed to the ability of the cardiovascular system to maintain life itself before any other bodily functions or work performance can be carried out. As such, the sequential environmental changes will restrict the number of suitable candidates to an even smaller number.

REFERENCES

(1) SCHAEFER, H.: Über die Sensibilität von Herz und Skelettmuskel und ihre Klinische Bedeutung. Klin. Wchnschr., 22: 553–560, 1943.

(2) LAMB, L. E., DERMKSIAN, G., AND SARNOFF, C. A.: Significant cardiac arrhythmias induced by common respiratory maneuvers. Am. J. Cardiol., 2: 563–571, 1958.

(3) RÜHL, A., AND THADDEA, S.: Anoxie und Milchsäurestoffwechsel von Herz und Lunge. Arch. exper. Path. u. Pharmakol., 191: 452–464, 1939.

(4) KOTTENHOFF, H.: Steigerung der Höhenfestigkeit durch Umstellung. Luftfahrtmedizin, 4: 294–313, 1940.

(5) GREENE, C. W., AND GILBERT, N. C.: Studies on the responses of the circulation to low oxygen tension. II. The electrocardiogram during extreme oxygen-want. Am. J. Physiol., 51: 181, 1920.

(6) GAUER, O.: Röntgenkinematographische Darstellung der Fliehkraftuirkung. Luftfahrtmedizin, 9: 121, 1944.

(7) GAUER, O., AND WEICKERT, H.: Das Elektrokardiogram des Menschen bei Fliehkraftuirkung. Luftfahrtmedizin, 9: 121, 1944.

(8) DERMKSIAN, G., AND LAMB, L. E.: Cardiac arrhythmias in experimental syncope. J. A. M. A., 168: 1623–1630, 1958.

(9) DERMKSIAN, G., AND LAMB, L. E.: Syncope in a population of healthy young adults; incidence, mechanisms, and significance. J. A. M. A., 168: 1200–1207, 1958.

(10) LENNOX, W. G.: Science and Seizures. New York, Harper and Brothers, 1941.

(11) BENSON, O. O., JR.: Coronary artery disease; report of fatal cardiac attack in a pilot while flying. J. Aviation Med., 8: 81–84, 1937.

(12) LAMB, L. E., AND KABLE, K. D.: Acute myocardial infarction in a twenty-one-year-old aviation cadet. J. Aviation Med., 8: 263–270, 1958.

(13) Committee on Prevention of Rheumatic Fever and Bacterial Endocarditis: Prevention of rheumatic fever and bacterial endocarditis through control of streptococcal infections. Mod. Concepts Cardiovas. Dis., 25: Suppl., 365–369, 1956.

23

NEUROPSYCHIATRY IN AVIATION

John C. Mebane, M.D.

The physician who lives intimately with aviation has a special regard for those phenomena which are the province of neuropsychiatry. The act of flying confronts him with a keen awareness of his surging emotions. If flying is a new experience for him, he may, like the air passenger, find it to be an encounter with the vast unknown. With time and greater familiarity, the physician acquires a particular appreciation of the intricate interplay of brain, body and machine which has enabled terrestrial man to conquer the force of gravity. Nervous and emotional reactivity have been so fundamental to aviation that there has been only a gradual crystallization of data in such form that one could say there existed a subspecialty of neuropsychiatry within aviation medicine (1). It is the purpose of this chapter to describe the impact upon man's nervous system of those stresses which are part of the act of flight. Aviation is a restless, demanding giant. Neuropsychiatry, to keep pace, must advance beyond phenomenology to direct all possible energy toward thwarting or softening the onslaughts of a new and unfriendly environment. Where this is not possible tools must be forged with which to identify the individual who is poorly equipped to deal with the stresses of aviation.

The neuropsychiatrist in aviation medicine is faced with complex questions. Neuropsychiatric disorders loom large as major obstacles in the path of successful adaptation to flying. In spite of the fact that emotional factors are of great importance, the clinician seldom finds them openly expressed. Disturbed emotions are hidden or expressed *via* the soma. Yet the neuropsychiatrist is asked to explore such disorders in terms of their effect upon the flyer's health should he continue to fly. The welfare of others, flying safety and the risk to expensive aircraft and equipment must also be considered. Such decisions are highly complex and sometimes unsatisfactory. Therefore, the neuropsychiatrist is usually asked to predict whether a potential flyer is predisposed to failure. In terms of overt illness, the neuropsychiatrist can act with confidence. The so-called borderline candidate is a severe test of his scientific and technical capabilities (2). Throughout the elaboration of neuropsychiatry in aviation, there has been steady pressure toward the establishment of standards by which to judge the fitness of the flyer for his duties. Such standards exist as an integral part of the enormous effort toward prevention which has become identified with aviation. Rigid standards, however, do not always do justice to the adaptive capabilities of man nor to the therapeutic advances of modern neuropsychiatry. It is appropriate and desirable, therefore, that knowledge from this special field of medicine be developed constantly to provide substance, direction and flexibility to the advance of aviation.

Neurologic Problems

The problems of a neurologic nature which assume special importance in aviation are those which result in a disturbance in the stream of consciousness. Such disturbances may attract little attention on the part of the busy physician in the everyday practice of medicine. In the field of aviation, however, impairment of consciousness under any circumstances becomes a matter of concern and the explanation for such episodes must be established whenever possible. An unconscious flyer severely compromises flying safety. This is certainly true of the solo flyer. However, it should be emphasized that as part of a crew the flyer with a disturbance of consciousness may interfere with controls, switches or otherwise add to the hazards of critical flying maneuvers or adverse weather conditions.

Flyers have no special immunity to neurologic disease and any large group will have its share of disorders of nerves and ganglia, and of vascular, inflammatory and neoplastic lesions of the central nervous system. Such disorders, once diagnosed, are managed clinically without special reference to the occupational group from which the patient arises. The mode of onset of neurologic disorders is of critical concern, however, inasmuch as there is frequently impairment of consciousness, this may be episodic, and probably will not be witnessed by the physician, not to mention the neurologist. The aviation medical practitioner is, therefore, concerned with matters of prompt recognition. The condition which must be frequently considered is epilepsy. A related problem is the differentiation of the various forms of cerebral dysrhythmia from the so-called syncopal reactions where impaired consciousness may be merely the end point in a highly complex and widespread breakdown of homeostatic mechanisms. An additional special concern is the evaluation of flyers who have suffered a disturbance of the nervous system at some time in the past and may seek to resume flying. The majority of such cases have suffered craniocerebral trauma and the presence of residual neurologic impairment must be considered.

Epileptic Disorders

Although epilepsy affects only about ½ of 1 per cent of the population approximately one-third of patients experience their first attack after reaching the age of 21 years. The physician practicing aviation medicine, therefore, must expect to encounter previously undiagnosed epileptics among flyers and must have a high index of suspicion of the protean manifestations of an epileptic seizure. It cannot be emphasized too strongly, however, that with seizures beginning in adulthood, the presumptive diagnosis is brain tumor until proven otherwise.

Seizure Patterns. Most epileptic seizures are of the major type. About two-thirds of these are preceded by some type of aura, frequently referred to the epigastrium. The aura may also be felt as a twitching or tingling in the periphery of one extremity. Occasionally, psychic auras of fright, or auditory or visual auras may be encountered. An epileptic cry often precedes the tonic-clonic seizure. In the usual case the victim foams at the mouth, may become deeply cyanotic, may bite his tongue or cheek or otherwise injure himself. The pupils are usually dilated and rarely react to light. The corneal reflex is abolished and the sphincters are relaxed. The seizure is followed by nervous exhaustion, deep sleep and hyporeflexia. A positive Babinski sign may persist for several hours, the subject may be unable to understand spoken words and may show facial weakness or nystagmus. A twilight state may ensue during which behavior is automatic and cannot be recalled later.

The major epileptic seizure is such a dramatic event that the physician is usually consulted unless such an attack is nocturnal or otherwise not witnessed by others. The patient's obvious helplessness is persuasive evidence that an incident of considerable importance has taken place. There are many seizures, however, where impairment is not so drastic and the patient may show amnesia, stubborn denial or rationalization regarding the disturbance. Such minor or partial seizures would obviously present a particular problem in flyers, and with the exception of petit mal, are likely to occur in older age groups. A wide variety of symptoms and signs may be noted, depending upon whether the seizure arises from a cerebral focus or from central integrating areas of the higher brain stem. There is frequently an aura preceding such minor seizures. This may be visual, auditory, gastric, olfactory or gustatory. Other forms of aura may be vertigo, a funny feeling in the throat, fear, paresthesias, nausea or a sensation of *déjà vu* or *jamais vu*. The motor manifestations of the seizure are varied and may include: incoordination, sudden loss of postural tone, negativism, staring, pushing, groping, searching, chewing, swallowing, spitting, smacking of the lips, myoclonic jerks, laughing, crying, rubbing, plucking, undressing, shouting, screaming or confused talking. The minor seizure may also be characterized by simple and abrupt fainting, sudden severe pain or vomiting.

Patients are often reluctant to discuss such bizarre episodes out of fear that the story will be misinterpreted as evidence of mental instability. Frequently, the minor seizure can be detected only by direct questioning. If one questions the patient carefully after an attack he is invariably found to be confused.

Photic epilepsy is a phenomenon which has been encountered rarely in flyers. Such attacks may result from the rays of the sun flickering through the rotating blades of a propeller. Equally rarely, a flyer will manifest photic epilepsy during electroencephalic screening including photic stimulation. In the absence of any clinical history of seizures such an occurrence makes the decision of flying fitness a difficult problem. Photic epilepsy is a possibility to be considered in unexplained helicopter accidents. At any rate, continuous flicker is an unpleasant experience, and helicopter crews should be shielded from overhead light during cross country flights.

SYNCOPE

VASODEPRESSOR SYNCOPE. This common type of syncope occurs under a wide variety of circumstances. The most frequent causes are fright, overpowering anxiety, sight of blood, pain, trauma, noxious agents and a variety of other stresses. The person who experiences such an attack often feels himself slipping away and may report that "everything went black" in contrast to the sudden loss of consciousness typical of an epileptic seizure. A fall in blood pressure occurs with dilation of peripheral and visceral blood vessels leading to pooling of blood, cerebral anemia and unconsciousness. Vasodepressor syncope occurs mainly in the erect posture and may be relieved in the recumbent position. A brief, usually mild tonic-clonic convulsion may be encountered, particularly if the subject is maintained erect.

ORTHOSTATIC HYPOTENSION. Cerebral anemia in this disorder results from failure of vascular reflexes to maintain peripheral resistance in the upright position. Loss of consciousness ensues if the process is not reversed by change of posture or muscular contractions, particularly of the lower extremities. Other stresses such as fatigue, chronic debilitating conditions, unfavorable body heat balance, vasodilating drugs and psychologic factors may contribute to the onset. Simple orthostatic hypotension tends to be repetitive, although it may be corrigible by a period of physical reconditioning. A closely related condition, chronic orthostatic hypotension, is the result of a defect in the autonomic nervous system producing continuous hypotension and frequent syncope in the upright position.

INTOLERANCE TO POSITIVE g FORCE. Centrifugal force directed footward produces cerebral anemia presumably by shifting blood to the splanchnic area and lower extremities. The degree of disturbance varies from confusion to abrupt loss of consciousness depending on the rate of onset, intensity and duration of positive g forces. Normal levels of tolerance have been established by repetitive centrifuge and in-flight tests on large numbers of personnel; however, these levels are variable depending on physical condition, knowledge of methods of increasing peripheral resistance by muscular contraction and emotional state. Cohen, Silverman and Zuidema (3, 4) have found lowered g tolerance to be closely related to increased anxiety and circulating blood epinephrine levels. Increased tolerance to g force was noted when the subject's emotional state was decisive, outward directed and associated with increased levels of blood norepinephrine. Sarnoff and the author (5) have correlated this finding with clinical studies of flyers who showed decreased *g* tolerance during episodes of anxiety.

HYPERVENTILATION. According to Engel (6) hyperventilation may lead to syncopal symptoms through at least four different mechanisms: decreased arterial carbon dioxide level, vasodepressor syncope, hysterical syncope and postural hypotension. The most frequent manifestations of hyperventilation are numbness and tingling of the hands, feet and face. Disturbances of consciousness are next in frequency, *e.g.*, dizziness, lightheadedness, giddiness or faintness. Tetany is seen in extreme cases. Emotional lability often accompanies the state of impaired consciousness. Wayne (7) has found that it is not possible to differentiate clinically between the symptoms of hyperventilation and hypoxia. Flyers should, therefore, be familiarized with such symptoms and trained to take corrective action even though unable to differentiate between the two. Hyperventilation has been suspected as a possible cause for critical deterioration of flying performance. Balke *et al.* (8) conducted in-flight sampling of expired air of jet pilot trainees and verified the existence of in-flight hyperventilation. Incidents of hyperventilation appeared to become more frequent with the increase in high performance capabilities of the aircraft flown. From an observational standpoint, experienced jet flyers are often aware of the anxiety of their passengers inasmuch as their rate of breathing is audible over the intercommunications system.

COUGH SYNCOPE. Derbes and Kerr (9) describe this phenomenon as a symptom complex characterized by the occurrence of loss of consciousness preceded by coughing. In certain instances there may be accompanying convulsions. From a collection of 290 cases, 97 per cent were men and 75 per cent of these were between 35 and 60 years of age. The peak incidence occurred in the fifth decade. The cough is usually dry, violent and frequently paroxysmal. The victim is usually a robust male possessed of a gregarious personality who overindulges in the pleasures of eating, drinking and smoking. He is subject to upper respiratory tract infections, often has pulmonary emphysema and sometimes bronchial asthma. The syn-cope tends to be sudden and totally unsuspected and injuries and accidents may occur.

THE OXYGEN PARADOX EFFECT. This condition is especially seen in young individuals who have exercised heavily and who may have been hypoxic for a period of time. When such a state is terminated by inspiration of rich oxygen mixtures, severe disturbances of consciousness have been known to occur. The role of hyperventilation in this phenomenon is difficult to assess inasmuch as it has been noted that the effect is more obvious if, during hypoxia, ventilation is voluntarily exaggerated. Although preliminary research has been done (10), no study of the incidence of the oxygen paradox effect has been carried out among flyers. Noell (11) has reported 2 cases from among 180 university students. Such a disturbance could be critically important to the flyer who discovers that he is hypoxic and abruptly switches his system to 100 per cent oxygen. The author examined 1 aircrew member who abruptly lost consciousness upon breathing 100 per cent oxygen after several minutes of an altitude chamber hypoxia demonstration. The episode was later reproduced during an electroencephalographic study. Unconsciousness accompanied by delta waves occurred when 100 per cent oxygen was administered after a period of breathing a 7 per cent oxygen mixture.

OTHER CAUSES OF SYNCOPE. There are many other conditions capable of interrupting the stream of consciousness, but for the sake of brevity only those have been chosen which are more frequent or else little known and deserving of consideration. The psychogenic seizure occurs in the immature, dramatic individual during an emotionally meaningful event. Such spells usually occur in the presence of others, the attack is bizarre and the subject is never completely unconscious. In the author's experience such reactions have been rare among flyers, and if psychic mechanisms operated, they were more likely to produce vasodepressor syncope such as fainting at the sight of blood.

Disturbances of consciousness have been observed in flyers who have performed the Valsalva maneuver too vigorously in flight, mistakenly believing that such a technique will counteract *g* force. Complete closure of the glottis markedly reduces venous return to the right side of the heart and ultimately impairs cerebral arterial circulation. The author has examined several flyers who experienced syncope after voiding an excessively full urinary bladder. Fatigue, ingestion of alcohol and recent awakening were factors in some of these men, but the syncopal mechanism nevertheless remained obscure.

DIAGNOSTIC PROCEDURES IN IMPAIRMENT OF CONSCIOUSNESS

Some episodes of impairment of consciousness in flyers may arise from an obvious cause; however, many of such disturbances are difficult diagnostic problems which require special diagnostic facilities. It is beyond the scope of this discussion to enter into an exhaustive analysis of the differential diagnosis of disturbances of consciousness. It is essential, however, to outline the various procedures which have been found valuable in obtaining a better understanding, if not always a specific diagnosis of the pathophysiologic mechanisms in individual cases.

A searching history of the episode of impaired consciousness and of pertinent background data is vital to diagnosis. This information must usually be gathered from witnesses, fellow flyers and family members as well as from the patient. Special attention should be directed to the family and birth histories and to the occurrence of infections in childhood.

Laboratory studies should include a hemogram, a serologic test for syphilis and a glucose tolerance test. The patient's psychosomatic response to venepuncture should be noted. Urinalysis, electrocardiogram and x-rays of chest and skull are also desirable. Clinical evaluation of cardiopulmonary status, a 3 minute orthostatic tolerance test, carotid sinus stimulation, breath holding in full inspiration and a cold pressor test may then be carried out. Simultaneous recording of the electrocardiogram may be useful with these tests. The tilt table may also be helpful as a stress inducing agent.

At this juncture it may be appropriate to conduct the psychiatric interview and to examine the patient neurologically. Clinical psychologic evaluation is frequently desirable, inasmuch as this group of flyer patients is characteristically defensive and all avenues of fact gathering must be called into use.

Electroencephalographic studies may be done at rest and during hyperventilation. A separate study of hyperventilation should be carried out in the fasting state. Tracings may also be recorded during hypoxia followed by rapid reoxygenation and during sleep and photic stimulation. Depending upon the particular case in question it may be helpful to conduct further studies in the altitude chamber recording brain, heart and respiratory activity simultaneously on different channels of the electroencephalograph machine. Where a problem of low g tolerance is suspected, in-flight and human centrifuge tests should be arranged. Powell et al. (12) have developed an elaborate series of tests to measure the effect of interaction of stresses which include hyperventilation, anxiety, hypoglycemia and prolonged exposure to low g force. Such ingenious efforts are characteristic of the work which is going forward in this field.

It should be emphasized that a battery of tests such as has been described here is an outgrowth of the rigid standards of military aviation medicine with regard to disturbances of consciousness. There is still much to be learned about limits of tolerance in the average man and control studies are still not adequate. For this reason, great caution must be exercised in evaluating the significance of findings from intensive studies such as those cited here.

MANAGEMENT IN DISTURBANCES OF CONSCIOUSNESS

Management in cases of unexplained impairment of consciousness begins with thorough diagnostic study. In some instances a disturbance will be uncovered which makes it obvious to all concerned that the subject cannot engage in active flying. In some cases the explanation will lie in what appears to be a reasonably circumscribed episode during which the victim was overstressed by subclinical disease, disturbed emotions, alcohol, drugs and fatigue. In such cases the psychiatric evaluation is often crucial in assessing the individual's likelihood of falling prey to the same stresses in the future. A particular challenge to expert opinion lies in the numerically few flyers who, having experienced an episode of impaired consciousness, emerge from intensive diagnostic studies with no evidence of disease or predisposition to such a disturbance. It is evident that the clinical disorders described here fall along a spectrum of flying fitness. In most instances the decision whether an individual may be permitted to engage in active flying cannot be a categoric one and must be based on many considerations. The proper handling of such cases probably rests not in blanket standards but in thorough diagnostic study, expert opinion and ultimate review by an authoritative board of experts. If standards regarding episodes of impairment of consciousness are too rigid, the flyer becomes understandably reluctant to discuss such problems with his physician. Every effort should be made, therefore, to handle each case on an individual basis.

CRANIOCEREBRAL TRAUMA

The rapid pace of our modern way of life, speeded along by motor scooter, automobile and aircraft has made high speed accidents and associated head injuries commonplace. An important part of neuropsychiatry in aviation lies in evaluation of the fitness of the flyer who has at some time in the past suffered the various complications of head injury. That this is not a simple matter is well known to physicians who have been placed under considerable pressure by the well motivated flyer who feels he has recovered adequately from head injury and demands permission to resume active flying. It is a part of good management in the early stages of such a patient-physician relationship to brief the flyer fully on the possible complications of head injury and on the precautions to be observed.

Post-traumatic epilepsy is a late complication of particular concern in the flyer who seems to be convalescing well after head injury. The incidence of seizures is directly related to the severity of the injury in terms of involvement of the cerebral cortex. At the time head injury occurs, the likelihood of post-traumatic epilepsy may be roughly gauged by such signs of damage as loss of consciousness, amnesia, hemiparesis, aphasia, focal seizures or localized electroencephalographic abnormalities. At a later date, despite the absence of these signs at the time of injury, brain damage may be detected in the form of brain atrophy on pneumoencephalographic examination. Post-traumatic epilepsy can develop without these findings, although their complete absence makes the diagnosis difficult to substantiate.

Walker (13) has found that post-traumatic convulsions usually begin within 2 years of head injury. If the interval is longer than this other causes should be considered. The incidence of epilepsy following closed head injury is approximately 3 per cent. An analysis of several reported series of cases of open head wounds revealed that approximately 30 per cent experience seizures. Walker found the incidence of seizures from one series to another to vary from 4.5 to 49 per cent where an open head wound had been sustained. The presence of infection following injury favors the development of seizures. Lesions located in or near the central sulcus also increase the chance of seizures; thus, parietal wounds are much more prone to have a complicating epilepsy that are frontal, temporal or occipital wounds.

Pneumoencephalography and electroencephalography are very useful in evaluating the extent of craniocerebral trauma. In closed head injury the pneumoencephalogram usually is normal or shows a symmetric dilation of the ventricles. According to Walker, 87 per cent of post-traumatic epileptics show an abnormal pneumoencephalogram. In cases of penetrating head injury, the findings may be bilateral ventricular enlargement with an outpouching at the site of the skull defect, unilateral ventricular enlargement with outpouching or simple unilateral ventricular dilation on the side of the lesion. These ventricular changes are not peculiar to post-traumatic epilepsy but can be found in a nonselected group of head injury cases. The incidence of severe ventricular distortion, however, is higher among those with seizures.

Electroencephalography at rest in acute head injury occasionally shows abnormal wave bursts such as occur in idiopathic epilepsy. These may be associated with convulsive attacks. When epilepsy has developed as the result of a brain injury the electroencephalogram is almost always abnormal. The changes are usually localized but a generalized disturbance is occasionally present. Focal delta activity, spikes or sharp waves, suggest brain damage. These are usually constant in location. A normal electroencephalogram does not rule out post-traumatic epilepsy. Walker reports normal tracings in 8 per cent of known seizure cases. When activating techniques are employed with electroencephalography, *e.g.*, hyperventilation, photic stimulation or intravenous metrozol, existing patterns may be exaggerated.

The seizure in post-traumatic epilepsy is focal in 80 per cent of cases. There may be a spread resulting in a generalized convulsion. It is not uncommon for these attacks to be in the form of petit mal or grand mal seizures without a localized aura. True Jacksonian seizures are rare. Those patients having no aura have a high incidence of frontal wounds; those with a motor aura, frontal and parietal injuries; and in the group with sensory auras, wounds predominate in the parietal region.

DETERMINATION OF FLYING FITNESS. As in the management of impairment of consciousness, individual consideration is desirable in rating the fitness of a subject to engage in active flying following a head injury. Certain complications clearly contraindicate active flying: persisting neurologic signs such as paresis, paralysis, sensory disturbances or convulsions. Personality changes or intellectual deterioration are incompatible with active flying. If the complication of head injury were simple unconsciousness or amnesia the length of time during which this existed should be determined as accurately as possible. The standards for flying fitness of the United States Air Force (14) regard unconsciousness or amnesia associated with head injury to be compatible with flying if the episode did not persist longer than 15 minutes. If unconsciousness lasted between 15 minutes and 2 hours the subject is suspended from flying duties and observed for 1 year. If amnesia persisted between 15 minutes and 4 hours a 1 year observation period is required. In flyers who have been unconscious more than

2 hours or amnesic more than 4 hours indefinite suspension from flying is in order. Post-traumatic headache if persistent longer than 3 months is also a basis for indefinite suspension from flying duties.

Occasionally, follow-up electroencephalograms in a flyer who has suffered head injury will show a dysrhythmic pattern. It is impossible in most of these cases to state whether this condition results from head injury or is merely a statistic variant not correlated with any clinical disorder. One solution to such a dilemma is in obtaining an electroencephalographic tracing on the flyer at the time he enters training. This tracing can then serve as a baseline for comparative studies in later years. Such electroencephalographic screening was found to be feasible on a large scale basis among U. S. Air Force flying trainees (15) and is worthy of consideration as part of the medical processing of career flying personnel.

PSYCHIATRIC ASPECTS

Psychiatric problems in aviation today combine ancient patterns of human emotional reactivity with many environmental stresses which are new and exciting. There was a tendency in the earlier days of aviation to formulate a novel version of psychiatry around such terms as aerosthenia, aeroneurosis and others. This is undesirable; such disorders can be adequately described and understood in the nomenclature of present day psychiatry. This is not altogether true of the stresses of flying in high performance aircraft and especially the stresses anticipated in space travel. Such undertakings involve adaptational responses which are a fascinating area for research in basic psychology.

COINCIDENTAL PROBLEMS

The psychiatrist who is consulted by flyers because of their emotional problems finds that the large majority of his patients suffer from disorders in which flying is more or less coincidental. Flying may have brought such individuals face-to-face with inner conflicts which dissipate the energy required for effective flying. Although it is tempting to fix responsibility upon the man's dramatic occupation, more detailed study usually brings out a far more complex situation, particularly with respect to the factors predisposing to breakdown within the individual. In a general way it can be said that the briefer the period of time a man has flown before he shows signs of maladaptation, the greater the likelihood that his failure is caused by intrapersonal conflicts. Conversely, true gross stress reactions are the lot of the experienced flyer.

Royal Air Force studies during World War II (16) provide some perspective of the magnitude of the flyer's internal problems: neuroses in flyers were equally distributed among men who had not flown on operations, men who had started their combat tour and men who had considerable experience in operations. Five per cent of cases arose in men who had not flown at all. Over half of all cases had not been exposed to more than slight stress while flying and nearly a third to none at all.

PSYCHOSIS IN FLYERS. Psychosis is an infrequent occurrence in which the stresses of flying do not appear to play a causal role. In a study of psychosis in 77 military flyers (17) the author found a somewhat higher incidence of nonschizophrenic psychoses than among psychotics drawn from a cross section of a general military population. The average age of the flyers was 28 years, as compared with 23 years for general military patients. The slightly older average age of the flyers, as might be anticipated, was accompanied by a comparably higher incidence of affective psychoses. Flyers in the third and fourth decades of life contributed an appreciable number of patients to this series. Although in general the patients showed a moderate degree of predisposition their records of past performance would not justify regarding them as failures of initial selection. Many had flown for several years and endured the rigors of combat. This study indicated that the psychotic flyer is a suicidal risk. There were two successful suicides in the group although neither involved an aircraft. Suicide by aircraft is well known, although fortunately rare, with the exception of combat flying where the occurrence may be more frequent than is generally appreciated. The earliest manifestations of psychosis in the flyer often lead him directly to seek the physician. In many cases, however, the physician is not consulted and a flyer in the prepsychotic borderland is a difficult management problem for operational and personnel authorities. The psychotic flyer is, of course, unfit for his usual duties. Following recovery from the psychotic episode, he often exerts great pressure upon medical authorities to restore him to flying. Because of the dangers of relapse, the difficulties in maintaining close supervision and the frequent desirability of keeping the patient on maintenance drug therapy, such individuals can be permitted to resume active flying only under very unusual circumstances.

PSYCHIC STRESSES OF FLIGHT

DANGER. Flying brings innumerable stresses to bear upon man's emotional and nervous apparatus, regardless of whether he is an air passenger or a professional flyer. Probably the greatest single threat in flying is its apparent danger to life and limb. The professional flyer knows that dangers are relative to many factors; type of flying and craft, maintenance, experience of the crew and so forth. The average air passenger does not make this distinction and harbors such interesting convictions as the belief that passenger cars are safer. He is sensitized to dramatic newspaper accounts of air tragedies and usually lacks specific information on accident rates. He makes no distinction between scheduled commercial passenger flying, military flying and private flying despite the fact that there are very important differences in risks. But most of all he is inclined to make the sweeping generalization that all flying is dangerous and carries the argument no further.

PHYSICAL DISCOMFORT. For the air passenger who flies infrequently, the odds are very much in favor of his never experiencing physical discomfort in the air. Nevertheless, the more one is exposed to flying, with the possible exception of commercial air travel, the greater grows his awareness of the associated physical discomforts. Discomfort associated with rapid ascent and descent is often more anticipated than realized. Some individuals are sensitive to this from the uncomfortable feeling they have learned to expect while riding in elevators. For them it is a pleasant surprise to discover that an aircraft can glide or climb through several thousand feet without their being aware of it. In some, changes in altitude may create middle ear or sinus pain of a very acute and distressing nature. The individual who is susceptible to motion sickness will find this discomfort sufficiently compelling to dissuade him from flying except under the most urgent circumstances. Other physical stresses which may exert considerable weight upon the individual's desire to fly include cold, noise and vibration. Long flights above 10,000 feet without adequate oxygen may be remembered because of the ensuing headache and nagging fatigue.

ENERGY DEMANDS. It is apparent from the physical stresses discussed previously that professional flying demands a considerable ability to expend energy and to tolerate discomfort. In addition to these necessities for individual adjustment, professional crews must show persistence, vigilance, accuracy, decisiveness, self control and presence of mind in a team work setting. The crew of a commercial airline must demonstrate leadership and consideration with regard to their passengers. Satisfactory demonstration of the qualities here noted is not a simple task under optimum flying conditions. Consider then the drain upon the crew of a United States Air Force Strategic Air Command bomber who carry out the following in a routine training mission; arise at 0300 hours, attend premission briefing and inspect the aircraft for 3 hours, takeoff after 1 hour's delay owing to weather conditions, fly for 10 hours during which two in-flight refuelings are accomplished, arrive over their base to encounter adverse weather conditions, attempt to land by ground controlled approach and ultimately receive orders to fly to another landing field an hour's distance. Upon landing the aircraft receives postflight inspection and servicing and the crew is debriefed. Only at this time are the men free to rest. Fatigue under such circumstances may be extreme. There are times in this type of flying, as in all others, when great effort must be expended to fight off boredom.

SPEED. With few exceptions the average individual is somewhat fearful of high speed and is not particularly attracted by the prospect of hurtling through space at several hundred miles per hour. A passenger on his first flight finds that there is little or no sensation of speed in flight principally because of the optical effects produced by the distance between the airplane and the ground or other fixed objects. This effect is increased with increase in altitude until a point is reached where there is no sensation of speed optically or otherwise. So strong is this conviction in some cases that passengers will sometimes think the aircraft has stopped in midair. This absence of a sensation of high speed is fortunate for it reduces an apprehension which would otherwise exist in many cases.

ALTITUDE. A particularly distasteful aspect of flight to the uninitiated is the prospect of leaving the earth and being high up off the ground. This might be expected inasmuch as everyone inherits a fear of falling and of high places. Here again the first flight is an illuminating experience for the anticipated sensation of height is entirely lacking. Our preconceived notions in this respect are based principally on having looked down from high buildings or other tall structures where an optical illusion exaggerates the psychic effect. This comes about by reason of the fact that when we look down the side of a tall building, for example, the walls appear to recede toward the vanishing point and the base of the building looks as though it were smaller than the top. In other words, we appear to be perched on the top of a truncated cone with the small end down which gives the impression of offering a relatively insecure support. In aircraft the situation is entirely different for in that instance there is no structural connection with the earth, there is, consequently, no optical illusion, and in fact there is little, if any, sensation of height in the ordinary sense of the word. That is, one can see that he is high up off the ground but there is no "feeling" of being high up. Another factor which influences this is that, again because of the absence of a structural link between the airplane and the ground, a person loses all conception of his gravitational relationship with the earth inasmuch as this is transferred more or less completely to the airplane. In other words, one gets the impression that if he, not the plane, should fall this would take place with reference to the airplane and not with reference to the earth.

PASSIVITY. A passive role in the face of environmental threats is a widespread source of anxiety. Yet the challenge of passivity must be met in some degree by passenger and professional flyer alike. The flyer is protected by extensive knowledge of the operation of the aircraft. Yet at times of sudden emergency he may find himself with few avenues of escape. Upon occasion he may have to deal with passivity as a flying instructor, allowing the trainee to take control and to work out his mistakes with a more intimate appreciation of dire consequences. Instrument flight is a particularly strong case in point: the well trained flyer knows that his life depends upon his heeding the messages brought to him by his instruments and must learn to disregard deep seated and compelling sensations which may conflict with this information. An aircraft in flight is the product of many hands and the flyer is inevitably vulnerable to the diligence and skill of the ground crew. Individual differences in ability to tolerate passivity have long been appreciated among combat aviators. The so-called "bomber pilot" is known for his steady, deliberate functioning while flying doggedly on a bomb run over a well defended target. The "fighter pilot," mercurial in his reactivity, must assume an active, aggressive role when threatened. The ability to be active in the face of danger has a high protective value. Grinker and Spiegel (18), among others, have noted that the less active members of a combat aircrew are more vulnerable to psychiatric breakdown. Occasionally, skilled pilots develop incapacitating anxiety when placed in a crew position from which they feel unable to exercise adequate control, for example, the rear seat of a jet bomber which is less well equipped with instruments and controls and where forward visibility is limited. A source of interest, and sometimes amusement, is the obvious discomfort seen among fighter pilots who must fly as passengers in the rear compartment of an aircraft. Problems of enduring passivity are great among air passengers who may know very little of what to expect on a routine flight, and are in constant readiness for the emergency that never comes. For them there may be silent terror at changes in aircraft altitude or engine speed while in flight.

SPACE FLIGHT. The stresses man will experience when he flies beyond the earth's atmosphere have become the objects of much speculation and intensive research. Simons' personal account (19) of the "Manhigh II" balloon flight to "hostile, unforgiving altitudes" in excess of 100,000 feet is a modern classic on this subject. Armstrong (20) has noted a peculiar and interesting psychologic reaction to high altitude flight. This is the tendency to conceive the airplane as being a wholly independent habitation or planet free of all earthly connection or relationship. This feeling becomes more and more fixed with increase of altitude and at extreme heights. When the earth is almost invisible through its ever present enveloping haze, this conception in some instances becomes absolute. The result is a profound loneliness accompanied by a state of mental depression and apprehension as though one were irrevocably separated from the earth and all its inhabitants. Clark and Graybiel (21) have recently reported this phenomenon which jet pilots have come to refer to by the term "break-off." This effect appears to be a minor factor in flight efficiency but might be important when coupled with other emotional reactions toward flight. Other stresses to be encountered in space have been studied by simulated means. Sensory deprivation might be encountered under some conditions of space flight and has been reviewed by Solomon et al. (22) using autobiographic, "brainwashing" and experimental data. Such data indicate that the stability of man's mental state depends upon adequate perceptual contact with the outside world. When deprived of such contact the following responses have been observed: intense desire for extrinsic sensory stimuli and bodily motion, increased suggestibility, impairment of organized thinking, oppression and depression, and in extreme cases hallucinations, delusions and confusion. Adjustment to zero gravity will be a major step for man in space. Gerathewohl (23, 24) found subjects experienced short periods of weightlessness with reactions varying from acute discomfort and motion sickness to feelings of restfulness and exhilaration. Oculoagravic illusions were observed leading to moderate disturbances in eye-hand coordination.

Positive Motivation for Flying

Aviation has become a major industry and in the process has come to offer a remunerative and interesting life to its members. A professional flying crew has a realistic expectation of a good salary, security with the company and prestige both within the organization and outside. The crewman is an important member of a team and is closely identified with it. There is the satisfaction which comes from intensive and continuous training and of the exercise of superior skill and judgment. For the military flyer there is the opportunity to participate in patriotic activity and to engage in a type of flying which is well in advance of civilian aviation. In these days of global flight the opportunity to travel is also a realistic inducement. As one descends the scale from commercial and military aviation to non-scheduled flying, flying schools and to less formally organized activities, such inducements decline accordingly and the satisfactions derived may be more purely personal in nature.

The scope of modern aviation far exceeds the expectations of the average citizen of a few decades ago. Such achievements as world travel on a routine basis have tended to obscure the deep emotional meanings which flying holds for the professional. Except for religion, flying has more profoundly fired the imaginations of great numbers of people than any other thing in history. Strangely enough it is probably our religious teachings which account, to a certain extent at least, for the average person's fascination with aviation inasmuch as almost all religions depict wings and ascent to the heavens as life's supreme spiritual reward. Thus, it is likely that man's inborn desire to fly is more of a spiritual than of a material nature for otherwise it would be difficult to fully explain the universal interest in aviation. Aggressive drives find great satisfaction in flying: conquest of time, gravity and weather; in wartime conquest of the enemy in aerial combat and bombardment. Certain

types of flying appeal to the gambler who gains unconscious gratification from cheating fate in his daily flying activities. Flying represents to some an escape from terrestrial conflicts. Problems of the work-a-day world recede in importance as one speeds aloft in a high performance aircraft. The harsh realities of earthly life become softened, remote, even unreal. The aviation world is exciting and stimulating. It is filled with contrasts only a flyer can appreciate. Life and death are sometimes only a second in time or a flick of the wrist apart. In a world whose frontiers are rapidly disappearing aviation represents an advance upon a new world with all the aspirations this implies.

The Professional Pilot

Candidates for flying training at military schools and at training schools for commercial pilots in this country are carefully selected both mentally and physically. Their interest in aviation is based on a more realistic and practical foundation and their ambition to fly is linked with a desire to learn a lifetime profession.

In spite of all the advantages possessed by this group, however, about 50 per cent of them are doomed to failure because of the presence or absence of certain inherent characteristics which are incompatible with the high standards of flying proficiency demanded by these schools. That is, most of the failed candidates could be taught to fly but not as well as is demanded for military and commercial flying and, hence, they are eliminated as soon as a decision has been reached in each case.

Upon completion of training the professional pilot enters a career which for convenience of discussion may be divided into four poorly defined psychologic periods.

In the first period we may expect to find a group of individuals to whom flying is an accepted sort of existence. The first few years of flying are glamorous ones and there are few inhibitions resulting from age or experience. Usually during this period there are no serious domestic or financial responsibilities to be concerned with and the dangers of flying exist in the mind of each individual only for the other fellow who is not quite so capable as he.

The second psychologic period in the life of the average pilot usually begins after 2 to 4 years of flying and may come about gradually or abruptly depending upon the circumstances. If his terrestrial and aerial existence pass without unusual incidents for the first few years the pilot gradually grows somewhat conservative, begins to realize his limitations and the limitations of airplanes from the structural, mechanical and performance standpoints and gains an appreciation of the uncertainty and hazards of bad weather and other unpredictable factors. In certain cases this change comes about rather abruptly and the precipitating cause can usually be attributed to one of two general circumstances. The most common is simply flying experience which sooner or later involves one or more narrow escapes, possibly a bad crash or in some cases one or more crashes and deaths involving other pilots who have been admittedly as competent as the individual concerned. The other common cause is the establishment of a home and the assumption of responsibility for a family. During this period the accumulated experiences and judgment of the individual increases his flying ability and he becomes a better and safer pilot.

The third psychologic period in the life of a pilot extends over a period of about 10 years and occupies roughly that part of the life span between the ages of 27 and 37. This period is characterized by a further increase in conservatism which balances any tendency to recklessness which may have existed in the earlier periods and, consequently, the pilot at this time is at the peak of perfection. However, this same period is also characterized by the fact that it involves various emotional adjustments which in a few instances are not successfully accomplished.

The fourth and final psychologic period in the life of the professional pilot occupies the time from about age 37 to the end of his flying career. If the individual has successfully passed through the preceding periods without having experienced any emotional difficulty he will enter this final period with perhaps a better mental attitude than is attained either before or after that time insofar as routine flying is concerned. As has been mentioned before, the safest years of a pilot's life begin at about age 38 and this is accounted for by his experience and the natural and acquired conservatism which normally increases with increasing age and sagacity.

Throughout the duration of this final period most individuals continue to fly without any apparent mental reservations and seem to be capable of going on almost indefinitely as far as their emotional equanimity is concerned and often do so until disqualifying physical defects intervene. There are others during this period, however, who gradually lose their desire to fly and the number of such individuals increases with increase in age. The reason that flying becomes distasteful in these cases may be because of assignment to particularly hazardous duty, inadequate compensation for the risks involved, the burden of administrative duties, lack of opportunity or time to maintain adequate flying proficiency, the repeated introduction of new and more complex flying equipment, the introduction of new flying techniques, a loss of self confidence or the gradual development of an undue conservatism. Regardless of which of the above factors is involved there is seldom, if ever, an outward manifestation of undue nervous or mental stress and the ultimate result depends almost entirely on the decision reached by the individual concerned. In certain cases the individual voluntarily gives up flying and devotes himself entirely to administrative work or engages in another occupation. Where such opportunity does not exist the individual is faced with the necessity of continuing his flying against his better judgment. In this event there may be no problem involved aside from the individual's distaste for his occupation but on the other hand there may be a falling off in the individual's flying ability. Where such cases occur it is impossible for medical science to offer much assistance for obviously the problem is not of a medical nature but rather a question of professional technical ability in aviation.

MALADAPTIVE REACTIONS

At the outset it must be emphasized that disruptive emotional reactions to flying are rarely expressed openly. Fear is hidden. Among air passengers overt symptoms are rare despite the fact that at times anxiety may be very great. Among flying trainees there are great prohibitions against washing out because of emotional unsuitability. The situation is the same with the professional flyer in whom emotional conflicts may have begun to interfere with performance. Strong defenses are erected against the direct expression of fear and the aviation medicine practitioner becomes sensitized to the psychic function often served by various somatic complaints to be described here. One large group is difficult to categorize: these are the individuals who would refuse to fly in an aircraft under any circumstances. In a sense, one cannot look upon them as maladapted inasmuch as they regard aviation as having no place in the neurotically restricted sphere of their lives.

SYMPTOMS OF DECOMPENSATION. When the stresses of flying are particularly great, as in military combat aviation, one can expect to see reactions with such prevalence that they are considered "normal." Hastings, et al. (25) observed this fact in their study of successful members of aircrew in the U. S. Eighth Air Force in World War II. Tension and anxiety were universal. Ninety-five per cent of the men developed definite stress reactions and 34 per cent suffered severely. These crewmen frequently and consciously showed aggressive behavior. Such outbursts usually occurred during periods of relative inactivity. Thirty-seven per cent of the men experienced episodic depressions often with a major self accusatory content. A rebellious attitude toward ground discipline and graphically obscene language were also part of their aggressive patterns. Virtually all said they were relieved of tension by actual combat no matter how dangerous or difficult it was.

Bond, in *The Love and Fear of Flying* (26) observed that the average flyer enters his profession with the outspoken conviction that it is not dangerous. As time goes on, evidence to the contrary is presented to him, and he next expresses himself by saying "It won't happen to me." As further time elapses, and as evidence continues to be presented depending upon the number of traumatic experiences undergone he may eventually develop a fatalistic attitude in which he says "It will happen to me, it's only a matter of time." As still more time elapses the fact that it does not happen, in itself, becomes as disturbing as would certain knowledge that death would occur at a certain time. When the individual has reached this frame of mind, he takes off on every flight with the expectation of disaster. If nothing disastrous occurs he eventually experiences a feeling of disappointment and guilt which may lead him to become careless and seemingly court death. An individual who is in this mental state is an optimum subject for the precipitation of an acute stress reaction. Bond cites as of special importance such factors as identification with a dead or wounded companion on the basis of unconscious aggression ("Thank God it was my friend and not me"). Closely knit crews favor this and Bond noted that many combat flyers learned that is was safer not to have any friends. It was extremely traumatic for the crewman to be intimately involved for many hours with a mutilated or dying man if strongly attached to him and endangered by his incapacity.

As the flyer passes through these stages toward eventual decompensation, the physician should look for tell-tale signs to assist him in early case finding: change in appearance, talk and behavior, loss of keenness for flying, loss of efficiency and alcoholic excess. Insomnia is a frequent accompaniment, often with vivid and terrifying dreams in which the flyer is the central figure watching his own death or injury. He may dream of midair collisions, of catching fire, spinning-in or being unable to land. Physical fatigue, weight loss and exaggeration of previously minor disabilities are common.

The flyer who is decompensating shows marked personality changes: he is introspective, feels different, inadequate and guilty. He shows a startle reaction to minor stimuli and meets his hostile environment with irritability. If overwhelmed by his feelings of guilt and inadequacy he may become deeply depressed. In general, the reaction takes a somewhat opposite form from the patient's usual personality.

PSYCHONEUROSES. Before proceeding to a

discussion of the various psychoneuroses mention will be made at this point of a condition which has been termed the gross stress reaction or acute emotional shock. Such a reaction results from a single terrifying experience and is manifested by the usual signs of terror which may persist for several hours following the experience and may result in a psychoneurosis. The signs usually seen are dilated pupils, violent tremors, speechlessness, cold sweats, shallow breathing, dazed or trancelike states, amnesia and general weakness or collapse.

The "traumatic neurosis," although not an accepted diagnostic term, is employed so often in medical parlance that is bears some discussion. As the term implies, this is a psychoneurosis arising out of an acute traumatizing situation. The clinical picture may be any one of the psychoneurotic reaction types although diffuse anxiety and phobic symptoms are most common. From a dynamic standpoint the ego is so overwhelmed by the acute trauma that it crumbles under the impact. Marked regression to a helpless state ensues and in the post-trauma period there may be a compulsion to repeat the experience in dreams or dissociative states. The "traumatic neurosis" tends to be fairly short lived and when it persists in later years it is usually because of an underlying character disorder, inadequate treatment at the time of the trauma, or both.

The dissociative reaction occurs when the psychic conflict is so great or the ego is so weakened that for a usually brief period behavior occurs which is not under conscious control. The acute anxiety overwhelms and temporarily governs the individual and the picture may resemble an acute psychosis. Generally, frank dissociative phenomena occur in young, suggestible and immature individuals. The most common form in the flyer is "freezing" at the controls and acute panic during the time of an emergency which may cost the life of the victim, an aircrew and an aircraft.

Extreme combat situations may produce a phenomenon which is seen less commonly in other flying situations: this is the phobia, a dramatically crippling reaction which is reminiscent of the reflex avoidance one finds

in experimental animals which have been trained and rewarded to carry out a task and then are punished and frustrated for following this same pattern. This "conditioning" process in the flyer may be sudden and overwhelming. It may, on the other hand, develop insidiously out of many lesser traumatic experiences, none of which, by themselves would be sufficiently intense to create an avoidance response. The reaction is characterized by irrational morbid fear of exposure to a feared object or situation. The latter may be sharply demarcated and encountered only in certain aspects of flight or it may be so diffuse that the flyer cannot go near a landing field. This fear response is primitive, rigidly stereotyped and not amenable to logical argument. In combat, phobic reactions may involve flak, searchlights, flying with a bomb load aboard, bailing out and the like. Among flyers as a group, claustrophobia, fear of heights and particular types of aircraft are most common. When encountered in a situation of lesser stress, as in commercial aviation, it is likely that the phobic reaction is not primarily related to flying, but is instead a chronic psychoneurotic disorder aggravated by a special situation arising in flight. Claustrophobic reactions to being enclosed in weather or darkness, to the wearing of oxygen masks or to being in an altitude chamber are rather common examples. A phobic response may be produced in a flyer who is placed in a crew position in which he feels his self reliance is compromised. Avoidance of flying over water is an interesting example of the irrationality of the phobia inasmuch as it may occur when the flyer clearly understands that there is safety while over water and away from enemy attack. Underlying the phobic response there is a common theme of obsessive need for control which is probably a prerequisite to the development of the reaction in all but the most severely traumatized cases.

The neurotic depressive reaction is characterized by feelings of dejection and hopelessness, poor sleep and loss of appetite and weight. There may be an associated agitation at times, but the picture is usually one of slowing of thought and action. Such reactions are seen commonly among combat flyers who see their comrades lost one by one. Strong group ties do not permit the conscious acceptance of the feeling of relief that it was the other fellow who was killed, not they. The tensions generated by this unconscious conflict may give rise to symptomatic acts of a self punitive nature and to feelings of guilt for still being alive which become a prominent feature of the depressive reaction.

PSYCHOSOMATIC DISORDERS. The psychophysiologic reaction patterns arise when unconscious conflicts and their associated anxiety are repressed and channeled into various bodily organ systems. The organ systems which are the targets of such bombardment may with time begin to undergo structural changes. All emotion has its physical reverberation, whether it be fear, rage, love or hate. These emotions are usually discharged although the degree and mode of discharge encounter many prohibitions in "civilized" cultures. Obviously, tensions accumulate if not discharged and manifest themselves in bodily symptoms. The psychologic disturbance underlying the physical symptoms is deeply repressed and, therefore, not readily recognized.

The psychosomatic diseases, especially certain types of cardiovascular disease and hypertension, are among the most costly and stubborn illnesses with which modern medicine is confronted. The flying environment places a great investment in stability of human performance under widely varying conditions and such stability often exacts its toll in the form of a psychophysiologic reaction. From a selection standpoint, were one to eliminate men who showed the psychologic tendencies toward such reactions, valuable manpower would be lost. It is the physician's task, therefore, to recognize the prevalence and early manifestations of these reactions and to handle comprehensively these patients who produce so much and complain so little.

Although categorized separately as a psychoneurosis, rather than one of the psychophysiologic reactions, the conversion reaction deserves special mention. The conversion reaction is closely related to the dissociative reaction. Instead of a gross disturbance of behavior, however, anxiety is bound down in disabling symptoms of predisposed or injured parts of the body usually under voluntary control. Common sites are the musculoskeletal system and, particularly in the flyer, the organs of special sense. If the conversion mechanism is successful, awareness of the provoking stimulus is lacking and the patient shows little anxiety or outward concern about his disability. The physician should consider a conversion reaction whenever he encounters blurring of vision, depth perception difficulties, vertigo, headaches, deafness or pain in the ears. Among the psychophysiologic reactions, there is not this solution to a well defined conflict; rather, the unresolved conflict continues and, although repressed, results in exaggerated physical concomitants of the initiating emotional state, for example, repressed anger leading to arterial hypertension.

Among the psychophysiologic reaction types, those affecting the gastrointestinal tract constitute a majority. The expression "aviator's stomach" has been employed to describe the symptom complex of mild, gnawing pain in the epigastrium, hyperacidity, gas formation and loss of appetite. Air sickness is a disorder which may be produced by one or several factors acting separately or together, however, psychic mechanisms must always be considered.

Headache in the flyer is a common complaint and psychogenic factors are of critical importance both in muscle contraction and in vascular headaches. Vascular or migraine headaches frequently do not run true to the classic picture and the physician should have in mind some of the salient features to aid him in diagnosis. The pain appears in acute attacks, is throbbing at the onset and later becomes steady. Its distribution is usually unilateral at least in the early stages; the intensity reaches a peak within a few hours and then gradually subsides. There may be associated labyrinth disturbance, anorexia, vomiting and transient visual distortions such as blurred vision, scotomata or hemianopsia. Tender cranial arteries may be felt in the area of pain. Irritability, photophobia, constipation or diarrhea, secondary scalp muscle contraction, acute unilateral conjunctivitis or pupillary dilation may appear 24 hours or more after the onset of headache. Often the patient has had headache for many years, his family has a history of similar headaches and his attacks seem associated with the fatigue of driving for some particular goal.

Tension or muscle contraction headaches characteristically have pain which is described as tightness or viselike pressure. The duration may be short, and the pain may shift from one site to another. The pain frequently changes in quality and intensity but is usually located in the occipital region. There may be associated tinnitus and vertigo. The pain may diminish considerably following muscle relaxation measures such as heat, massage and intravenous barbiturates. Tension headache in the flyer should be looked upon as a clear-cut indicator of acute stress and exploratory and ventilative psychotherapy directed toward current life situations affords considerable relief in most cases.

The physician's time is well invested in these patients because they are the conscientious, hard working, self driving, undemanding individuals who make dependable pilots. Relieved of their distressing symptoms they become even more efficient. A certain amount of conservatism is indicated in the migraine sufferer, however, inasmuch as his flying fitness may be hampered by visual scotomata. If migraine headaches are frequent, if they incapacitate the individual temporarily for his usual pursuits, if he requires regular medication and, particularly, if his vision is impaired during the headache, he should not be permitted to fly. This is not to imply that such an individual cannot resume flying at a later date after the precipitating causes of his migraine have been isolated and treated. The trained flyer who has migraine is seldom a chronic sufferer and his prognosis is favorable when compared with the general group of individuals afflicted with migraine.

ILL DEFINED REACTIONS A disorder may arise under certain conditions of flight which is suggestive of a dissociative reaction. Among the causative factors are overattentiveness to the instruments of flight, the hypnotic effect of the drone of the engines, the monotony of the radio beam and other sounds. The pilot under such circumstances may become inattentive to the attitude and orientation of the aircraft. This phenomenon is sometimes referred to as "autohypnosis." In contrast to this reaction, "fascination" has been defined by Clark (27) as a condition of heightened attention in which the pilot fails to respond adequately to a clearly defined stimulus situation in spite of the presence of necessary cues and knowledge of the proper response. An example of pilot fascination might be found in the flyer who becomes so absorbed in his radar scope as he homes-in on his target that he fails to pull out in time and a collision occurs. "Target fixation" has been thought to occur in gunnery practice when the flyer rams his target or pulls out too late to clear the ground. Ali (28) found in a study of such accidents among flyers in the Pakistan Air Force that "fixation" occurs in the last planes strafing a target in trail. As successive planes strafe the target, the dive angle becomes steeper so that the last aircraft is in a very unfavorable position to pull out. The last flyers, therefore, find themselves caught in a dilemma between physical impossibilities and their own compulsivity and eagerness not to abort a target run.

ETIOLOGY OF MALADAPTIVE REACTIONS

Unravelling the causes of maladaptive reactions among flyers may at times be relatively simple and attributable to a single overwhelming episode. Such cases are dramatic and impressive, but for the most part not typical of the reactions usually encountered. The physician must approach each case on an individual basis and attempt to assign relative weight to each of three important contributing factors: primary load factors associated with conditions of flight, secondary load factors which are the area of environmental support to the flyer and, finally, the personality of the flyer himself as noted previously among the problems coincidental to flying. Depending upon many conditions, the relative importance of each of these factors waxes and wanes; this is particularly true in military aviation which often experiences dramatic changes in all three factors over very brief intervals of time. In this regard, Sarnoff has made an important contribution to the understanding of psychiatric disorders in flyers in the very comprehensive case studies in "Medical Aspects of Flying Motivation" (29).

PRIMARY LOAD FACTORS. These are factors inherent in the flying situation itself which may operate to produce psychic decompensation. Bond has observed that many of these factors are particularly disturbing because the flyer suffers enforced passivity; he cannot always prepare for them nor can he rely on corrective action if necessary. Catastrophes are especially traumatizing, including crippled aircraft, engine failures, fire in the air, horrifying sights, personal losses or injuries, loss of important leaders, unavoidable or unexplainable accidents unrelated to pilot error, immersion in the sea or any event which corresponds with the specific fears of the individual. Physical factors adding to the primary load are fatigue, loss of sleep, inactivity, cold, heat, high altitude flying and uncomfortable personal equipment.

Scheduling of flights and weather conditions also add to the primary load. Anticipation of a difficult flight or a combat mission is worse than the flight itself. For this reason, last minute cancellation and repeated cancellations are especially stressful. Proficiency in weather flying requires a fortuitous combination of experience and on-going training in the absence of significant distractions from other areas of the flyer's life. True "sharpness" in weather flying is probably achieved by the flyer as readily as is surgical "sharpness" in the physician. For the flyer who is weak in this aspect of flight it is not difficult to imagine the conflict produced by assignment to flying in an area with characteristically difficult flying weather.

For the military flyer there are many other burdens. Enemy defenses, including heavy flak and fighter opposition. Crew position may be particularly stressful when a crewman is assigned to a position which conflicts with his need to be active and to meet environmental threats aggressively. The Royal Air Force in World War II found a direct relationship between the incidence of neurosis attributed to flying duties and the duty assignment: air gunners were most vulnerable, pilots and navigators least. Grinker and Spiegel made similar observations regarding the United States Air Force.

SECONDARY LOAD FACTORS. These are the factors in the flyer's environment which motivate him negatively and lessen his feeling of support. Such factors lower the flyer's resistance to the stresses of his duties. Among these are lack of effective leadership, lack of confidence in other crew members or key personnel, poor or inadequate crew training and discipline or other defects in the over-all personnel program. For the military flyer important contributions to the secondary load are made by world political conditions, the presence or absence of war, the attitude of the public toward the armed forces and the support provided his family.

AIR TRANSPORATION OF NEURO-PSYCHIATRIC PATIENTS

Strickland and Ferris (30) have reported a study of 2879 patients flown by the Military Air Transport Service. Among the group symptoms during flight were reported in only 10.2 per cent. No serious reactions occurred and no symptoms were reported which were considered to have altered the prognosis of any patient. The number with somatic symptoms was 4.5 per cent which was within the range of expectancy for well individuals traveling by air. The total percentage of psychologic symptoms was 5.7 per cent and the majority were caused by disturbed behavior on the part of patients with major psychoses. The study tended to disprove that psychoneurotics are more susceptible to motion sickness than the average person. As only 8 proved epileptics were transported, an opinion could not be advanced as to whether or not they are more prone to have seizures during flight than at other times. Of course, such an accomplishment as this was not achieved without careful training and assignment of medical and flight crews. Patients must be classified according to their condition and hospital facilities must be available during stop overs. The medical crew must also be familiar with the judicious use of sedatives, tranquilizers and restraints.

Tillisch *et al.* (31) reported two patients flown by air after cranial operations who suffered severe nausea and vomiting. One patient who flew 48 hours after a lumbar puncture had not only severe nausea and vomiting but marked exacerbation of headache with dyspnea and cyanosis. It was concluded that as a general rule patients with a recent cranial operation or cerebrospinal fluid puncture should not fly.

Preventive Psychiatry in Aviation

Preventive medicine in aviation today might be regarded somewhat facetiously as a continuous campaign to make improbable disabilities and losses impossible. As a "battle of statistics" it may lack the drama of an acute emergency in clinical medicine. But still, if one cites psychiatric selection methods as part of a preventive program, there is excitement in the strides which have been made since 1916 when the incidence of neuroses in pilot trainees in the U. S. Army Air Corps was 50 per cent and 90 per cent of accidents were the result of pilot error. If prevention at times seems tedious, the physician can derive some inner comfort from the knowledge that his efforts have on innumerable occasions kept difficult situations from deteriorating rapidly.

In prosecuting the preventive campaign the physician finds himself in an unusual position with respect to the individual flyer. If he adheres to the basic operating principle that no one has an inherent right to endanger the lives of others, and if he believes that the operation of an aircraft under any conditions can be a source of danger to others, then he becomes a highly influential agent in the determination of flying qualifications for the population at large. It follows that certain risk categories will be established and individuals within these categories will be denied the privilege of flying. Once placed in this position the physician encounters innumerable pressures both from individuals and from the vexing medical problems they pose; *e.g.*, the flyer who faints would seem to be a hazard in flight. But suppose he has never fainted before and the episode in question occurred under considerable stress? How much risk is involved in allowing the man to continue to fly? Ob-

viously, the physician cannot make a persuasive argument to the laity in terms of individual cases. But when he cites reductions in accident rates brought about by rigid standards of physical fitness, he is on firmer ground. The physician who has actually seen flyers lost through accidents caused by physical defects will also approach his duties with a clearer perspective. Nevertheless, prevention may at times seem a thankless task despite its tremendous importance. The achievement of a sound philosophy of preventive medicine and psychiatry obviously requires understanding, conviction and maturity on the part of the physician.

The physician who is interested in preventive psychiatry as applied to such groups as the personnel of a commercial airline company finds his duties highly complex and often rather remote from clinical medicine. This has been brought into bold relief as preventive psychiatry as a program has developed during recent years in industry (32) and in the armed services. It has been customary in the past when discussing preventive psychiatry to become involved in esoteric discussions of morale, leadership and group dynamics. As experience has grown, certain clear-cut practices of management have emerged which provide a reasonable assurance of good morale when incorporated into an on-going personnel program. This has the advantage of providing a reasonably enduring cushion against the various stresses of duty in a way that is less susceptible to the presence or absence of inspiring leadership. Morale and productivity can then be maintained on a rather steady level. It is evident from this discussion that the physician must necessarily become intimately concerned with policies and practices of the personnel department. He must meet problems at their source rather than later when illness results. In so doing, the physician becomes closely allied with many who, despite their lack of medical or psychiatric training, are in a position to make important changes in the flyer's working environment. The clinically trained physician is in danger of feeling lost under such circumstances and requires moral support from members of his profession. A sound background in preventive medicine will permit him to act with confidence when he finds basic principles of prevention being ignored. Nevertheless, his role is that of a team worker, and except for strictly medical considerations, he finds himself contributing to a personnel program for which he does not have primary responsibility.

THE ORGANIZATION

The nucleus of a program in preventive psychiatry rests in the policies and activities of the organization as they affect the individual's welfare, his feeling of security, productivity and self satisfaction. The program administered by a commercial airline company or an airforce may have implications for mental health which are staggering. On first inspection, however, the measures which carry such weight would not seem to have very much to do with psychiatry as the clinician might think of it.

ENGINEERING. The primary flying load for the flyer is directly proportional to the actual conditions under which he carries out his duties. The care with which aircraft are designed and tested and the degree to which human engineering factors are considered are, therefore, of vital importance. The physician has an important contribution to make in focusing attention upon human engineering problems from the earliest phases of design of new aircraft, as well as in research and design of protective flying equipment. Finally, the flyer needs the assurance that his aircraft and equipment are being maintained with thoroughness and efficiency.

TRAINING. Good training means emotional preparedness. The ability to respond immediately in an emergency may well be lifesaving. As mentioned previously, one of the most threatening aspects of the flyer's environment is the ever present danger of suddenly enforced passivity. To anticipate danger with purposeful familiarity is a result of good preparation. Training, not just in operating the aircraft, but in handling passengers, escaping from aircraft and in survival techniques provide inestimable emotional support. Most fear is fear of the unknown. Good training can identify and dispel many needless fears. Because effective

training involves emotional readjustments the timing of the various steps in the training program should be closely observed. Training should be sufficiently vigorous and realistic to screen out men who are not equipped to carry the load. It should not be so arduous, however, that it overstresses otherwise healthy crewmen.

SCHEDULING. Proper apportionment of the flying load is of great importance both in the flyer's daily routine and in long range planning. The stresses of particular flights should be studied from the standpoint of their length, frequency and the hazard involved. Crews should be afforded relief for short periods during flight for moving about, eating and taking refreshments. Crew stop overs on long flights should be timed adequately, quarters should be comfortable and there should not be too many outside distractions to compete with the flyer's need for relaxation. Stressful flying assignments should have a definite duration with the assurance of rotation to more favorable duties upon completion. Such rotation policies require careful training and supply of replacement crews who are capable of stepping in and taking over difficult flying assignments with a minimum of disruption of established routines.

INTERNAL CORRECTIONS. The organization should possess an alert agency designed for the specific purpose of trouble shooting, isolating sources of difficulty and correcting them with as little delay as possible. Inasmuch as many such problems involve the human factor to a high degree, the physician can provide much assistance to such an agency. Machinery should exist for hearing the grievances of individuals and for handling problems in a tactful, fair manner. A particularly important function of such an agency is responsibility for investigating aircraft accidents. Few things can be quite so disturbing to the flyer as an unexplained accident and he deserves to know the details of all unusual occurrences as quickly as these are recognized. Anonymous reporting of incidents in flight should also be encouraged provided the rights of the individual will not be compromised. The physician can assist training authorities by following closely those flyers who have

experienced an accident. Getting such individuals back to their duties at the appropriate time will require understanding of
the emotional reactions produced by the
event and the degree to which the flyer has
succeeded in overcoming them.

OTHER PERSONNEL POLICIES. An effective
organization retains its members over long
periods of time. The stability gained from
this feeds back automatically in terms of
benefits to the organization and the accomplishment of its mission. The problem of
utilization of personnel becomes particularly
pressing as the professional aircrew member
approaches the retirement years. The so-
called aging pilot is a challenge to the wis-
dom of the organization inasmuch as the
differences between actual age and functional age may be considerable from person
to person. Generally, a reasonable retirement
age must be established by the company
which will not remove capable, productive
flyers from their duties prematurely. Upon
retirement from active flying, such individuals need the assurance of being placed
so as to continue to contribute to the organization in terms of the experience each
has accumulated. Conversely, the organization has the difficult problem of screening
its personnel so that seniority does not become the only basis for advancement to
greater responsibility both in flying and
ground positions. A particular personnel
program which deserves the support of the
physician is financial protection for the
flyer who becomes disqualified from his
duties because of illness. Obviously, flyers
will be reluctant to seek early medical assistance for disabilities if they have reason to
believe that their income will be jeopardized.
The aviation medical officer is in a much
better position to sell the concept of preventive medicine if his flyers know they
will not be penalized for requesting early
treatment. Such protection should certainly
include emotional problems since not to provide this simply drives such problems into
the "somatic underground." This is not to
imply that the physician will reward failure
and assumes that the medical expert is
qualified to assist the organization in handling personnel problems appropriately
where medical aspects are secondary.

THE PHYSICIAN'S CONTRIBUTION

Every aspect of the aviation medical
officer's duties contributes to good morale
and mental health among his flyers. The
physician need not practice psychiatry and
certainly does not have to be a psychiatrist
to render support to a preventive psychiatric
program. Whether he is inspecting crew
rest quarters, attending a flying safety meeting or examining crews on the flight line
he is boosting the morale of his men. The
physician must observe the flying situation
closely and fly often enough to assess primary load factors. He should mix freely in
the crew rooms, the hangars and in the
air. In informal meetings he can observe
individual crews and evaluate their adjustment. The physician should maintain close
liaison with operational, training and personnel members so as to implement his own
contributions to a preventive program;
however, this intimate relationship should
be outside the knowledge of the crews insofar as possible.

SELECTION. A comprehensive program in
preventive psychiatry logically begins with
selection of the right man for the right job.
It is important, therefore, that the physician
learn those qualities which make a successful flyer, and learn to recognize them among
the applicants whom he examines. Combined
with this empathic understanding must be
skill in interviewing technique and a knowledge of the uses and limitations of various
psychologic tests. Although a vital part of
the preventive program, initial selection
techniques should never be regarded as
vitiating the importance of long term medical maintenance and other measures designed to utilize to the maximum those
individuals who possess certain basic qualifications.

OUT-PATIENT CARE. In a medical program
with a preventive orientation there seems
to be an inherent danger that the individual
may be lost among statistics. Professional
flyers are healthy people whose major contact with the physician is on an out-patient
basis. The physician finds himself challenged
to match the thoroughness and efficiency of
aircraft maintenance in caring for his flyer
patients, yet still preserve an individual
orientation and an awareness of the preva-

lence of emotional disturbances in dispensary work.

SUSPENSION FROM FLYING. An area in which the physician's work has many direct and indirect implications for the emotional welfare of the group is in his handling of medical suspensions from flying duties. Removal from flying often presents an emotionally charged situation, certainly where the problem is psychiatric. When medical action to suspend a flyer is taken there must be sound reasons for doing so. The physician will be hurt, and his men will also suffer, by a reputation for grounding too strictly or too leniently. If the flyers know that the doctor wants to keep them flying and to clear up their problems before grounding is necessary they are not likely to avoid him or seek treatment elsewhere.

TEACHING. The physician has many opportunities to address large or small groups of flyers. These occasions may range from flying safety meetings to presentations of first aid techniques. It becomes evident rather quickly to the physician that his teaching duties rank on a par with his clinical responsibilities. As a teacher he will find that his flyers are inordinately interested in psychology. In informal sessions this is noted in numerous questions centering on psychologic problems. Spontaneous discussions at such times can be meaningful and corrective to the participants and can be utilized very effectively by the discerning practitioner. Understandable explanations of such phenomena as anxiety, its purpose and its manifestations, can be made. Environmental stresses can be discussed together with their impact on the flyer and their role in the formation of symptoms. The aviation medical specialist finds his flyers as a group to be keenly intelligent and able to utilize a sensible presentation of psychiatric problems.

THERAPY

EMOTIONAL REACTIONS OF AIR PASSENGERS. Fear is a very prevalent reaction among air passengers but usually remains hidden. The aircraft commander and his crew are the chief bulwarks against overt expression of fear by serving as calm, efficient examples to the passengers. Simple, well timed greetings, warnings and explanations allow the passenger to relax, to prepare for rough weather ahead or to anticipate a change in engine speed as the case may be. The appearance of the Captain will often serve to reassure the passengers. Distractions such as meals, reading material and conversation also dilute the stress the particular individual experiences. Rarely, a passenger may become sufficiently anxious to indicate a visit by a physician during a stop over. Mild sedatives at such times usually enable the passenger to continue his trip. Anxious passengers may tend to hyperventilate and then become acutely disturbed with the onset of symptoms typical of this disorder. The aircrew should be trained to look for this and to instruct the passenger in breath holding or rebreathing by means of a paper bag.

GROSS STRESS REACTIONS. The treatment of this condition is rest in hospital with narcosis for 24 to 48 hours. Sodium amytal is the drug of choice. The physician caring for a flyer shortly after an accident may find himself on the horns of a dilemma in providing adequate treatment for the flyer, yet still permitting accident investigation authorities an opportunity to gain information. There is no simple solution to this problem; however, the physician should monitor all such activities and insure that unnecessary questioning and delay of treatment do not take place. Where gross stress reactions respond rapidly to treatment, the question of when flying should be resumed is of importance. Although each case must be judged individually it is believed that the following general rule should be observed. Assuming that the patient has suffered no injury he should be allowed to fly again as soon as he appears to have regained his composure. After a flight or two it may then be desirable to insist on a rest for a week or 10 days. It is generally unwise to keep the patient away from flying for some time following a terrifying experience. He may develop excessive anxiety owing to the prolonged period of worry concerning his reactions to a return to flying. Once a flight has been made, however, the patient can be allowed further time for complete recovery with the knowledge that he has, and therefore can, fly without any difficulty.

THE CONSULTING PSYCHIATRIST. Whenever possible it is desirable for primary control of emotional problems in the flyer to rest with his own aeromedical practitioner. The latter is more accessible, communication is more rapid and appreciation of the background in the particular case is greater. Further, the flyer maintains contact with his work surroundings and continues to feel a part of his group. Referral to the consultant may carry with it the implication that the problem is too complex and serious for one's personal physician to manage. If the flyer feels unconscious guilt about his inability to function, referral to the specialist may encourage the fixation of symptoms as an excuse for failure. The specialist in aviation medicine should, therefore, be prepared to conduct out-patient exploratory and supportive psychotherapy as the need arises in his flyers. This should be done under the supervision of a consulting psychiatrist who can maintain contact with each case and who is familiar with the flyer's environment. In addition to working with the flyer's intrapersonal difficulties through psychotherapy the practitioner in aviation medicine is in a position to manipulate the environment. It may be justifiable to treat the patient by interview psychotherapy while allowing him to continue to carry out his flying duties. In some cases a change to less arduous or hazardous flying may be indicated; brief leaves may be given or an initial period of rest followed by a program of reconditioning.

The consulting psychiatrist, in addition to supervising out-patient psychotherapy conducted by the aviation medical specialist, should arrange to treat more difficult and serious cases. The same environmental manipulative measures are available to him; however, he will be more concerned with such questions as job changes, permanent suspension from flying and hospital treatment. At times the consultant, because he is not so personally involved in the organization, may be best suited to treat emotional problems in executives and other key personnel where the aviation medical practitioner feels himself to be too much a "member of the family." Nevertheless, to function most effectively, the consultant should also have a very intimate understanding of the organization and its inner workings.

THE USE OF DRUGS. A useful general rule is that the flyer who needs to take medication is not fit to fly. This is not to imply that the occasional use of medications is incompatible with flying. If the physician becomes too restrictive in this matter he simply cuts himself off from the flyer and his problems. Among the analeptic drugs, caffeine and dexedrine are well known and may be valuable in combating the fatigue of a long mission. Methylphenidate (Ritalin) is a newer compound which possesses a more sustained action with less gastrointestinal and cardiovascular side effects than dexedrine. Needless to say, medication should not be used in flight until test doses have been given to personnel on the ground and the subjects closely observed for their reactions. The proper dosage and time of administration for the individual should be established as closely as possible. Finally, stimulants should not be given to flying personnel to be used at their discretion but should be issued as needed under the direction of a physician.

It is highly questionable whether sedatives or tranquilizers have any role in flying as such, with the possible exception of their use to insure adequate rest on the part of the flyer after a long mission.

PROGNOSIS IN PSYCHIATRIC ILLNESS

Information regarding the consequences of psychiatric illness in the flyer has been gained chiefly from military experience in World War II and the Korean Conflict. As noted previously, assessment of the flyer's readiness to resume flying duties following a period of decompensation is a matter which requires keen observation on the part of the physician. In such decisions he is torn between an optimistic desire to get his men back in the air again and concern lest the flyer find himself too abruptly in another situation in which an overload of anxiety will cost him his life. Bond has emphasized the importance of avoiding further trauma during the recuperative period when the ego is weakened and less resistant. Significantly, however, only the most neurotically predisposed flyers show serious disintegration as a result of a single accident. During the Korean conflict cases of psychoneurosis were for the most part restored to flying duties as quickly as possible. Their intensive training and experience were regarded as adequate to enable them to overcome whatever stresses they might encounter in combat operations. From a standpoint of flying safety these men were regarded as, if anything, safer flyers than their colleagues. Whether they were as effective in their duties is not known. It is difficult to evaluate the worth of such a policy because of the lighter stress load of the Korean campaign when compared with the stresses in various theaters in World War II. Among medical observers of this policy in Korea it was the author's impression that most felt such a viewpoint was realistic and successful.

The Royal Air Force in World War II found that the determining prognostic factors in flyers who broke in combat were the degree of neurotic predisposition and the proximity of the treatment facility. The degree of hazard and stress encountered in the operational tour did not affect the prognosis for full flying duties. For the entire Royal Air Force, 22.5 per cent of men who had broken were restored to full flying duties. When treatment was carried out by the unit medical officer, however, 35 per cent of a group of 286 cases were returned to full flying. Suspension from flying was necessary in 20.5 per cent and "executive flying" was permitted in 31.5 per cent. Treatment results of a neuropsychiatric treatment center were reported on a large group of crewmen who had completed more than 100 operational flying hours. Of the group, 48 per cent were restored to full duty and 12 per cent to limited flying. Within this group were 272 men who showed no predisposition to neurosis. Among them 71 per cent returned to full flying duties as compared with only 14 per cent of men who were judged to be severely predisposed to neurosis.

Hastings, Wright and Glueck divided the men who broke into categories of operational fatigue and psychologic failure. Of the operational fatigue cases, 70 per cent treated by narcosis therapy returned to combat flying. Of 26 psychologic failures similarly treated only 19 per cent returned to combat.

Grinker and Spiegel found that two-thirds of flying officers returned to the United States during World War II for convalescence were returned to full flying duty. Among a group of flying enlisted men only 23 per cent returned to full flying, apparently because of lower selection standards, less understanding of the need for early treatment, less personal attention from the flight surgeon and absence of a long term interest in aviation.

Treatment results during 1951 of the Korean campaign revealed that 74.5 per cent of psychiatric cases returned to full flying duties. This somewhat better figure than World War II would appear to be the result of the lighter operational load and also of medical support which had profited from the lessons of World War II.

Long term follow-up evaluation of the effects of combat induced psychologic reactions is beclouded by changing cultural and medical standards of diagnosis and treatment. Among World War II returnees, the most frequently persistent symptoms were restlessness, irritability, aggressive behavior, fatigue, insomnia, anxiety and personality changes. Carlson and Rafferty (33) found that 53 per cent of flying officers were well enough not to visit a physician during a 4-year period after their World War II reaction. The duration of symptoms before diagnosis and treatment were found to have a direct bearing on the persistence of residual effects.

The author has reported findings in 100 military flyers who were neuropsychiatric problem cases. Combat experiences in this group were of minor importance (34). Of the group, 40 were regarded as representing primarily psychiatric problems. From a standpoint of prognosis, 16 were medically disqualified from flying and 14 continued or resumed their flying duties. In 10 cases, administrative handling was recommended.

In summarizing the data available on the matter of prognosis in the flyer who has experienced psychiatric illness it is evident that the picture is far from discouraging. If the over-all medical program is alert to the importance of early treatment, if the basic orientation is preventive and functions closely with the organization in pursuing an effective program of selection and utilization of the individual flyer, then prognosis in individual cases is quite favorable indeed.

REFERENCES

(1) MEBANE, J. C.: Neuropsychiatry for the Flight Surgeon. Randolph Air Force Base, Texas, School of Aviation Medicine, USAF, 1956.

(2) MEBANE, J. C.: Psychiatric standards. In Symposium on Physical Standards and Selection. Randolph Air Force Base, Texas, School of Aviation Medicine, USAF, 1957.

(3) COHEN, S. I., SILVERMAN, A. J., AND ZUIDEMA, G. D.: Physiologic stress response evaluation by focused interviewing. A. M. A. Arch. Neurol. & Psychiat., 76: 670–674, 1956.

(4) SILVERMAN, A. J., COHEN, S. I., AND ZUIDEMA, G. D.: Psychophysiological investigations in cardiovascular stress. Am. J. Psychiat., 113: 691–693, 1957.

(5) SARNOFF, C. A., AND MEBANE, J. C.: Episodic psychogenic G force intolerance. J. Aviation Med., 29: 287–290, 1958.

(6) ENGEL, G. L.: Fainting: Physiological and Psychological Considerations. Springfield, Illinois, Charles C Thomas, 1950.

(7) WAYNE, H. H.: Clinical differentiation between hypoxia and hyperventilation. J. Aviation Med., 29: 307–316, 1958.

(8) BALKE, B., WELLS, J. G., AND CLARK, R. T., JR.: In-flight hyperventilation during jet pilot training. J. Aviation Med., 28: 241–248, 1957.

(9) DERBES, V. J., AND KERR, A.: Cough Syncope. Springfield, Illinois, Charles C Thomas, 1955.

(10) SHIRLEY, R. C.: The Paradoxical Effect of Oxygen in Aviation Medicine. Is It a Problem in the United States Air Force? Unpublished Training Report. Randolph Air Force Base, Texas, School of Aviation Medicine, USAF, 1956.

(11) NOELL, W.: The post-hypoxia paradox effect. In German Aviation Medicine, World War II, Vol. I. Washington, D. C., Government Printing Office, 1950, pp. 487–492.

(12) POWELL, T. J., CAREY, T. M., BRENT, H. P., AND TAYLOR, W. J.: Episodes of unconsciousness in pilots during flight in 1956. J. Aviation Med., 28: 374–386, 1957.

(13) WALKER, A. E.: Posttraumatic Epilepsy. Springfield, Illinois, Charles C Thomas, 1949.

(14) Medical Examination. Air Force Manual 160-1. Washington, D. C., Department of the Air Force, 1953.

(15) HABERER, E., AND SARNOFF, C. A.: Mass Electroencephalographic Testing. Randolph Air Force Base, Texas, School of Aviation Medicine, USAF, to be published.

(16) Air Ministry: Psychological Disorders in Flying Personnel of The Royal Air Force, Investigated During the War 1939–1945. Air Publication 3139. London, His Majesty's Stationery Office, 1947.

(17) MEBANE, J. C.: Psychosis in military flyers. J. Aviation Med., 27: 390–396, 1956.

(18) GRINKER, R. R., AND SPIEGEL, J. P.: Men Under Stress. Philadelphia, Blakiston Co., 1945.

(19) SIMONS, D. G.: Pilot reactions during "man-high II" balloon flight. J. Aviation Med., 29: 1–15, 1958.

(20) ARMSTRONG, H. G.: The Principles and Practice of Aviation Medicine, Ed. 3. Baltimore, The Williams & Wilkins Co., 1952.

(21) CLARK, B., AND GRAYBIEL, A.: The break-off phenomenon. J. Aviation Med., 28: 121–126, 1957.

(22) SOLOMON, P., LEIDERMANN, P. H., MENDELSON, J., AND WEXLER, D.: Sensory deprivation; a review. Am. J. Psychiat., 114: 357–363, 1957.

(23) GERATHEWOHL, S. J.: Personal experiences during short periods of weightlessness reported by sixteen subjects. Astronautica acta, 4: 204–207, 1956.

(24) GERATHEWOHL, S. J., STRUGHOLD, H., AND STALLINGS, H. D.: Sensomotor performance during weightlessness; eye-hand coordination. J. Aviation Med., 28: 7–12, 1957.

(25) HASTINGS, D. W., WRIGHT, D. G., AND GLUECK, B. C.: Psychiatric Experiences of the Eighth Air Force, First Year of Combat (July 4, 1942 to July 4, 1943). New York, Josiah Macy, Jr., Foundation, 1944.

(26) BOND, D. D.: The Love and Fear of Flying. New York, International Universities Press, Inc., 1952.

(27) CLARK, B., NICHOLSON, M. R., AND GRAYBIEL, A.: Fascination: a cause of pilot error. J. Aviation Med., 24: 429–440, 1953.

(28) ALI, M.: Personal communication.

(29) SARNOFF, C. A.: Medical Aspects of Flying Motivation. A Fear of Flying Case Book. Randolph Air Force Base, Texas, School of Aviation Medicine, USAF, 1957.

(30) STRICKLAND, B. A., AND FERRIS, C.: The Effects of Air Transportation on Various Clinical Conditions. Reactions of Psychiatric Patients to Air Transportation. Randolph Air Force Base, Texas, School of Aviation Medicine, USAF, 1954.

(31) TILLISCH, J. H., STOTLER, J. F., AND LOVELACE, W. R., II.: Study of the effects of airplane transportation of 200 patients. J. Aviation Med., 14: 162–172, 1943.

(32) ROSS, W. D.: Practical Psychiatry for Industrial Physicians. Springfield, Illinois, Charles C Thomas, 1956.

(33) CARLSON, W. A., AND RAFFERTY, J. S.: Follow-up Study of Neuropsychiatric Cases Which Appeared Before the First C.M.E. Randolph Air Force Base, Texas, School of Aviation Medicine, USAF, 1949.

(34) MEBANE, J. C.: Clinical neuropsychiatry in aviation medicine; a survey of 100 military problem cases. J. Aviation Med., 26: 471–478, 1955.

24

AVIATION DENTISTRY

Lucian Szmyd, D.M.D
Clarence M. McCall, Jr. D.M.D.

Aviation dentistry is concerned with the effects of oral diseases and dental treatment on the capabilities of flying personnel. Conversely, it is concerned with the effects of flight on the teeth and related structures. The problems in aviation dentistry fall into two general groups: some are strictly dental problems related to flight; others are so closely allied to medical problems as to affect the general health of aircrew members. Effective resolution of these problems requires that all physicians and dentists be aware of their interdisciplinary relationship and the need for close liaison.

Experience has demonstrated the importance of dental health in any aircrew effectiveness program. Such a program imposes specific responsibilities on both the flight surgeon and the dental surgeon. The flight surgeon should realize that oral health is basic to the safety, comfort and efficiency of aviation personnel; he can maintain proper medical administrative control only by understanding the effects of oral disease and dental treatment procedures on aircrew effectiveness. The dental surgeon likewise should be cognizant of the total physical demands on the flyer and should be keenly aware of his responsibility for keeping the flight surgeon informed on dental health matters.

A study has been made of such problems as qualifications for flying training, aerodontalgia, dental implications in aerotitis media and dental identification of air crash victims. Service to the flight surgeon has been improved by continued investigation into the ways oral surgery and restorative, periodontal and prosthetic dentistry relate to flight. The work of the physician in taking care of dental emergencies has been outlined (1) and, more recently, drugs commonly used in dentistry but contraindicated in flight have been re-evaluated. The problems of evacuating maxillofacial patients by air will continue to be of interest. Each innovation, whether in the field of therapeutics, aircraft potentialities or logistics, presents new areas for research and clinical achievement by aviation dentistry.

DENTAL EXAMINATION

The dental examination of candidates for flying training is directed toward the detection of dental defects which are likely to handicap the individual for satisfactory performance of flying duties or which would require extensive interruption of flight training for their correction. Standards are patterned after the dental criteria employed in the United States Air Force (2). It should be emphasized that disqualifying dental defects will often be of a temporary or remedial nature. The candidates should be informed of any substandard conditions which may be brought up to standard by elective dental treatment.

Procedure

The oral tissues should be examined by inspection and palpation supplemented by roentgenograms of all teeth and supporting structures. Electric and thermal viability tests should be performed when degenerative changes in the pulpal tissues are suspected. Study models are recommended when detailed information concerning jaw and tooth relationships is desired.

Interpretation of Findings

Candidates for flying training should have eight serviceable, vital, permanent teeth in each of the upper and lower arches, exclusive of third molars, so positioned as to retain and adequately stabilize bridges or partial dentures. These teeth should be functionally opposed by natural teeth or by artificial teeth on serviceable bridges or partial dentures. An elongated or malposed natural tooth which cannot be brought into functional occlusion with either a natural or artificial opposing tooth or one which demonstrates marked destruction of supporting tissues should not be considered a functional tooth. Malocclusions severe enough to affect the individual's health and conditions requiring continued orthodontic treatment should be considered disqualifying.

The following dental conditions should also be considered disqualifying until corrected: (1) extensive caries and defective restorations including bridges and partial dentures; (2) diseases of the jaws or associated structures, such as cysts, tumors, chronic infections and severe periodontal conditions; (3) temporomandibular joint disturbances; and (4) ununited fractures of the maxilla or mandible.

RESTORATIVE ASPECTS

Aerodontalgia

Aerodontalgia is defined as toothache provoked by lowered barometric pressure during flight or during simulated flight. Aircrew effectiveness is reduced by aerodontalgia inasmuch as personnel having this type of pain are frequently incapable of performing their duties. The flight surgeon must have an adequate knowledge of this problem in order to facilitate diagnostic and corrective measures.

Aerodontalgia is a condition intimately related to pre-existing dental pathology and usually represents an acute exacerbation of subclinical symptoms (3). Changes in atmospheric pressure aggravate the impaired circulation in irritated or diseased pulps and may lead to early manifestations of inflammatory and degenerative changes in the pulpal and periapical tissues (4). Low temperature, varying oxygen percentages, vibration and motion in space appear to play no role as activating factors.

It has been postulated that dental restorations may be displaced during flight by the expansion of gases entrapped under fillings. Experiments in which air bubbles were produced under fillings failed to substantiate this concept. The teeth are subjected to three distinct abnormal variations in environment during high-altitude flights: (1) decreased barometric pressures, (2) increased oxygen percentages and (3) lowered atmospheric temperatures. Research has shown that these environmental factors have no adverse effect on normal teeth and dental restorations (5).

The initial reports of the incidence of aerodontalgia were compiled early in World War II when dental service was not yet available for the large number of flight trainees. At that time toothache ranked fifth in frequency of all complications from exposure to low barometric pressures with an average incidence of 1 to 2 per cent (6). With present day dental diagnostic and treatment methods and more effective preventive programs only an occasional case of aerodontalgia is encountered. Aerodontalgia rarely occurs at the altitudes utilized by commercial aircraft.

Experience has shown that certain findings are peculiar to aerodontalgia. The tooth pulp is usually viable when pain occurs during ascent and nonviable if pain occurs during descent. Pulpal degeneration with periapical involvement is generally considered as the causative factor when pain persists after flight. A repeated flight or the utilization of a single altitude chamber flight is seldom helpful in establishing a diagnosis inasmuch as the patient may experience one painful episode without recurrence. Toothache may occasionally show a remarkable constancy in the altitude at which it becomes manifest. Pain is often relieved as ground level is approached. On descent, the toothache may subside at the same altitude at which pain began.

Etiologic factors in toothache at ground level should also be suspected in diagnosing aerodontalgia. Offending teeth are localized by employing the usual dental diagnostic procedures which include history, oral examination, roentgenograms and viability tests. Recently restored teeth, deep seated restorations, defective restorations, restorations without underlying base materials and carious teeth should be ruled out.

Treatment of aerodontalgia does not vary from therapy rendered for toothache at ground level. Prevention of aerodontalgia is based on maintenance of high standards in restorative dentistry.

Referred pain from unerupted or partially erupted third molars and from aerotitis media may complicate the diagnosis of aerodontalgia. Pain may appear in the teeth of the upper jaw as a result of maxillary aerosinusitis. This is more likely to occur in the molar and premolar teeth whose apices with corresponding vessels and nerves may be separated from the sinus cavity only by the Schneiderian membrane and, thus, be exposed to pressure changes within the sinus. This pain usually occurs on descent and often continues at ground level. The patient may reveal a history of chronic sinusitis or acute nasopharyngitis.

Cooperation between flight surgeon and dentist is indicated when a differential diagnosis must be made of aerosinusitis, aerotitis media or aerodontalgia.

Periodontal Aspects

There is no reliable evidence that flight conditions are etiologically related to periodontal disorders. Dental questionnaires received from 200 Army Air Force dental surgeons indicated a higher incidence of periodontal disturbances among flying personnel (7). This report suggested that lack of proper oral hygiene, fatigue, inadequate diet, nervous tension, excessive use of alcohol and tobacco, anoxia, reduced atmospheric pressure and the effects of frequent absences from the home base were etiologic factors.

It is difficult to conceive of any special environmental conditions peculiar to present day flying which would exert a deleterious effect on periodontal tissues. An increased incidence of acute ulcerative gingivitis (Vin-

cent's infection) and other gingival disturbances among flyers can be explained through neglect of oral hygiene and laxity in maintaining high standards of general health. The value of instruction in oral hygiene practices and periodic oral prophylaxes cannot be overemphasized. The physician should stress the importance of good oral care and should insure that aircrews carry with them aids for oral hygiene.

Dental pressure habits, such as grinding or clamping of teeth, lip biting and cheek sucking, have been noted among flyers. These manifestations of tension contribute to the development of periodontal and temporomandibular joint disturbances. It is doubtful that temporomandibular disorders are more prevalent in aircrew members than in any group of comparable background but when present they jeopardize aircrew effectiveness. The crews of future high performance aircraft may be exposed to psychologic stresses which further accentuate the psychosomatic aspects of temporomandibular disorders. Changes in body positions of personnel in such aircraft may also impose additional physical stresses on the temporomandibular joint and contiguous structures.

It is important for the flight surgeon to be cognizant of the early signs and symptoms of temporomandibular joint disturbances inasmuch as these conditions are more amenable to treatment in the beginning stages. Early clinical symptoms may include temporal and postauricular headache, earache, tenderness and trismus of the masticatory and cervical musculature, tinnitus, crepitus, clicking, popping, pain and swelling in the temporomandibular joint region with limitation or alteration in the pattern of jaw movement. Patients may experience locking of the mandible or difficulty in bringing the teeth into tight occlusion. The habit of bruxism is a common finding. Pain is usually unilateral and is not limited to the region innervated by the trigeminal nerve. The head, neck and shoulder may also be involved. These symptoms appear to be unrelated and diagnosis is further complicated by underlying psychosomatic factors.

Painful episodes may follow a yawn, difficult tooth extraction or other wide opening movements of the mandible. Chronic headaches, clicking in the joint and locking of the condyle commonly precede pain in the temporomandibular joint. Palpation of the masticatory muscles may reveal the presence of spasm and tenderness.

Dental consultation is particularly valuable in the establishment of a differential diagnosis. Treatment may require psychotherapy, drug therapy and physiotherapy and will probably involve all the dental subspecialties. Experience has demonstrated the advisability of preceding other forms of treatment with conservative periodontal therapy.

Prosthetic Aspects

Phonetics

It is essential that flying personnel speak intelligibly because improper enunciation over communication systems may jeopardize the safety of the aircraft. A variety of speech defects may be produced by faulty partial or complete dentures. The most common phonetic difficulty is mispronunciation of "s" and "sh" sounds. Speech discrepancies may be detected by requiring the examinee with prosthetic replacements to repeat phrases involving these consonants, *e.g.*, "Sixty-six ships sailed the Mississippi."

The initial period of awkward and indistinct speech is a major problem for aircrew members with new dentures. A technique for artificial denture construction has been devised to eliminate this lengthy period of speech adjustment (8). This technique is based on analysis of pre-extraction or past artificial denture speech and determination of individual tongue-palate relationships. Correct consonantal speech is insured which enables the flyer to enunciate clearly from the time of denture insertion.

Denture Retention

Interest in the effects of rapid acceleration, deceleration and changes in atmospheric pressure on the retention of artificial dentures has been stimulated by reports of difficulty in wearing dentures during flight. These reports concerned aircrew members who were forced to remove dental appliances because of discomfort or instability. Loss of denture stability during flight may compromise the safety of the aircrew.

The available information concerning the problem of denture retention at altitude is based on research utilizing extraoral measuring equipment (9). This methodology is questionable because the wide mouth opening necessary for extraoral testing devices relaxes facial muscles which normally exert favorable retentive forces on the denture. An intraoral measuring device which does not interfere with these retentive forces is necessary to make a valid study of denture retention under varying barometric pressures. No clear-cut criteria relative to denture stability in flight are now available.

The advent of improved oxygen equipment has diminished the problem of pain and trauma incident to pressure on the cheeks from tight masks. Irritation of the oral tissues may be the result of impingement between the mask and the prosthetic appliance. Many such cases have been successfully resolved through a cooperative effort of dentist and flight surgeon in contouring the denture and fitting the mask.

Until a more realistic investigation of these problems can be accomplished no additional recommendations can be made other than to require the highest standard of perfection for dental prosthetic restorations.

Oral Surgery Aspects

Drug Therapy

The flight surgeon maintains administrative control of flying personnel receiving medication which may compromise aircrew efficiency and safety. Three such drug groups frequently prescribed for flying personnel undergoing dental treatment are the narcotics, antihistaminics and tranquilizers.

Investigation of the time cycle for postextraction pain suggests a method for diminishing the problem of medical administrative control of oral surgical patients receiving narcotics. The pain time cycle follows a relatively uniform course with the necessity for controlling severe post extraction pain usually confined to the day of surgery. The routine prescription of narcotics beyond this period is unwarranted.

Research has failed to substantiate early

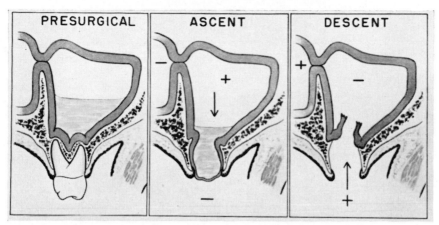

FIG. 133. Maxillary antrum; postextraction complications

reports of the therapeutic efficacy of the antihistaminics and tranquilizers in controlling postextraction sequelae (10, 11). Recent dental studies indicate that drowsiness is a common complication of antihistaminic therapy and that tranquilizing drug administration prolongs the postextraction convalescent period. In view of these findings the use of present day tranquilizers and antihistaminics for the control of postextraction sequelae in flying personnel does not appear to be indicated.

Postextraction Complications

Physical factors encountered during flight may adversely affect the postoperative course of certain oral surgical patients. Surgical removal of maxillary posterior teeth often necessitates the loss of considerable alveolar bone and may deprive large areas of antral membrane of bony and soft tissue support. Whenever the antral membrane is exposed or perforated in a surgical procedure the patient should be cautioned not only against sneezing and blowing of the nose but also against air travel (12). When the maxillary sinus is normal and the ostium is patent, differences in pressure between the air within the sinus cavity and the surrounding atmosphere are brought into equilibrium quickly and uneventfully at a rate depending on the size of the ostium and the extent of change in barometric pressure. Obstruction of the ostium by redundant or hypertrophied tissue, anatomical deformities, polyps, mucus or purulent exudate may delay or prevent

equalization of pressure, resulting in herniation or perforation of the Schneiderian membrane at the extraction site (fig. 133). Roentgenograms should be obtained to evaluate the presence of infection or other abnormalities when the integrity of the maxillary sinus is jeopardized during tooth extraction.

Secondary hemorrhage incidental to dental surgery may be brought about by variation in barometric pressure during flight. Individuals with oral bleeding invariably swallow blood increasing their susceptibility to nausea and vomiting. Blood in oxygen equipment will seriously impair its efficiency. Clinical experience indicates that flying activity should be routinely restricted for 48 hours following tooth extraction and the patient re-examined before return to duty. Resumption of flying duties should also be delayed when dental treatment requires the postoperative use of surgical or periodontal packs.

Administrative control of flying personnel is also required in cases of alveolar osteitis (dry socket). This complication of tooth extraction is incompatible with the performance of flying duties. The site for which alveolar osteitis shows a marked predilection is the mandibular third molar area. Alveolar osteitis is characterized by pain, swelling, trismus, fever and general malaise. It is important to note that clinical manifestations may be delayed until the fourth postoperative day. Treatment requires approximately 10 days during which time the patient is unfit for flying duties.

Dental Aspects of Aerotitis Media

Aerotitis media is a frequent source of discomfort and temporary hearing loss caused by failure to ventilate the middle ear during flight. Early investigators believed that malposition of the mandible was an etiologic factor in the development of this entity (13–15). Condylar displacement or hypotonicity of masticatory and tubal muscles in subjects with mandibular overclosure was thought to result in anatomical inhibition of the opening mechanism of the eustachian tube. Therapy was directed toward restoration of normal vertical dimensions. Consistent results have not been obtained with this approach.

A more recent concept of dental implication in aerotitis media is based on neuromuscular relationships within the masticatory system. It has been suggested that neuromuscular imbalances may be reflected from the masticatory muscles to the tensor veli palatini muscles through the trigeminal nerve which is their common source of innervation. Spasticity and fatigue in these muscles can impair ventilation of the middle ear.

Under this premise, treatment is directed toward correction of the etiologic factors involved in the neuromuscular imbalances. Dental therapy includes resolution of gingival inflammation, relief of occlusal interferences and replacement of missing teeth. Restoration of lost vertical dimension, previously suggested as treatment for aerotitis media, is also a therapeutic measure for the relief of neuromuscular disturbances and should be considered in the over-all evaluation.

Air Evacuation of Maxillo-facial Patients

Extensive research in the areas of motion sickness, mechanical phases of air transportation and physiologic factors in flight has brought about advancements in the techniques of air evacuation of patients with maxillofacial injuries (16). Experiences under combat conditions have proven the value of temporary stabilization, control of motion sickness, quick release mechanism of jaw fixation and therapeutic measures such as elective tracheotomy, restoration of blood volume and Levin tube feeding for the maintenance of airway, hydration and balanced diet.

Temporary stabilization of facial fractures expedites procedures whereby the patient can be transported for definitive treatment with a minimum of secondary trauma. It also reduces the need for nursing care, improves morale, simplifies feeding and promotes patient comfort. Intermaxillary fixation supplemented by a head bandage for support of the mandible is a method of choice in attaining temporary stabilization. A head bandage (fig. 134) alone will provide gross stabilization of the fractured elements when a dentist is not available or limited armamentarium precludes stabilization by intermaxillary traction.

A basic problem in the evacuation of maxillofacial patients stems from the fact that the jaws are immobilized. Such patients may experience serious respiratory difficulties resulting from aspiration of vomitus incident to motion sickness. Although almost anyone can be made sick when the intensity, duration and nature of the motion are adequate, a patient is more susceptible to air sickness than is a well person.

The flight surgeon's evaluation and preparation of the maxillofacial patient for evacuation includes a consideration of the physi-

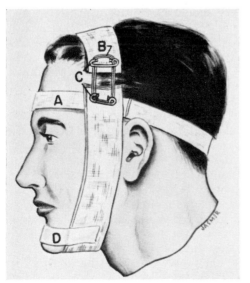

Fig. 134. Emergency head bandage. *A*, gauge; *B*, elastic band; *C*, safety pins; *D*, adhesive tape.

cal and physiologic aspects of flight. The following therapeutic measures greatly reduce the incidence of motion sickness and contribute to the physical well-being of the maxillofacial patient:

1. Information should be obtained regarding the patient's susceptibility to motion sickness. This knowledge is helpful in predicting the incidence of air sickness.

2. Preflight lavatory hygiene aids in preventing the accumulation of gas in the bowel. Expansion of this gas at altitude may cause marked intestinal distension.

3. The patient's fracture diet is modified to limit intake of "gas forming" foods such as milk, carbohydrates and carbonated drinks.

4. Evacuation of the maxillofacial patient is delayed when turbulence is forecast.

5. Emergency equipment provided for the flight should include a mechanical suction and a tracheotomy set.

6. Indoctrination prior to take off will alleviate apprehension or fear of flying.

7. The patient is placed low in the litter block in a location over the wing. The supine position reduces air sickness by abolishing excitation of the utricle. The prone or lateral position is used when edema or hematoma involves the floor of the mouth or when other conditions predispose the patient to the development of respiratory difficulties.

8. The patient is shifted to a position favorable for swallowing during in-flight meals. Decreased air density at altitude reduces the effectiveness of the cough mechanism and may prolong efforts to clear the respiratory passage should a small amount of food be inadvertently aspirated.

9. Antimotion sickness drugs are administered orally or parenterally; they include: meclizine hydrochloride (Bonamine); diphenhydramine hydrochloride (Benadryl); cyclizine hydrochloride (Marezine); promethazine hydrochloride (Phenergan); and dimethydrinate (Dramamine).

Air sickness in a patient has a psychologic effect on the other passengers and will frequently be followed by their sudden illness. When symptoms of drowsiness, pallor, cold sweating and nausea, which usually precede vomiting, are observed by the medical flight personnel, therapeutic measures are instituted. Loosening tight belts, massaging the abdomen, adjusting pillows to minimize lateral head motion, requesting patient to keep eyes closed, mild medication, reassurance and use of oxygen during flight are effective procedures for the alleviation of air sickness.

Occasionally, maxillofacial injuries will be immobilized by the use of wires rather than elastic bands between the maxilla and mandible. This practice is hazardous and such patients are not transported unless the "tie wires" between the jaws are removed before flight or replaced by elastics. Removal of intermaxillary immobilization wires jeopardizes the integrity of the mandible and may lead to serious complications. The upward and inward pull of the elevator muscles and the downward and backward pull of the depressor muscles on the fractured elements may disrupt their continuity. Intramaxillary wiring on the maxilla and mandible should not be depended upon to overcome this muscle pull. Collapse of the osseous structures supporting the tongue and soft tissues in the floor of the mouth may lead to serious respiratory embarrassment.

When substituting elastics for intermaxillary "tie wires," cut only one wire at a time and replace it immediately with an elastic band. Bandage scissors suitable for cutting elastics and wires should be available to both the patient and the medical attendant.

A quick release mechanism for jaw fixation provides an additional safety factor in the air evacuation of maxillofacial patients. One technique for rapid release of jaw fixation utilizes a strong cord which is passed through the lumen of each intermaxillary elastic band (fig. 135). A second method for effecting quick release of jaw fixation employs a 15-gauge needle. The blunted needle is passed through alternate maxillary and mandibular elastic loops. A strong cord is tied to the

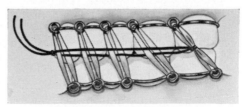

Fig. 135. Quick release mechanism; rip cord

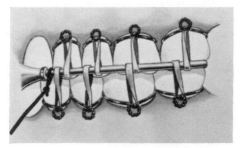

FIG. 136. Quick release mechanism; needle type.

needle hub and taped to the patient's cheek (fig. 136).

DENTAL IDENTIFICATION

The dental identification is an invaluable aid for identifying deceased persons or verifying other methods of identification. Accurate dental identification is possible because the human dentition resists the destructive forces involved in aircraft accidents and the existence of identical dentitions is extremely improbable. The dental identification record is a chart of all fillings, missing teeth, prosthetic appliances, bridges and dental anomalies. These records should be made for all persons who are required to fly. It is especially important to maintain current dental records for personnel on flying status.

The physician may be required to identify the remains of air crash victims by comparing dental findings charted at the scene of the accident with original dental records. Identification is facilitated when the pre-existing dental identification records are available at the postmortem examination. When such records are not immediately available the mouths of deceased persons are charted for later comparison with original dental identification records. Essential armamentarium for the postmortem dental examination includes adequate illumination, mouth prop, tongue blade, gauze and mouth mirror.

The examiner performing the dental identification must be familiar with certain basic information concerning dental terminology and the materials utilized in dentistry. The complete normal human dentition consists of 32 teeth. The location of individual teeth is established by assigning them numbers from 1 to 32 in the manner indicated in table 74.

Another method frequently used in the designation of tooth location divides the dental arches into four quadrants. Teeth are numbered from the midline to the third molar as follows:

Maxilla

$$\text{Right} \frac{8\ 7\ 6\ 5\ 4\ 3\ 2\ 1 \mid 1\ 2\ 3\ 4\ 5\ 6\ 7\ 8}{8\ 7\ 6\ 5\ 4\ 3\ 2\ 1 \mid 1\ 2\ 3\ 4\ 5\ 6\ 7\ 8} \text{Left}$$

Mandible

The maxillary right first molar would be identified by the sign 6| the sign |1 designates the mandibular left central incisor.

The clinical crowns of the teeth are divided into five surfaces (fig. 137).

1. *Occlusal*; the biting surface (in anterior teeth this is termed the incisal surface).

TABLE 74
Numbers of the Teeth Establishing Location

Tooth	Maxillary		Mandibular	
	Right side	Left side	Right side	Left side
Third molar	1	16	32	17
Second molar	2	15	31	18
First molar	3	14	30	19
Second bicuspid	4	13	29	20
First bicuspid	5	12	28	21
Cuspid	6	11	27	22
Lateral incisors	7	10	26	23
Central incisors	8	9	25	24

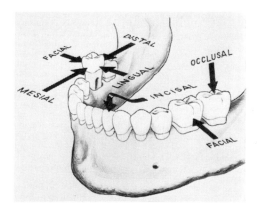

FIG. 137. Designation of tooth surfaces

2. *Facial*; the surface contacted by the lip or cheek.

3. *Lingual*; the surface in apposition to or contacted by the tongue.

4. *Mesial*; the surface or interproximal area facing the anterior midpoint of the dental arch at the median sagittal plane.

5. *Distal*; the interproximal surface facing

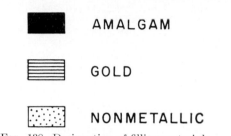

FIG. 138. Designation of filling materials

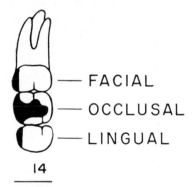

FIG. 139. Charting of an amalgam restoration

away from the anterior midpoint of the dental arch.

The following abbreviations for tooth surfaces are frequently encountered on dental identification records: M, mesial; I, incisal; O, occlusal; D, distal; F, facial; and L, lingual. When two or more tooth surfaces are involved the abbreviations may be combined; for example: MO, mesio-occlusal and MOD, mesio-occlusodistal.

The three most common filling materials used in dentistry are:

1. Amalgam, a silver- to black- colored alloy.

2. Gold, in the form of cast inlays and crowns.

3. Nonmetallic materials, silicates, porcelains and plastics.

Symbols are used on dental records to denote the type of filling material. Gold is designated by a series of parallel lines, amalgam by a solid black color and non-metallic materials by stippling (fig. 138). The location and type of each filling in the mouth is charted on the dental identification record by drawing the outline form of the restoration and then filling it in with the symbol appropriate for the particular filling material used (fig. 139). Decayed teeth are designated by outlining the area involved. An "X" is used to denote missing teeth.

Missing teeth are usually replaced by

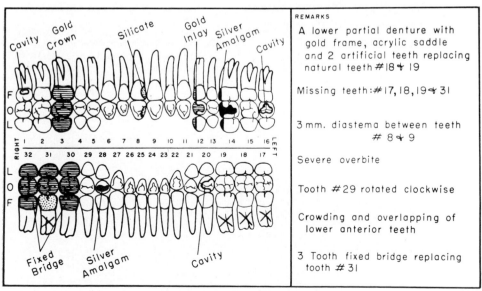

FIG. 140. Sample dental identification record

fixed bridges, partial dentures or full dentures. These prosthetic appliances are described as to location and composition under "Remarks" on the dental identification record. The materials commonly employed to construct prosthetic replacements are acrylic resins, gold and chrome-cobalt alloys. Inscription of the owner's name on the prosthetic appliance is an effective adjunct to dental identification and is recommended for flying personnel with partial or full dentures.

Charting is facilitated by marginal notes relative to dental findings such as cavities and filling materials. The "Remarks" section may also be used to note the presence of abnormalities, e.g., mottled enamel, malocclusion, supernumerary teeth and exostoses.

A completed dental identification record is presented (fig. 140).

RESEARCH

Research activity is stimulated by the environmental and psychologic factors which the transition to high performance aircraft may impose on the basic problems of aviation dentistry. Investigations presently being pursued include: the role of salivary analysis in stress determinations; psychologic aspects of temporomandibular joint disturbances; and the relation between dental findings and aerotitis media. The resolution of these problems will form a significant contribution to the care and welfare of aviation personnel.

REFERENCES

(1) Emergency Oral Medicine. Randolph Air Force Base, Texas, Air University, School of Aviation Medicine, USAF, 1957.
(2) Department Of the Air Force: Medical Service Medical Examination. Air Force Manual 160-1B. Washington, D. C., Government Printing Office, 1957.
(3) BURKET, L. W.: Oral Medicine. Philadelphia, J. B. Lippincott Co., 1946.
(4) ORBAN, B., AND RITCHEY, B. T.: Toothache under conditions simulating high altitude flight. J. Am. Dent. A., 32: 145–180, 1945.
(5) ARMSTRONG, H. G., AND HUBER, R. E.: Effect of high altitude flying on human teeth and restorations. Dent. Digest, 43: 132–134, 1937.
(6) DE VOE, K., AND MOTLEY, H. L.: Aerodontalgia. Dent. Digest, 51: 16, 1945.
(7) Flying and dentistry, Air Surgeon's Bull., 1: 1–4, 1944.
(8) ALLEN, L. R.: Improved phonetics in artificial denture construction. J. Prosthetic Dentistry, 8: 753–763, 1958.
(9) SOGNNAES, R. F.: Studies on Aviation Dentistry. Ottawa, Canada, Associate Committee on Aviation Medical Research, National Research Council of Canada, 1944.
(10) SZMYD, L.: A clinical evaluation of an antihistaminic preparation in oral surgery. Oral Surg., 9: 928–931, 1956.
(11) SZMYD, L., McCALL, C. M., AND ENRIGHT, E. T.: Tranquilizing drugs in oral surgery. J. Oral Surg., 16: 310–313, 1958.
(12) SZMYD, L.: Oral surgery complications caused by flight. U. S. Armed Forces M. J., 8: 264–270, 1957.
(13) COSTEN, J. B.: A syndrome of ear and sinus symptoms dependent upon disturbed functions of the temporomandibular joint. Ann. Otol. Rhin. & Laryng., 43: 1–15, 1934.
(14) WILLHELMY, G. E.: Ear symptoms incidental to sudden altitude changes and the factor of overclosure of the mandible; preliminary report. U. S. Nav. M. Bull., 34: 533–541, 1936.
(15) LOWRY, R. A.: Loss of intermaxillary distance: effect on aviators and relief by interdental splint. U. S. Nav. M. Bull., 37: 367, 1939.
(16) SZMYD, L.: Air evacuation of maxillofacial injuries. A. M. A. Arch. Surg., 74: 809–813, 1957.

25

TOXICOLOGY IN AVIATION

John E. Boysen, M.D.

The toxicologic nature of the aviation environment includes those chemical products carried on, or as a part of, the aircraft. No sharp dividing line can be established academically, so arbitrarily this chapter will set this "line" at those factors occurring or likely to occur in the aircraft during flight or in taxiing operations. Occupational exposures to potentially toxic chemicals will not include those occurring during shop maintenance operations or other types of ground operations. The discussion will be limited to chemical stress factors and not those resulting from mechanical or physical agents or to biologic agents which are discussed in other sections of this text.

The Problem of Chemical Toxicity

The extent to which chemical stress factors have caused or contributed to aircraft incidents or accidents has never been precisely determined although some attempts have been made. In November 1955 a Joint Committee on Aviation Pathology was created by the Secretary of Defense of the United States to study methods of improving histopathologic and biochemical procedures which will demonstrate antemortem existence of hypoxia or dangerous concentrations of toxicologic chemicals. The members of this committee are appointed from the Armed Forces Institute of Pathology, the U. S. Army, Navy and Air Force, as well as the British Royal Navy, British Royal Air Force and the Royal Canadian Air Force. Autopsy specimens from all aircrew victims of

aircraft accidents are sent to the Armed Forces Institute of Pathology for study.

Data concerning aircraft incidents have been compiled by the CAA (1) for the past few years. These data refer only to U. S. civil air carrier aircraft reported in the Summaries of Daily Mechanical Reports (CAR 40 and 41). Table 75 contains a compilation of such incidents for the period of July 1954 to July 1957. Of a total of 162 incidents, 126 occurred during flight of which only 70 were severe enough to convince the pilot that he should make an unscheduled landing. It will be noted that no attempt has been made to include possible or known causes of fatal aircraft accidents in this series.

In a study of physiologic factors in aircraft accidents in the U. S. Air Force, Konecci (2) reported that "factors affecting the normal physiologic state of the pilot or crew are contributing causes rather than primary causes of major aircraft accidents. A few physiologic conditions like hypoxia and vertigo/disorientation were primary causes." In this study he reported a series of 332 major aircraft accidents during the calendar year of 1956. These factors were broken down into three categories of "definite," "probable" and "possible." These data are included in table 76. It will be noted that a number of these factors are directly or indirectly related to chemical toxicologic effects. It should be obvious that many of these have not been proven by exhaustive chemical analyses of body fluids or of the cabin environment immediately prior to the

TABLE 75

Incidents of Smoke or Other Atmospheric Con-
taminants in Scheduled Air Carrier Aircraft
(July 1954 to July 1957)

Source	Number of Incidents	Occur-ring in Air	Unsched-uled Landing
Radio and electronic equipment	38	30	12
Electrical equipment	63	48	27
Compressor-supercharger	13	11	9
Heater	18	17	12
Miscellaneous	30	20	10
Total	162	126	70

accident. It is entirely possible that many chemical toxicants may have been present in sufficient quantity to produce deleterious effects upon the aircrew without their presence being made known to any of the aircrew and certainly not to subsequent investigators. One cannot but wonder if the incidence of toxicologically significant amounts of noxious chemicals may not have contributed to the accidents which actually had as their primary cause, a "physiologic malfunction" of any one of the aircrew members.

In the majority of investigations of major aircraft accidents, "pilot error" has been assessed as a major cause. Obviously, this is a complex factor involving, primarily, training and experience. The question is raised, especially when dealing with experienced pilots, as to what factors caused the lack of good judgment or orderly reflexive reaction to an emergency situation. Could not a toxic chemical in the cabin environment have produced this unfavorable, though minor, physiologic or psychologic malfunction? Alcohol and carbon monoxide from smoking are well known for their effects upon the higher cortical centers of the brain which, when disturbed, can produce a significant decrease in efficiency involving discrimination, exercise of good judgment, etc.

Although a high degree of suspicion that chemical agents have contributed to specific aircraft accidents or incidents the proof is exceedingly difficult. Unequivocal proof would require chemical analysis of the cabin air at the time of, and preceding, the accident

(or under simulated circumstances) and chemical analysis of tissue fluids of the aircrewmen concerned at the time of the accident. Obviously these conditions are virtually impossible to meet. The first condition is impossible in fatal air crashes when the airframe is demolished unless automatic analytic equipment were installed which survived the crash. In aircraft incidents not resulting in a crash, the circumstances of flight can often be repeated and the suspected agent evaluated. The second condition is undoubtedly the most practical because it can be accomplished even in fatal crashes except when complete disintegration occurs. The finding of toxic chemicals in blood or other tissue fluids in sufficient quantities to produce a given malfunction or clinical entity is the most direct and in-

TABLE 76

Physical and Physiologic Factors in 332 Major
Aircraft Accidents in the U. S. Air Force
(1 Jan. to 31 Dec. 1956) *

Factors	Causes and Contributing Causes			
	Definite	Probable	Possible	Total
Fire in flight†	59	12	5	76
Restricted or hampered vision	58	12	5	75
Smoke in cockpit†	37	18	5	60
Vertigo/disorientation†	4	18	24	46
g-Forces	8	14	17	39
Hypoxia	4	10	16	30
Noxious fumes†	9	7	11	27
Vibration or noise	5		20	25
Fatigue†	3	4	6	13
Acrobatics	6	7		13
Decompression	2	3	7	12
Physical disturbance†			11	11
Carbon monoxide†	1	1	7	9
Hyperventilation			4	4
Incapacitation†			3	3
Language barrier		1	1	2
Air sickness†			1	1
Inadequate nutrition		1		1
All other combined	13	3	14	30
Total	209	111	157	477

* From Konecci (2).

† Conditions in which chemical toxicants could have acted as primary or contributing factors.

criminating evidence that could serve to establish it as an etiologic agent.

It appears necessary then that one can only approach this problem of toxic chemicals in aviation, as one would in any other occupational setting, with a thorough understanding of toxicologic principles followed by specific and detailed knowledge of the potentialities of specified chemical agents involved in the aviation environment. The following sections of this chapter will discuss these two features.

PRINCIPLES OF TOXICOLOGY IN AVIATION

There are certain fundamental and basic principles concerning the "life cycle" of chemical agents which must be known and understood if logical and effective measures are to be taken to control exposure, to prevent harmful effect, or finally, to treat those individuals who have absorbed quantities in excess of that which is within the capability of the individual to tolerate. This understanding must include a knowledge of the environment—its chemical composition, quantitative as well as qualitative, the mode of absorption into the body, its fate within the body, the effect of the chemical or its detoxification products upon tissues, organs, or physiologic systems and finally the mode and effects of elimination from the body.

Occupational toxicology differs in many respects from forensic toxicology. This is particularly true in the rather restricted occupational environment of aviation. These differences consist primarily of: the portal of entry, the time-dose relationship and the number of chemical agents involved.

In forensic toxicology the most important and most frequent portal of entry involved is the gastrointestinal tract. Suicidal attempts with bichloride of mercury taken orally is a good example. Inhalation is of secondary importance and absorption through the skin of minor significance. Conversely, in an occupational environment, the respiratory tract is by far the most important with the skin next in order of importance and the gastrointestinal tract of minor significance. Also in an occupational environment one or more portals are very likely involved. In addition to inhaling air contaminated with a toxic agent, the skin is exposed to the same environment and, in

addition, a small amount may be entering the gastrointestinal tract as a result of food contaminated by dirty hands. The relative clinical significance of these differences can be illustrated in mercury poisoning, for example. Mercury in sufficient quantities in the blood stream is capable of causing a renal failure. If it had gained access to the body *via* the respiratory tract one would not expect to see the symptoms and signs of severe gastrointestinal irritation seen when the toxicant was ingested.

The second major difference is that of the time-dose relationship. In forensic toxicology one generally is dealing with a single massive dose which, as one would expect, gives rise to an acute intoxication of a typical type. On the other hand, in an occupational environment, the dosage is generally small but continues over a long period of time—perhaps 8 hours a day, 5 days a week, for weeks, months or even years. One would, therefore, expect that the majority of cases of occupational intoxications would be of a chronic nature. Obviously there are exceptions. Because aircrews do not spend a "40 hour week" in their airborne environment, one also could logically expect that any adverse effects encountered by aircrews would tend to be more of an acute or subacute nature unless complicated by an environment to which they are exposed while on the ground.

The third important difference between forensic and occupational toxicology is that the former usually deals with only one chemical compound or formulation, the latter with a varying mixture. Although there is always a tendency to simplify, to select one chemical and attempt to attribute all symptoms and findings to it is rarely possible. The effects of exhaust gases is a good example. The thermal decomposition products are composed of carbon monoxide, aldehydes and other substances. It would be foolish to expect to find a syndrome attributable to only one of these compounds when other compounds are known to exist in significant quantities.

The Environment

"The reactions between a living man and the atmosphere about him are so immediate, so continual and so much a matter of course, that the normal individual passes days, even years, without a thought of breathing. Several times each day he thinks of food and not infrequently of digestion. He is interested in the principles of elimination; he gladly accepts scientific knowledge and takes elaborate precautions in food and drink. But of of respiration and gaseous substances which he takes into his body through his lungs he is generally oblivious" (3).

At altitudes beginning about 10,000 feet most human begins cease to become oblivious of their breathing atmosphere. The increasing lack of oxygen serves as a reminder as breathing becomes faster and more difficult as the altitude increases. Aircrews are well aware of the effects of hypoxia. Contaminants of this atmosphere are not so easily recognizable unless other signs of irritation become noticeable. Contamination of breathing atmospheres at altitude has not been as thoroughly studied as that at sea level. However, some extrapolations can be made which may be considered quite valid. Fortunately, for aircrews the use of oxygen through a mask has served as a protective device and has undoubtedly contributed to the saving of many lives which otherwise might have been lost owing to fatally toxic cabin environs.

Toxic chemical substances in an aircraft cabin environment may have their origin in fuels or exhaust gases, from deicing agents, from lubricants or hydraulic fluids or even from material carried as baggage or freight. Or, they may arise from the increased vaporization of materials at altitude o from thermal decomposition occurring during a fire involving any materials carried aboard or an integral part of the aircraft, i.e., electrical insulating materials or upholstery fabrics. Subsequent sections of this chapter will be devoted to a more detailed discussion of the precise nature of these chemical substances and the effects which might be expected.

The environment with which we are concerned in aviation medicine is an extremely dynamic one. It is capable of extreme variations in short periods of time. For purposes of this discussion "the environment" will be considered to be that volume of air contained within the aircraft cabin. Rapid changes in chemical composition of this environment can be caused by: (1) changes in cabin altitude; (2) ventilation rates, especially when pressurization is being utilized and (3) in-

troduction of foreign chemical agents into the environment by mechanical failure such as leakage of hydraulic lines, fuel lines, superchargers or heat exchangers or by fires of electrical equipment or upholstery materials. The use of fire extinguishing agents produces an added factor. An oxygen system constitutes an auxiliary and at times a completely separate environment insofar as breathing is concerned. This is also is a potential source of respiratory contamination.

In order to understand the true impact of potentially toxic chemicals in this environment the parameters of that environment must be defined quantitatively. It is not enough to merely establish the presence of a known toxicant as one might do with a biologic agent. Chemical agents do not have the power of reproduction!

What are these parameters of the aviation environment? Obviously the most important single factor is the amount of the toxicant available for absorption. This is generally expressed in terms of concentration of the material in air (milligrams per liter or "parts per million"). A second factor concerns the physical nature of the chemical. Is it an inert gas such as oxygen or carbon monoxide which crosses the alveolar barrier according to the gas laws or is it a reactive gas such as HCl which combines with the moisture on the bronchial walls and produces varying degrees of irritation? Perhaps it may be in the form of a vapor, a fume or a suspended particulate. If the latter, the particle size is of extreme importance for the size will determine whether it gains access to the alveoli or whether it is detained by the nasal cilia to be subsequently swallowed. Its solubility determines its ultimate fate. Water soluble substances gain access to the blood stream rather readily through the respiratory barrier but with difficulty through the skin. The reverse is generally true in the case of fat soluble substances. Fat soluble substances generally tend to become highly concentrated in the organs and tissues in the body which have a high fat content, notably the central nervous system.

The extent to which a given enclosure is contaminated can be calculated if certain factors are known. The following formula (4) can be used to determine the extent of contamination of an aircraft cabin in the event of accidental or intentional release of carbon dioxide from a fire extinguisher or other devices. The formula was originally used to estimate the concentration of carbon monoxide by internal combustion engines in relatively small enclosures such as in garages; however, it is equally applicable to an aircraft cabin.

$$C = \frac{100K(1 - e^{-Rt})}{RV}$$

where C equals per cent contaminant after time t; R equals air changes per hour; t equals time in hours; V equals volume of enclosure in cubic feet; K equals volume of contaminant liberated (cubic feet per hour); and e equals the base of the natural system of logarithms.

In industrial situations it has been found useful to establish certain maximum concentration values which are known or believed to be "safe." These are known as maximum allowable concentrations (MAC) or maximum tolerable levels. Certain governmental agencies have established these by law for use in regulating working conditions in civilian industry. The application of these values to any given situation in an aviation environment especially at altitude must be made with a thorough understanding of all of the factors involved, including the premises upon which these values are based. The basic premise upon which "MAC's" have been established is that exposure to an agent at a given level of concentration for periods of 8 hours daily for a working life of 30 years will produce no demonstrable ill effect. The critical factor determining this level in certain chemicals is the acute toxic effect it may produce. For example, carbon monoxide is not known to have a chronic effect. Therefore, its "MAC" is based entirely upon its ability to produce changes under conditions of short duration exposures. On the other hand, radioactive isotopes, for the most part, have been assigned MAC's which are based upon long term chronic effects. These values have been developed and, therefore, predicated upon the assumption that the worker is at sea level. Any significant degree of altitude has not been considered. There is some evidence that certain substances are more toxic at altitude but this evidence is sketchy

at best. The most extensively studied compound is probably carbon monoxide.

From all the evidence available it seems reasonable to conclude that any substance which significantly impairs any link in the oxygen mechanism (the hemoglobin of the blood, respiration, circulation, permeability of cellular tissues or the oxidative mechanisms within the cells) would also be more toxic at altitude. Some examples of this would be carbon monoxide which affects the oxygen carrying capacity of hemoglobin, the sulfa drugs which also interfere with hemoglobin by producing methemoglobin and the anesthetics which are believed to inhibit the oxidative activities of nerve cells.

There can be little doubt that the MAC's are valuable "bench marks" but one must not make the mistake of drawing conclusions or making predictions based upon this one figure without taking into consideration the time of exposure. Although the MAC of carbon monoxide may be 50 p.p.m. this does not mean that an exposure of a few seconds to concentrations of even 20,000 p.p.m. will produce any demonstrable effect. (This is the concentration of CO in one puff of cigarette smoke!) This concept has a direct bearing in the majority of aircraft operations. Most flights are of relatively short duration and frequency. Incidents during flight are also of relatively shorter duration. For example, if a fire is noted aboard the aircraft, it will very likely be extinguished in short order so the concentration of the extinguishing agent will build up suddenly and diminish suddenly after use because of the relatively rapid ventilation of the aircraft. Similar changes will occur in the concentrations of any of the thermal decomposition products of such a fire.

Absorption

In the aviation environment by far the most important route of entry of toxic chemicals is *via* the respiratory tract. Of secondary importance is the skin and thirdly the gastrointestinal tract. It must not be forgotten, however, that part of the material entering the respiratory tract may be entrapped in the secretions of the trachea, bronchi, etc., moved in a retrograde manner by ciliary action and will eventually be swallowed and, thereby, become absorbed through the gastrointestinal tract.

It is not surprising that the pulmonary tissues comprise an important avenue of entry when one considers that the blood capillary area is of the order of 100 square meters as compared to the total skin surface area of the average man of only 2 square meters. In addition to this, entry through the pulmonary parenchyma provides the shortest route to the heart and brain without benefit of detoxification by the liver before recirculation occurs.

Chemicals may be present in the breathing atmosphere in the form of gases, fumes, mists, vapors or dusts. Dust particles with a diameter greater than 10 microns rarely arrive at the alveolar barrier. They are arrested by the mucous secretions of the upper respiratory tract to be removed by ciliary action and subsequently swallowed. Those less than 10 microns are phagocitized, enter the pulmonary lymphatics and eventually the hilar lymph nodes. Gases, fumes, mists and vapors may enter the alveoli and pass into the alveolar capillaries in accordance with definite physicochemical laws. The rate of diffusion through the pulmonary barrier depends upon the relative partial pressures in the alveolar air, on the one hand, and that in the capillary blood on the other. On the capillary side of the barrier the instantaneous partial pressure of the gas or vapor in the blood is determined by its solubility in the blood. The blood in the capillaries is continuously replaced by fresh circulating blood until the blood returning from the body tissues has become saturated. If this particular dissolved gas is readily soluble in the tissues or certain organs or underoges rapid detoxification, the blood returning to the lung will contain little of the dissolved gas. Consequently, the time required to reach saturation will be relatively long. Insoluble gases will reach blood saturation in a relatively short period of time. The rate of circulation will also be a factor.

Henderson and Haggard (5) have deduced a rather simple formula which describes the absorption of inert gases through the lung:

$$t_x = 2.303 \log_{10} \frac{1}{1-x} \cdot \frac{(BK + L)W}{LB}$$

where t_x equals the time required to reach certain fraction, x, of blood saturation; B equals circulation rate (number of liters or kilograms of blood flowing through the lungs per minute); K equals the coefficient of distribution of gas between equal volumes of pulmonary air and blood; L equals pulmonary ventilation in liters per minute; and W equals body weight in kilograms.

From this it can be readily seen that other factors remaining constant the time required to reach a given degree of blood saturation is: (1) proportional to the weight of the individual, (2) inversely proportional to the rate of circulation and (3) inversely proportional to the effective pulmonary ventilation.

One can readily understand then, that a given concentration of a toxic gas in an aircraft cabin may be quite innocuous to a passenger at rest but significantly toxic to the steward who is exerting himself physically in the performance of his normal duties. On the other hand, this same concentration of gas may be innocuous to a large man but harmful to a small man or child each of whom are undergoing the same physical activity.

The mechanism of absorption described above will be entirely different if the chemical involved exerts a local reaction. For example, some of the acid gases (sulfur dioxide, chlorine), in concentrations sufficiently high, will produce a severe irritant action on the mucosae of the pharynx, trachea, etc. This may produce profuse quantities of mucus which tend to dissolve the gas so effectively that it never reaches the alveoli. Therefore, any effects these gases exert will result from their local action.

Absorption through the skin and through the gastrointestinal tract are not significant portals of entry in the "flight environment." Although there are potential sources of trouble resulting from spillage or spraying of hydraulic fluids or anti-icing agents on the hands, face or clothing the exposure at its worst will be relatively short, insofar as absorption of the chemical into the blood stream. Local effects of such accidents constitute another problem. Chemical burns, for example, are a distinct possibliity. Similarly, irritants, acids or alkalies in the form of liquids, mists or vapors gaining access to the conjunctiva or cornea may be disastrous if vision is impaired even though insignificant quantities of the material have been absorbed by the blood stream.

The Syndrome of Chemical Intoxication

The clinical picture resulting from exposure to toxic chemical agents will vary depending upon (1) the concentration of the chemical whether entering the body *via* the respiratory, dermal or gastrointestinal portal and (2) the site of action. The site of action may be (a) at the point of entrance (portal of entry), (b) a specific organ, cellular system, a metabolic process or enzyme system or (3) at the site of excretion.

Some substances presenting themselves at the portal of entry in low concentrations will be absorbed through the barrier without disturbing these tissues. If sufficient amounts of the chemical reach other specific tissues or organs of the body organic changes will occur and a typical clinical picture will present itself. On the other hand, if the concentrations are high enough the tissues at the portal of entry may be irritated to such a degree that the chemical is rejected and little or no systemic absorption will take place. Examples of these conditions occur in the case of many of the pulmonary irritants. Many of the acid gases are so irritant to the upper respiratory tract that the individual escapes from the environment before any damage can occur to the alveoli and certainly before any absorption has occurred. On the other hand, phosgene or nitrogen dioxide resulting from fuming red nitric acid (a rocket fuel) have little upper respiratory irritant properties but will cause a severe pulmonary edema if exposure is sufficient. Dilute solutions of bichloride of mercury can be retained in and absorbed by the gastrointestinal tract and result in a typical renal failure syndrome. On the other hand, a concentrated solution will be so irritating to the gastric mucosa that vomiting may occur promptly, thereby preventing significant absorption and subsequent renal damage.

Regardless of the portal of entry, once a toxic chemical passes this barrier it enters the circulating blood and tends to become fairly uniformly distributed to all of the tissues of the body. Because of the nature of the chemical itself it will have some predelection to certain organs or tissues. This selective absorption will continue as long as absorption into the body occurs and will tend to decrease the concentration in the circulating blood. As a general rule, many of the fat soluble compounds tend to accumulate in the nervous system because of its high lecithin content (tetraethyl lead, anesthetic agents). In many, an attempt is made by the liver to detoxify the agent and excrete it through the biliary and gastrointestinal tracts. The chlorinated hydrocarbons, *i.e.*, carbon tetrachloride, are typical. If sufficient amounts have been absorbed, acute yellow atrophy will occur. Carbon monoxide, which affects the transport of oxygen *via* hemoglobin, produces hypoxia. Cyanides produce a similar picture but by means of a different mechanism, *i.e.*, tissue respiration.

Mercury is probably the classic example of a chemical producing symptoms which arise from action on the portal of exit or excretion. The damage to the kidney is chiefly tubular and is, therefore, manifested by the presence of casts, albumin and oliguria leading to a typical renal failure syndrome. Uranium poisoning is another example of damage to the portal of exit.

The clinical syndromes produced by exposure to and absorption of relatively high concentrations of toxic chemicals for short periods of time are well understood. When the concentration is low the picture may be more obscure. There is good evidence to believe that the early effects produced by low concentrations are independent of the chemical constitution of the foreign substance. A wide variety of materials of radically different chemical nature have been studied extensively. The signs and symptoms produced are remarkably similar and consist of unusual fatigue or irritability, headache, nausea, anorexia, palpitation, precordial pain, vertigo, pain or numbness in the extremities and dyspnea on exertion. The most pronounced clinical findings include pulse pressure changes, fall in venous pressure, reduced muscle tonus, changes in pulse rate, diminution in voltage of T-waves in the electrocardiogram, sometimes an increased

P-R interval and decreased resistance to stress.

"It is important to realize that there is no great difference between the results of continued exposure to chemicals in intensities short of those causing acute organic injury and the results of prolonged exposure to cold, to lack of oxygen, or to excessive physical labor or, indeed, to the early stages of infectious or metabolic diseases. Even when we pass from the stage of functional changes involved in the 'adaptation syndrome' to a state of actual organ damage, there is really no fundamental difference between the damage produced by chemicals and that caused by other types of disease. A chemical, like an infecting organism, may select one organ for its most pronounced action. Often it is more selective than an infecting organism, but the pathologic changes produced do not differ fundamentally from those already noted in infectious diseases. However, since even in obvious poisoning, the functional derangements produced by the chemical are still important, injudicious chemotherapy may be harmful in chemical poisonings to an extent which we are all apt to overlook when, in infectious diseases, we aim to destroy the infecting agent" (6).

The syndromes produced by relatively high concentrations of toxic chemicals for short periods of exposure vary with the chemical compound or combination of compounds concerned. The symptoms as well as clinical findings and laboratory findings will depend upon the organ or organ system of primary involvement which is fairly specific for each compound. A more thorough discussion of these differences will be included in a subsequent section of this chapter dealing with specific chemical compounds and formulations.

Diagnostic Criteria

The proper diagnosis of occupational diseases caused by excessive absorption of toxic chemicals is extremely important not only where the adequate treatment of the individual is concerned but because of the implications such a diagnosis may have upon modification of airframes, or associated equipment, upon development of protective measures or devices to prevent future recurrences and lastly upon compensation claims. There are a few general principles that should be followed scrupulously in order to avoid the pitfalls which in the past have been the source of considerable embarrassment to otherwise astute clinical diagnosticians.

CAUTION. This is without a doubt the most important of all of the diagnostic rules, for with the exercise of extreme caution the criteria which follow will also be met. As has been previously pointed out many chemical intoxications present clinical syndromes which are very similar to those produced by bacterial or other biologic agents or to those conditions which are of a degenerative nature.

THE CAUSATIVE AGENT MUST BE PRESENT IN THE ENVIRONMENT IN SUFFICIENT QUANTITY TO PRODUCE THE SYNDROME. It is quite obvious that an agent can hardly be incriminated if it were not available for absorption. In spite of this simple concept, the history obtained from an individual patient often erroneously indicates the presence of a specific chemical which does not, in fact, exist in that environment. There is a tendency to assume that all painters are exposed to lead. In these modern days there are many paints which contain no lead whatsoever, consequently the abdominal cramps of such a painter could not justifiably be ascribed to lead. The actual quantity of toxicant in the environment must be sufficiently great in order that the amount absorbed will exceed the ability of the body to excrete it. The determination of these quantitative values—the concentration of a toxicant in the environment—is information which can be obtained from an industrial hygiene survey. Care should be exercised to insure that these values represent as close as possible the true values at the breathing level of the individual concerned.

THE TIME-DOSE RELATIONSHIP MUST BE ADEQUATE. With absorption, detoxification and excretion occurring simultaneously the resultant of these processes must be sufficiently high to produce the syndrome in question. This obviously means that the dosage-time factor must be of an order of magnitude which will result in the "deposition" in the body of significant quantities of the agent.

THE AGENT MUST BE CAPABLE OF PRODUCING THE SYNDROME. The symptom complex produced by relatively small amounts of certain chemical agents may often be nonspecific and easily confused with other agents, chemical or biologic, or even with conditions unrelated to environment. However, where large doses are involved many of the chemicals produce a specific combination of symptoms and clinical and laboratory findings. For example, the organic leads, of which tetraethyl lead is the prime example, has never been known to produce anything but a specific type of encephalopathy whereas inorganic lead rarely, if ever, produces such a picture except in children.

TIME BETWEEN EXPOSURE AND APPEARANCE OF SYMPTOMS MUST BE ADEQUATE. This is directly related to the previous criteria. In general the greater the amount of material absorbed in a given time, the shorter the latent period before the onset of symptoms. There are some exceptions such as in the case of metal fume fever in which the symptoms almost invariably appear some 8 hours after cessation of exposure. The sequence of events should be known in each specific chemical just as the incubation periods of infectious diseases is known.

OTHER CAUSES FOR THE CONDITION MUST BE RULED OUT. Although a high degree of suspicion may be centered upon one or more chemical constituents in an individual's occupational environment, every effort must be made to eliminate normal degenerative processes, infectious diseases and even other chemical toxicants. Not infrequently it has been found that agents, encountered in the hobby workshop at home, were the actual etiologic agents rather than those in the occupational environment.

Control of Potential Chemical Hazards

The control of chemical hazards follow the same general principles in aviation as in any ground operation in the shops or in industry. The most important and the most effective point of control is at the source. Sometimes this may be virtually impossible. In emergencies mechanical failure may occur in which case the control measures will need to be applied to the individual.

Source control must begin on the drawing board. During the earliest phases of design and during development of an aircraft, measures must be taken to prevent toxic agents from gaining access to the crew or passenger compartments. Ventilation systems must be so designed that there is virtually no likelihood of "bleed air" from the engines making

its way through heat exchangers into the cabin. Pressure differentials must be worked out so that exhaust gases in the slip stream do not gain access to the fuselage. The type and amounts of fire extinguishants must be such that fires in flight can be extinguished without exposing the crew or passengers to toxic quantities of the agent. If all of the potentialities of chemical toxicity are not studied and measures taken early in the development of the aircraft, expensive remodification may become necessary.

In order to provide for emergencies during flight, when a control failure has occurred, certain personnel protective measures and devices must be available. Fortunately, the most important and most effective device, the oxygen mask, is generally available for reasons other than protection from chemical agents. The FAA requires that all aircrew be provided with readily available masks in all air carriers. Emergency type oxygen masks for use with a continuous flow oxygen system are available for the passengers. Little if any protection has been made available or found necessary for protection of the eyes in the event that agents having a lacrymation capability find access to the cabin environment.

Medical Control Measures

ENVIRONMENTAL CONTROL. This is normally the function of industrial hygiene engineers who are equipped to gather samples of dusts, vapors, fumes or gases in the working environment for eventual chemical or physical analysis. The results of such a survey or investigation will provide a quantitative concept of the breathing environment under actual conditions of operation. The concentration of toxic gases, the identification of unknown gases, the particle size of dusts and other pertinent findings can thereby be learned. Based upon this information, practical and logical decisions can be made which should result in modification of equipment, changes in operating procedures or any other combination of measures designed to protect the health and efficiency of the personnel who may be involved.

PREVENTIVE MEDICAL MEASURES. The ultimate test of the effectiveness of mechanical devices or other control procedures is the prevention of absorption of toxic chemicals to the point of harmful effect. This level of harmful effect in many cases is below that of actual clinical disease. Subclinical disease may often have a detrimental effect upon efficiency which is most important when one is concerned with the performance requirements of aircrewmen. The detection of subclinical disease is not often easy; however, with the use of periodic physical examinations and associated chemical analyses of pertinent body fluids a trend or level of absorption can be established. Although it is not within the scope of this brief resume to discuss the details of each of the possible chemical intoxications in aviation and their subclinical or clinical characteristics, it is important that certain principles be observed. First, the physician charged with these responsibilities should obtain an intimate knowledge of the work environment. He should know what chemical compounds are actually or potentially present. He should know the nature of these compounds, their physical state, their chemical properties and any other pertinent characteristics. This information must be obtained first hand with the aid of the technical knowledge and skills of other disciplines.

Periodic physical examinations too often become a routine chore with little purpose other than fulfilling a directive or meeting a requirement of some other sort. The nature of the examination should be tailored exactly to the nature of the hazard to which the particular individual is exposed. After one understands the metabolic "life history" of a given chemical the necessity for analyses of certain body fluids which may indicate increasing levels of absorption, for example, will become self evident. Because the amounts of material being dealt with in these circumstances are generally in micro quantities it is imperative that well equipped laboratories provide the results. Errors which might be acceptable in other clinical laboratory fields cannot be accepted in this situation.

The frequency of periodic physical examinations should be determined by the nature and extent of hazard. Where the materials present in the environment are of an extremely hazardous nature the periodicity of examination should be more frequent. Similarly, if control measures have not been too

effective or are questionable the frequency should increase. Another point that is often overlooked is the selection of personnel to be examined. It is not always necessary or even wise to do mass examinations. If one knows the work situations, as he should, he will know the individuals who are, in fact, subjected to the greatest hazard either because of their exposure to higher concentrations or because of their exposure for longer periods of time to equal concentrations. By making these selections one can be reasonably certain that others are receiving a lesser degree of exposure and are, therefore, relatively unlikely to suffer even subclinical disease. Furthermore, the work load entailed in doing the examinations will be kept to a reasonable level.

The purposes of this type of "physical examination" is not intended to replace the normal routine physical examination whose sole purpose is to uncover the usual types of degenerative or other nonoccupational diseases. Whether they are combined is a matter to be decided by the responsible examining physicians.

The final point to make is the importance of correlating the results of environmental analyses with those of the analyses of body fluids and other clinical findings. If there is no correlation, and this is consistent in repeated analyses, another source of exposure outside the work environment should be sought. Not infrequently the source of dangerously high levels of absorption have been found in the home hobby shop of men who may or may not have received any exposure to the incriminated chemical in their occupational environment.

POTENTIAL TOXICOLOGIC PROBLEMS

Fuels and Propellants

Aviation fuels, in a very general sense, include the fuels used in combustion engines, the "jet fuels" used in turbine engines and the propellants used in rocket engines or JATO engines. These will be discussed separately.

AVIATION GASOLINE. The principle constituents of aviation gasolines include various aliphatic and aromatic hydrocarbons (table 77). Although other constituents such as tet-

TABLE 77

Chemical Composition and Other Properties of Aviation Fuels†

Composition	Octane Rating				JP-4	JP-5
	80	91/96	100/130	115/145		
Isopentane (per cent)	15 to 20	15 to 20	15 to 20	15 to 20		
Alkylates (per cent)	30 to 40	30 to 40	30 to 40	30 to 40		
Aromatics (benzene, toluene, xylene) (per cent)	3 to 15	3 to 15	3 to 15	3 to 15	20	20
Straight run gasoline (paraffin series) (per cent)	25 to 52	25 to 52	25 to 52	25 to 52	50	50
Olefins (C_5 and up) (per cent)					5	5
Mercaptan sulfur (per cent)					0.005‡	0.005‡
Total sulfur (per cent)	0.05‡	0.05‡	0.05†	0.05‡	0.4‡	0.4‡
Additives						
Corrosion inhibitor (per cent)					0.007‡	0.007‡
Tetraethyl lead (TEL) (ml., per U. S. gallon)	0.5	4.6	4.6	4.6		
Tricresylphosphate (ml. per U. S. gallon)				0.1 to 0.12		
Kerosene (per cent)					30	30
Reid vapor pressure (p.s.i.)	5.5 to 7.0	5.5 to 7.0	5.5 to 7.0	5.5 to 7.0	2 to 3	0
Flash point (°F.)	30 to 40				0	140
Freezing point (°F.)	−76	−76	−76	−76	−76	−40
Explosive range (per cent)					2 to 10	2 to 10
Dye	Red	Blue	Green	Purple		

* From Henderson and Haggard (5).

† Octane ratings are those of military specifications (Mil-F-5572). Commercial fuels are essentially the same (ASTM D910-48T), *i.e.*, red, 80/87; blue, 91/98; green, 100/130; purple, 115/145; plus an additional one, brown, 108/135. Tetraethyl lead (TEL) content is the same except: 91/98 contains 2.0 ml. per gallon; 100/130, 3.0 ml. per gallon; and 108/135, 3.0 ml. per gallon.

‡ These percentages are "by weight"; all others "by volume."

raethyl lead and tricresyl phosphate which are in themselves quite toxic are found in certain aviation gasolines, they are not under ordinary conditions of use of great significance from a toxicologic standpoint.

The opportunity or likelihood of exposure of aircrews or passengers in flight is not great. Mechanical failure of distribution lines or of the ventilation system does provide a theoretic possibility but this has not been found to be significant in the past. The opportunity for difficulties following exposure to gasoline or its vapors on the ground or in the fuel handling procedures prior to flight are much greater but are not appropriate to this discussion.

Toxicity. On contact with the skin gasoline causes a local irritation owing to the defatting action of the chemical. Repeated contact may result in sensitization. Exposure to gasoline vapors in high concentrations may result in systemic effects from the nar-

cotizing properties of the hydrocarbon of which it is composed. The syndrome produced is not dissimilar to that of alcoholism. Concentrations of 0.26 per cent for a period of 1 hour will cause a "drunken" state. The usual symptom complex consists of excitement, disorientation, nausea, visual and hearing disorders and if exposure is sufficiently long or the concentration sufficiently high may result in unconsciousness, convulsions and death. It is generally believed that concentrations should not exceed a maximum of 0.03 to 0.10 per cent for continuous exposure. Concentrations of 1.3 to 6 per cent are within the explosive range.

AIRCRAFT GAS TURBINE FUELS. These are the so-called "JP" fuels. The original three fuels (JP-1,2 and 3) are various mixtures of straight run gasoline (containing no lead) and "cracked" kerosene. The problems associated with the handling of these fuels is essentially no different than those associated

TABLE 78

*Rocket Propellants—Solid**

Chemical Compounds	Code Number			
	JPL-100-L	JPL-125	JPL-118	AN-509
KClO₄	47.12			
NH₄ClO₄	21.15	56.0	57.0	75.0
Thiokol P-3†	28.85	41.0	30.0	
Paraquinone diox-amine	1.92	2.0	2.0	
Diphenylquanidine	0.95	1.0	1.0	
Fuel (G.S.-1)‡				24.64
1-Hydroxycylohexyl hydroperoxide				0.31
Lecithin				0.05
Cobalt naphthenate				0.01
Tertiary butyl cate-chol				0.03

* Composition equals percentage by weight.

† Liquid polymer of dichlorodiethyl formal (98 per cent) and 1,2,3-trichloropropane (2 per cent).

‡ Fifty per cent styrene and 50 per cent A-10 (adipic acid, maleic anhydride, diethylene glycol).

with ordinary aviation fuel. The one principal difference is the absence of lead and aromatic amines in the JP fuels. The more recent and more commonly used jet fuels, JP-4 and JP-5, are not significantly different from a toxicological viewpoint. Their composition is listed in table 77.

ROCKET PROPELLANTS. The development of rocket engines has required the development of a new variety of fuels other than those derived from petroleum. There are two general types: liquid propellants and solid propellants. The only type used in civil aviation in the United States is the solid propellant employed in a JATO unit. These propellants consist of potassium chlorate, engine oil and tar. Some of the propellants are listed in tables 78 and 79.

Conditions of Exposure. From the standpoint of aircrews and passengers in flight the possibility of exposure to either the propellant itself or to the exhaust gases therefrom is rather remote, probably of the same magnitude as that of exposure to exhaust gases in piston engined aircraft. Normally, JATO units are carried on the undersurface of the wing and outboard a significant distance. For the sake of completeness a brief description of some of the pertinent toxico-

logic considerations is, however, deemed appropriate.

Toxicity. The solid propellants have essentially the same properties insofar as their toxic potentials are concerned. The chlorates, potassium chlorate ($KClO_4$) and ammonium chlorate (NH_4ClO_4) are both powerful oxidizing agents. They are extremely irritating to the skin and are capable of causing severe burns on contact. They both constitute a dangerous fire and explosion hazard. During use, *i.e.*, after firing, the gases which are discharged in the process of combustion consist primarily of sulfur dioxide (SO_2), hydrogen sulfide (H_2S), hydrogen chloride (HCl) and carbon monoxide (CO). Exposure of experimental animals to this mixture of exhaust gases has produced a pathologic picture which might easily have been predicted after knowing the individual constituents. These effects consist of a tracheitis, pneumonitis, pulmonary hemorrhage and pulmonary edema. In some animals showing no other signs of pathology the blood was cherry red in color and was found to contain carboxyhemoglobin of the order of 40 to 50 per cent saturation. Severe conjunctivitis was also noted.

The concentrations of each of these contaminants resulting from the combustion of a 400 gram charge of JPL-126 into a 20 cubic meter chamber resulted in the following: H_2S, 1.21 mg. per liter; SO_2, 0.50 mg. per liter; HCl, 1.22 mg. per liter; and CO, 1.75 mg. per liter. This would indicate that a significant risk could occur if conditions of humidity, wind and distance from the detonation were favorable (7).

TABLE 79

Rocket Propellants—Liquid

Primary Compound	Oxidizer
1. Liquid hydrogen or alcohol or other hydrocarbon	Liquid oxygen
2. Aniline or furfuryl alcohol or xylidine or petroleum hydrocarbons or hydrazine	Fuming nitric acid
3. Permanganate or hydrazine hydrate or hydrazine	Hydrogen peroxide
4. Nitromethane	

Red Fuming Nitric Acid is the oxidizing agent generally in use rather than "white." The former contains dissolved oxides of nitrogen (nitrous fumes); the latter contains very little. The dissolved oxides of nitrogen are evolved as reddish-brown fumes with small amounts of acid vapor. Nitric oxide is fairly rapidly oxidized to nitrogen dioxide (NO_2), which readily polymerizes to nitrogen tetroxide (N_2O_4). The inhaled fumes at body temperature consist of approximately 30 per cent NO_2 and 70 per cent N_2O_4. Nitric oxide (NO) is primarily a cerebral depressant and is capable of forming methemoglobin. Contrariwise, nitrogen dioxide and nitrogen tetroxide, probably as a result of their ability to form nitric acid on contact with water, are local irritants. Consequently, contact with the skin will result in severe acid burns. Contact with the cornea may produce corneal changes with permanent visual impairment and if inhaled a series of rather distinct clinical pictures will be evident. These may be summarized as follows:

1. Irritant gas type; pulmonary edema after a latent period of a few hours and death in 1 to 2 days. This picture is almost identical to that seen in phosgene poisoning.

2. Reversible type; dyspnea, cyanosis, vomiting vertigo and sometimes unconsciousness with recovery.

3. Shock type; rapid onset of suffocation, convulsions and cessation of breathing.

4. Combined type; cerebral symptoms develop early but subside after removal from the fumes. After a latent period of a few hours pulmonary edema develops. This is probably the result of exposure to relatively high concentrations of nitric oxide mixed with relatively high concentrations of nitrogen dioxide and nitrogen tetroxide.

Hydrazine is a colorless, fuming liquid which is extremely caustic, unstable and highly explosive in vapor form. It is soluble in water. Both the anhydrous form or the hydrate are used as propellant components. The principal actions of hydrazine following absorption in sufficient quantities consist of (1) convulsive seizures, (2) severe hypoglycemia and (3) marked hemoconcentration resulting in circulatory shock. Both renal and hepatitic damage may also be produced. The excretion of urine is greatly accelerated and will continue until the amount of body water has been severely reduced. Evidence of hydrazine absorption can be made by determining the hydrazine nitrogen concentration in urine. Because of its caustic nature, contact with the skin or other exposed surfaces can cause extremely severe alkali burns and severe irritation of the pulmonary tract. An MAC of 5 p.p.m. has been suggested.

In some propellants a mixture of aniline, hydrazine and furfural alcohol is used. There is good experimental evidence that any physiopathologic effects of exposure and subsequent absorption of the vapors of this mixture would be primarily those of aniline, *i.e.*, methemoglobinemia with resultant decrease in oxygen saturation. The odor of this mixture resembles that of aniline and is detected at a level of 4 to 10 p.p.m. This should serve as a warning of the presence of acutely dangerous concentrations but not of those concentrations which would be hazardous for prolonged or repeated exposure.

Boranes. A considerable interest has recently been shown in the use of various boranes for use as rocket propellants. Three of these compounds; diborane (B_2H_6), pentaborane (B_5H_9) and decaborane ($B_{10}H_{14}$) are of particular interest. The first one mentioned is a colorless gas, the second a colorless liquid and the third occurs as colorless needles. These compounds all are extremely toxic and have been described as being even more toxic than hydrogen cyanide. Diborane's characteristic effect following inhalation is the production of pulmonary edema, probably the result of the local action of the diborane itself in spite of the ease with which it hydrolyzes to boric acid. On the other hand, the primary effects of both the penta- and the decaborane is upon the central nervous system. Experimental animals become progressively weaker, incoordination ensues, tremors develop, followed by convulsions and death. MAC values have been suggested to not exceed 1 p.p.m. for acute exposures. Limited experimental work (8) has been done to determine the odor detection level. This was found to be between 2 and 4 mg. per cubic meter for the di- and pentaboranes, and 0.3 mg. per cubic meter for decaborane. This would lead one to conclude that odor may provide an adequate warning in the case of decaborane but certainly not in the other two.

In recent subacute and chronic inhalation studies of pentaborane at levels of 0.2 and 1.0 p.p.m. it was concluded that the concentration should be kept below 0.2 p.p.m. for prolonged or repeated exposure. In one group of investigations at this level it was found that the experimental animals showed a loss of appetite, weight loss, apathy, docility, decreased physical activity and muscle tremors. There was some evidence of liver damage as measured by the bromsulfalein test. At

TABLE 80

Formulations of Typical Hydraulic Fluids and Lubricants

Type	Chemical Composition	
	Compound	Per cent
Hydraulic fluids		
PRL-3169	Ethyl dibromobenzene	82.5
	Aroclor 1248	10.1
	Acryloid HF 55	3.9
	Mineral oil base stock	3.1
	Paranox 441	0.4
PRL-3209	Ethyl dibromobenzene	79.4
	Aroclor 1248	9.7
	Acryloid HF 55	3.6
	Calcium cetyl phenate (60 to 70 per cent)	3.0
	Mineral oil base	2.9
	Tricresyl phosphate	1.0
	Paranox 441	0.4
PRL-3039	Di-secondary amyl sebacate	88.0
	Di-2-ethylhexyl sebacate	5.3
	Acryloid HF 25	5.2
	Tricresyl phosphate	1.0
	Phenothiazine	0.5
	Silicone DC 200	0.001
Lubricants		
Mil-L-17535	Di-isoamyl adipate	96.65
	Barium petroleum sulfonate	3.00
	Phenothiazine	0.35
Mil-L-7808	Bis (2-ethylhexyl) sebacate	94.5
	Tricresyl phosphate	5.0
	Phenothiazine	0.5

the present time there appear to be no specific laboratory analyses which would serve as an index of incipient chronic pentaborane intoxication.

Lubricants and Hydraulic Fluids

This group of compounds and formulations will be discussed together because the basic chemical structure of most of the formulations are essentially similar (Fig. 78). In general, they consist of a base oil plus certain other chemical compounds which improve certain properties of the formulation for a specific purpose, one of which is the inflammability. The base oil may be naturally occurring (*i.e.*, petroleum or castor oil) or a synthetic oil (*i.e.*, bis-2-ethylhexyl adipate, or azelate, di-isoamyl adipate, etc.). In most formulations the "base oil" will occur in a concentration of 80 to 90 per cent. The remainder will consist of such chemicals as tricresyl phosphate, 1 to 5 per cent, phenothiazine, 0.5 per cent; and numerous other compounds in quantities which are not sufficient to contribute significantly to the toxicity of the compound. The variety of formulations used for purposes of lubrication and for operation of hydraulic control systems is so extensive that the toxic nature of any one will differ from that of others. It is, therefore, imperative that the specific lubricant or hydraulic fluid be made known before any conclusions are drawn implicating any specific compound as an etiologic agent.

MODE OF EXPOSURE. The probability of being exposed to lubricants during the operation of an aircraft is very remote except in case of breakdown of a ventilation system which allows air from the engine into the system. If that should happen the oil itself would probably not be involved but rather its thermal decomposition products. The probability of exposure to hydraulic fluids is another matter. Normally from 15 to 55 gallons of hydraulic fluid are carried on an aircraft. This fluid will be enclosed in a system operating at pressures of 1500 to 3000 p.s.i. Many of the lines of the hydraulic system will traverse the crew compartments so any leak in the system, in the line itself or at a joint will produce either atomization and mist formation or a stream of the fluid itself. The nature of the exposure will then obviously be one involving inhalation and perhaps skin contact, on the one hand, and skin contact only in the latter instance. The possibility of eye contact also exists.

TOXICITY. A considerable amount of experimental work has been done on this group of compounds and various combinations in order to determine their toxicologic properties. The results of these studies would tend to indicate that all of the synthetic base oils will readily pass through the dermal barrier, are capable of producing degenerative changes in the liver, brain, kidney and heart, pulmonary hyperemia and pulmonary edema. Erythema, hardening and cracking of the skin will result from prolonged contact. Some irritation of cornea and conjunctiva could occur from an accidental splash in the eye. These remarks apply specifically to the "sebacates," adipates and azelate. Ethyl dibromobenzene and its formulations in mist form are somewhat more toxic than certain of the aliphatic esters. The vapors of tetrachlorotetrafluoropropane appears to be more toxic than the more common chlorinated hydrocarbon solvents. The chemicals, such as tricresyl phosphate which are contained in many of the formulations apparently add very little, if any, to the toxicity of the formulation.

The toxicity of thermal decomposition products of this group of synthetic materials (9) is primarily the result of the breakdown products of the aliphatic esters (for example, di-2-ethylhexyl sebacate). Comparatively, the toxicity of these synthetics is probably a little less than twice that of the paraffinic hydrocarbon lubricating oils. Fogs formed at 550 or 400° F. were much less toxic than those formed at 600° F. The materials produced by thermal decomposition of both the hydrocarbon and the synthetic esters consist primarily of aldehydes, carbonyls, carbon monoxide and undecomposed particulate matter.

Fire Extinguishing Agents

There undoubtedly is no ideal and universal fire extinguishing agent for aircraft. The problems of providing an agent which will quickly extinguish a fire regardless of the nature of the burning material is the first hurdle. The second problem is to find one which has little or no physiologic effect on the human being who may be in the vicinity. Not only is the effect of the material itself of importance but the effect of its decomposition products is of even greater importance primarily because these thermal products are generally far more toxic than the extinguishant itself.

Water, of course, is the oldest and perhaps the best known fire extinguishing agent. It has the unfortunate limitations of weight, relatively high freezing point (important in aviation) and is ineffective in both electrical (class C) and flammable liquid (class B) fires. Carbon dioxide has been extensively used in aviation but it also is not to effective in extinguishing fires of combustible materials such as paper, textiles, etc. It has a toxicity factor which is significant in the enclosed space of an aircraft cabin whereas this would not be important in fighting a fire in an open area. The third "group" of agents include the halogenated hydrocarbons, the principal ones of which include carbon tetrachloride, methyl bromide and monochloromonobromomethane (commonly known as "CB"). A partial list of this group of agents which have undergone toxicologic investigations are included in table 81.

The choice of agent for specific applications has been based upon four factors: (1) the efficiency of the agent as an extinguishant, (2) the toxicity of the agent *per se*, (3) the toxicity of the thermal decomposition products and (4) the quantity to be used. Obviously the efficiency of the agent as an extinguishant is of primary importance. If the quantity necessary to stop a fire is small enough so that the total quantity liberated into the cabin of an aircraft, for example, cannot reach toxic concentrations then a relatively more toxic agent can be successfully used. In simple terms this was the reason that monochloromonobromomethane ("CB") was adopted for many applications in the aviation industry and aboard aircraft in particular.

Regardless of the agent, aircrews and passengers can be exposed to these agents following the use of portable extinguishers in either the aircraft cabin or in cargo compartments. Most aircraft are also equipped with automatic or semiautomatic fire extinguishing systems located near or in the engine nacelles and also in cargo compartments. From the former it is possible for the agent

TABLE 81
Relative Toxicity of Fire Extinguishants*

Compound	Undecomposed		Decomposed	
	mg. per liter	*p.p.m.*	*mg. per liter*	*p.p.m.*
Tetrafluormethane (CF_4)	3220	895,000	3220	895,000
Carbon dioxide (CO_2)	1180	656,000	1240	690,000
Methyl iodide (CH_3I)	22	4,000	350	60,000
Perfluoromethylcyclohexane ($C_6H_{11}CF_3$)	1170	82,000	120	8,000
Dibromodifluoromethane ($C_2H_2F_2Br_2$)	210	23,000	110	12,000
Bromotrifluoromethane (CF_3Br)	5070	834,000	90	14,000
Ethyl bromide (C_2H_5Br)	660	148,000	75	17,000
Methyl bromide (CH_3Br)	23	6,000	65	16,000
Monobromomonochlorodifluoromethane (CF_2BrCl)	2200	326,000	50	8,000
Monobromomonochloromethane (CB) (CH_2ClBr)	340	64,000	22	4,200
Dibromotetrafluoroethane ($C_2F_4Br_2$)	1340	132,000	17	1,700
Dibromodifluoromethane (CF_2Br_2)	470	55,000	16	1,900
Dibromotrifluoromonochloroethane ($C_2F_3ClBr_2$)	280	25,000	8	700
Carbontetrachloride (CCl_4)	180	29,000	2	300

* The figures in this table are "approximate lethal concentrations" for 15 minutes of exposure in rats. They are arranged in the order of increasing toxicity (reading from the top down) of the decomposed vapors which tends to approximate the conditions likely to prevail in a fire excluding the contribution of toxic products originating from thermal decomposition of materials other than the extinguishing agent itself. Adapted from Medical Division Research Report No. 23; "An Investigation of the Toxicity of proposed Fire Extinguishing Fluids," October 1950.

to gain entry into the ventilation system of the cabin itself through heat exchangers.

In the event of overexposure, the effect upon aircrewmen or passengers will obviously depend upon the chemical nature of the agent, its concentration and the total time of exposure. For the purposes of this discussion it will be necessary to eliminate from consideration any mention of the toxic thermal decomposition products of upholstery fabrics, electrical insulation, metals or other materials which may be involved in any fire aboard the aircraft. These will be discussed in a separate section of this chapter.

Carbon dioxide occurs normally in the breathing atmosphere in concentrations of about 0.5 per cent. It can be tolerated at concentrations of 3 per cent and even for 5 to 10 minutes at 5 per cent. At concentrations of 20 to 25 per cent few would remain conscious longer than 1½ minutes. Symptomatically, the individual would be observed to increase his rate and depth of breathing, his conjunctivae would be injected, respiration would become increasingly difficult, he would note unusual sensations of taste and smell, headache, vertigo, lack of judgment, weakness, incoordination and fi-

nally collapse. Actually this is a picture of hypoxia with the added factor of respiratory center stimulation caused by an increased carbon dioxide tension.

Insofar as acute exposures (short term, high concentration) to the halogenated hydrocarbons the toxicologic actions are primarily of a narcotic nature. Their primary action is upon the central nervous system. Some of the commonly used anesthetics, *i.e.*, chloroform, ethylene, etc., are closely related chemically to this group of agents. If exposures are sufficiently severe, *i.e.*, long term at low concentrations, they will produce hepatic and renal damage. However, the problem concerning the flight surgeon is one of short term exposures in flight. High concentrations may be sufficiently severe to produce narcosis but more frequently and more likely will be the lesser exposure which will result only in minor(?) aberrations of physiology and, therefore, of behavior which may have a detrimental effect upon the pilot who is in control of the aircraft.

Antifreezing Agents

This group of agents includes deicing fluids, coolant fluids and antidetonant injection (ADI) fluids. They will be discussed together because the chemical formulations of all three contain common chemical compounds. Deicing fluids are used to keep windshields, carburetors and propellers free of ice. They consist of various combinations of ethyl alcohol, isopropyl alcohol, methyl alcohol, propylene or ethylene glycol and water. ADI fluids are used in the fuel of combustion engines to improve performance for short periods of time. They are injected into the combustion mixture when required. They consist of such mixtures as methyl alcohol 50 per cent in water, or equal parts of methyl and ethyl alcohol 50 per cent in water. Coolant liquids for use in liquid cooled engines are almost a thing of the past. Ethylene glycol and water was used most commonly.

Although a potential danger of exposure to these compounds does exist it is not great. First, relatively small amounts of these materials are carried aloft. Fifty or 60 gallons of ADI fluids may be carried and lesser amounts of the deicing fluids. Secondly, most of the compounds with the exception of methyl alcohol, ethylene glycol and to some extent ethyl alcohol are of a low order of toxicity. The alcohols of a higher molecular weight are relatively more toxic but at the same time decrease in volatility as the molecular weight increases. This latter fact actually decreases the resultant toxic potential.

The usual cause of exposure to any of these agents in an airborne aircraft is a rupture of a line or of a joint in the line which permits a spray under pressure to enter the environment of the cabin. This creates both an inhalation hazard and also a hazard from skin contamination.

The dangers of exposure to methyl alcohol are the result primarily of inhalation of the vapor or of a mist. The effect of high concentrations would primarily be that of a narcotic although less than that of ethyl alcohol. The difference between the concentration required to produce narcosis is not much less than that which would prove fatal. Visual disturbances including blindness can result from lower concentrations repeated over an extended period of time. The MAC is generally accepted as 200 p.p.m. (260 mg. per cubic meter). Concentrations

of 30,000 to 50,000 p.p.m. for 30 to 60 minutes are considered to be dangerous.

The effects of absorption of ethyl alcohol through the respiratory tract are similar to those encountered after ingestion. In addition, as one might well expect, some irritation of the mucous membranes and of the upper respiratory tract occur in addition to the headache, dizziness, tremors, nausea and eventually narcosis. The early effects of low concentrations or short duration, high concentrations of the vapor may include a decrease in the powers of concentration and alertness which may have an extremely profound effect upon the successful operation of an aircraft. A concentration of 1000 p.p.m. (1900 mg. per cubic meter) is the accepted MAC.

Ethylene glycol has a low vapor pressure which would probably not be capable of producing a concentration higher than 110 p.p.m. even in an enclosed space. This concentration would not be expected to have any effect upon a man exposed for 8 hours daily for months. However, it must be remembered that under the circumstances prevailing in an aircraft in flight the conditions may be somewhat different. The compound may be liberated in the form of a fog, mist or spray in which case the amounts available for absorption would greatly exceed that available from the vapor itself. In addition, the decrease of atmospheric pressure at altitude will tend to increase vaporization. Propylene glycol has a similar action to that of ethylene glycol but is far less toxic. It is considered comparable to glycerin when taken by mouth.

The toxicologic action of ethylene glycol which is representative of most of the group is threefold in order of importance: (1) renal, (2) necrosis of the liver and (3) central nervous system depressant. Irritation of the pulmonary tissues has followed exposure to high concentrations of the vapor. The material apparently selects the convoluted tubules of the kidney and results in suppression of urine, uremia and death.

Insecticides, Herbicides and other Agricultural Chemicals

Aircrews and passengers in aircraft may be exposed to agents used as insecticides, herbicides, fungicides and other agricultural chemicals in three different ways, *i.e.*, during disinsectization of aircraft engaged in international operations, from cargo being carried aboard the aircraft or during aircraft spraying operations.

Both the International Sanitary Regulations of the World Health Organization and the regulations of U. S. Public Health Service provide for disinsectization of aircraft before takeoff or at some time prior to landing. During this period both the aircrew and the passengers will be subjected to insecticide exposure. Disinsectization is conducted with the use of an insecticidal aerosol dispensed in the amount of not less than 5 grams of the formulation for each 1000 cubic feet of enclosed space (USPHS) or 10 grams per 1000 cubic feet (WHO). If a formulation containing 3 per cent by weight of DDT were used, the concentration of DDT which would result would be approximately 10.5 mg per cubic meter if the WHO regulations are followed and about 5.3 mg. per cubic meter for the USPHS. The recommended threshold limit value for DDT is 1 mg. per cubic meter. It must be remembered that this latter figure is predicated upon an 8 hour exposure per day. The actual duration of exposure during an insectization procedure is only of the order of 5 to 10 minutes so the risk is virtually nonexistent when handled properly. At the present time the accepted formulations (10) of insecticides used are contained in table 82.

It is possible that aircrews and passengers will be exposed during flight to these materials carried in the cargo compartments in the event of accidental rupture or spillage of a container. The risk of such an accident is very remote, however, because the shipping regulations provide for methods and materials for packing and crating which have been most successful in preventing such accidents.

The third mode of exposure to this group of agents occurs during crop spraying operations so obviously this does not involve passengers. Aircraft spraying of insecticides, fungicides, herbicides or fertilizers is generally performed by small, slow flying aircraft equipped with tanks containing the agent plus the necessary associated equipment for producing the desired spray, mist or fog. Intoxication of pilots engaged in these operations has occurred not infrequently. In some instances it resulted from repeatedly flying through a previously laid fog; in others, it was produced by careless handling procedures during tank filling operations.

Although there are a large number of chemical compounds and a much greater variety of chemical formulations encountered as insecticides, fungicides, etc., they may be classified into essentially three groups: (1) chlorinated hydrocarbons, (2) phosphate esters and (3) miscellaneous. The chlorinated hydrocarbons are the only ones used for the disinsectization of aircraft and this has been limited to the use of DDT in the formulations noted in table 82. This group includes all related compounds having chlorophenothane as their chemical prototype. In addition to DDT (2,2-bis-*p*-chlorophenyl-1,1,1-trichloroethane), dieldrin, endrin, aldrin,

TABLE 82

Formulas for Insecticidal Aerosols: G-382, G-651, G-1152 and G-1029

Component	High Pressure Aerosols		Medium Pressure Aerosols	
	G-382	G-651	G-1152	G-1029
	per cent by weight			
Pyrethrum extract (20 per cent pyrethrins)	5.0	6.0	5.0	6.0
DDT	3.0	2.0	3.0	2.0
Cyclohexanone	5.0		5.0	
Lubricating oil (SAE 30)	2.0		2.0	
Aromatic petroleum derivative solvents				
Velsicol AR60 or Socony Vacuum 544G		8.0		6.0
Velsicol AR50 or Socony Vacuum 544C				2.0
Trichlorofluoromethane (Freon-11 or Genetron-11)			25.5	25.2
Dichlorodifluoromethane (Freon-12 or Genetron-12)	85.0	84.0	59.5	58.8

heptachlor, chlordane and toxaphene are representative.

The phosphate esters or organic phosphates include such compounds as parathion, systox (demeton), TEPP (tetraethylpyrophosphate), Trithion, Phosdrin, thimet and others. These have only been encountered in the spraying operations of the agricultural industry.

The miscellaneous group includes DNOC (dinitro-o-cresol) used as a herbicide, phenyl mercuric acetate, nicotine, sulfur dust and many others. They also would be encountered only in an agricultural application.

The chlorinated hydrocarbons gain access to the tissues of the body by inhalation, ingestion and through the intact skin. Their actions are similar and vary only in degree depending upon the variation in chemical and physical properties, i.e., solubility in water or fat, vapor pressure, etc. Their primary action is one of central nervous system stimulation. Secondarily, they are capable of producing degenerative changes in the liver, kidney and brain. Consequently, exposure to high concentrations for relatively short periods can produce a syndrome of anorexia, excessive salivation hyperirritability, tremors terminating in convulsions, coma and death from respiratory failure. If the exposure is to lower concentrations over a longer period of time the signs of central nervous system involvement will not be as prominent although muscular incoordination, headache, nausea or vomiting, hyperirritability, insomnia, weight loss and convulsions might be noted. Evidence of damage to the liver, kidneys and brain should also be expected. An enlarged liver resulting from fatty degeneration may be noted. The electroencephalogram may demonstrate diffuse cortical discharges which is particularly significant in the presence of a previously normal electroencephalogram. Differential diagnosis in cases of intoxication by chlorinated hydrocarbons is often difficult but is aided by the absence of fever, changes in blood chemistry or blood counts, including the differential white cell count, and in blood pressure. Another point to keep in mind is that if the symptoms persist for more than 1 week after removal from exposure, the cause is probably not a chlorinated hydrocarbon. Treatment is primarily supportive, i.e., control of convulsions with barbitals, such as pentothal and phenobarbital, and a high protein diet with amino acid supplements.

The phosphate ester group of insecticides are capable of entering the body either through the pulmonary tract, the gastrointestinal tract or through the intact skin. They are metabolized to substances which actively inhibit the cholinesterase enzymes. The cholinesterase enzymes of the central nervous system are the only ones of importance in this reaction, however, because it is believed that the acetylcholinesterase enzyme contained in the red blood cells closely parallel the central nervous system enzyme. Therefore, the erythrocyte enzyme activity is the one used as a measure of anticholinesterase activity. The symptomatic level is believed to be approximately a drop of 30 per cent of normal. Excessive absorption produces a picture of intense parasympathetic stimulation resulting in weakness, unsteadiness, blurred vision, headache, nausea and a feeling of tightness in the chest. This is rapidly followed by vomiting, abdominal cramps, diarrhea, profuse sweating, tremors, dyspnea and, finally, coma, convulsions and death. The pupils of the eye are pin point and nonreactive. The development of this syndrome, if absorption has been great enough, occurs very rapidly thereby making active treatment mandatory. It is extremely important to begin atropinization quickly and in large doses. Atropine should be administered either intramuscularly or intravenously in doses of from 2 to 6 mg. every 15 to 30 minutes until full atropinization is established as noted by the pupillary dilation and dryness of throat. A total of 20 to 30 mg. may be needed during the first 24 hours. Termination of exposure should perhaps have been mentioned first for emphasis. It is important not only to remove the patient from the locale of exposure but exposure must be halted by removal of all clothing followed by a thorough cleansing of the entire body with soap and water to eliminate a possible opportunity to absorb more of the agent through the skin.

Thermal Decomposition

The chemical changes produced by subjecting any of the material carried aboard an aircraft to temperatures above normal operating temperatures (less than 100° F.) may and usually does produce profound changes in the toxicologic hazard of that environment. These chemical changes are those of rapid oxidation which, if complete, have as their end products carbon dioxide and water. However, complete oxidation is rarely if ever achieved so the end products generally consist of carbon monoxide, aldehydes, various other intermediates depending upon the chemical nature of the source plus lesser amounts of carbon dioxide and water.

The temperatures to which a chemical substance is subjected will have a direct bearing upon the type and amount of certain decomposition products. For example, the fogs formed from di-2-ethylhexyl sebacate (synthetic lubricant) at 400 and 550° F. were much less toxic than those formed at 600° F. This same type of change occurs when Teflon or Kel-F, used as an insulation for electrical wiring, is heated above 752° F.

High temperatures occur normally in aircraft operations during the combustion of fuels or propellants and abnormally in overheating of electrical equipment; in mechanical breakdowns which allow burning of lubricating oil and in actual conflagration of any of the various components of the airframe or its cargo. The folllowing discussion will briefly cover the nature of these products of thermal decomposition as well as their source and will be followed by a more detailed discussion of the toxicologic properties of the principle decomposition products.

PETROLEUM PRODUCTS. Gasoline, jet fuels and the naturally occurring lubricating oils are, for the most part, mixtures of various aliphatic hydrocarbons. Thermal decomposition of this group of compounds occurs during normal combustion of the fuel and accidentally when failure of the lubrication system allows lubricating oils to enter the combustion chambers or to be sprayed on the external surfaces of a hot engine. The amount of oxygen present for oxidation will determine the relative amount of certain decomposition products. For example, during takeoff when the fuel mixture is set at "rich" the fuel to air ratio is increased (decreased oxygen) as compared to cruise. The concentration of carbon monoxide in the exhaust gas has been found to be 8.75 per cent compared to 3 per cent (by weight),

respectively. Carbon dioxide, on the other hand, shows the reverse relationship as one would expect: 10 *versus* 15 per cent. Other products, such as methane, butylene, oxygen and hydrogen, will also be found in the exhaust gases in small quantities, plus nitrogen and water (70 and 9 per cent respectively).

Lubricating oils, both the paraffinic hydrocarbons and the esters (synthetics), decompose under high temperatures to form a mixture of aldehydes, carbonyls, carbon monoxide and undecomposed particulate matter. This statement would also apply to most of the hydraulic fluids because their basic chemical compositions are very similar.

FIRE EXTINGUISHING AGENTS. Carbon dioxide does not decompose when exposed to high temperatures, consequently there is no alteration in its toxicity when utilized to extinguish a fire. This is a distinct advantage when compared with certain of the halogenated hydrocarbons. This is one of the factors which has virtually eliminated the use of carbon tetrachloride as an extinguishant aboard aircraft. It decomposes to form one of the most toxic of the carbonyls, phosgene. Other halogenated hydrocarbons also form some carbonyls during pyrolysis but in quantities which are not so significant. The pyrolysis products of methyl bromide do not increase the toxicity of the agent greatly but its toxicity is so much greater in the undecomposed state than most of the other hydrocarbons that it has been largely discarded in American aircraft.

PROPELLANTS. The thermal decomposition products of the perchlorate type propellants used in JATO assist devices consist of hydrogen sulfide (H_2S) sulfur dioxide (SO_2), hydrogen chloride (HCl) and carbon monoxide (CO). Particulate matter is also discharged which gives it the character of a smoke. According to some experimental work these particulates did not contribute to the overall toxicity so they may be disregarded. Fundamentally the toxicity of H_2S is about twice that of SO_2, which is twice that of CO. HCl is not toxic although it is quite irritating. From experimental work on animals it would appear that the principal effect of this mixture of gases is the result of the CO component.

PLASTICS. Many different types of plastics are used in the fabrics and upholstery materials of aircraft cabin interiors. Similar types of materials are widely used as insulation for electrical wiring. The plastic employed may include certain polyester resins such as styrene, urethane, the epoxy resins, the phenolic resins or Kel-F and Teflon. The latter two are used principally for electrical insulation.

In general, these materials are essentially inert at normal temperatures. However, at high temperatures a breakdown does occur. In the case of Kel-F and Teflon the decomposition products consist of strong acids (expressed as HF), an equal concentration of ionizable fluorides plus a significant quantity of finely divided particulate matter. In infrared studies it was suggested that the products were probably perfluoroisobutene and oxygen difluoride. In experimental studies involving fairly high concentrations to these decomposition products the subject animals developed typical signs of pulmonary edema or a chemical pneumonitis and diffuse degeneration of the brain, liver and kidneys. This is a similar picture seen in the cases involved in such fires as the Coconut Grove fire in Boston in 1942. Similar findings might be expected in an uncontrolled fire involving modern aircraft upholstery or drapery materials.

Carbon Monoxide

CO is the most commonly encountered toxic gas in the environment of aircrewmen and passengers alike. It is almost always present in varying concentrations in the combustion of fuels (exhaust gases), lubricants or practically any material carried aboard an aircraft in the event of a fire. Exhaust gases are commonly used to provide cabin heat through the use of heat exchangers. Properly maintained heat exchangers will not permit leakage of exhaust gases into the ventilation system. Failures have occurred when connections or parts of the mechanism have been subjected to excessive vibration, wear or aging which have produced cracks or other avenues of cross flow to occur. Instances of contamination have also occurred as a result of gases in the slip stream gaining access to the aircraft cabin owing to pressure differentials in the ventilation portals.

The atmospheric concentration of carbon monoxide is usually expressed at "parts per million" or as a percentage. The maximum allowable concentration in aircraft, depending upon the agency concerned, varies from 40 to 100 p.p.m. (0.005 to 0.010 per cent). The most practical method for making this determination is a device made by the Mines Safety Co. (U. S. A.). It uses a colorimetric indicating gel devised by the National Bureau of Standards. The method depends upon a color change from yellow to green in the sensitive portion of a glass tube through which a measured volume of air is passed. The degree of color change is compared with a standard to determine the concentration of carbon monoxide. Care must be exercised in making the test in order to obtain a sample from the actual breathing atmosphere of the individual or the working area of the individual concerned.

In case of known or suspected exposure, the most significant finding is the carbon monoxide content of the blood. This value represents the actual resultant absorption of the gas in a given period of time regardless of varying concentrations of the gas in the immediate atmosphere and of other variables affecting the rate and extent of absorption. The most reliable method of determining saturation of blood carboxyhemoglobin is the method of Van Slyke. Roughton and Scholander have also developed a microchemical technique.

As will be discussed later, carbon monoxide can be assumed to be in equilibrium between alveolar air, arterial blood and venous blood. From these assumptions, verified by experimental results, a method was developed which utilized alveolar air passed through the Mine Safety appliance device and thereby determining the concentration directly. From this can be calculated the saturation level of carbon monoxide in the blood.

ABSORPTION. When carbon monoxide in the air is inhaled the carbon monoxide reaching the alveoli tends to pass through the alveolar walls into the capillary or arterial blood in the same manner as oxygen. After gaining entrance into the blood stream it rapidly enters the erythrocytes where it combines with hemoglobin in the same manner as oxygen does. Insignificant amounts are held in solution in the serum.

There is one very important difference between oxygen and CO in respect to its ability to combine with hemoglobin. CO combines from 210 to 250 times more easily. This combination is determined by the partial pressure of each gas independently, taking into account the so-called "distribution coefficient" of 210 to 250. This relationship can be expressed mathematically as follows (11):

$$\frac{\text{per cent Hb CO}}{\text{per cent Hb O}_2} = M \frac{\text{pCO}}{\text{pO}_2}$$

in which M equals the distribution coefficient; pCO and pO_2 equal the partial pressures of CO and O_2, respectively; and per cent Hb CO and Hb O_2 equal the blood saturation of CO and O_2, respectively. This will serve to illustrate the reason that a concentration of 0.084 per cent CO in air will produce an amount of carboxyhemoglobin in the blood equal to the amount of oxyhemoglobin produced by a concentration of 20.9 per cent oxygen in air ($M = 248$).

The rapidity with which the hemoglobin becomes saturated with carbon monoxide is determined by the partial pressure (pCO) of carbon monoxide, the volume of inspired air per unit time (duration of exposure), the rate of the blood circulation and the amount of hemoglobin available for combination.

TABLE 83

Application of Hill's Equation to Oxyhemoglobin Dissociation Curve Data on Human Blood at pH 7.4 and 37° C.

pO₂	Per Cent Saturation
2.1	2
3.8	4
5.5	6
8.2	10
10.9	15
13.4	20
17.9	30
22.0	40
26.3	50
31.1	60
36.1	70
45.7	80
51.7	85
61.4	90
75.0	94
87.7	96
113.0	98

* From Roughton (12).

The partial pressure of CO (pCO) in a given environment, other factors remaining constant, determines the degree of saturation. The concentration or partial pressure of the gas in the lung varies with altitude. Because the partial pressures of carbon dioxide and water in the lung remains essentially constant, the relationship between concentration or partial pressure of CO in the atmosphere and at the alveolar wall will vary in the following manner.

$$\text{pCO} = \frac{\text{per cent CO}}{100}(P_B - 40)$$

where P_B is the barometric pressure in mm. of Hg at the altitude in question and 40 is a numerical factor which assumes a constant respiratory quotient, a partial pressure of water vapor of 47 mm. of Hg and a constant pCO_2. Under the same circumstances and assumptions the partial pressure of oxygen can be determined from

$$\text{pO}_2 = (0.185 \times P_B) - 37$$

The combined effect of the partial pressures of carbon monoxide and oxygen will determine the amount of carboxyhemoglobin and oxyhemoglobin present at equilibrium. The balance of the hemoglobin will exist as reduced hemoglobin. For example, at 20,000 feet ($P_B = 349$ mm. of Hg.), the pO_2 would be 27.6 mm. of Hg and the pCO_2 would be 0.062 mm. of Hg. Their combined effect would be their arithmetic sum, taking into account the "M factor," the distribution coefficient, which in this instance will be taken as having a value of 210, thus:

$$(\text{pO}_2 + M\text{pCO} = \text{p (CO} + \text{O}_2))$$

$$27.6 + (0.062 \times 210) = 40.6 \text{ mm. of Hg}$$

A partial pressure of 40.6 mm. of Hg of oxygen (or O_2 and CO combined) would produce a total saturation of 74 per cent of the available hemoglobin (table 83). From this can be deduced the portion of hemoglobin saturated by CO by use of the following formula:

$$\text{per cent Hb CO} = \frac{M\text{pCO}}{\text{pO}_2 + M\text{pCO}}$$

$$(\text{per cent Hb CO} + \text{per cent Hb O}_2)$$

Example:

$$\text{per cent Hb CO} = \frac{(210 \times 0.062)}{27.6 + (210 \times 0.062)} \quad (74)$$

$$= 24 \text{ per cent}$$

The volume of air coming in contact with the alveolar walls has a direct relationship with the rate of absorption. As the rate of respiration increases, the volume of air made available per unit time increases along with the absolute amount or number of carbon monoxide molecules. Coincidently, the circulatory rate also increases, thereby making more reduced hemoglobin available per unit of time. The practical significance of this point is that the time required to reach maximum saturation of carboxyhemoglobin is decreased during exercise or during hyperventilation from any cause.

A fourth factor having a direct effect upon the rapidity of saturation is the absolute amount of hemoglobin available in the circulating blood. For example, a normal human adult has approximately 16 grams of hemoglobin per 100 cc. of blood. The time required for 50 per cent saturation with carboxyhemoglobin would obviously be shortened considerably if this individual had had a hemoglobin level of 10 grams per 100 cc.

This latter factor is of considerable importance if one is dealing with a case of simple anemia being exposed to significant quantities of carbon monoxide in which case the anemic individual would be affected much faster than an individual with a normal hemoglobin level.

The effects of absorption of carbon monoxide are primarily owing to the replacement of oxyhemoglobin with carboxyhemoglobin in the erythrocytes. If this were the only effect, one would expect the same response in an individual at sea level whose blood had a carboxyhemoglobin saturation of 60 per cent as in one whose oxyhemoglobin saturation was 40 per cent owing to anemia. However, this is not the case. Haldane once stated that "miners may do their ordinary work though their hemoglobin percentage is reduced to half by ankylostomiasis whereas a person whose blood is half saturated with CO is practically helpless."

Carboxyhemoglobin tends to shift the oxygen dissociation curve to the left, thereby decreasing the ability of the blood to release its oxygen at the tissue level. This becomes extremely critical during periods of excessive demand during exercise or simple hypoxia when the normal resting reserves have been expended. The oxygen dissociation curve of a simple anemia is shifted to the right of normal, is sigmoid in shape but flattened leaving little reserve but is capable of releasing oxygen at tissue level at a much higher pO_2.

The rate of absorption of carbon monoxide in man, taking into account three of the four major variable factors, i.e., time of exposure, ventilation rate and atmospheric concentration, has been well illustrated in the graph shown in figure 141. The degree of saturation of carboxyhemoglobin (sea level) can be determined by estimating the ventilation rate, drawing a horizontal line to the point interrupting the time of exposure, drawing a vertical line to the atmospheric concentration curve. The horizontal intercept gives the degree of saturation.

The symptomatology of CO poisoning related to blood saturation is shown in table 84. It should be stressed that these apply only to sea level and not at altitude. If an individual is exposed to identical concentrations of CO at sea level as compared to an exposure at altitude, the degree of saturation with CO will be identical assuming all other factors are constant except the partial pressure of oxygen. On the other hand, the signs and symptoms he will exhibit will be much more pronounced at altitude. This change is primarily the result of increasing hypoxia caused by decreasing pO_2 values as higher altitudes are reached. Diringshofen and Hartmann have shown (table 85) the proportions of Hb O_2, Hb CO and reduced Hb at various concentrations of CO at altitudes from sea level to 8000 meters. One will note from this table that at any given concentration of CO, the level of Hb CO decreases slightly as higher altitudes are reached and that the level of Hb O_2 decreases to a much greater extent which explains the fact that the symptom at higher altitudes are much more severe than the concentration of Hb CO would indicate.

It has been demonstrated by Armstrong and Heim that hypoxia resulting from an oxygen saturation of less than 88 per cent

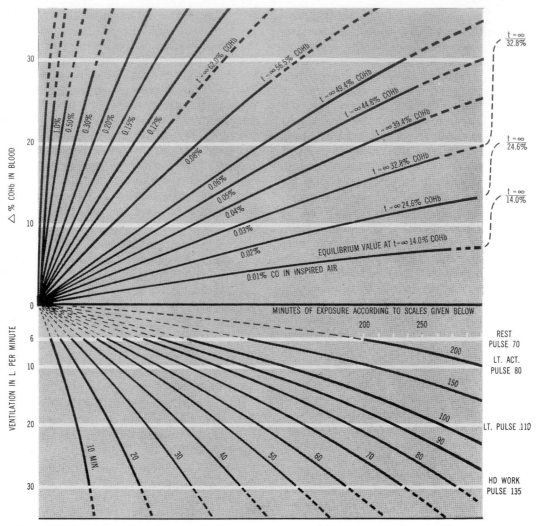

FIG. 141. Uptake of CO by man in various percentages of CO and rates of ventilation.

To use this chart, first determine the approximate ventilation and, having fixed this point upon the ordinate scale of ventilation, draw a horizontal line to the right intercepting the time curves (marked 10, 20, 30, etc.). The intercepts define the time scale for the ventilation in question; a vertical line, raised from the desired time of exposure on this time scale up to the proper curve in the upper quadrant, gives on the ordinate scale, the increase of per cent COHb resulting from this time of exposure. The curved lines in the lower quadrant are time lines; *i.e.*, all points on the 20 minute line are 20 minutes. The solid portions of the curves in both the upper and lower quadrants show the region covered by experimental data; the dotted portions are extrapolations. The equilibrium values which each curve approaches and which would be reached at infinite time are indicated after the symbol $t = \infty$. (From Forbes, W. H., Sargent, F., and Roughton, F. J. W.: The rate of carbon monoxide uptake by normal man. Am. J. Physiol. **143**: 594–608, 1945. Reprinted with the permission of the authors and publisher.)

results in a series of subjective manifestations considered dangerous in flying personnel. These consist of lowered attention, difficulty in concentration and retention, slight muscular incoordination, sleepiness and mental and physical lethargy. Obviously, such a hypoxic hypoxia is equally

dangerous whether caused by a lowered pO_2 or an increased pCO.

Carbon Dioxide

Carbon dioxide is used extensively in its gaseous form as a fire extinguishing agent and in its solid form (dry ice) as a refrigerant

TABLE 84

Symptoms Developed with Various Concentrations of CO in the Blood

Per Cent CO in the Blood	Symptoms
0 to 10	None
10 to 20	Tightness across forehead, possibly slight headache, dilation of cutaneous blood vessels
20 to 30	Headache, throbbing in temples
30 to 40	Severe headache, weakness, dizziness, dimness of vision, nausea and vomiting, collapse
40 to 50	Same as 30 to 40 with increased pulse rate and respiration and more possibility of collapse
50 to 60	Syncope, increased respiration and pulse, coma with intermittent convulsions, Cheyne-Stokes' type of respiration
60 to 70	Coma with intermittent convulsions, depressed heart action, possibly death
70 to 80	Weak pulse and slowed respiration, respiratory failure and death

for cargo. In either of these instances it can gain access to the passenger or crew compartments and has, under unfavorable conditions of ventilation, increased in concentration significantly enough to cause difficulty.

Carbon dioxide has ordinarily been thought to act purely as a simple asphyxiant, which is likely true in low concentrations (below 5 per cent). But at concentrations of 5 to 10 per cent and above it acts as a narcotic, which is apparent from studies in which the pO_2 of the breathing mixture was maintained at normal sea level values, while the concentrations of CO_2 were increased.

The generally accepted MAC in industry is 0.5 per cent. However, higher concentrations can be tolerated without impairment for short periods. The relationship of symptomatology to concentration and time of exposure is depicted in the time concentration curves of King (fig. 142). The "Bodily compensatory reactions—perception" occur at concentrations from 1 to 2.5 per cent depending upon time of exposure. Under these conditions an individual will notice air hunger to an intense feeling of suffocation, increased rate of respiration and circulation. From these concentrations to a level of 7 per cent concentration, again depending on time of exposure, the discomfort of breathing will be distracting and impairment of vision and hearing will occur. Higher concentrations will lead to convulsions, loss of consciousness and eventually death if time of exposure is sufficiently long. It is generally accepted that concentrations of 7 to 10 per cent will cause unconsciousness in some individuals in a few minutes and concentrations much above 10 per cent in less than a minute.

The concentrations above are expressed as "dry" carbon dioxide in the ambient air at

TABLE 85

Proportions of HbO_2, $HbCO$ and Reduced Hb in Volume Per Cent with Various Concentrations of CO at Altitudes from 0 to 8000 Meters

Height	With Normal Air		With 0.0025 Per Cent CO in the Air			With 0.005 Per Cent CO in the Air			With 0.01 Per Cent CO in the Air			With 0.02 Per Cent CO in the Air			With 0.03 Per Cent CO in the Air		
	HbO_2	Reduced Hb	HbO_2	HbCO	Reduced Hb	HbO_2	HbCO	Reduced Hb	HbO_2	HbCO	Reduced Hb	HbO_2	HbCO	Reduced Hb	HbO_2	HbCO	Rebuced Hd
0	95	5	92	3.5	4.5	89.3	6.7	4	83.5	12.5	4	74.7	22.3	3	67.7	30.3	2
1000	94	6	91.1	3.4	6.0	88.4	6.6	5	82.7	12.3	5	74.0	22.0	4	67.0	30.0	3
2000	92	8	89.2	3.3	7.5	86.5	6.5	7	81.8	12.2	6	73.2	21.8	5	66.3	29.7	4
3000	88	11	86.3	3.2	10.5	84.2	6.3	9.5	80.0	12.0	7	72.4	21.6	6	65.6	29.4	5
4000	85.5	14.5	82.9	3.1	14.0	81.0	6.0	11.5	77.5	11.5	9	70.5	21.0	8.5	64.2	28.8	7
5000	81	19	79.1	2.9	18.0	77.2	5.8	17.0	74.0	11.0	12	67.8	20.2	12.0	62.5	28.0	9.5
6000	76	24	74.2	2.8	22.0	73.5	5.5	21.0	70.5	10.5	17	64.7	19.3	16.0	60.1	26.9	13.0
7000	70	30	68.9	2.6	28.5	67.9	5.1	27.0	65.7	9.8	24	61.6	18.4	20.0	57.3	25.7	17.0
8000	62	38	61.7	2.3	36.5	61.4	4.6	34.0	60.0	9.0	31	57.0	17.0	26.0	53.2	23.8	23.0

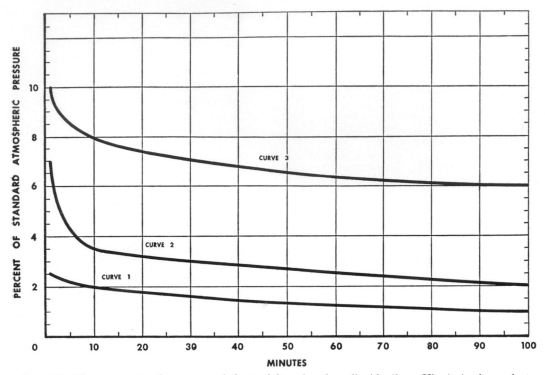

FIG. 142. Time-concentration curves of the toxicity of carbon dioxide (from King). As drawn here, the area between curves 1 and 2 corresponds approximately to the area in the diagram of King labeled *bodily compensatory reactions—perception*; the area between curves 2 and 3 to the area labeled *distracting discomfort, at or near tolerance limits—deterioration*; and the area above curve 3 to the area labeled *dizziness, stupor, unconsciousness*. (From *Aviation Toxicology* (11). Reprinted with the permission of the authors and publisher.)

sea level. This is the data which would normally be provided by an industrial hygiene laboratory. In order to understand and use such data one must interpolate the analytic data into physiologically equivalent data.

The gaseous exchange between the body and the ambient environment is primarily a function partial pressure differentials in the "body," *i.e.*, alveolar pCO_2 and the ambient air. The mean alveolar pCO_2 at sea level is approximately 36 mm. of Hg varying from 30 to 48 mm. of Hg. These levels vary with rate and depth of respiration, exercise, etc. When the concentration of CO_2 in the inspired air added to that already present in the alveoli exceeds the pCO_2 on the arterial side of the alveolar barrier, despite physiologic mechanisms to eliminate CO_2, the symptomatology of CO_2 poisoning become apparent. This level has been determined to be in the 4 to 7 per cent concentration in the inspired air or when the combined pCO_2

(alveolar) exceeds a level of the order of 50 mm. of Hg. What is this physiologically equivalent to at altitude?

If an air sample is taken at an altitude of 18,000 feet, and found to have a concentration of 10 per cent, what is its partial pressure? From this its "equivalent" at sea level can be deduced as well as the expected symptomatology. When the ambient air is inspired the gaseous mixture becomes saturated with water vapor, which exerts a partial pressure of 47 mm. of Hg. The barometric pressure at 18,000 feet is 379 mm. of Hg. When subtracting that portion exerted by water vapor the balance is 332 mm. of Hg. So, if 10 per cent of the ambient air is composed of CO_2, its partial pressure is 10 per cent of 332 or 33.2 mm. of Hg. Mathematically this can be expressed:

$$pCO_2 = \text{per cent } CO_2 \ (B_p - 47)$$

where pCO_2 equals the partial pressure of CO_2 (wet); per cent CO_2 equals the concentration CO_2 in ambient air; B_p equals the barometric pressure at altitude in question; and 47 equals the partial pressure of H_2O vapor in the lung.

Using the same formula and transposing, one can determine the concentration of CO_2 in ambient air at sea level to which this 10 per cent CO_2 at 18,000 feet would be equivalent

$$\text{per cent } CO_2 = \frac{pCO_2}{(B_p - 47)}$$

Substituting:

$$\text{per cent } CO_2 = \frac{33.2}{(760 - 47)}$$

$$= 4.6 \text{ per cent}$$

Therefore, all factors being similar, an individual being exposed to 10 per cent CO_2 at 18,000 feet would be expected to develop the same symptomatology as an individual exposed to 4.6 per cent CO_2 under the same conditions at sea level. This fact has been well proven experimentally.

In the past aircraft incidents have occurred in which CO_2 from fire extinguishers or dry ice carried as cargo were incriminated. A flight surgeon may be asked to estimate the maximum quantity of dry ice which could be carried without endangering the crew or passengers. The factors which must be determined are the volume of the cabin space, its rate of ventilation, and the rate at which the CO_2 is released whether from an extinguisher or vaporized from solid CO_2. In order to simplify the problem, it may be assumed that the rate of release is within a minute or 2 of the entire amount of CO_2 available, and that the rate of ventilation is nil. This would be to assume the worst possible conditions—and certainly provides a safety factor of significant magnitude.

For example, if one would accept a maximum concentration of 3 per cent CO_2 at sea level in an aircraft with a 1000 cubic foot cabin, how much dry ice could be carried at 10,000 feet altitude at a temperature of 25° C.? A concentration of 3 per cent CO_2 at sea level is equivalent to:

$$\text{per cent } CO_2^a = \frac{\text{per cent } CO_2^s(B_p^s - 47)}{(B_p^a - 47)}$$

where B_p^s equals the barometric pressure at sea level (mm. of Hg); $B_p^a{}_2{}^a$ equals the barometric pressure at altitude; per cent CO: equals the per cent CO_2 in inspired air at altitude; and per cent CO_2^s equals the per cent CO_2 in inspired air at sea level. Substituting:

$$= \frac{3.0(760 - 47)}{(523 - 47)}$$

$$= \frac{3.0(713)}{476}$$

$$= 4.5 \text{ per cent at 10,000 feet}$$

In a cabin of 1000 cubic feet, this would represent a volume of carbon dioxide of 45 cubic feet at a temperature of 25° C. and at the 10,000 feet altitude. Correcting this to standard conditions:

$$45 \times \frac{(273)}{(298)} \times \frac{(523)}{(760)} = 28.4 \text{ cubic feet}$$

where $\frac{(273)}{(298)}$ equals the temperature correction factor (°A.) at 25° C.; and $\frac{(523)}{(760)}$ equals the pressure correction factor (mm. of Hg) at 10,000 feet. This is equal to:

$$28.4 \times 28.3 = 814 \text{ liters}$$

$$(1 \text{ cubic foot} = 28.3 \text{ liters}$$

or

$$\frac{814}{22.4} = 36.3 \text{ moles}$$

$$(22.4 \text{ liters} = 1 \text{ mole})$$

or

$$36.3 \times 44 = 1597 \text{ grams}$$

$$(\text{molecular weight of } CO_2 = 44)$$

or

$$\frac{1597}{453.6} = 3.5 \text{ pounds}$$

$$(1 \text{ pound} = 453.6 \text{ grams})$$

At first glance, 3.5 pounds may seem to be an extremely small quantity of dry ice to produce a concentration of 3 per cent calculated "dry," and at sea level equivalent. In a practical situation one must remember that this was assumed to be the amount "instantaneously" vaporized, so if the rate of vaporization is taken into consideration, the amount permitted will be considerably larger. If it vaporized at a rate of 10 per cent per hour, for example, one could begin with 35 pounds, neglecting such factors as the ventilation rate of the cabin, as well as the rate of disbursion throughout the cabin environment. Cabin ventilation rates are generally fairly high, providing an additional safety factor.

Aldehydes

This group of compounds is encountered as a product of incomplete combustion of lubricating oils or petroleum fuels and could possibly be produced in a cargo compartment fire in which fats, oils or glycerin were heated to a sufficiently high temperature. The principal member of this group is acrolein (propenal, CH_2CHCHO). Another is acetaldehyde (ethanal, CH_3CHO). Acrolein is the irritant commonly noted in the exhaust gases emanating from automobiles.

Acrolein vapor is only slightly soluble in water but it is extremely irritating to the eyes and upper respiratory tract. It is immediately detectable by odor at a concentration of 1 p.p.m., intensely irritating at 5.5 p.p.m. and lethal in a short time at 10 p.p.m. In addition to the severe lacrymation, salivation, burning and itching of the eyes and nose, sneezing and coughing may occur if exposure is prolonged or the concentration is high. Pulmonary edema is possible. It is also said to possess narcotic properties. However, the acute and severe onset of the upper respiratory tract involvement would probably overshadow any narcotic effects under normal conditions of exposure. The MAC is generally taken to be 0.5 p.p.m.

Acetaldehyde is very soluble in water which aids in producing severe irritation of the conjunctivae and the mucous membranes of the upper respiratory tract. Conjunctival burns have been known to occur. Its MAC has been set at 200 p.p.m.

Carbonyls

Phosgene ($COCl_2$) is one of the most common of the carbonyls which is formed during the combustion of carbon tetrachloride or other chlorinated hydrocarbons in a flame or in contact with a very hot metal. This circumstance is most commonly produced when using a carbon tetrachloride fire extinguisher to extinguish a fire in a small confined enclosure which permits the build-up of a high concentration of the gas.

Phosgene is freely soluble in water. It quickly hydrolyzes to hydrochloric acid and carbon dioxide. It is probable that this production of HCl is the principal cause for the severe irritant action upon the respiratory tract. In its gaseous form it quickly reaches the lower portions of the respiratory tract, i.e., the alveoli, before the major hydrolysis takes place. For this reason, comparatively little irritation of the upper respiratory tract occurs before a significant irritant action of the pulmonary parenchyma has already occurred. This then results in a delayed but severe type of pulmonary edema. The action of phosgene resembles in many ways that of nitrogen dioxide.

At a concentration of 1 p.p.m. the gas is barely detectable; at 2 p.p.m. it is moderately strong and is irritant to the eyes, nose and throat. It is said to be dangerous to life at 12.5 p.p.m. for a 30 to 60 minutes exposure and rapidly fatal at 90 p.p.m. One p.p.m. is equal to 4.05 mg. per cubic meter at 25° C., 760 mm. of Hg. Although the effects of phosgene at altitude have not been studied it is reasonable to expect that any effects would be related directly to the concentration of the gas at any given altitude.

Oxygen Contamination

With the advent and extensive use of pressurized aircraft the need for oxygen breathing systems has been confined largely to use during emergency conditions when the cabin air is known or believed to be contaminated or when pressurization is accidentally lost. These remarks apply to commercial carriers for the most part other than normal military transport aircraft where the conditions of flight require the use of oxygen continuously. Oxygen is also used to some extent in private flying and obviously for medical purposes during the transport of patients requiring it.

Although the probability of contamination of oxygen systems with toxic chemicals is not great it is a potential source of trouble and has caused some difficulties in the past.

Potentially toxic substances may be introduced during the manufacture of the oxygen and during its transfer to pressurized cylinders. The present methods of manufacture and the controls exercised in order to insure established standards of quality make this a very remote possibility indeed. A far greater danger occurs during or prior to the "filling operation." During maintenance or repair of an oxygen system the oxygen lines, joints and regulators are removed and cleaned. Solvents such as trichlorethylene are commonly used. If this chemical or any other used for this purpose is not thoroughly removed from the system, enough material may remain and enter the stream of oxygen as it is inhaled. Following cleaning and reassembly, the system is purged with nitrogen or compressed air in order to clear out any volatile substance which may remain. It is then filled with oxygen. When done efficiently the possibility of contamination is extremely remote. Although not strictly a toxicologic problem a number of instances have been reported in which the system was purged and filled with nitrogen. Fortunately, in those cases reported the error was discovered before critical altitudes were reached.

Objectionable odors have frequently been encountered in oxygen breathing systems. These have usually been caused by deteriorating rubber and other substances emanating from the rubber or plastic materials which are exposed to the oxygen stream. Probably the most frequently reported odor is that of one of the mercaptans, a sulfur compound having an odor similar to hydrogen sulfide (rotten eggs!). These have never been known to be in a sufficiently high concentration to be toxicologically significant but have been of psychologic significance. The concentration necessary to produce nausea and even vomiting is extremely low as one might well imagine. The practical importance of this cannot be overemphasized.

The Challenge of the Future

The technologic developments of the past have been entirely responsible for the present status of aviation. With each new advance, with each new chemical, measures have had to be devised to protect man from any adverse effects these materials might have if they become absorbed. Control measures have been devised and established or installed. The future promises an even more rapid rate of advance. Many new chemicals for use as fuels or propellants are being developed and studied. Nuclear reactors to serve as basic power plants are in the early stages of development. Many will have tremendous toxicologic potentialities. Ozone, a powerful oxidizing agent and an extremely toxic substance even in low concentrations, is being studied. Other oxidizers such as oxygen difluoride and trioxydifluoride are in a similar class.

The future of aviation is dependent upon the close cooperation of many technical disciplines if its advancement is to be rapid and orderly. As new chemical substances are developed in the laboratory, substances which theoretically promise to perform more efficiently and effectively a particular function must have their toxicologic properties determined in order that effective and economic control devices or measures can be devised and instituted for the protection of aircrews, passengers and ground operations personnel. The thorough understanding of the toxic properties and control features are an essential part of the many so-called "human factors," which contribute to the safety of flight.

REFERENCES

(1) Aviation Toxicology Bulletin, Nos. 11–16. Washington, D. C., Medical Division, Office of Aviation Safety, CAA, 1954–1957.

(2) Konecci, E. B.: Physiologic factors in aircraft accidents in the U. S. Air Force. J. Aviation Med., 28: 553–558, 1957.

(3) Henderson, Y., and Haggard, H. W.: Noxious Gases and the Principles of Respiration Influencing Their Action. New York, Reinhold Publishing Corporation, 1943, p. 13.

(4) Jones, G. W., Berger, L. B., and Holbrook, W. F.: U. S. Bureau of Mines Technical Paper No. 337. Washington, D. C., 1923.

(5) Henderson, Y., and Haggard, H. W.: Noxious Gases and the Principles of Respiration Influencing Their Action. New York, Reinhold Publishing Corporation, 1943, p. 78.

(6) Foulger, J. H.: Pathologic Physiology—Mechanisms of Disease. Philadelphia, W. B. Saunders Co., 1950.

(7) Feinsilver, L., MacNamee, J. K., Mc-

GRATH, F. P., AND OBERST, F. W.: Inhalation Toxicity of Combustion Products of Perchlorate Fuel Propellants. U. S. Army Chemical Corps, 1950.

(8) KRACKOW, E. H.: Toxicity and Health Hazards of Boron Hydrides. U. S. Army Chemical Corps Medical Laboratory Special Report No. 8. U. S. Army Chemical Center, 1951.

(9) TREON, J. F., CAPPEL, J. W., CLEVELAND, F. P., LARSON, E. E., ATCHLEY, R. W., AND DENHAM, R. T.: Toxicity of products formed by the thermal decomposition of certain organic substances. Am. Indust. Hyg. A. Quart., 16: 187–195, 1955.

(10) International Sanitary W.H.O. Regulations. Geneva, World Health Organization, 1957.

(11) Committee on Aviation Toxicology, Aero Medical Association: Aviation Toxicology. New York, Blakiston Co., 1953.

(12) ROUGHTON, F. J. W.: Handbook of Respiratory Physiology. Randolph Air Force Base, Texas, School of Aviation Medicine, USAF, 1954, chapter 5.

26

AIRCREW MAINTENANCE

Benjamin A. Strickland, Jr., M.D.

Aircrew maintenance, which is also frequently referred to as an aircrew effectiveness program, may be defined as those measures usually of a preventive nature, employed to keep flying personnel in good health and at the peak of efficiency at all times, under all circumstances and especially in connection with their flying. The practice of aviation medicine may be considered to reach its zenith when it achieves a comprehensive state of aeromedical effectiveness of pilots and other aircrewmen. Aircrew maintenance, properly practiced, evaluates and monitors the whole man in his total environment and applies the full resources of aviation medicine to the operational requirements of the flyer.

Underlying Principles

At the present time human factors concerning aircraft design, cockpit configuration, comfortization and other bioengineering aspects are receiving marked emphasis. Many aircraft manufacturers have added aeromedical physicians to their staffs who are actively consulted by aeronautical engineers. These developments greatly enhance aircrew maintenance programs by obviating some of the unsatisfactory design characteristics sometimes embodied in aircraft. Graybiel (1) has made a major contribution to aircrew effectiveness by his concept of man the instrument and man the individual as applicable to problems involving aircrews. In this concept it is pointed out that many of the critical problems have moved from the dispensary into the cockpit and that the aeromedical physician should follow. His premise is that the most urgent problems are no longer medical in the usual meaning of this term but center around the task in the aircraft. Here the distinction between man the instrument and man the individual becomes artificial. It is emphasized that the solution of the problems, which involves many agencies with interlocking interests, suggests the need of greater coordination. Graybiel's conclusion is that aeromedical personnel, with a firm appreciation of what is truly involved in "success in flying" can make an important contribution at both the working and advisory levels. This involves vital segments of aircrew maintenance activities in which the opportunity exists to identify and evaluate, under actual operational situations, many of the significant problems.

Intimate day-to-day health surveillance of flyers is usually possible in the military services but practically impossible in commercial aviation and among the thousands of private flyers throughout the world. Hence, effective care-of-flyer measures vary widely in quality and quantity. Nonmilitary flyers are not usually situated so that their health maintenance can be frequently monitored by flight surgeons and they must turn to their family physician for routine medical care. Hence, there is a real need for them to be thoroughly indoctrinated and trained, insofar as is possible, on self monitoring of their fitness to fly. A great part of the health effectiveness program of the flyer depends primarily on the degree of aeromedical discipline that he is able to exert on his own behalf. This principle is applicable to both military and civilian flyers.

Common sense application of preventive aeromedical principles is the basic ingredient of aircrew maintenance. Only the physician who has acquired necessary knowledge in the specialty of aviation medicine is fitted to practice in this area. The care of the flyer begins when he presents himself as an applicant for flying training. At this time it should be possible to eliminate all who are, or are likely to become, mentally, physically or temperamentally unfitted for aviation. The original examination for flying is discussed elsewhere, however, the initial impression made by aeromedical personnel on the examinee has far reaching implications. The career of a flyer in regard to his own efficiency and effectiveness may be moulded to a considerable extent by a proper introduction to the medical aspects of his part in aviation. The tenor of this first contact with aeromedical procedures may have a profound influence on how carefully he acquires and heeds vital indoctrination. Future attitude and stimulation of interest toward good aeromedical hygiene can be either enhanced or degraded for his entire career at the time of the original examination for flying.

During the career of a flyer, whether it lasts only a few years or until retirement age is reached, he must face constant changes in himself and changes in the types of aircraft he is called on to operate. The human organism is dynamic not static. Aeronautic development is dynamic not static. Hence, aircrew maintenance must be ever changing and pace must be kept with advances in the biologic and the aeronautical sciences. Aging in the flyer must be carefully evaluated as it affects his aircrew performance. Personal hygiene and health habits must be monitored. His mental and emotional equanimity should be assessed and kept at an optimum level insofar as is possible. From the foregoing it can be seen that the goal of aircrew maintenance is to assist the flyer in keeping himself physically, mentally and operationally fit to fly.

In prosecuting an effective program of aircrew maintenance the objectives should be the achievement and continuation of maximum potential in the following areas:

1. Periodic medical examinations
2. Maintenance of mental health and physical fitness
3. Medical aspects of flying safety
4. Prolongation of effective flying careers
5. Prevention, diagnosis and treatment of disorders and injuries peculiar to aviation
6. Human factors in aeronautical design
7. Air rescue and survival
8. Protective and emergency equipment
9. Aeromedical indoctrination and training

Certain of the above are discussed in separate chapters in this volume. The reason for this is that developments in recent years have been so multitudinous and of such magnitude that certain areas of aeromedical knowledge formerly very limited in scope have now become of major significance and, hence, require specialized discussion.

The varied types of flying and aircrew duties have become exceedingly diverse. The airline pilot, the civilian test pilot, the military pilot, the private flyer and many other types of flying personnel, all should receive the benefits of medical aircrew maintenance. The private flyer in effect carries out his own aircrew maintenance program except for his periodic medical examination for flying required by FAA regulations. The airline pilot and the civilian test pilot are under the aegis of company flight surgeons. Aircrew maintenance of these is a combination of self maintenance on the part of the individual flyer, care by the family physician and limited supervision and guidance from the company medical authorities.

Direction and top level supervision by a physician trained and experienced in aviation medicine is an essential element of health maintenance of flyers. In commercial airlines this is accomplished by the airline medical director and his staff. In the military services it is carried out by the Surgeon General of the respective service concerned and experienced flight surgeons at various echelons of command. Policy making and advisory functions are important aspects of this top level organization. Directors of operations frequently consult aeromedical personnel concerning both medical and nonmedical problems. The observation of Ogle (2) that those in aviation medicine should seek to be a part of the solution rather than a part of the problem is paramount. This should obviously apply at all levels but is particularly appropriate in policy making matters.

The manner in which the flight surgeon carries out his scope of responsibilities is one of the major determinants of the quality of any aircrew maintenance program. A good aircrew maintenance program at operational level will promote greater motivation, esprit and confidence among flyers. For example, the pressure under which an all weather interceptor pilot works is of such nature that a close psychologic appreciation and understanding is required. The pilot himself and the squadron commander both need the advice and help of a competent flight surgeon who functions in the role of a wise family physician. The squadron commander needs the advice of this experienced technician in providing preventive maintenance for his crews as is done by aircraft maintenance personnel for the aircraft. Clinical care of the hospitalized flyer is an important aspect of the duties of the flight surgeon and this should be carried out on a cooperative or collaborative basis with hospital personnel.

PERIODIC AND SPECIAL MEDICAL EXAMINATIONS

A periodic medical examination is a diagnostic survey of the physical and mental status of the flyer with particular reference to his effectiveness as a pilot or crew member of an aircraft. The purpose of such an examination is to determine the presence or absence of any physical or mental abnormalities. It should be designed to detect early or insidious evidence of disease processes of any type whatsoever. The goal should be preventive in nature to obviate any decrement on his effectiveness as a flyer.

In safeguarding the health and effectiveness of flyers a periodic medical survey performed by a physician trained in aviation medicine is essential. Such an examination must provide an accurate estimate of the physical and mental status of the individual as of a given time. In addition, it must furnish a prognostic picture which will enable the airman himself as well as operational supervisory personnel to be reasonably certain of his fitness as an aircraft operator. The dynamic nature, *i.e.* one of constant change, of normal aging processes necessitates both a retrospective and a prospective analysis of findings.

It is interesting to speculate on what percentage of aircrew members of commercial airlines and of the military services would voluntarily seek periodic medical examinations if such were not mandatory. Aeromedical physicians have ventured the opinion that only the psychosomatic neurotic or the hypochondriacally inclined would do so. Estimates of biometricians as to the percentage of males in the general population between the ages of 21 and 65 years who secure, on their own initiative, an annual health check-up by a physician vary between $\frac{1}{2}$ and 1 per cent.

If the aeromedical practitioners will become better acquainted with their examinees by spending as much time as possible "on the line" many advantages will accrue. It will be found that the flyer will be appreciative of a good periodic medical examination instead of wanting to get it over as quickly as possible. By knowing the flyer well, both as his physician and as a friend, the periodic examination will be greatly enhanced in value and significance as well as properly received.

In commercial aviation and in the government services, periodic medical examinations are required annually. Special examinations for flyers may be required at any time for many reasons such as following a serious illness or after major surgery.

The value of the annual medical evaluation depends in large part on proper orientation of the flyer who is being examined. The purpose of the procedure must be explained clearly and simply in lay terms and all factors which might create misunderstanding must be clarified. The examinee should be informed what an annual examination will include, what it can and cannot do and what he can do to make the examination more profitable. The complete health record of the examinee should be reviewed by the flight surgeon prior to the reporting time of the examinee and items requiring special attention should be noted.

Even in this era of public enlightenment on medicine frequent instances occur in which laymen are deplorably unorientated on medical procedures. This can be overcome by properly informing the examinee concerning the import and significance of his annual medical examination. One method of advantageously accomplishing this has been by the use of information letters. Usually the aircrew member is notified in writing that he is scheduled to report at a certain time for his annual medical evaluation. It is easy to arrange for inclusion of an information letter orientating him on exactly what can be expected from the interview and examination. Each of the laboratory and diagnostic procedures should be explained in lay terminology. There are still laymen who are under the impression that the only purpose of a urinalysis is to detect venereal disease. A simply stated explanation should be included in the information letter concerning what the medical examination *per se* will not reveal. It should be stressed that detection of many disorders depends in large part on the frankness and honesty of the examinee. Most disorders can be detected if the physician is alerted by the examinee and, conversely, a large list of diseases can be concealed if the examinee fails to mention his symptoms. Therefore, time can be saved in the actual interview by the dissemination of prior instructions to the individual who is being examined. He should be prepared in advance to actively cooperate during the interview.

In the information letter which is sent to the individual prior to his examination a listing of symptoms oftentimes serves the purpose of indicating to the layman clues which should be reported to the flight surgeon at the time of the interview. A suggested list for inclusion in the information letter is as follows:

1. Any blood discharged from the body in stools, urine, or sputum
2. Any dizziness or loss of consciousness
3. Any abrupt or unexplained change in weight
4. Any change in bowel habits, or abnormality in color or consistency
5. Any change in sleeping habits, as, for instance, requiring additional pillows
6. Unexplained fatigue or weakness
7. Any persistent, unexplained headache
8. Persistent cough

9. Pain or difficulty associated with normal body functions—swallowing, urinating, having a bowel movement, etc.
10. Persistent, unexplained "indigestion" or recurrent abdominal pain
11. Chest pain
12. Any mass or lump, in any location
13. Any sore on the skin or in the mouth which does not heal
14. Swelling of joints or extremities
15. Any other symptom which has caused concern

The content of the closing portion of this orientation letter should stress that the primary responsibility for keeping himself healthy rests with the flyer. He should be impressed with the fact that he should take the initiative in reporting symptoms which will lead to detection of diseases in their early stages. It should be pointed out that any of the symptoms listed above should actually be reported as soon as they are noted. It should be stated that the annual medical examination will supplement his own health vigilance by ruling out any insidious diseases. Finally, the statement should be included that the annual medical evaluation provides an excellent opportunity for the flyer to review his health status and to secure medical advice on problems of health and hygiene.

Experience has indicated that at least 15 minutes should be allocated for an interview with the examinee as the initial step. Careful inquiry should be made concerning the interval history since the last examination. In the present decade the annual medical examination of flyers has been revised considerably. Paper work has been reduced allowing more time for a purposeful health interview with the examinee. Many unproductive portions of the examination have been eliminated. For example, the determination and recording of data on height, color vision, color of hair and other characteristics which can be assumed to be essentially unchanged through the years has been discarded.

A typical annual examination as utilized by a leading airline includes the usual general physical examination with eye tests and audiometric tests. Additional procedures employed are a 6 foot roentgenogram of the chest, electrocardiogram, red and white blood cell counts, hemoglobin, urinalysis, blood serology and a serum cholesterol in selected cases. On the electrocardiograph the standard chest leads plus V-1, V-3 and V-5 tracings are routine. Other laboratory procedures are done when specifically indicated. The medical director of this particular airline states that plans are underway to perform tests for serology and serum cholesterol on alternate years.

As an example of the annual physical examination for flying personnel utilized in the military service, the United States Air Force employs the following:

1. A statement by the examinee about his health since the previous examination

2. Chest x-ray

3. Examination of the urine for albumin and sugar

4. Hemoglobin determination

5. Dental examination

6. Electrocardiogram when indicated (required for those over 40 years of age)

7. Digital examination of the rectum including the prostate in males, when indicated (required for persons over 40 years of age)

8. Pelvic examination and examination of the breasts in females when indicated (required for those persons over 30 years of age who may be required to undergo examination)

9. Height and weight

10. Blood pressure and pulse (sitting)

11. Measurement of uncorrected and corrected visual acuity, distant and near, is performed on all personnel. In addition, heterophorias, depth perception and accommodation is measured on all aircrew and air traffic control personnel

12. Respiratory and cardiovascular systems

13. Audiogram

14. Extremities

15. Review and discussion

16. Detailed study where indicated

The original examination for flying, being designed for young applicants, has stringent standards to insure prolonged occupational usefulness. Some of these provisions do not take into account the physiologic changes occurring as the flyer grows older, such as mild presbyopia, which do not warrant removing him from flying duty. In addition, aircrew members, who are not pilots, such as navigators and flight engineers need not meet the strict standards required of pilots. As a practical means of taking these factors into consideration, the procedures utilized by one of the military services is noteworthy. In this system different classes or categories of medical standards for flying are utilized. One category includes standards for individuals applying for flying training as aircrew members. Other categories prescribe somewhat relaxed standards for graduate and experienced pilots and other aircrew members. For example, older pilots with many years of flying experience and thousands of hours of flying time who have a limited reduction in visual acuity, which is correctable, can be qualified. For such aircrew members the criterion for medical standards is assurance that physical condition permits maintenance of flying efficiency, safety and preservation of the person's well being. A third category, which specifies substantially low standards, may be allowed for certain aircrew members and all others not in primary control of the aircraft.

For certain minor defects found on examination of aircrew members, which according to the stated standards are disqualifying, the custom has been to grant waivers in selected cases. This practice is based on the premise that flying experience in a graduate pilot compensates for certain minor physical defects. It is not known how much defect in the older pilot can be offset by his experience and judgment but certain statistics indicate that the accident rate of older pilots with waivered defects is lower than that of younger healthy pilots. In other words, each time an older pilot is permanently grounded he must be replaced by a younger one and it is enigmatic whether or not safety has been increased unless it is shown that the defect in the older pilot is more dangerous than the inexperience of the younger one.

In conducting the physical examination of graduate aircrew personnel the detection of disqualifying defects is but one of the many factors to be considered. Of prime importance is the detection of incipient processes which, while not disqualifying, may lead to serious consequences unless corrective measures are instituted. The results of such examinations should be compared with previous ones in order that progressive changes may be noted. When a defect is found during the examination an effort should be made to determine its genesis and etiology. It should be analyzed as to whether it originated as a result of mode of living, from flying, from lack of proper exercise or diet or from other causes which are capable of regulation.

In the event a disqualifying abnormality is found which will require a long period of time for correction or which is permanently disqualifying it should be evaluated on an individualized basis. Every effort should be made to satisfy the unfortunate flyer concerned as to the correctness of diagnosis and as to the fact that the defect does constitute a definite flying hazard. If the diagnosis is questioned the flyer should not only be allowed, but encouraged to seek the opinion of qualified consultants. To convince a flyer that a defect, short of serious illness or injury, is dangerous in the air is not usually an easy task. Such grounding incurs a marked loss of income for the military flyer and a total loss of income for the civilian pilot. Therefore, in certain instances they may be expected to appeal to higher medical authority, to independent medical sources or to legal sources for relief. This obviously necessitates the most profound consideration of his findings by the flight surgeon to obviate the possibility of a faulty diagnosis or improper interpretation of standards.

The procedure of using waivers for the purpose of continuing the flying careers of aircrew members with minor defects which do not meet stated standards, must be accorded careful consideration. One must be certain that duty performance and flying safety are not compromised. When a waiver is required full use will be made of consultations. All waivers previously granted for nonstatic defects must be reappraised at the time of the re-examination. If indicated a specialist's report will be accomplished to reflect current evaluation with regard to progression. The examining flight surgeon recommends a waiver when appropriate as a part of the report of medical examination. This request for waiver is evaluated by supervisory aeromedical personnel who have been given authority to grant waivers, such as the FAA, the central office of an airline medical department or major command flight surgeons in the military services.

Certain disqualifying abnormalities of major significance in flying are waivered only under exceptional circumstances. Complete data on such cases should be forwarded to the highest medical authority of the organization, company or government service concerned for review and consideration. Such conditions are:

1. Any loss of consciousness, regardless of duration or circumstances
2. Any malignant disease
3. Any convulsive seizure
4. Gastrointestinal hemorrhage, gastrectomy or gastroenterostomy
5. Any disease or defect of the eye or adenexa which might threaten normal binocular vision
6. Visual acuity defects in either eye exceeding 20/100, correctable with lenses to 20/20
7. Recurrent spontaneous pneumothorax
8. Pulmonary segmental resection or other intrathoracic surgery
9. Any heart disease, including paroxysmal arrhythmias, electrocardiograph abnormalities and suspected coronary insufficiency
10. Systolic blood pressure findings consistently greater than 170 mm. of Hg or diastolic readings greater than 100 mm. of Hg
11. Any peripheral nerve disorder resulting from disease or trauma, excluding Bell's palsy
12. Any craniocerebral injury
13. Any encephalitis, encephalopathy or central neurologic disability
14. Chronic alcoholism or other disease, the proximal cause of which is alcoholism
15. Suspected or attempted suicide
16. Any psychosis
17. Diabetes mellitus
18. Fenestration operation for otosclerosis
19. Neurosyphilis
20. Surgical removal of herniated nucleus pulposus with or without spinal fusion
21. Any controversial condition which it is felt necessary requires a decision by the ultimate medical authority

As an example of the proper management of flyers who have had major surgery performed the method of dealing with thoracic surgery cases is a good illustration. The appraisal of fitness to fly following thoracic surgery is much more than observing the status of wound healing. Decreased barometric pressure experienced in flying imposes stress upon ventilation and respiration. Aircrew members who have undergone wedge resection, segmental resection, lobectomy or combined abdominothoracic surgery require extremely careful consideration before return to flying status. The prerogative of returning to flying those individuals in whom thoracotomy has been performed should be vested in the best experienced opinion available such as the Chief Medical Director of an airline or the Physical Standards Division of the Surgeon General's Office of the military service concerned. Expert opinion of those qualified both in aviation medicine and chest surgery indicates that particular ventilatory tests need not be specified. Flyers who have undergone chest surgery can be evaluated by comparing a pre- and postoperative set of spirometric findings. Copies of spirograms should be available with the complete medical examination findings.

In evaluating postoperative chest surgery cases a careful resume of the specific comments pertaining to deformity of chest, wound healing, pain on motion of chest and symmetry of thoracic movement are essential items to be covered. Postoperative fluoroscopic and radiographic studies are important. Detailed determination of the position and movement of mediastinum, position and movement of diaphragm and position, shape and movement of thorax is of value. A radiologic description of lungs, pleurae and intercostal spaces should be included. When the case has been completed a detailed summary including specific comment on the factors previously mentioned should be compiled. In certain situations it may be desirable to subject the recovered thoracic surgery case to an altitude chamber flight for purposes of evaluating his responses. However, one must remember that such a procedure is not a substitute for careful clinical evaluation concerning fitness to fly. Furthermore, great care should be taken not to expose any such case to the rigors of an altitude chamber flight until the best possible evaluation of his fitness for such a procedure has been made by clinical methods. Under certain circumstances, a chamber flight may be a logical intermediate step

between clinical qualification for flying and actual flight to considerable altitude involving accelerative forces and other stresses of flights.

In cases which deal with problems in internal medicine among aircrew members, gastrointestinal disorders are perhaps the best examples. When a flyer has peptic ulcer careful evaluation is necessary. Following necessary treatment on a nonflying status, careful consideration must be made of his crew status, type of aircraft normally flown, operational conditions and other factors. The type of flying assignment to which he may return—transport, fighter, airline, ferrying—may necessitate different handling. Different operational conditions, such as diet availability while on duty, irregularity of rest and others, must also be considered. Opinions vary, but 2 to 5 months after successful treatment is considered as necessary for observation before return to flying status. However, sound clinical judgment should determine the basis for cure and return to flying duties rather than an arbitrary time limit. Full utilization of adequate consultation is essential and the most experienced aeromedical opinion must be sought before return to flying.

AEROMEDICAL INDOCTRINATION AND HEALTH TRAINING

In achieving success in flying a vital factor is knowledge and understanding on the part of the flyer of the physiologic changes encountered in flight. In addition, he must be indoctrinated and trained in the use of protective equipment and apparatus which will enable him to withstand the physical and mental stresses of flight. Further, the flyer must know the basic principles of adequate first aid, survival under adverse conditions and, finally, the principles of daily hygienic living.

In 1942 the military services instituted an altitude training program aimed at indoctrinating all aircrews in the physiologic aspects of flight. Major emphasis was placed on oxygen requirements and equipment, particularly the proper use of oxygen masks. Since its inception physiologic training efforts have been monitored and promoted by those engaged in aviation medicine. Actually, responsible for providing this instruction are aviation physiologists assigned to physiologic training units. Flight surgeons provide medical and technical supervision required in implementation of adequate physiologic training. Initial crew member training in this field is conducted during the flying training courses for future pilots and other crew members. Upon completion of pilot or other crew member training the need for continued study and review of protection at altitude is essential for continued success of the operational aircrew. Hence, refresher physiologic training is conducted at periodic intervals for all rated personnel This refresher training is a very important part of aircrew maintenance. It includes several hours of lectures and demonstrations and an altitude chamber flight to simulated high altitude followed by a rapid decompression. Often included in the refresher training is ejection seat training and night vision training.

Rapid advances in aircraft design, oxygen apparatus and protective equipment necessitate frequent revisions of refresher physiologic training for graduate pilots and aircrew members. The advent of jet transports for commercial airlines poses new aircrew maintenance problems for airline aeromedical personnel. A jet airliner which will cruise at 30,000 feet or more must have a flight crew trained in the use of oxygen equipment in event of failure of pressurization systems. One major airline has already sought indoctrination in the low pressure chamber for crews who will be flying jet transport aircraft. Special training must be made available on how the entire crew of a commercial airliner can cope with explosive decompression. The pressure ratio of 8.6 p.s.i. in the jet propelled airliners, in event of failure of the system, might well result in a disturbing situation.

Included in flight physiology refresher courses is a review of the condensed and essential elements of the instructional material of the original training in aviation physiology. Emphasis on new equipment and new methods should be effected. Usually, several or all of the following subjects are covered in refresher courses:

1. Physiologic effects of altitude
2. Oxygen equipment
3. Cabin pressurization and rapid decompression
4. Pressure breathing
5. Principles and problems of vision
6. Atypical sensory phenomena
7. Noise, vibration and ultrasonic phenomena
8. Physiologic effects of speed
9. Acceleration
10. Escape from aircraft
11. Emergency procedures
12. Prechamber flight indoctrination
13. Toxic gases and special weapons

Refresher training should be adapted to the type of requirements with which the trainees are faced. For example, pilots of jet fighter type aircraft will require different refresher instruction than aircrews of troop carrier transports. By the same token every effort should be made to arrange schedules for refresher training so that aircrews comprising a given class of trainees are utilizing the same type of aircraft.

Inasmuch as airline flyers do not receive their initial flying training from the company but have usually attained the status of a graduate pilot at the time of employment, no assurance can be had that they are properly indoctrinated in aviation physiology. Hence, it is highly advisable that an aeromedical indoctrination program be included in their flight crew training. McFarland (3) describes an adequate aeromedical course and adds that, in his opinion, every transport pilot should be thoroughly indoctrinated in a low pressure chamber.

In the military services refresher courses consist of 4 hours of instruction and two simulated flights in the low pressure chamber. The first of the two chamber flights includes ascent to 43,000 feet using 100 per cent oxygen during which various demonstrations and practice are utilized. The second flight involves a rapid decompression from 8000 to 30,000 feet and specifies that oxygen masks will be secured in place after decompression has occurred.

Some operational commands in the military services have felt the need for refresher indoctrination courses as often as once yearly. The reason for this more frequent scheduling is the high performance characteristics of aircraft utilized which fly at speeds well above Mach 1 and at altitudes in excess of 40,000 feet. Talbot (4) has observed that hypoxia and spatial disorientation and, to a lesser extent, decompression sickness and hyperventilation are continuing threats to flight safety and crew effectiveness. He concludes "reported . . . experiences firmly support present policy that requires thorough refresher training of jet aircrew personnel in flight physiology and protective equipment every eighteen months."

In addition to formal refresher training supervisory operational personnel and flight surgeons should utilize every available opportunity to augment the preparedness of flyers. Dissemination of information in booklets, circulars and home reading courses are valuable media. Flight manuals for pilots of commercial airlines should include a section on flight physiology and first aid. Military aircrews can be given information through informal talks and demonstrations in connection with flying safety meetings, mission briefings and other occasions when unit assembly is held. The flight surgeon has an excellent opportunity to remind and refresh his clientele during his activities in connection with the monitoring of protective flying equipment, at the time of the annual medical examination and on various informal occasions.

Flying safety publications are numerous in all branches of flying, both military and nonmilitary. Flight surgeons should utilize such to the utmost. It will be found that operational supervisors and flying safety agencies will welcome with enthusiasm contributions on aeromedical subjects adapted for aircrew consumption. For example, the sensory illusions of flight, a resume of a hypoxia incident or the dangers of self medication in flyers are particularly appropriate for inclusion in flying safety publications. Refresher indoctrination should include appropriate topics described in other sections of this chapter and in other chapters of this volume.

One of the greatest contributions that can be made toward accident prevention as a part of aircrew maintenance is vigorous and constant attention to training and indoctrination in oxygen discipline. Aeromedical personnel must positively avoid complacency regarding this subject. In military flying during recent years hypoxia continues to be a major problem. For example, during an 18 month period 59 fatal aircraft accidents were experienced by the United States Air Force with a "cause undetermined" classification. In this series the altitude of the aircraft immediately before the accident and other significant indications, pointed to hypoxia as the most likely cause. Various observers have noted that about 1 in 10 flyers will experience some degree of hypoxia in flights of 1 hour or more when cockpit conditions are equivalent to 25,000 feet or more. This occurs even though masks are worn and the flyer feels he is familiar with oxygen equipment. Experience has shown that poorly fitting masks, valves in masks stuck open, leaks in the oxygen system, defective regulators, accidental disconnection of oxygen hose or other avoidable conditions are the factors usually involved. Thorough and constant oxygen indoctrination and training will help obviate such occurrences. Many apparently competent flyers seem to forget that the most effective preventive factor of hypoxia is full use of cockpit pressurization to the maximum of which the system is capable. Instances of unexplained accidents have been recorded in which the pressurization system was known to be inoperative prior to takeoff and fatalities resulted from diving in from high altitude without attempts to recover control. It is probable that hypoxia was the primary difficulty.

Flight surgeons should constantly re-evaluate the status of training on oxygen use and equipment of aircrews under their care. Masks should be periodically inspected for proper fit and evidence of deterioration. Nonmedical personnel responsible for inspection, maintenance and servicing of oxygen systems in aircraft should themselves be indoctrinated in low pressure chambers on modified plans, preferably to 20,000 feet to illustrate the dangers of improper servicing of oxygen systems.

Routine refresher altitude chamber training and indoctrination can be adequately given by nonphysician personnel trained in aviation physiology. However, the best preventive practices dictate that a flight surgeon should function on a standby status when chamber flights are underway. This means an "on call" status for the flight surgeon rather than his being physically present at the chamber. Crew members who appear for chamber flights should of course be cleared by the flight surgeon. In addition, those scheduled for pressure suit indoctrination should be evaluated by the flight surgeon for pulmonary conditions, history of decompression sickness, abdominal hernia or obesity. It is considered highly desirable that the flight surgeon actually be present at the chamber when partial pressure suit indoctrinations are underway as this involves very high altitudes. When ejection seat indoctrination is scheduled those with a history of injury or surgery of the back or neck should also be cleared by the flight surgeon.

In addition to the physiology of flight *per se*, refresher training is essential to include reviews of basic principles and orientation in the newer aspects of the following:

1. Noxious gases and vapors
2. Effects of temperature
3. Injuries in aircraft accidents
4. Psychologic aspects of flight
5. Protection in aerial combat
6. Medical aspects of flying safety

The flyer, whether he functions as a commercial airline pilot or as the sole crew member of a supersonic jet fighter must know first aid and emergency medical care. Aircraft accidents sometimes occur where medical aid may take many hours or even days in reaching the scene. When a flyer escapes from a disabled aircraft by parachute he must know enough to adequately handle any injuries sustained when leaving the aircraft or incurred on contact with the ground. Injuries and other conditions may occur during flight and the aircrewman must know how to cope with such until the aircraft can land and medical assistance obtained. Particularly in military aviation during wartime the occupants of the aircraft may sustain wounds as a result of enemy action. The success of an air mission, or at the very least, the successful return of aircrewmen from a mission will often depend on the knowledge and training in first aid. Refresher training in this area must be frequent enough to insure a satisfactory level of proficiency. Members of aircrews need a practical knowledge of the proper first aid treatment of the following:

1. Fractures: one method of immobilizing

each of (a) upper extremity, (b) lower extremity and (c) spine, should be known
2. Flesh wounds
3. Burns
4. Hemorrhage
5. The tourniquet
6. Shock and use of morphine
7. Chest wounds
8. Abdominal wounds
9. Head injury
10. Frostbite
11. Heat stroke and exhaustion
12. Resuscitation   (Holger - Nielsen method)

In programs covering the above topics 5 or 6 hours has proven sufficient. Every possible effort should be made to adapt the training to the audience and to be certain that it is understood. Demonstrations are essential and use of moulages has been found highly valuable. Practice by the aircrews receiving the training should be mandatory. Indoctrination should encompass prevention of disease and injury under survival situations, use of protective equipment, basic sanitation and principles of hygienic living described in other portions of this chapter. Military aircrews will require indoctrination and training in medical aspects of atomic, biologic and chemical warfare. For example, orientation of aircrews on flash burns of the retina as the result of an atomic explosion is highly appropriate. For all aircrews, whether military or nonmilitary, adequate indoctrination and refresher training should be given concerning drugs and flying, diet and nutrition, alcohol and tobacco, exercise and rest, physical and mental fitness and other aspects of personal hygiene. In addition, health factors in tropic and arctic climates and effects of heat and cold should be included.

DRUGS AND THE FLYER

Any agent or substance capable of altering the physiologic and psychologic processes of the flyer is of vital importance to those who practice aviation medicine. Hence, drugs and medications, whether used prophylactically, therapeutically or for other reasons, require special consideration. Many drugs decrease the ability of the human organism to withstand stresses and to compensate for adverse influences such as are encountered in flying.

Conversely certain drugs have been found to have stimulating effects which, under certain circumstances, mobilize the reserve mechanisms of the body to withstand unfavorable environmental factors. Inasmuch as flying effectiveness depends to a major extent on an optimum degree of psychosomatic fitness, it is axiomatic that the mere existence of the need in a flyer for drugs should raise serious doubts as to his fitness to fly at such a time. In other words, if a flyer is not well enough to fly without the support of drugs, he should not fly until the condition requiring drugs is eliminated. Furthermore, it is considered undesirable by many to attempt to extend, through the use of drugs, the tolerance or endurance of a healthy flyer who is properly maintained through good aeromedical practices.

If a given drug could be expected to act solely to correct an abnormality, halt or destroy an infecting organism, alleviate a given symptom or group of symptoms or produce a desired prophylactic response, without side effects, flying performance and efficiency might not be impaired. However, such not being the case, those engaged in aircrew maintenance must exert the closest possible monitoring and medical supervision over drugs and medications taken by flyers. Particularly important is the problem of self medication. The only recourse here is a vigorous information and orientation program aimed at the flyer himself. He must be positively made aware of the fact that the taking of self prescribed medication may impair his flying performance with possible dire consequences.

Commonly used household medications, such as aspirin, nasal decongestants used as nose drops, cathartics and vitamin preparations, should be discussed with flyers. Many airmen, for example, do not realize that certain nose drops can produce tachycardia, tremors, incoordination and visual disturbances. Additionally, physicians not familiar with aircrew requirements may not assess such factors when prescribing drugs.

In monitoring routine medical care of airline pilots, it is necessary that the best possible indoctrination of the flyer regarding effects of drugs and medications be attained. It is necessary, as pointed out earlier, because airline flight crews generally utilize their family physician for routine medical care. Such physicians may or may not be familiar with the decrement on flying performance imposed by certain medications and drugs. An additional safeguard can be achieved by securing from pilots the name and addresses of their family physician. Airline flight surgeons can then send to these practitioners a letter outlining the adverse effects during flight caused by certain drugs with the request that they be used with caution and their effects explained in detail to the airman. Because of the constant and large output of new drugs, periodic efforts of this type will be wise.

The flight surgeon must keep current on new drugs so that flying safety will not be compromised by the prescription of little known medications. He must always consider individual susceptibility and hypersensitivity. The public press abounds in sensational descriptions of new medications and the flight surgeon must inform airmen concerning effects and dangers of such. Contraindicated for individuals on flying duty are tranquilizers, antihypertensives, anticholinergics, antihistamines and other drugs affecting the psychomotor and sensory functions.

Flyers should be especially warned concerning self medications containing antihistaminics. Individual response to this type of drug varies considerably ranging from lack of effect after an average dose to marked drowsiness and even mental depression. Depth perception is adversely affected and the vestibular apparatus is depressed. Ashe (5) cites experimental work which shows that this group of compounds in effective doses significantly reduces perceptual motor skills. There are other side effects of the antihistaminics which need not be enumerated here but which add up to the conclusion that they should not be used by personnel involved in operational flying.

The antibiotics are extremely valuable in reducing time away from flying duty as a result of infectious processes. Inasmuch as these drugs are not generally accessible for self medication the flight surgeon can usually control their use. However, streptomycin, dihydrostreptomycin and chloromycetin require special consideration in aviation medicine. The first of these may produce vertigo, deafness and other symptoms of eighth nerve damage. Although much less toxic, dihydrostreptomycin should be used with great care in aviators. Other antibiotics should be substituted if at all possible and any airman who has received therapy with these two drugs should be carefully evaluated before return to flying duty. Chloromycetin may be damaging to the blood forming system and, consequently, may affect the oxygen transport mechanisms. Aircrewmen who are treated with this drug should have careful hematologic studies both before and after such therapy and before return to flying. Generally, except in urgent operational situations such as combat flying, aircrewmen should be excused from flying duties when antibiotic therapy is utilized.

Certain amphetamine drugs are sometimes used to decrease or delay fatigue and drowsiness in situations where prolonged flight duty is necessary. This practice must be kept under close and constant control and vigilance of the flight surgeon. Such a drug is indeed a "two edged sword." It has been found that amphetamines induce a diminished sense of fatigue and will delay its onset for periods up to 4 hours. In addition, central stimulation is produced increasing alertness and postponing performance decrement. The well known adverse effects of this family of sympathomimetic drugs, although less for dextroamphetamine in relation to its central stimulation potency, are very significant among flyers. One must weigh the risks of performance impairment caused by in-flight fatigue against the risks of adverse effects inherent in these drugs. They should never be used routinely but only when decrement of performance is impending. Thorough orientation of aircrews who may be given these drugs is essential and trial administration to each flyer prior to use in flight is highly desirable. The use of these stimulating drugs has not been a suspected or proven factor in aircraft accidents. Fatigue, however, is listed by Konecci (6) as a contributing factor in 47 accidents during the years of 1955 and 1956. Stimulants should never be substituted for proper nutrition, adequate rest and proper sleep. Concrete evidence that drugs and medications *per se* have been the direct causes of aircraft accidents does not exist; however, some fatal accidents attributed to

pilot error have been suspected as implicating self medication by airmen. This is borne out by the following condensations of reports which might easily have resulted in fatal accidents:

Case 1. Pilot took off feeling "not too good but good enough to fly." He had consulted the flight surgeon on the evening prior to the incident about a head cold. He was advised that if certain medications were given to him that it would be necessary to ground him and was instructed to contact the flight surgeon the following morning if he were scheduled to fly. Pilot, nonetheless, contacted a friend and obtained some Benadryl capsules (50 mg.) and other capsules from a box. Instructions on box stated "do not fly for 24 hours after taking." Pilot took medications. The next morning on gunnery hop he flew into banner doing class "C" damage to aircraft. Return to base and landing were uneventful. He stated, when he broke off target, he felt he would easily clear same as he completed his gunnery run. Subsequent discussion with pilot brought out statement, "I've learned my lesson now. Somehow, I thought you doctors were exaggerating the effect of these drugs on the body." Pilot did not report to flight surgeon immediately after incident. His commanding officer stated that pilot's sensorium seemed clouded and slightly hazy after landing when he questioned him. The flight surgeon felt that, although the medication taken may not have been the primary causative factor of the incident, it was, in his opinion, a contributing factor.

Case 2. A physician prescribed Piperazine Citrate in the usual dose for a flyer's family for the purpose of eradicating pinworms. Inasmuch as such therapy should be administered to the entire family at the same time, the father who was a pilot, took the medication along with the others. After several days of therapy and not having been seen by a flight surgeon—nor having been removed from flying status—this officer prepared to take off on a flight. While performing his preflight check he noted some blurring of vision and upon looking out at the tower, he saw two of them! Needless to say he aborted the flight and reported to the flight surgeon. Commonly available information on this drug indicates that an occasional patient may experience urticaria, vomiting, blurred vision or general muscular weakness. In the ordinary patient, these are not serious. However, the potential threat to flying personnel warrants their temporary suspension from flying status during the treatment period.

The latter story illustrates again the importance of careful surveillance of the drugs which are prescribed for flying personnel, especially by physicians who may not be familiar with their aeromedical implications.

Any detailed discussion of the many classes of drugs and the legion numbers of individual compounds is not feasible here. It is sufficient to reiterate that an essential responsibility of those engaged in aircrew maintenance is constant vigilance concerning drugs and medications. Constant stress should be accorded to the doctrine that even though the drug or medication itself may not be deleterious in flying, the underlying cause for which the drug is used is important. Self medication cannot be completely eradicated among flyers but the precautions necessary to prevent untoward events can be made familiar to all.

DIET AND NUTRITION

In maintaining the health of flyers an important facet is proper nutrition through optimum dietary intake. Along with proper exercise and rest an adequate diet is essential in flying efficiency. Aeromedical support of aircrews will, therefore, involve surveillance whenever possible and guidance through perennial indoctrination concerning their nutrition and dietary habits. This is necessary for many obvious reasons but is not accomplished easily. In the military services certain situations lend themselves to actual supervision of dietary intake. For example, the flight surgeon of an aircraft carrier at sea or one with a tactical unit subsisting in a field mess while on maneuvers can function thusly. Contrariwise, an airline flight surgeon who has no such opportunities, must depend largely on indoctrination and dissemination of information for the monitoring of nutrition and diet of airmen. There are two basic factors in diet and nutrition of aircrews; namely, (1) what they eat while on duty and (2) what they eat while off duty. Inasmuch as the great majority of aircrews are married and eat most of their meals at home, it is essential to orient the wives of flyers as to proper nutritional practices. This will accomplish much in flyer fitness as well as increase rapport with the clientele of the flight surgeon.

A certain amount of aeromedical supervision over dietary intake while on duty can be effected by checking menus of in-flight meals and company operated eating facilities. Generally, however, aircrew personnel of all types will have to be relied upon to select their own food wisely. In order for this to take place the airman must have sufficient knowledge on diet and nutrition which he can apply in his daily living. To provide him with this practical understanding is the responsibility of aeromedical personnel.

The old adage that "we are what we eat" is particularly applicable to the nutrition of aircrews. A biologic machine such as the human body requires better than ordinary management of fuel replenishment in order to cope with the stresses of flying. In addition to the necessary caloric intake derived from proper proportions of fat, protein and carbohydrate, mineral and vitamin content are particularly important. For example, vitamin A is of particular significance inasmuch as good night vision is important in aircrews. McFarland (3) gives a comprehensive resume of diet and nutrition in aircrew maintenance which is an excellent source of indoctrination material.

Obviously important is the long range cumulative impact on flying effectiveness of adequate diet and proper nutrition in airmen. Susceptibility to many disease processes and adjustment to the normal changes of aging is greatly influenced by daily practices in this area over long periods of time. However, in the profession of flying the short range aspects of preventing decrements in aircrew performance owing to the immediate state of nutrition has received much attention. Conditioning of aircrew personnel through proper preflight, in-flight and postflight feeding is accorded special emphasis in the military services. Therefore, at this point preflight and postflight feeding will be discussed in some detail.

Preflight feeding may be arbitrarily considered to include the food ingested during the 24 hours preceding actual performance of flying duties. A more limited approach would be consideration of the last meal or food intake prior to flight duty. Certain items of food and drink have effects lasting many hours not compatible with optimum physical and mental efficiency. It is, therefore, reasonable to deal with preflight feeding as covering the two or three meals and other food eaten prior to flying.

As a general rule aircrew personnel should partake of a freshly prepared and properly balanced meal of foods compatible with flying an hour or 2 prior to takeoff. This meal should be had under pleasant unhurried conditions which will promote desirable relaxation and proper digestion. Such a meal should be based on a daily caloric intake of from 3000 to 3600 calories depending on age, physical characteristics and length of time before the next meal. Inasmuch as only light to moderate physical exertion is involved in flight duties one should eat to fly the aircraft not to carry it. This is particularly important in individuals who are inclined to obesity. They frequently rationalize that the preflight meal must be large for various reasons. It is unwise for pilots of high performance aircraft to eat a huge meal just prior to takeoff. Inhibition of digestive processes may occur and mental faculties may be dulled. Other adverse effects may supervene, such as expansion of gases in the gastrointestinal tract owing to decreased barometric pressure. Noise and vibration encountered in flight may cause a slowing of digestion. If a combat aircrewman on alert status is subject to fly on a moment's notice, food and drink ingested for several hours prior to assumption of duty should be carefully selected. In addition to the reasons cited above certain foods or very heavy meals may cause overloading of excretory organs and hamper flight efficiency in other ways. Preflight meals should be moderate in size, bland, palatable, easily digested and satisfying.

Present day military aircrews, because of the types of aircraft utilized or specific operational conditions encountered, may require specific diet control. This is to prevent or reduce flatulence and improve crew effectiveness at high altitude. When such is necessary individual food tolerances and preferences must be taken into account. As an example of the dietary procedures advocated in a combat ready operational situation the following is cited (7):

"Total daily food intake should usually include items from all of the following food groups:

Leafy, green and yellow vegetables	One or more servings daily, some raw, some cooked
Citrus fruits, tomatoes or salad greens	One or more servings daily
Other fruits, other vegetables and potatoes	Two or more servings daily
Milk and milk products	At least a pint of milk (for adults) or equivalent in evaporated or dried milk, cheese, ice cream or in cooking
Meat, poultry and fish	One or more servings daily
Peas and nuts	Two or more servings weekly
Eggs	Four or more per week; one or two daily preferred
Bread, flour, cereal (whole grain, enriched or restored)	Two or more servings per day as needed
Butter, fortified margarine	One or 2 ounces per day
Other foods as needed for energy requirements	

The following are foods to be avoided:

a. Greasy foods and any others containing excessive amounts of fats

b. Highly concentrated carbohydrate foods

c. Highly seasoned foods and condiments (including catsup, chili sauce, garlic, mustard, meat sauces, etc.)

d. Gas forming foods. The foods most commonly considered to be "gas-forming" are: raw apples, melons, dried beans, peas and lentils, broccoli, cauliflower, cucumbers, parsnips, rutabagas, radishes, turnips, onions, green peppers, garlic, cabbage, brussel sprouts, kohlrabi and sauerkraut. These and high roughage foods should be avoided whenever possible during a period of about 24 to 48 hours prior to flight. This follows from the fact that food usually requires about this long to pass through the intestinal tract

e. Foods high in roughage. Foods high in roughage which should be avoided in preflight meals are: bran products, celery and berries

f. Any food idiosyncrasy of the individual, which will include foods which are unduly laxative or known, from experience, to be particularly gas forming even though perhaps not listed above

g. Alcohol or carbonated beverages. It is important for pilots not to drink alcoholic beverages for 12 and preferably 24 hours prior to alerts or flights. The dulling of mental faculties can, of course, have the gravest consequences. Carbonated beverages should be avoided for one or two hours before flying"

Special crew conditioning diets are sometimes resorted to during periods of stressful combat flying or prior to long training flights. This may be accomplished by providing "training tables" for specific aircrews in the same manner as used by athletic teams.

Rarely is it necessary to utilize such practices more than a few days or, at most, a few weeks in the most unusual situations. Occasional observers in past years have proposed the utilization of specific diets to increase altitude tolerance. These efforts were based on the premise that diets with high carbohydrate content should increase the partial pressure of oxygen in the lungs. In addition, the rapid and easy assimilation of carbohydrates, providing ready glucose to the brain, enhances psychomotor performance. McFarland (3) reviews this subject thoroughly and concludes that any such benefits have been minimized in importance because of pressurization of aircraft. Inasmuch as aircraft have come to commonly operate at very high altitudes, an increase in ceiling of 1000 to 2000 feet, which might be obtained by special diets, is of no practical consequence.

The work of Lawton (8) has received considerable attention from supervisors of operational flying. He felt that relative hypoglycemia might be the etiologic component of certain low altitude near accidents and cited case reports, two of which follow:

Case 1. A student pilot became unconscious while flying with an instructor at an altitude of 8000 feet. After the plane was landed by the instructor, the flight surgeon studying the cause of the student's failure did a 6-hour glucose tolerance test and at the end of 3 hours the blood sugar was reported as 53 mg. per 100 ml.

Case 2. A young pilot flying solo in a jet plane reported blacking out for a short period at an altitude of only 1700 feet. On recovering he found himself at an altitude of only 200 feet but was able to make a safe landing. This individual also was given a 6-hour glucose tolerance test and at the end of 3 hours a low point of 63 mg. per 100 ml. was reported.

Lawton's opinions are based on the fact that when blood sugar levels drop to around 70 mg. per 100 ml. or lower in the average well nourished individual, profound central nervous system symptoms may occur. When hypoxia, decompression sickness or severe *g* forces are superimposed it is likely that many unexplained accidents might be accounted for. Because high carbohydrate meals result in relatively rapid dissipation of satisfactory blood sugar levels because of fast absorption and quick utilization of glu-

cose, Lawton (8) advocates a preflight meal of high protein content. This is based on the often forgotten fact that in normal metabolism proteins are converted to amino acids which in turn evolve gradually into glucose, thus maintaining safe blood sugar levels from meal to meal. With aeromedical monitoring of preflight meals, particularly breakfast, and a vigorous indoctrination program the accident rate in the Flying Training Air Force underwent a considerable reduction when Lawton's concepts were implemented.

In certain types of military operations it is necessary to keep flyers on extended alert periods. This sometimes involves requiring the aircrewman to be physically present at a readiness facility for many hours ready to "scramble" at an instant's notice. Obviously the flyer should have had a thoroughly proper and adequate meal prior to this duty. However, feeding during these alert periods is very important and a properly operated flight line kitchen is essential. This facility need not be elaborate but should be kept clean, operated efficiently and the foods available should be fresh and well prepared. It is not necessary to provide elaborate menus in such facilities. High protein foods such as tasty meat sandwiches with plenty of meat in them, milk, fruit juices and similar items should suffice. Snacks obtained at a flight line food facility should not be used as a substitute for an adequate preflight or postflight meal. This will require constant vigilance by the flight surgeon.

Because of the physically sedentary nature of the duties of aircrews in general, obesity control is a recurring problem. Perhaps the most frequently requested waiver among flyers over 35 years of age, except for presbyopia, is overweight. The management of such cases is essentially the same as in nonflyer segments of the general population. However, care must be exercised in such regimens for aircrewmen who continue their flying during weight reduction programs. Obviously drugs should not be used to effect weight reduction among flying personnel unless they are removed from flight duty. A positive policy on obesity among aircrews is necessary. Wives of flyers, in addition to orientation on diet and nutrition as it affects her husband's flight efficiency, should be thoroughly briefed on control of obesity and their help enlisted. This has been found to be a potent source of assistance when they are made to realize that the family income may be reduced by removal from flying status for obesity. Another approach consists of instituting low calorie menus at dining facilities utilized by aircrew personnel. Such menus for appropriate flyers are usually arranged by suggesting eliminating certain items which are being served and having them take larger portions of low calorie items on a given menu.

Postflight feeding of aircrews should, within reason, cater to the personal preferences and tastes of the individual. Recognizing that the exigencies of flight duty frequently disrupt and modify personal eating habits, the postflight meal should be a repast to be pleasantly anticipated. It should be such as to contribute definitely to morale and a sense of well being in the flyer who has returned from a successful flight. Even though inflight feeding has been much improved in recent years it will be found that postflight feeding is still important. In the military services this "human refueling," especially in combat operational flying, should receive careful aeromedical supervision. It should be designed and planned to compensate for any in-flight periods of a marked nutritional deficit (9). Good postflight feeding will stimulate valuable physiologic processes as well as enhancing esprit de corps. Time between missions may actually be reduced, if necessary, when a completely optimal nutritional state is maintained. After landing, aircrews should be provided with refreshment and nourishment without too much delay. In many situations, such as interrogations, "debriefing" and other postflight duties, it is desirable to provide milk, fruit juices, coffee, nonalcoholic beverages and similar items for aircrews before or during such periods. Certainly, attention to nourishment should not be long delayed after a mission is completed. Returning aircrewmen will usually welcome such which would be followed later by a complete meal. It has been found that relaxation from tension and the psychic stress of fatiguing flight duties is greatly promoted by eating.

ALCOHOL AND THE FLYER

Flying while under the influence of alcohol has never constituted a significant problem in aviation. However, flying while suffering from a hangover caused by the after effects of alcohol is of some significance and has been occasionally implicated in aviation accidents. To obviate this various recommendations concerning time interval between drinking and flying have been advocated. Certainly no harm can come from taking one or two moderate drinks before the evening meal and then operating an aircraft the next morning. This is not true when the individual imbibes repeatedly throughout the evening and night and then flies early the following day. For this reason various airline companies and military units have established rules concerning time between drinking and flying. This time period has varied between 24 and 12 hours. Obviously any regulation regarding this is difficult to monitor or enforce. Some observers have felt that if not more than 4 ounces of whiskey or equivalent amount of alcohol is taken it appears safe to fly after 12 hours. However, general unanimity of opinion exists that if more than this amount is ingested, at least 18 and probably 24 hours should elapse before flying. The body of an average sized individual can burn about $\frac{1}{3}$ fluid ounce of pure alcohol per hour. It is concluded that flyers should be advised not to fly until 24 hours after the last drink containing alcohol. It is advisable to include a presentation on alcohol as a part of indoctrination and training of flyers. Excellent detailed material for this purpose has been set forth by McFarland (3).

In the military services the flight surgeon may have numerous opportunities to observe the drinking habits of flyers under his jurisdiction. Whenever excessive drinking is noted in an aircrew member an attempt should be made to ascertain the cause. For example, in combat flying situations overindulgence in alcohol may be the first sign of operational fatigue. Aeromedical personnel should not be reluctant to exercise a definite but not overly aggressive approach on the subject of alcohol and flying. However, such actions should be effected in most instances in an unobtrusive manner without endangering the rapport between the flight surgeon and the flyer. Military commanders should be advised concerning such problems among flying personnel of their unit or organization.

During and since World War II there came into vogue the practice of providing for combat aircrews a postflight drink of whiskey or other alcoholic beverage. The basis for this was the relaxant effects of alcohol following missions involving danger and unusual tension. The usual dose was about 2 ounces of whiskey which was consumed in the presence of those dispensing it. No instances are on record indicating adverse results of this practice. However, it has been pointed out that some individuals with a tendency toward instability are not benefited in that they may take several more unnecessary drinks from other sources following the one which was dispensed. In addition, individuals who had never previously drank were thought to have been influenced to begin using alcohol. Therefore, many experienced flight surgeons feel that the use of postmission whiskey should be carefully monitored. Specifically, those flyers who desire to be so accommodated should perhaps be required to request such in contrast to the questionable practice of offering spiritus frumenti on a routine basis to all. Care should be exercised to preclude dispensing of mission whiskey to crew members who have recently received amphetamine drugs. Similarly, where the barbiturates are used following missions the flight surgeon should be vigilant to the combined effects of these drugs with alcohol.

Use of Tobacco

Moderate use of tobacco has never been conclusively demonstrated to impair health. This applies to flyers but they should be made aware of the harmful effects of excessive smoking on their fitness to fly. First of all the irritant effect of tobacco smoke in excessive amounts on the respiratory passages and lungs is of significance. This may be of major concern among flyers who have to breathe oxygen continuously while flying. It is easy to imagine the difficulties that a pilot on 100 per cent oxygen during an entire flight would have if he were afflicted with a severe cigarette cough. The gastrointestinal system is altered in its functioning to some extent by smoking. The subjective sensation of hunger is diminished in many individuals probably by the inhibition of gastric contractions. An increase in saliva is produced. Peristalsis of the intestines is usually increased. Appetite is dulled. This last point may be of occasional importance among flyers in whom a weight gain is indicated. The cardiovascular system is affected in various ways by smoking but in otherwise healthy flyers these effects are of little, if any, practical significance.

The use of tobacco by flyers is obviously impossible to monitor. Orientation on the deleterious effects on flyers of excessive smoking should be included in any well rounded indoctrination program. In this presentation it is well to cover (1) the effects on altitude tolerance caused by inhalation of tobacco smoke, (2) the effect on night vision and (3) other physiologic effects of smoking. When very excessive smoking is observed in flyers it is usually a sign of extreme emotional tension or other psychic disturbances and efforts should be made to reach the underlying cause.

Among aircrew members little appreciation or understanding is apparent concerning the reduction in altitude tolerance resulting from smoking during flight. Experimental studies have conclusively shown that the carbon monoxide level it builds up in the blood can reduce altitude tolerance by as much as 5000 feet. This results from inhalation of carbon monoxide from smoking with a decrease in altitude tolerance which can become quite critical especially when combined with hypoxia incident to failure of oxygen equipment.

Reports of fatal accidents seem to indicate that the pursuit of the smoking habit in high performance aircraft has considerable hazards. In one accident a pilot was seen by his wingman to remove his oxygen mask and smoke at least two cigarettes at 17,000 feet. It was revealed at the accident investigation that the pressurization system of the aircraft was faulty, the cockpit pressure apparently being the same as that outside the aircraft. Muscle tissue analysis revealed a carbon monoxide saturation of 48 per cent. The findings of the investigation board opined that part of the carbon monoxide was derived from smoking. The inhalation of this carbon monoxide by the already hypoxic pilot may have contributed to further reduction of the oxygen saturation of the blood sufficiently to result in incapacitation.

Similar instances of this nature have been observed and smoking branded as a probable cause factor. Hence, it is desirable that the dangers associated with smoking in aircraft in flight be brought to the attention of all pilots. Aeromedical physicians should place increased emphasis on the subject of smoking in flight with special reference to the additive effects of hypoxia and carbon monoxide. Mention should also be made at flight safety meetings and at other opportunities concerning the influence that smoking has on night vision. It is well known that the ability to see at low levels of illumination is markedly decreased by smoking. It has been shown that the smoking of three cigarettes can produce the same total effect on vision as is experienced by ascent to 8000 feet altitude without oxygen.

Exercise and the Flyer

Physical fitness of those who fly is of real importance in aircrew effectiveness. Although muscular development *per se* is of limited practical significance among flyers the achievement and maintenance of good muscle tone is rewarding in many ways. For example, military flyers can wear and use their personal and protective equipment with less discomfort if they have good muscle tone. Airline pilots after flights of several hours duration will find themselves less fatigued in the gluteus maximus regions if their bodies are not soft and flabby. All flyers should be strong enough to cope with the extreme physical demands in survival situations on land and sea. Military flyers must be adequately fit to withstand the rigors of escape and evasion. For example, those who were physically fit were more often successful in returning to their units after going down on the "hump" route over the Himalaya Mountains during World War II. General job efficiency of aircrews is enhanced through the benefits of a proper amount of exercise. Obesity control programs in addition to diets should include properly designed exercise measures.

An optimum state of physical fitness in flyers has definite favorable results. In addition to the well known improvements in general physiologic and metabolic processes, attributes of special importance to flyers are influenced considerably. Mental alertness is facilitated. Stamina and endurance are increased. Fatigue is postponed. Tension is reduced. Motor skills and neuromuscular coordination are improved. McFarland (3) observes that in airline pilots emotional tension is relieved and general well being is improved by exercise. He states that such benefits are far out of proportion to the actual amount of exertion involved and concludes that a program of regular exercise should be required of airline pilots. The physically fit flyer is better suited to cope with emergencies requiring rapid and accurate coordination. Such a situation may involve a sudden requirement to do several things very rapidly such as feather a propeller, turn on a fire extinguisher, increase or alter power to other engines and so on *ad infinitum.* Exercise will build up stress tolerance as shown by the larger adrenals seen at autopsy in athletes dying in accidents. McGuire (10) has estimated that there are 23 major metabolic alterations produced by exercise which will operate to the individual's advantage in stressful situations. Many deleterious physical states are prone to occur in the physically unfit flyer. Faulty posture has been cited by some as being responsible for such symptoms as backache, chronic fatigue, constipation, varicose veins and others. Lack of condition with consequent poor muscle tone is probably the primary culprit and poor posture the result rather than the cause in many cases. Low back pain is seen frequently in pilots and is often owing to lack of tone in supporting muscles rather than other reasons.

Exercise which produces extremely strenuous exertion should be generally avoided in aircrewmen. A moderate program over an extended period of time will produce desirable results in general flying efficiency and in increasing stress tolerance.

Indoctrination, training and health information programs for flyers should emphasize the value of good physical fitness in promoting flying efficiency. Research data and physiologic principles should be adapted for aircrew orientation and explained comprehensively. Flight surgeons at the time of the annual medical examination should be on the lookout for signs of physical deterioration resulting from lack of exercise. This procedure presents a particularly good opportunity for the flyer to be counseled on physical fitness.

In the military services the flight surgeon in his aircrew maintenance duties can often actively assist in effecting a physical fitness program. Generally he should avoid being made responsible for such programs but should act in an advisory capacity. He should make a concentrated effort to educate flying personnel in the need for a good level of physical fitness as achieved through exercise. As monitor of the health and welfare of a group of flyers he should remember the secondary benefits such as improved morale, relief of boredom and injection of variety in the daily cycle of sleep-eat-fly-eat-work mode of living. Aeromedical personnel must be cognizant of the specific needs of their charges concerning physical conditioning. A jet interceptor squadron would require a different program than one for aircrews of the Military Air Transport Service. Fighter pilots oftentime prefer more competitive, more athletic physical training programs. Flyers who are utilizing high performance aircraft such as the "Century" series of jet fighters should take daily physical conditioning exercise. This will enhance tolerance to intense g forces, increase respiratory efficiency, and produce other advantageous results. Organized sports and games in which the flight surgeon participates are much better received by flyers than calisthenics. Recreational types of exercise are always more popular.

Re-establishment of physical fitness in flyers following illness or injury should receive special attention by the flight surgeon. Nonmedical supervisors of physical fitness should receive individualized advice concerning these cases. Remedial exercises after discharge from the hospital will often speed return to flying duty. Emphasis should be placed on the advantages of a definitely planned physical rehabilitation regimen

rather than relying on the flyer himself to recover completely on a leave status.

SLEEP AND REST

As in any occupation which requires better than average physical and mental fitness sleep and rest are important to the flyer. Inasmuch as physiologic and psychic recuperative processes vary in each individual and are influenced by many factors the amount of rest and sleep needed by flyers cannot be arbitrarily determined. Some find that rest without sleep may provide some restoration from fatigue for limited periods. Others require actual sleep and gain little benefit from bodily rest without sleep. The state of emotional tension is directly involved and profoundly influences rest and sleep. When the symptom of insomnia is present in a flyer every effort should be made to ascertain the underlying cause and corrective action taken. Prolonged lack of sleep in flyers adversely affects the higher mental processes such as memory and alertness, both so important in aircrew duties. Further, altitude tolerance has been shown to be lowered by excessive and prolonged loss of sleep. Although many flyers must actually sleep to obtain necessary relaxation and rest after flying, it is important to recognize the value of rest in the recumbent position even if the individual does not fall asleep. Pilots of high performance aircraft who have been confined to cramped cockpits and wearing cumbersome heavy protective equipment while flying are greatly refreshed by reclining in a horizontal position. However, when fatigue among flyers requires special consideration, sleep *per se* is important. Many studies have shown that physical fatigue may be greatly alleviated by a brief nap but that mental fatigue is not significantly reduced without a relatively prolonged period of sound sleep.

Disturbances among airmen of their individual rest and sleep habits owing to speedy passage through time zones is important in aircrew effectiveness. This upset of diurnal rhythm has been analyzed by Strughold (11). From 2 days to 1 week may be necessary for the flyer to adjust his physiologic and psychic rest and sleep cycles if he flys, for example, from California to England. In the average flyer gradual adaptation to the new schedule is usually reached without too much difficulty.

Rest and sleep factors in nonmilitary flyers cannot usually be observed and supervised. As in other aspects of aircrew maintenance the only recourse open to aeromedical effort is education through indoctrination and training avenues of approach. Mention of rest, sleep and relaxation should always be made when personal hygiene for flyers is discussed.

Among military flyers the flight surgeon often can take positive steps to facilitate adequate rest and sleep of aircrew personnel. For example, flyers on alert status should be allowed to sleep when the operational situation permits and they are not actively engaged in mission functions. The flight surgeon should see that comfortable cots or beds are provided in such instances. Obviously such a policy would be particularly applicable for crews on night alert status between midnight and dawn. The diurnal sleep and fatigue cycle of crew members during this period has been found to be particularly important. In addition, operational readiness exercises which sometimes last from 48 to 72 hours should be monitored by the flight surgeon to see that adequate sleep is had in order to maintain maximum aircrew effectiveness.

The cumulative need in flyers for prolonged opportunities to secure needed rest and relaxation should be a subject of special aeromedical attention. Airmen engaged in active air operations should avail themselves of their full allocation of vacation and leave time. This is generally from 15 to 30 days each year with full pay. It has been found that individual duty performance is improved when flyers take sufficient leave at one time, such as from 10 to 30 days. For them to adequately profit from a temporary respite from flying duties and a change in environment, flight surgeons should advise at least a 10 day vacation every 6 months.

When flyers are subjected to any extraneous physiologic strains, adequate rest and recuperation before performing flight duty should be insured by the flight surgeon. An example is found when aircrew personnel are requested to make blood donations.

It is well recognized that donating blood imposes some degree of embarrassment, for a varying period of time, upon the donor's physiologic resources. Although regenerative processes compensate quite well after a few days, the loss of a pint of blood may still be significant for a longer period when combined with the stresses of flight. Especially among aircrew members of high performance aircraft, such as single seat jet types, any compromise of peak physiologic fitness appears highly undesirable. Therefore, pilots should not be used as blood donors. Nonpilot crew members, particularly combat crews in the military services, should not ordinarily donate blood. Exceptions may be made in unusual circumstances where a rare blood type is involved, or in an unusual emergency. Individuals donating blood should not perform flying duties for a period of at least 72 hours following the donation. Even in the event of tremendous needs of blood reserves such as in wartime only noncritical crew members, those who are not "cockpit personnel" should be used as blood donors.

PROGRAMS FOR AIRCREW MAINTENANCE

In this final section there will be outlined the essential ingredients of an aircrew maintenance program. It is up to the flight surgeon to accomplish these objectives as head of the aircrew maintenance team. Some of these objectives can only be reached through sagacious advice and recommendations to operational supervisory personnel and to the flyer himself. In the military services this will involve a very close working relationship between aeromedical personnel and the commanders of flying units, usually squadron or group commanders. However, as has been emphasized elsewhere the key to good aircrew maintenance is the closest possible friendly relationship with the flyer but with careful avoidance of an oversolicitous attitude. The following is an example of the scope of duties of a military flight surgeon in an acceptable aircrew maintenance program.

General Activities of the Squadron Flight Surgeon

The general activities of the squadron flight surgeon encompass a dynamic approach to prevention of aircraft accidents and a constant alertness to medical aspects of flying readiness. He is intimately familiar with the unit combat mission. He must be intimately familiar with the physical and mental stresses to which aircrew members are subjected. These stresses must be evaluated in the light of the ability of the aircrewmen to cope with them. Complete knowledge is essential concerning conditions in the assigned aircraft relating to health, comfort and safety. Aircraft oxygen systems must be studied by the squadron flight surgeon. Adequacy of personal equipment for a specific mission must be insured with cognizance taken of the peculiar features of a specific mission, *i.e.*, duration, altitude and underlying terrain. Continuous observation of the general state of physical and mental health of each crew member must be maintained. An attitude of friendly counsel rather than oversolicitous supervision is essential in the flight surgeon-crew member relationship. Squadron flight surgeons should actively perform the following functions and duties:

1. Confer at least once weekly with the squadron commander concerning: (a) aeromedical problems pertaining to the aircraft, aircrew and operational missions, (b) general medical and morale problems within the squadron, (c) specific problems of individual aircrew members, and (d) specific flying safety programs with medical implications.

2. Undergo the physiologic training refresher course as required of aircrews.

3. Obtain issue of a complete set of personal and protective equipment similar to that of tactical aircrews of the squadron.

4. Participate in at least one operational flight per month in assigned tactical aircraft. Flight surgeons assigned to squadrons equipped with single seat jet aircraft should participate by flying in a similar two seated type aircraft, at least once monthly.

5. Spend a minimum of 4 hours per week at the squadron operations building and in the squadron area ("on-the-line") with the personnel of the squadron, carrying out the following purposeful and objective pursuits: (a) Attend squadron meetings and mission briefings. At least once weekly present periodic short talks of an informal type at these meetings on flying safety and aeromedical subjects. (b) Be available in the squadron operations building just prior to and immediately after squadron briefings and meet-ings for informal conferences, interviews, etc., with flying personnel of the squadron. (c) Personally participate in the physical training program of the squadron at least twice weekly. (d) Make periodic visits, at least once weekly, to the protective equipment locker rooms or issue room at the time the pilots are taking out and donning such equipment prior to flying. (e) Become familiar with cockpit configuration, oxygen systems, protective and escape devices and other features pertaining to human factors in assigned aircraft. (f) Accompany flight leaders to their aircraft periodically for familiarization and orientation purposes pertaining to operational characteristics of assigned aircraft. (g) Become familiar with technical orders pertaining to personal and protective equipment such as oxygen masks, protective helmets, *g* suits, partial pressure suits, etc. (h) Make periodic checks on morale and medical aspects of working conditions of squadron ground crews, particularly aircraft crew chiefs and other personnel who are members of the squadron tactical elements. (i) With the squadron commander, inspect the personal and protective equipment of all pilots at least once each 6 months, checking for proper fit, adequacy and condition; this inspection to be performed with the pilot actually wearing his equipment.

6. Supplement the annual physiolgic training with demonstrations and talks on physiology of flying once each 6 months. Participate in the formal squadron training program at least once each 3 months with instruction to flying personnel on self help emergency first aid, medical aspects of escape and evasion, the psychologic and physiologic aspects of aviator's vertigo (disorientation) and other pertinent subjects concerning medical training of aircrews.

7. Conduct the annual physical examination for flying on aircrews of the squadron or squadrons to which he is assigned as flight surgeon.

8. Prepare medical reports and review and comment on investigations pertaining to aircraft accidents involving personnel of squadron or squadrons to which he is assigned as squadron surgeon.

From the above it can be seen that the military flight surgeon has multitudinous responsibilities.

Functions of Supervisory Aeromedical Personnel

There are additional aircrew maintenance functions which should be effected by appropriate supervisory aeromedical personnel. Some of these are:

1. Insure that each operational flying unit has a flight surgeon assigned to it by name.

2. Establish a separate sick call for flying personnel. This does not preclude an appointment system for flying personnel.

3. If necessary, reschedule medical service activities, such as sick calls and ward rounds, in order to make it possible for medical officers assigned as squadron or unit flight surgeons to perform their aeromedical duties. This means that they should be available to participate in squadron or unit activities and be present in the squadron area at the time of mission briefings, squadron periods and other squadron activities.

4. Insure that periodic examinations are conducted adequately and that reports are prepared and forwarded promptly.

5. Inspect flight line ambulance equipment with particular emphasis on standard operating procedures, frequent test runs and close supervision of personnel and equipment. Materiel shortages, such as ambulance radio equipment and appropriate grid maps, should be noted and reported promptly. Practice crash alerts should be conducted a minimum of once every 2 months and a crash ward or other standby type of emergency facility maintained.

6. Conduct preventive medicine surveys among flying personnel and facilities. Particular attention should be given the industrial hygiene program with evaluation of noise hazards and precautionary measures in utilization of toxic solvents and fuel.

7. Monitor all aeromedical aspects of flying safety programs.

8. Exercise careful medical supervision over escape and evasion exercises involving flying personnel.

9. Insure proper space, equipment and personnel in the flight surgeon's section for providing over-all aeromedical mission.

10. Ascertain proper practices concerning adequacy, indoctrination and use of ear defenders by personnel exposed to excessive noise levels.

11. Make frequent checks of administrative handling of removal from and return to flying status and of the granting of waivers concerning aircrewmen.

12. Review the flight surgeon's medical files, charts, statistical records and reports for completeness and accuracy.

13. Monitor the physical fitness program for all flying personnel.

14. Check adequacy of alert facilities reference sanitation, feeding, recreation, rest, comfort and noise.

15. See that immunizations on all flying personnel are kept current.

16. Provide the operations officer with a list of all personnel required to wear spectacles while flying.

17. Insure that aeromedical personnel have adequate reference material and library including medical journals.

Aircrew Maintenance of Airline Flyers

An aircrew maintenance program for airline flyers is by necessity somewhat different from that in the military services. Reasons for this have been cited previously. The two principal methods in which aircrew maintenance is effected in aircrews of airlines is through the periodic medical examination and through dissemination of information to them concerning their health and welfare. Stratton (12) emphasizes prevention in the maintenance of airline pilot personnel. In his concept the surveillance of flyers to assist them in reaching retirement age in good health is a major contribution of the annual or special medical examination. By recording findings over several years, a base or norm is established for the individual. This serves as a means to properly evaluate any deviation from the recorded base and is, thus, a major factor in maintenance. He states that a good prevention program should include:

1. Advice to pilots regarding the use of certain drugs from which problems might arise.

2. Advice regarding the donation of blood.

3. Avoidance of excessive weight through a correct diet and proper exercise; hazards of obesity.

4. Advice on other benefits of exercise, rest and sleep, information on sleep and rest cycles.

Inasmuch as close observation of airline flyers by company flight surgeons is not usually feasible, Stratton indicates that close cooperation between the check pilot and the flight surgeon is important in recognition of disorders such as neuropsychiatric disorders. As an index of effectiveness of aircrew maintenance in commercial aviation, his study showed that in a 6 year period only 7 out of 893 pilots were released for medical reasons, representing 1.6 men per thousand per year.

Those in flying safety and in research and development as it concerns human factors have mentioned the possibility of establishing crew conditioning and control centers. Such an activity, probably many years off, would have crews carefully checked both subjectively and objectively prior to very demanding missions. It is conceivable that ingenious physiologic and psychologic procedures and instrumentation could indicate the state of functional readiness in a crew member.

What are the end results of good aircrew maintenance in terms of aircrew effectiveness? Efficient accomplishment of required functions in flying is the result. This means that the competent flyer must do more than muddle through without accidents. Certainly accident prevention is among the very foremost objectives of aircrew maintenance. However, in order to rise above mediocrity in flying efficiency he must achieve and maintain adequate fitness to meet with real success in his profession. An unfit flyer is an unsafe flyer and an unsuccessful flyer. The goal of aircrew maintenance is a fit flyer.

REFERENCES

(1) GRAYBIEL, A.: Problems involving the pilot and his task; the changing emphasis in aviation medicine. J. Aviation Med., **27:** 397–406, 1956.
(2) OGLE, D. C.: Management of aviation medicine. U. S. A. F. M. Service Digest, **6:** 14–20, 1955.
(3) McFARLAND, R. A.: Human Factors in Air Transportation, Occupational Health and Safety, Ed. 1. New York, McGraw-Hill Book Co., Inc., 1953.
(4) TALBOT, J. M.: Unexplained aircraft accidents in the U. S. Air Forces in Europe. J. Aviation Med., **29:** 111–116, 1958.
(5) ASHE, W. F.: Drugs: are they friend or foe of the aviator? *In* Proceedings of the Aviation Medicine Symposium on Toxic Hazards in Military Flying and in the Aviation Industry. Headquarters A.M.C., 1957.
(6) KONECCI, E. B.: Physiologic factors in aircraft accidents in the U. S. Air Force. J. Aviation Med., **28:** 553–558, 1957.
(7) Aircrew diet control. Surg. Bull., A. D. C., 5–7, 1957.
(8) LAWTON, W. H.: Physiological investigations in the flying safety program of the flying training Air Force. U. S. Armed Forces M. J., **8:** 937–944, 1957.
(9) Flight Surgeon's Manual. Air Force Manual 160–5. Washington, D. C., Government Printing Office, 1954.
(10) McGUIRE, T. F.: Personal communication, 1958.
(11) STRUGHOLD, H.: Physiologic day-night cycle after long distance flights. Internat. Record M. & General Practice Clin., **168:** 576–579, 1955.
(12) STRATTON, K. L.: Medical care of airline pilot personnel. J. Aviation Med., **25:** 630–636, 1954.

27

CIVIL AVIATION MEDICINE

Ludwig G. Lederer, M.D.

The federal agency responsible for civil aviation in the United States has recently been completely reorganized and given a new title. The previous organization was composed of the Civil Aeronautics Administration (CAA) and the Civil Aeronautics Board (CAB). The new organization is known as the Federal Aviation Agency (FAA) and has taken over the responsibilities of the CAA which has been abolished. However, in this Chapter and in Chapter I the term CAA will still be used when discussing the activities of that agency while it was still in existence and the term FAA will be used to refer to the activities of the present agency which came into existence on 1 January 1959.

In the reorganization mentioned above the Office of the Medical Director was also reorganized and given a stature commensurate with its work load and responsibilities. Under the CAA the Medical Director operated a small division under the Director of Flight Safety. In the new FAA the Medical Director reports directly to the Administrator of FAA and has the title of Civil Air Surgeon. His office has been greatly expanded and now consists of four divisions which in turn are divided into 14 branches.

Just prior to the establishment of the FAA two separate committees made a detailed study of the CAA medical activities and submitted reports containing a number of sweeping recommendations. The agencies involved were the Flight Safety Foundation and the Aviation Medicine Committee of the American Medical Association. Later in this Chapter the highlights of the recommendations of these two agencies will be outlined and briefly discussed.

FAA FLIGHT EXAMINATIONS

Examinations given to airmen in Civil Aviation may be separated into those required by law and those given by organizations or conducted voluntarily. In the early portion of this chapter we shall deal only with those physical examinations required by law.

Physical examinations for airmen in the United States have been required by law since 1926. The Air Commerce Act of that year stated that "the Secretary of Commerce shall by regulation provide for the periodic examination and rating of airmen serving in connection with aircraft of the United States and submit qualifications for such service." This provided the statutory authority for the physical examination of civilian pilots.

The first medical director to implement this regulation was Doctor Louis Hopewell Bauer, who resigned his commission in the Medical Corps of the United States Army in November 1926 to assume duties in the aeronautics branch of the Department of Commerce. The duties assigned to Doctor Bauer were primarily to formulate standards for these examinations and to select designated examiners to perform these examinations efficiently and competently.

Much of the early history of Civil Aviation Medicine is described in Benford's *Doctors in the Sky* (1). The original problem of formulating physical standards and selecting

530

designated medical examiners is still a problem plaguing the Federal Aviation Agency. As recently as 1958, the Civil Aeronautics Administration appropriated a sizable sum to the Flight Safety Foundation to restudy this problem.

Preceding the passage of the Federal Aviation Agency in 1958 the regulations pertaining to physical standards for airmen were promulgated by the Civil Aeronautics Board and implemented and administered by the Civil Aeronautics Administration (CAA). These regulations were administered by the Medical Division of the CAA under part 29 of the Civil Air Regulations (2).

The physical standards for airmen have been the subject of much review and comment during the last 30 years. These standards were originally drawn up as minimum standards necessary to operate aircraft in a safe manner. The standards were divided into three classes. Class I encompasses the airline transport pilot. Class II includes the commercial pilot (for hire class). Class III covers the student and private pilot.

The examinations for classes I and II vary but slightly and are conducted by designated government examiners, usually private physicians who have had aviation medical training and who are appointed on a yearly basis according to geographic need by the medical department of the Federal Aviation Agency. Class III examinations can be administered by any physician at the present time; however, the report of the Flight Safety Foundation (3) recommends that all civil airmen should be examined by designated examiners.

The application and interpretation of the physical standards for all three classes are watched carefully by several special interest groups. The Air Transport Association is interested in the scheduled transport pilot. The Aircraft Owners and Pilots Association is interested in the private and student pilot and the Airline Pilots Association is interested in these standards as they affect all pilots, especially airline transport pilots.

These organizations referred to above are interested in keeping their pilots in flying status. They are watchful of any changes in physical standards which would cause an unnecessary hardship in maintaining flying

status. Physical standards for airmen, therefore, are open to modification in relation to aging and also as the judgment, skill and experience of the pilot make up for certain physical deficiencies. As an example, a modification for the standards relating to blood pressure requirements was adopted by CAA and applies to airline pilots 30 years of age or over whose cardiac and kidney conditions, after complete cardiovascular examination, are shown to be normal (table 86).

CONDUCT OF THE PHYSICAL EXAMINATION FOR AIRMEN

The procedure and conduct of the physical examination for civil airmen does not vary much from that described in previous chapters of this book. There are some modifications which should be mentioned. The examination of the eyes has been simplified so that optical measuring machines such as the Keystone Orthorater and the American Optical Sight Screener can be utilized. Although these machines cannot measure prism divergence, this is not too important in the phoria examination for civil airmen.

The medical department of the Civil Aeronautics Administration has issued a guide for medical examiners (4) which sets forth the standards and guide lines for the conduct of the physical examination for all three classes of airmen. The forms necessary for these examinations may be obtained from any CAA (FAA) office in any city in the United States and its possessions. The certificate issued by the examiner is valid, if passed, for 6 months for the airline transport rating; 1 year for the commercial pilot; and 2 years for the student and private pilot.

It is interesting to note that an added

TABLE 86

Class I Adjusted Blood Pressure Requirements

Age Group	Maximum Readings (Reclining Blood Pressure in mm. of Hg)		Adjusted Maximum Readings (Reclining Blood Pressure in mm. of Hg)	
	Systolic	Diastolic	Systolic	Diastolic
20 to 29	140	88		
30 to 39	145	92	155	98
40 to 49	155	96	165	100
50 and over	160	98	170	100

requirement states that a holder of a license shall not exercise the privileges of his license during any period when such holder is aware of any decrease in medical fitness which might render him unable to meet the medical requirements for the issue or renewal of his license.

International Standards for Airmen

The International Civil Aviation Organization, the so-called United Nations of Aviation with headquarters in Montreal, Canada, has promulgated standards and recommended practices for personnel licensing (5). A full time medical advisor is in residence for this organization. Proposals for changes in standards or recommended practices with regard to physical requirements may originate within the organization or can be contributed by member states. This information is circulated to the various member states, comments are obtained from interested parties and a meeting is held to discuss these changes if enough opinion warrants the occasion.

FUTURE TRENDS IN CIVIL AVIATION MEDICINE AND PHYSICAL STANDARDS

For nearly all of its 30-odd years of existence the medical division of the CAA was denied a location of importance within its own organization. It was looked upon as a certifying division which had no direct access to the top echelon. It was not kept abreast of similar aviation medical functions in the armed forces. Within the past few years, however, instances of sudden incapacitation while flying as a result of organic medical conditions have focused a new light of importance to medical functions in the certification of airmen.

The recent report of the Flight Safety Foundation (3), which has studied intensely all functions of the division of aviation medicine in CAA, specifically refers to recommendations needed to improve CAA medical functions. These are:

I. The term "Medical Qualification" should be used instead of "Physical Standards."

II. New "Medical Qualifications" should be adopted. The principal changes needed are:

A. All differences between class I and class II be eliminated.

B. More complete visual testing be required for class III; in fact there should be the same requirements as for classes I and II except that the visual acuity for uncorrected vision could be at a lower permissible level.

C. The measurement of depth perception should be retained.

D. Hearing qualification should be strengthened to hearing of whispered voice at 15 feet instead of 8 feet.

E. For all three classes, under general physical conditions, two grounds for denial of a certificate without recourse to appeal be mandatory; these are:

1. Diabetes mellitus requiring insulin or other hypoglycemic drugs for control; and

2. Established history or diagnosis of a myocardial infarction or angina pectoris or other evidence of coronary artery disease which may reasonably be expected to lead to myocardial infarction.

F. A new requirement is recommended; namely, an electrocardiogram at the time of issuance of original license in classes I and II, at age 40, and once per year after age 40.

G. A new requirement for a chest X-ray at the time of original issuance of any medical certificate for all classes, I, II and III.

H. A hemoglobin measurement to be required at the time of each examination.

I. Under nervous and psychiatric disorders, the following grounds for denial without recourse for appeal should be mandatory; history of hospitalization for established diagnosis of:

1. A psychotic disorder.

2. A severe psychoneurotic disorder.

3. Epilepsy.

4. Alcoholism.

5. Drug addiction.

III. No sound basis exists at this time to justify any further change in medical qualifications applicable to airmen in jet and turboprop transport operation.

IV. Periodicity of time intervals for examinations shall remain the same in all classes.

V. Present provisions for physical deficiencies wherein skill, judgment and experience compensate for existing physical deficiency, part 29.5, Civil Air Regulations, should be retained.

With respect to medical certification procedures, the FSF report (3) recommends that all three classes of airmen should be examined only by designated government examiners. They further recommend that these examiners should, in the event of newly designated individuals, show some degree of specialization in that they should be members of the American Board of Preventive Medicine (certified in Aviation or Occupational Medicine) or a similar specialty rating in Internal Medicine or have the equivalent in training or professional competence. The examiners should be well versed in CAA examination requirements and procedures, should demonstrate a willingness to follow them, possess the necessary facilities and equipment properly to conduct CAA examinations, and be willing to participate in periodic specialized training activities as conducted or suggested by CAA and otherwise show evidence of a continuing interest in aviation medicine.

It is further recommended in the FSF report (3) that:

1. The CAA medical division should maintain a continuous check on the performance of all designated examiners, with appropriate correction of mistakes or withdrawal of designation if necessary.

2. Medical examination forms for class I and II airmen should be revised to include more medical history.

3. The CAA Guide for Medical Examiners (4) should be revised, brought up to date, simplified and be so arranged as to furnish material new in the field of aviation medicine to the designated examiner.

4. A list of competent medical consultants should be maintained and utilized for special medical problems centrally in the CAA medical division and also on a regional level.

5. Improvements should be made in the record keeping system and sampling should be made from time to time of current records and findings compared to records of previous examinations on the same individuals.

6. Administrative procedures should be set up to correlate performance of pilots with operational people. This would be important in considering the issuance of medical certificates with "operational limitation."

7. A study should be made covering a representative cross section of designated examiners on the costs of conducting CAA medical examinations in order that there may be a realistic understanding of the relationship between what the CAA is asking medical people to do and the fees being received. The question of who pays the examination fees when an individual fails to pass an examination was not considered in these recommendations.

8. In appeal cases, because of the highly technical character and the special preparation needed for these cases, a closer liaison between the General Counsel and the Medical Division is recommended, perhaps even by the assignment of medicolegal personnel to specialize in these cases. It was also recommended that the CAA should make more use of expert medical witnesses in appeal cases.

9. Medical participation in accident investigation is highly recommended; however, this may require consideration of permissive legislation.

10. As to medical research, it is recommended that increased attention should be given to medical factors directly related to safety in civil aviation for passengers as well as air crews. Some of this may appropriately be carried on within the CAA organization or delegated to universities and other research agencies on a grant-in-aid basis. Further, in the field of suggestive re-

search, major attention should be given to cardiovascular conditions, diabetes and mental disorders—their possible relation to accidents—and to specific medical conditions present under the practice of issuing limited medical certificates and also to the question of permitting corneal lenses to be worn.

Aid of Other Agencies to Improve CAA Medical Procedures

In 1957 legislation was introduced in the Congress of the United States under Senate Bill 1045 to create a separate and distinct office of Aviation Medicine within the CAA structure. The Secretary of Commerce, after Congressional hearings were held, appealed to the American Medical Association for advice in this matter. A Committee on Aviation Medicine was formed as a subcommittee to the Council on Industrial Health. This Committee met frequently, conferred with all interested parties and seriously considered all of the recommendations of the FSF report (3). In general, the Committee endorsed the FSF-CAA report, with some amplifications. Some of these are:

I. Medical standards
A. Class III applicants should not have vision poorer than 20/200 without correction in each eye providing that correction is brought up to 20/20 or better in one eye and 20/30 in the other by corrective lenses, correcting lenses to be worn while exercising the privileges of an airman's certificate.
B. Hearing qualifications for classes I and II. If the applicant does not meet the standard of spoken voice in normal conversational tones at 15 feet, an audiometric examination shall be given. The applicant may qualify if the hearing loss in either ear is no greater than 25 decibels in any of the three frequencies of 500, 1000 and 2000 cycles per second.
C. That an electrocardiogram be on file on each airman holding a class I or class II certificate at the time of original issuance or at the time of promulgation of this directive.
D. The chest X-ray shall apply to clas-

ses I, II and III at the first examination or after promulgation of the regulation.
II. Regarding the study recommended by FSF on the costs of conducting CAA medical examinations with a view toward making the fees paid for the examination realistic, it is a further recomendation that the fees should be commensurate with the extent of the examination required.
III. With respect to appeal cases, a recommendation was made that special problems may arise in that the appeal cases are usually held at a "place convenient to the applicant's place of residence or employment." A comparison here was made between this legislation and Food and Drug Administration legislation under Section 502j of the United States Food and Drug Act, wherein cases of a serious nature are not heard at the convenience of the appellant.
IV. The Committee on Aviation Medicine of the American Medical Association was also vitally interested in the organizational setup of the new Federal Aviation Agency and the chain of command between the administrator and the head of the medical department. The duties and responsibilities of the medical director were also of prime interest to this Committee. The Committee was assured by representatives of the Federal Aviation Agency that the Civil Air Surgeon (formerly the medical director of CAA) would answer directly to the administrator of the Federal Aviation Agency. The Civil Air Surgeon is to be responsible for the development and projection of aviation medical policies, standards and practices; directs Medical Department programs relating to physical qualifications, training and selection of aviation personnel; and the aeromedical aspects of aircrew, aircraft safety and equipment. He coordinates Federal Aviation Agency aeromedical programs within the other Government agencies, civilian organizations and foreign governments.

It is indeed interesting to note that the Office of the Civil Air Surgeon in the first six months of 1960 has been elevated to the status of a bureau within the Federal Aviation Agency. It is now known as the Bureau of Aviation Medicine. The head of this bureau is still known as the Civil Air Surgeon.

With respect to some of the recommendations made by the FSF, the Bureau of Aviation Medicine of the FAA, with excellent support from the Aerospace Medical Association and the Committee on Aviation Medicine of the American Medical Association, has been able to put into law the recommendations regarding:

1. Absolute disqualification for diabetics requiring insulin or proven myocardial infarction, psychotic disorders, epilepsy, alcoholism, and drug addiction.
2. All aviation medical examiners for all three classes of licenses are now designated by the FAA.
3. Age sixty (60) as a mandatory retirement age for all air carrier pilots.
4. Medical participation in accident investigation has been accomplished and together with the CAB, a Human Factors Team has been organized.
5. Visual standards have been liberalized to exclude most of the phoria testing.
6. ECG requirement has been emplemented.

This indeed marks progress in aviation medicine to date. However, a word of caution is in order. Although the regulatory function and research requirements have made great strides within the FAA, the judicious application of the regulations will depend upon astute, mature clinical judgment. The respect of the pilot personnel for good clinical judgment on the part of the FAA staff is not only necessary, it is mandatory.

MEDICAL ASPECTS OF COMMERCIAL AVIATION

Although some airlines have been in operation for 30 years or more, the adoption of the Civil Aeronautics Act of 1938 was the birth date of most airlines now operating in the United States. As airlines grew in size and personnel, or because of the epidemiologic aspects of overseas operation, medical departments were formed.

Airlines can be separated into international, transcontinental, regional, sectional and intrastate carriers.

Table 87, tabulated by the Air Transport Association of America, shows the phenomenal growth of the airline industry.

It is indeed interesting to compare the percentage increase especially in daily seats available and the number of passengers carried in the last 20 years.

Even though the airline industry has grown so greatly, only the six largest carriers have an organized medical facility or department. These are, in alphabetical order, American, Capital, Eastern, Pan-American, Trans-World and United Airlines. Many of the smaller airlines have a medical consultant, some medical facilities for the care of injured employees but no organized medical program as such.

The first publication dealing with the medical aspects of the health and efficiency of civil airmen was perhaps a document prepared by McFarland (6), who was the coordinator of the medical program for Pan-

TABLE 87

Growth of U. S. Air Carriers (20-Year Period)

	1938	1958	Per Cent Increase
Number of airlines	23	53	130
Cities served	286	706	147
Airplanes in service	345	1,829	430
Seats available (daily)	4,800	94,200	1863
Cruising speed (fastest transport)	220 m.p.h.	360 m.p.h.	64
Number of passengers carried	1,306,000	49,339,000	3678
Number of people employed	13,300	138,000	938
Average fare in cents per revenue passenger mile	5.32	5.42	1.9

American Airways System. In this treatise, Doctor McFarland covered various subjects, such as the nature and causes of fatigue in airline pilots, the effect of high altitude in lack of oxygen, the importance of diet, the role of physical exercise and relaxation, the effects of alcohol, the influence of smoking, the care of one's health in the tropics, the use of the eyes at night and in bright sunlight and a short chapter on "How Long Can the Airman Fly." Two other textbooks by Doctor McFarland have now become standards in the field of commercial aviation (7, 8). Many articles have been published pertaining to commercial civil aviation medicine. Most of these can be found by consulting the bibliography of the *Journal of Aviation Medicine*. Some of these articles refer to pertinent problems in commercial aviation medicine, and others to the philosophy and organization of commercial aviation medical setups. The interest and scope of aeromedical problems in civil aviation has widened considerably in the last few years. This is evidenced by the formation of the following organizations which have some medical function relating to civil commercial aviation medicine.

I. National
   A. Federal Aviation Agency (formerly CAA and CAB)
   B. Air Transport Association of America
   C. Air Line Pilots Association
   D. American Medical Association Committee on Aviation Medicine
   E. Aerospace Medical Association
   F. American Board of Preventive Medicine
   G. Civil Aviation Medical Association

II. International
   A. International Civil Aviation Organization
   B. International Air Transport Association
   C. International Federation of Air Line Pilots Association
   D. International Board of Aviation Medicine
   E. Airline Medical Directors Association
   F. Aero Medical Associations, AGARD French speaking branch, etc.

   G. International Congress of Aviation Medicine, etc.

A reference to the international scope of aviation medical activity can be found in the August 1958 issue of the *Journal of Aviation Medicine* on the "President's Page."

The medical examiner for the airlines works directly for the management of the airlines and a much more comprehensive health maintenance type and pilot type physical examination is conducted at company expense.

The pilot examination in airlines that have a medical department is quite comprehensive, especially for the initial or pre-employment pilot physical. This is necessary because the airline desires only the best of personnel and intends to spend much time and money on training and transitioning from one type of aircraft to another. It is also a well known fact that aging is incessant and it is the desire to pick applicants with physical standards far above the minimum FAA type standard so that after 30 years or so of flying they can still pass the FAA class I type of physical examination necessary to exercise their airman's certificate. For these reasons, selection examinations include mental testing such as an I.Q. test, a personality evaluation test, such as the Humm-Wadsworth or the Minnesota-Multiphasic Personality Inventory, and some type of mechanical aptitude test. The medical history is quite extensive and searching and the physical examination includes a neurologic survey, as well as such laboratory tests as a complete blood count, blood cholesterol, urea nitrogen, nonprotein nitrogen, nonfasting blood sugar, a chest X-ray, electrocardiogram, blood serology and complete urinalysis. The usual extensive eye, ear, nose and throat examination is also performed.

The interval of examination is usually once per year for the airline type of examination conducted by the airline physician and once every 6 months for class I conducted by the designated FAA medical examiner. Other individual operating crew members also take the FAA physical examination at less frequent intervals. The flight engineer qualifies once per year. With the advent of more and more aircraft operating within the United States, another category of airmen deserves some attention and description. This is the tower control operator. The tower control operator in some of the major cities in the United States is responsible for the control of departing and arriving aircraft, and as such, has a very responsible position. In some busy airports, the magnitude of landings and takeoffs has reached one in every 24 to 30 seconds. The working conditions and environment placed on the tower control operator has led to a special study conducted by the Flight Safety Foundation and reveals many interesting deficiencies in the work environment of this individual (9). The recommendations made in this report are such that if properly adopted by the Federal Aviation Agency, the working environment of the tower control operator will be made much more in keeping with industry practice.

CHARACTERISTICS OF COMMERCIAL AIRCRAFT

It is interesting to note that the first airliner or transport type aircraft specifically constructed for passenger use within the United States was the original Douglas DC-3. Its counterpart, the C-47, was known as the "workhorse" of the Air Force. Other aircraft developed during and after World War II were primarily patterned after the Douglas DC-4, the first four engine airliner. The DC-4, although not pressurized, showed some advantages in passenger carrying capacity. However, it was not until the development of the Douglas DC-6 that pressurization and other passenger comforts were added to the average airliner in the United States. The Douglas DC-7, the Boeing Stratocruiser and the Lockheed Constellation, all four engined aircraft, likewise were pressurized and had better ventilation rates than their predecessors. Two engine aircraft like the Martin 202 and the Convair 240 produced later versions with pressurization and were called Martin 404 and Convair 340 and 440, respectively.

An interim type of aircraft utilizing a jet type engine but with reduction gear hookup to conventional propellers—the prop-jet or turboprop—is now being widely utilized in commercial aviation. The first aircraft of this type was the Vickers Viscount widely operated in Europe since 1950 and now operated extensively in North America by Trans-Canada, Northeast, Continental and Capital Airlines. The American version of this type of aircraft is the Lockheed Electra. A larger version is the Bristol (English) Britannia. Aeromedical aspects of the Viscount turboprop were described by the writer in 1956 (10). Advantages of this aircraft over existing conventional piston type aircraft are less vibration and noise in flight and slightly better cabin pressurization levels.

The first pure jet commercial aircraft was the Comet I, II and III operated by British Overseas Aircraft and manufactured by DeHaviland in Great Britian. This operation was described by Whittingham in 1954 (11). Unfortunately this aircraft did not survive the effects of metal fatigue owing to the high differential in cabin and ambient atmospheric pressure and this episode was aptly described as the Comet disaster by Armstrong et al., in 1955 (12).

The Comet IV, a new version by DeHaviland, the Boeing 707, the Douglas DC-8 and the Convair 800 and 880 are now the new types of all jet passenger aircraft which will be used in commercial aviation.

The problems associated with all jet operation are not too great as far as passenger and crew operation is concerned. The advantages are:

1. Simpler aircraft to operate manually for crew members; fewer control panel switches and gadgets.

2. Less fatigue in crews owing to less noise and vibration in flight.

3. Less chance of motion sickness in passengers as the result of less turbulence at higher altitudes.

4. Less interference with physiologic time clocks for both crews and passengers owing to shortened flight time.

The disadvantages are:

1. Crews must "think ahead of aircraft"; no chance for "going around again" owing to fuel consumption problems.

2. Some resistance to passenger acceptance owing to "oxygen drills" to combat emergencies caused by sudden decompression.

3. More hazard to cabin attendants if "change of direction" occurs when attend-

ants are serving or walking or on "dive" maneuvers caused by increased speed.

4. Humidification problems in American built jets because of dryer cabin air. The English jet has humidification apparatus to artificially charge the cabin air with moisture.

5. Atmospheric glare during daylight flight owing to less dust particles at 35,000 to 45,000 feet.

Pressurization in Commercial Aircraft

The most important contribution to passenger comfort in air travel was the development of the pressurized cabin designed to "keep the passenger as near to sea level" or the altitude of destination as possible. The altitude to which passengers are exposed is dependent on two factors, namely, actual altitude of flight and pressurization of the aircraft. This subject as a means of real passenger comfort has been discussed by the writer (10), by Kidera (13) and by Schreuder (14).

Ideal pressurization, a Utopia in aviation medicine, is difficult to obtain. This would mean no change in differential pressure to the passenger or such gradual change from the altitude of origin to the altitude of destination that any change would go unnoticed physiologically.

Conventional aircraft mentioned previously in the piston engine category are pressurized by means of superchargers discharging air into the cabin maintaining a maximum pressure of 4.16 pounds per square inch for the Douglas DC-6 and up to 5.16 p.s.i. for the DC-7 (13). The Lockheed (Super) Constellation has somewhat the same range or perhaps slightly better, 5.36 p.s.i. pressurization. The turboprop aircraft have increased this pressurization level to a maximum of 6.5 p.s.i. but for safety and to keep metal fatigue at a minimum and because of short haul operation they actually use only 5.5 p.s.i. as an operational optimum (fig. 143).

The pure jet aircraft mentioned previously maintain a cabin pressure of 8.0 to 9.0 p.s.i. This is necessary because the operational optimal altitude owing to high fuel consumption for the larger of these aircraft will be at or near 40,000 feet. This means that actually the pure jet will be able to give the passenger an 8000 foot cabin at 40,000 feet, the turboprop will give the passenger a 2500 foot cabin at 20,000 feet and the conventional piston aircraft will give a 5000 foot cabin at 20,000 feet. These are, of course, maximum figures. For many flights where high altitudes for the aircraft are not necessary the cabin can in

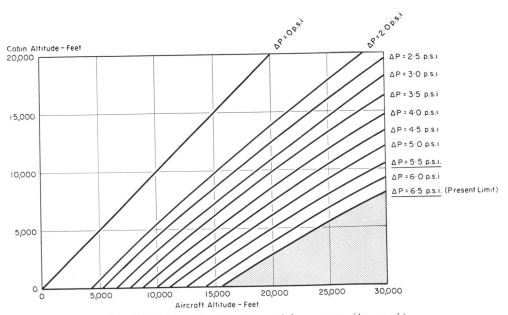

Fig. 143. Values of cabin differential pressures. (Δp = p.s.i.)

many instances be maintained at or near sea level or adjusted to destination pressures.

VIBRATION CHARACTERISTICS OF COMMERCIAL AIRCRAFT

Vibration is often referred to in aeromedical literature because of its importance to passenger and crew comfort. However, there is very little scientific data available of the vibration constants or levels of present commercial type aircraft. The Chief, Airframe and Equipment Branch of the Civil Aeronautics Administration (15), stated:

"The Civil Air Regulations do not contain specific detail requirements for maximum allowable vibration and noise levels for the pilot's compartment or the passenger cabin. The regulations do however contain a qualitative requirement, covered in section CAR 4b, 350 (g): 'Vibration and noise characteristics of cockpit appurtenances shall not interfere with the safe operation of the airplane.' Compliance with this requirement has been determined by CAA test pilot's qualitative observations of the vibration and noise levels during the flight tests associated with the type certification program. As a result of this approach to the requirements, we have no data available in regard to the noise or vibration levels in existing transport type aircraft."

Although some manufacturers of commercial aircraft have such data, it is not readily available. We must, therefore, look to the contributions of military aviation medicine for some of the basic work in this field.

In the classic work reported by Getline (16) on vibration tolerance levels of military aircraft, the unit of measure used was displacement in thousandths of an inch at cycles per second of frequency of motion. In Getline's first figure on subjective responses to vibration (fig. 144), three curves are drawn which were established by Goldman (17). Curve I defines a level at which vibration is perceived by the average individual, curve II defines a level of unpleasantness to vibration perceived and curve III represents a level where the subject refused to tolerate exposure to vibration after a short period of time. Medical literature, however, in the field of calibrated ballistocardiography deals primarily with displacement as a unit of measure of motion. This unit of measure is usually in

thousandths of an inch per second displacement at natural body frequency which is normally 4.3 cycles per second. The author has superimposed on this chart a figure of a heart at the level of average normal displacement of 0.0022 inches at a natural body frequency of 4.3 c.p.s. (18) which falls below the line of curve I. In general, this is true inasmuch as the motion of the average normal heart is imperceptible to most individuals. In figure 145, Getline has plotted the vibration data of several types of aircraft. The author again has superimposed the heart symbol and the mark V for the vibration constant for the Viscount average cruise level. Black dots indicate aircraft from which complaints of vibration were received, blank circles represent aircraft acceptable from a vibration standpoint. It will be noted in this graph that nearly all of the dark dots are reported by conventional piston propeller driven aircraft or helicopters, except for two jet types. Getline explained this as follows: both were F-84 jets, one had a structural failure in a motor mounting, the other was considered a poor production model. All other jet aircraft were rated as tolerable as regards vibration and many of the jets were in the lower levels of inches of displacement and lower frequencies in cycles per second. A

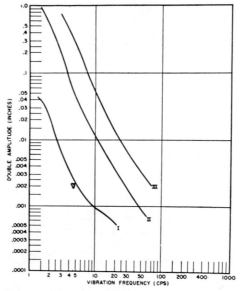

FIG. 144. Subjective responses to vibration. (From Getline, after Goldman.)

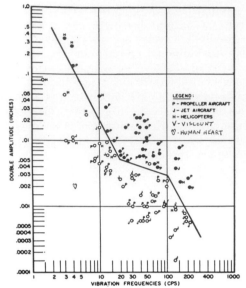

Fig. 145. Vibration tolerance curve for military aircraft. (From Getline.)

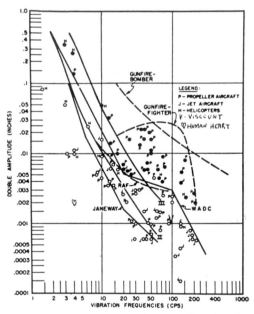

Fig. 146. Summary of aircraft vibration data. (From Getline.)

line separating those aircraft in which vibration was a complaint and those in which it was not became the Wright Air Development Center tolerance curve for military aircraft.

In figure 146, Getline has drawn from left to right four other curves relating to the establishment of vibration tolerance criteria. These are (1) Janeway's "comfort level," a standard of the automotive industry; (2) Goldman's middle curve which establishes a level of intolerance to vibration; (3) requirements established by the Ministry of Aircraft Production, RAF; and (4) the vibration response in the seat frame of a fighter aircraft while 0.50 caliber machine guns are fired from a turret. The author has again superimposed the symbols of V for Viscount vibration level and the displacement average figure for the human heart beat. Note that the WADC curve for the most part is below Goldman's curve III; this can be interpreted that some aircraft above Goldman's curve III could be tolerated for short periods of time with respect to vibration discomfort.

Vibration in all propeller driven aircraft, engineers generally agree, originates from the tips of the propellers of the inboard engines. The number of motor mounts present makes no difference. The figure for frequency in cycles per second (c.p.s.) are calculated at higher cruising speeds by multiplying the motor r.p.m. times propeller reduction ratio times number of propeller blades divided by 60 (c.p.s.) (19). The study of vibration in commercial type aircraft is important with respect to the inducement of passenger and crew fatigue. The clinical effects of vibration of small amplitude, however, are as yet not determined; but we do know that if we can keep the vibration amplitude down we are progressing in the right direction with respect to adding to crew and passenger comfort.

In recent years, helicopters have been used for commercial air transport. Referring back to the Wright Air Development Center vibration tolerance curve, it was noted that the helicopter created vibration characteristics of greater displacement in inches at variable frequencies of cycles per second. From this data, it is unlikely that long trips in helicopter aircraft are conducive to passenger comfort.

PROBLEMS OF NOISE IN COMMERCIAL AVIATION

With the advent of turbine type engines the entire aircraft industry, both manufacturing and transportation divisions, has been faced with a noise problem. Noise levels are present in turn around procedures on the ramp, in run up procedures for maintenance purposes and in engine test cells. Perhaps the first organized hearing conservation program in commercial aviation aside from that developed in the United States Air Force was done at Capital Airlines as it began to realize it had a noise problem in the operation of the turboprop Vickers Viscount airplane. Adequate directions for organizing a hearing conservation program are quoted in Air Force Regulations No. 160-3, 29 October 1956, which was used as a pattern in the development of the hearing conservation program at Capital Airlines. The preliminary work done by Capital Airlines in the United States correlates very well with the Air Force findings, namely, that individuals with previous ear trouble or damage are most prone to show hearing losses when subjected to continuous high intensity noise levels or with noise levels in the higher frequency ranges of cycles per second, which are commonly found in the turbine type engine. The greatest noise problem in the Rolls Royce Dart 510 engine occurs in the frequency of 2400 to 4800 cycles per second. With the utilization of more and more pure jet type aircraft it can be correctly stated that noise will be the greatest problem as far as commercial aviation is concerned. In addition to hearing conservation programs, which must be adequately developed, monitored and put into operation, an educational program as far as community noise levels are concerned is also in order. For details the reader is referred to a chapter on noise in this text.

Toxicologic Hazards in Commercial Aviation

With the utilization of jet type aircraft, different types of fuels, synthetic oils and other toxicologic hazards are being encountered. A book on toxicologic hazards in aviation was published by the Aero Medical Association from material developed by the Civil Aeronautics Administration. Turbine engine powered aircraft in commercial aviation in the future will present other toxicologic problems. First and foremost

among these will be the effect on personnel of synthetic fuels and high grade kerosenes as regular fuels for aircraft. The problem of handling methanol for water injection systems is another personnel hazard in this type of motor maintenance. Other health maintenance problems in commercial aviation medical divisions concern themselves with the annual examinations of gas tank workers where leaded gasoline is used. The determination of lead levels in blood and the removal of these individuals from such work when these levels become excessively high is necessary for good health maintenance. Sand blasting personnel and electroplating shop workers, because of the use of hazardous chemicals, are also subject to annual periodic health maintenance examinations.

Handling Hazardous Material Aboard Commercial Aircraft

In the last 10 years, the development of certain types of atomic energy material consisting of radioisotopes with extremely short half-lives has presented a problem of quick transportation. This material is usually transported from points of manufacture to areas of clinical usage by commercial carriers. The adequate packaging in order to protect cargo handlers, crews and passengers has been an aeromedical problem. This has been solved very adequately by having airline medical directors meet with atomic energy officials, inspect areas of manufacture of this material in atomic energy plants and to offer recommendations on proper packaging and handling.

With the manufacture of vaccines for certain disease entities such as poliomyelitis and Asian flu, similar problems were met and dealt with by airline medical men in commercial aviation. The carrying of etiologic agents is vital for the public health by commercial aircraft carriers. This is necessary because some of the material used in the manufacture of vaccine will not live for any appreciable length of time. Rules and regulations for the carrying of this type of material are issued by the Restricted Articles Tariff Section of the Air Transport Association of America. The proper and logical handling of these areas of hazardous material has resulted in an advance in public health not known before and with adequate safety to air crews, aircraft and passengers.

DISCOMFORT STUDIES IN COMMERCIAL FLIGHTS

As early as 1939 Colonel Arnold D. Tuttle, the late Medical Director of United Airlines, and two of his associates, Doctor George J. Kidera, present Medical Director of United Airlines and the writer, conducted intensive studies on passenger discomforts encountered in commercial aircraft flights. The writer continued these studies (19) and during 1946 compiled data in one airline on 1,120,977 passengers. He found that on an average, in 18 per cent of the trips flown some medical discomfort occurred. This discomfort involved an average of 1.16 per cent, or 12,903 of the passengers flown. Of the discomforts experienced for the year, 77 per cent were attributable to motion sickness. Of the motion sickness encountered, 60 per cent occurred in the adult female, about 25 per cent occurred in the adult male, and about 15 per cent occurred in children both male and female. The other discomforts which were commonly encountered were: approximately 6 per cent earache, about 8 per cent headache, about 3 per cent temporary deafness and approximately 5 per cent common colds. It can be seen from this study that the primary discomfort is motion sickness, that it involves principally the adult female passenger and that the other common discomforts were earache, headache, temporary deafness and colds. This study indicated that the medi-, cations needed to curb passenger discomfort, in the order of importance, are: (1) effective motion sickness remedies, (2) headache remedies, (3) earache remedies, (4) cold remedies or alleviating agents of the symptoms of a cold and (5) something to relieve temporary deafness owing to descent and blockage of the eustachian tubes. This study was conducted with DC-3 and DC-4 nonpressurized aircraft. In recent years, other studies have shown that the percentages of discomfort are still relatively the same; however, with the acquisition and intelligent use of pressurized aircraft and high wing loading principles and the fact that pressurized aircraft can fly at higher altitudes and thus avoid turbulence, the total discomfort figure in commercial aircraft flights at the present time is somewhere near $\frac{1}{2}$ of 1 per cent of passengers carried.

Motion sickness remedies, within the past 5 years, have been perfected to the point where very effective remedies are now available to the public for over-the-counter sale. Nearly all writers agree in the field of motion sickness that results are best obtained when the remedy is taken 15 to 20 minutes before boarding the vehicle causing motion. It is important, therefore, that the passenger obtain and consume an effective dose before boarding the aircraft. The motion sickness remedies of choice are: cyclizine hydrochloride (Marezine), in doses of 50 mg. for short flights inasmuch as this drug acts for approximately 4 hours and causes the least amount of drowsiness. For longer flights, Meclizine hydrochloride (Bonamine) is recommended in doses of 25 mg. and 50 mg.; however, this drug causes more drowsiness. In individuals who need effective sedation plus a motion sickness remedy, like cases of angina pectoris and individuals with gall bladder disease wherein vomiting might reactivate illness, the drug dimenhydrinate (Dramamine), in doses of 50 mg., and promenthazine (Phenergan), 25 mg. are recommended.

Other factors play a part in inducing motion sickness such as vision and ventilation. Odd forms of motion to which one is not accustomed is also a factor such as pitch, roll, scend and yawing. From our studies (19) we found that motion sickness is more prevalent during daylight hours compared to night flights. In a study made on DC-3 aircraft we found that seating played a very important part in the induction of motion sickness. In a group of 4274 cases of motion sickness studied, we found that the two window seats immediately aft of the left wing of the aircraft showed the highest incidence of motion sickness. Figure 147 shows a layout of the seating pattern in a DC-3 aircraft. The percentages appearing below seats 1, 4, 7, 10, 14, 17 and 20 indicate the incidence of motion sickness observed for these seats when motion sickness occurred. The less frequent cases of air sickness are

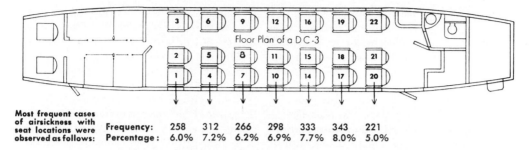

Most frequent cases of airsickness with seat locations were observed as follows:

Frequency:	258	312	266	298	333	343	221
Percentage:	6.0%	7.2%	6.2%	6.9%	7.7%	8.0%	5.0%

Motion sickness was distinctly greater in incidence in the left-hand window seat of the DC-3 type airplane, as shown in this diagrammatic sketch of the seating arrangement of the DC-3 with percentage of airsickness seen in each seat indicated. The data for these percentages are based on well over 5,000 cases of motion sickness.

Less Frequent *Cases of* *Airsickness*	SEAT NUMBER	FREQUENCY	PERCENTAGE
	18	184	4.3%
	15	182	4.2%
	12	181	4.2%
	19	177	4.1%
	16	171	4.0%
	6	170	3.9%
	2	167	3.9%
	5	167	3.9%
	11	154	3.7%
	3	152	3.5%
	21	146	3.4%
	9	141	3.2%
	22	128	2.9%
	8	123	2.8%
		4274	

FIG. 147. Over-all incidence of motion sickness seat numbers in DC-3 type aircraft.

shown also in figure 147 for the other seats when motion sickness occurred. The writer feels that the Civil Air Regulations which call for banks and turns to the left accounts for the high incidence of motion sickness occurring on this side of the aircraft. The effect of motion is further increased immediately aft of the trailing edge of the left wing as one views the ground terrain rapidly slipping by and creating a form of physiologic nystagmus which may help to initiate vestibular reflexes to initiate the motion sickness syndrome.

PASSENGERS AS MEDICAL ENTITIES

Aside from the apparently well passenger, an airline, because of its common carrier status, often carries for hire individuals with known medical entities.

Some of these entities can well be classified as physiologic, such as early infancy, pregnancy and congenital malformation as lung atresias, congenital heart malformations, etc. The rules and regulations adopted by most airlines have been published (20) and are well known to airline medical men. In chapter 28 of this text "Airomedical Evacuation," is discussed more fully. In other publications (21) the writer has covered other medical conditions of travel and air travel.

A new booklet, "Criteria for Passenger Flying", has been formulated by a special committee of the Aerospace Medical Association whose Chairman was Dr. Otis B. Schreuder, Medical Director of Pan American Airways. This booklet will be published and distributed to all interested physicians as a joint effort of the committee on Aerospace Medicine of the American Medical Association and the Aerospace Medical Association.

The average medical director, not having his office at the airport proper, very seldom sees many of these cases. The passenger relations and ticketing personnel do see these cases. A practical guide should be provided so that they can deal intelligently with the passenger obviously ill, regarding his condition to travel. In cases of doubt, medical advice should be sought. In many cases a telephone conversation with the passenger's doctor will do. Of course, more information is gained if the airline medical consultant speaks with the family doctor. United Airlines has stated that in every case where a medical doubt existed and where a doctor was contacted, no complications occurred en route that necessitated a nonscheduled landing because of medical difficulty with a passenger.

Although there are no set rules and regulations for the responsibility of the medical director to the critically ill passenger, nevertheless, it could be looked upon as the duty of any physician to do the proper thing at the right time for any critically ill person. Cabin attendant personnel are briefed during their training course on sudden medical emergencies, which includes insulin shock, epileptiform seizures, cerebralvascular accidents, myocardial infarctions, pulmonary and other emboli and hyperventilation syndrome (22). Although cabin attendant personnel are not professionally trained, the ability to recognize a serious medical condition from one not so serious is important. In all instances we ask that the captain be informed when a potential or actual medical emergency exists. Pilot personnel assist with oxygen administration and arrange by radio communication for ambulance facilities and a physician to meet the aircraft, when possible, and also plan unscheduled landings. In many instances the pilot or captain may magnify a simple medical emergency. Sometimes the captain is quite demanding in having a doctor meet the aircraft. This problem is being dealt with by the Airline Medical Directors by having a series of informative articles appear in the Airline Pilots Association News regarding these situations. If the airline captains were a little more informative in their communications when a critical medical situation exists, it would help the local people to have the right type of aid present. As an example, one airliner had a sudden

decompression; the captain radioed for a doctor but gave no details. The doctor appeared but unhappily forgot his otoscope.

The last instance in which the airline of the writer had an acute myocardial infarction aboard, the passenger was in a hospital bed 43 minutes from the time of the initial attack and he was covered with therapeutic levels of oxygen all the way including his ambulance ride. In this airline, we have two outlets on the oxygen carry around bottle; one delivers oxygen levels comparable to sea level conditions and the other outlet, marked with a distinctive color, is a so-called therapeutic outlet which delivers 8 liters per minute.

Oxygen Requirements in Commercial Aircraft

For approximately 10 years, each commercial aircraft operating above 8000 feet of actual altitude was required to have oxygen aboard for at least 10 per cent of the number of passengers carried. Crew oxygen regulations are more severe and require that any crew member shall use oxygen when operating for more than $\frac{1}{2}$ hour at or above 10,000 feet actual altitude. Oxygen regulations have been covered in the Civil Air Regulations in part 4B and part 40.

With the operation of commercial jet aircraft, oxygen requirements have become more severe because of the eventuality of sudden decompression occurring at altitudes of 25,000 feet or above. For this reason, the Civil Air Regulations were changed to combine previous regulations in a more functional manner. Oxygen will now be provided for 10 per cent of passengers above 10,000 feet of operation and for 100 per cent of passengers above 14,000 feet giving a flow to supply an equivalent of oxygenation of 10,000 feet actual altitude. These are minimum regulations and some airlines will exceed these requirements and provide a 5000 foot equivalent oxygen supply. Full 100 per cent oxygen can be obtained for any period of time if arrangements are made prior to flight with most airlines for particular medical cases.

It is the responsibility of the medical director to arrange for good medical care for emergencies in every city in which his airline operates. In order to accomplish this, we use physicians known as medical line consultants. They are selected by having the local station manager submit the names of two or three physicians who have been contacted and state that they are available for such services. The medical director investigates their professional qualifications and designates one or more as a medical line consultant. These doctors are not on the payroll of the company, they are not eligible for special privileges like courtesy passes and they work strictly on a fee per case basis. Very often designated CAA medical examiners are used for this purpose.

In the event that the passenger is unconscious or seemingly dead, we deplane the passenger into a waiting ambulance, inasmuch as really no one aboard the aircraft, except a physician who may be traveling as a passenger, can legally pronounce the passenger dead. At times physicians who are traveling as passengers are willing to give a professional opinion regarding death; however, when the physician is told that if he does give such an opinion he will have to wait with the body and transmit his information to the coroner or medical examiner at the location where the aircraft is making a landing, the physician usually declines any professional opinion in order not to interrupt his trip. The way in which we handle this situation may leave some questions in doubt in the minds of the reader; however, one must realize that the medical director has the responsibility not only for proper disposition of the dead or dying passenger but also not to unduly inconvenience the other passengers who are traveling at the same time. We further feel that this procedure is correct because in instances where the passenger may be seemingly dead, immediate transport to a hospital for resuscitation is of primary importance. On the other hand, if the passenger is dead, he will be pronounced dead on arrival by competent hospital professional help who are well versed with the final procedure of processing a death certificate.

With respect to the passengers who are obviously dead owing to major aircraft accidents the responsibility of the medical director is two fold. First, he has the obligation to see that the passenger is accurately identified. This is important from several

medicolegal aspects; insurance, death benefits, etc. The other obligation which the medical director has is to provide, in a very judicious manner, the most humanitarian way of handling and informing the next of kin regarding the death of the passenger.

Regarding the first function, the accurate identification of the dead, the medical director must work closely with the local coroner or medical examiner. Because of several jurisdictions of police powers in some areas, this may take some finesse. In some instances the coroner may delegate and accept the findings of the medical director without doing the work himself. The death certificates, however, must be executed by the coroner or medical examiner.

In recent aircraft accidents, owing to the increased speed of aircraft now available and the type of fuel used, many of the dead passengers are quite mutilated and some are burned beyond ready recognition. Where finger prints are available the local police authorities will aid in checking prints and with the assistance of the Federal Bureau of Investigation many identifications can be made quite rapidly, especially in males. In some recent accidents we have had to go to teeth identification (23). It is now becoming a MUST for the airline medical director to have an accurate knowledge of dental anatomy (see chapter 24). This should include old and new terminology of teeth, teeth surfaces and types of fillings. The utilization of x-ray facilities of the teeth and bone joint areas, such as the sternoclavicular joint, can be valuable information as to sex and age. Complete autopsies of the remains and chemical analysis of brain, lung, liver, kidney, urine and blood are now becoming routine. These tissues and body fluids are quick frozen with CO_2 ice. Cooperation is readily given by the Armed Forces Institute of Pathology, Section on Aviation Pathology. Biochemical tests are made by this facility which can give valuable information as to the presence or absence of alcohol, therapeutic levels of drugs, carbon monoxide and evidence of hyperventilation and whether or not the body was exposed to fire while still alive.

With respect to the handling of relatives, it is our custom to try to see that no immediate next of kin views the remains. We find that the shock to the average layman is quite severe. Passenger service personnel help out here. We try, when the family insists, to let someone view the remains who is one step away from the next of kin. Personal effects found on the body are shown to the next of kin and very often aid in "ready" identification.

In summary, it might be noted that in commercial aviation medicine, the duties and responsibilities of the airline medical director are primarily to maintain high standards of selection and maintenance of airline personnel, including flight crews and ground personnel, in addition to his responsibility to the passenger. Organizations such as the Airline Medical Directors Association and the section of airline medicine in the Aero Medical Association at their annual meetings, concentrate on problems which are faced by the airline medical director. At the present time, symposia are being held in the Airline Medical Directors Association at annual meetings, on the causes which can result in sudden physical incapacitation in the cockpit. It is very apparent to the airline medical director that the greatest causes of attrition of pilot personnel are in the following order:

1. Personal automobile accidents
2. Cardiovascular disease
3. Neuropsychiatric diseases
4. Degenerative diseases, such as hypertension, diabetes, etc.

The airline medical director is also used for consultation and advice for in-flight problems, feeding problems, etc., within his own airline by the various operational departments. In general, the airline medical director feels that as a flight surgeon he is in reality an epidemiologist, a public health expert, an aerologist and above all an astute clinician of flying personnel, their families and an occupational physician to support ground personnel needed to maintain his aircraft.

As regards the future of aviation medicine pertaining to commercial aviation, the economic outlook is not too bright. The acquisition of high performance aircraft will be a very expensive proposition and in some instances, because of economic pressure, airlines will tend to minimize their medical

functions. The medical department is classified as a nonincome producing facility. Every effort should be bent to prevent this because, with the utilization of high performance aircraft, medical problems will increase. The proper selection and training of flight crews and the maintenance of personnel handling these aircraft will cover many medical aspects. In support of this, the Committee on Aviation Medicine of the American Medical Association's Committee on Industrial Health has come forth with a statement recommending that the operators of all high performance aircraft (nonpropeller driven) should have excellent medical facilities immediately available at all times.

REFERENCES

(1) BENFORD, R. J.: Doctors in The Sky. Springfield, Ill., Charles C Thomas, 1955.
(2) Part 29, Physical Standards for Airmen. Washington, D. C., Government Printing Office, as ammended 1 Oct. 1949.
(3) Medical Aspects of Civil Aviation. Flight Safety Foundation—Civil Aeronautics Administration Medical Study, Report No. 2. New York, Flight Safety Foundation, 1958.
(4) Guide for Medical Examiners, U. S. Department of Commerce. Washington, D. C., Civil Aeronautics Administration, 1954.
(5) Personnel Licensing, Annex I. International Standards and Recommended Practices. Montreal, Canada, International Civil Aviation Organization.
(6) MacFARLAND, R. A.: Keeping Fit for Flying. An Analysis of Important Factors Influencing the Health and Efficiency of Civil Airmen. New York, Pan American Airways System, 1943.
(7) MacFARLAND, R. A.: The Human Factors in Air Transport Design. New York, McGraw-Hill Book Co., 1946.
(8) MacFARLAND, R. A.: Human Factors in Air Transportation. Occupational Health and Safety. New York, McGraw-Hill Book Co., 1953.
(9) Physical Qualifications of Air Traffic Control Personnel. Flight Safety Foundation—Civil Aeronautics Administration Medical Study Report No. 1. New York, Flight Safety Foundation, 1958.
(10) LEDERER, L. G.: The aeromedical aspects of turbo-prop commercial aircraft; a study of Viscount passenger operations in the United States. J. Aviation Med., 27: 287–300, 1956.
(11) WHITTINGHAM, H. E.: Aeromedical problems of jet passenger aircraft. J. Aviation Med., 25: 440–450, 1954.
(12) ARMSTRONG, J. A., FRYER, D. I., STEWART,

W. K., AND WHITTINGHAM, H. E.: Interpretation of injuries in the Comet aircraft disasters. Lancet, 1: 1135–1144, 1955.

(13) KIDERA, G. J.: Medical and surgical considerations in selecting airline passengers. New York J. Med., 58: 853–858, 1958.

(14) SCHREUDER, O. B., AND CONSTANTINO, J. G.: Transportation of patients by commercial airlines. J. Aviation Med., 26: 184–188, 1955.

(15) VOLLMECKE, A. A.: Personal communication.

(16) GETLINE, G. L.: Vibration Tolerance Levels in Military Aircraft Supplement to Shock and Vibration. Bulletin No. 22. U. S. Navy Research Laboratory, 1955.

(17) GOLDMAN, D. E.: Mechanical Vibration and Its Effects on Man. Lecture and Review Series No. 52-1, U. S. Naval Medical Center, 1952.

(18) SMITH, J. E., LEDERER, L. G., AND MANDES, J. C.: Evaluation of the calibrated displacement, velocity and acceleration ballistocardiograph in angina pectoris. Am. Heart J., 49: 344–359, 1955.

(19) LEDERER, L. G., AND KIDERA, G. J.: Passenger comfort in commercial air travel with reference to motion sickness (part of a symposium on motion sickness). Internat. Rec. Med. & Gen. Practice Clin., 167: 661–668, 1954.

(20) LEDERER, L. G.: In CONN, H. F., ET AL.: Current Therapy. Philadelphia, W. B. Saunders Co., 1951, pp. 631–635.

(21) LEDERER, L. G.: In CONN, H. F., ET AL.: Current Therapy. Philadelphia, W. B. Saunders Co., 1951–1959, see Sections on Aviation Medicine, Motion Sickness and Disorders Associated with Travel.

(22) LEDERER, L. G., AND KIDERA, G. J.: Hyperpneic tetany in commercial aircraft passengers. Proc. Soc. Exper. Biol. & Med., 5: 1946.

(23) GONZALES, T. A., VANCE, M., HELPERN, M., AND UMBERGER, C. J.: Legal Medicine: Pathology and Toxicology, Ed. 2. New York, Appleton-Century-Crofts, Inc., 1954, chapter 3.

28

AEROMEDICAL EVACUATION

Harry G. Armstrong, M.D.

In the United States, patients may be air evacuated by three different means depending on the circumstances. Military patients and their dependents are flown in air evacuation aircraft of the military services while civilian patients may use either the regularly scheduled commercial airlines or chartered civilian transports. Each of these three methods differs from the others in certain respects and it is important that these differences are understood.

Military aeromedical evacuation efforts in the United States date back to 1910 and those interested in this story are referred to an excellent historic review of the subject by Guilford and Soboroff (1). During World War II, even though it was not officially considered to be the primary method of patient movement, some one and one-third million sick and wounded military patients were flown by the U. S. Air Corps and it was demonstrated beyond question that a patient who could be moved by any means could be moved as safely and much more efficiently by air. This fact gained official recognition in 1949 when the Secretary of Defense directed that the evacuation of all sick and wounded in the military forces of the United States, both in peace and war, would be accomplished by air when practical and not otherwise medically contraindicated.

The responsibility for this evacuation of military patients was delegated to the Military Air Transport Command of the Air Force, which is composed of both Air Force and Navy transport units, except that in areas not served by that command the military service concerned is given the local responsibility. Counting from the time accurate records were initiated at the beginning of World War II, the Air Force evacuated its 2,000,000th patient on 23 February 1954.

This effort is conducted on a highly organized basis and the military services have not only a tremendous background of experience but also specially adapted aircraft, well trained and experienced air and aeromedical crews and certain especially designed items of medical equipment to assist in carrying out their mission.

In contrast to the military situation described above, the air evacuation of patients in civil life, except in major disasters, depends on arrangements made on an individual basis by the physician or patient concerned. If it is decided that the patient should travel as a passenger on a commercial airline then the following considerations must be taken into account.

Patients suffering from active tuberculosis or from any infectious or contagious disease are prohibited by law from traveling on public conveyances including aircraft. In addition, certain patients may also be prohibited from travel on a commercial airline by a regulation of the Air Transport Association of America which reads as follows:

"Participating carriers will refuse to carry or will remove en route any person whose status, age, physical or mental condition is such, in the opinion of the participating carrier, as to render him incapable of caring for himself without assistance, contributing to the discomfort of, or making himself objectionable to, the other passengers or involving any hazard or risk to himself, to other persons, or property." This regulation refers to the unattended patient. If the patient is accompanied by an attendant who will be responsible for caring for him en route then most airlines will interpret the above regulation in terms of this arrangement.

In addition, if prior arrangements are made most air carriers will allow a blind passenger's "seeing eye" dog to travel in the passenger compartment if the latter is properly muzzled and secured on a short leash. Wheel chair patients will generally be carried if prior arrangements are made to load and unload the patient. It may be possible to arrange for transport of litter patients on litters specially designed for the specific aircraft concerned which are available through the traffic department of the airline concerned. Most patients wearing plaster casts will be transported provided the casts are not of such size or shape as to prevent the passenger from being accommodated by the regulation seat. Patients with diabetes mellitus will be accepted if they can give their own insulin or will not need insulin during the flight. In all cases if the patient is obviously ill or severely incapacitated the airline will require a certificate from the attending physician both as to the details of the illness suffered and releasing the airline from any responsibility for the case. The airline stewardesses, although no longer required to be registered nurses, are usually well trained in first aid and have available on the aircraft a small first aid kit. Oxygen, with the necessary regulators and masks, is also carried routinely and is available to any passenger requiring its use.

Where it is thought that oxygen or other special attention might be required by a patient the attending physician should so state in a letter addressed to the flight stewardess but presented first to the ticket agent who will determine whether or not the services requested can and will be made available. Necessary arrangements should be made to have the patient at the airport well in advance of takeoff time if loading is a problem or so that they may be given the most desirable seat. Special attention should also be given for arranging necessary assistance at the patient's destination—a matter which is frequently overlooked.

The use of chartered aircraft for the movement of patients is normally devoted to cases not acceptable to the airlines, where the point of origin or destination is not serviced by an airline, in certain emergencies and disasters, where the patient is not ambulatory or is critically ill. In arranging for the use of such aircraft it may be advisable, if pertinent, to inquire as to whether the aircraft is equipped and the crew qualified for night and weather flying, whether the aircraft has provisions for adequate cabin temperature control, whether the cabin door is adequate to admit a stretcher case and, finally, whether or not the cabin is adequate in size to accommodate the patient or patients plus the necessary medical attendants and medical equipment.

Suitable aircraft are available for charter at almost all airports and there are several hundred such craft scattered throughout the United States which are specially equipped for the aeromedical evacuation of patients on a charter basis. The latter usually consist of one or two engine transports capable of accommodating 2 to 5 seated patients or 1 to 2 stretcher cases. Most of these are provided with stretchers, oxygen, bed pans, urinals, emesis basins, blankets, sheets, pillows and in-flight suction apparatus. All of these aircraft are licensed by the FAA and have met the required air worthiness standards. Larger aircraft are available, up to and including commercial airliners and helicopters can also be employed. The principal disadvantage of chartered aircraft is the higher costs but they have the distinct advantage of complete flexibility of operations including a flight pattern tailored to the patient's needs and usually any patient will be accepted if accompanied by a physician's certificate.

GENERAL CONSIDERATIONS

The question as to whether or not a patient should be transported by air or by other means should, of course, be based on the welfare of the patient. Due principally to the fact that aircraft accidents are featured in the news the average person has a grossly exaggerated idea of the dangers of flying. As a matter of actual fact the most recent figures show that, on a passenger mile basis, flying on a commercial airliner is three to four times safer than riding in one's own automobile. The environment of an aircraft cabin is generally equal to that of one's home or a hospital ward in that it is well ventilated, temperature controlled and free of dust and dirt. The great advantage of aeromedical evacuation, of course, is the shortened time element not only in emergencies but in practically all instances. Obviously a patient that is en route for 4 hours by air can be expected to arrive in a more rested condition and in better shape than if he had traveled 30 to 40 hours by surface means. Another important point in this connection is the shorter period of time that a patient is out of touch with a physician and with needed hospital care. On this basis the more serious the illness the greater the indication for movement by air.

In reviewing the literature on aeromedical evacuation one is struck by the reversal of attitude over the years. In earlier times papers on this subject consisted principally of dire warnings of the ill effects of flying on patients while the more recent literature consists largely of reports of no or minimal reactions. Also one finds many reports in the literature of laboratory studies on the effect of altitude on patients which are grossly misleading owing to the fact that extreme altitudes were used or sudden hypoxia induced allowing no time for the body to make the usual physiologic adjustments as actually occurs in flight. Both May (2) and Friedberg (3) have questioned the practicality of these findings and have placed this matter in its true perspective. Some individuals have perhaps also been confused by descriptions of the very elaborate preparations and equipment necessary to move critically ill patients by air by overlooking the fact that the same preparations would be necessary for movement by any other method.

Although aeromedical evacuation has all the advantages cited above there are conditions peculiar to flight that may have an adverse effect on certain clinical states and this question will now be discussed. The conditions peculiar to flying which are of concern to us here are three in number and consist of air sickness, the mechanical effects of decreased atmospheric pressure, and hypoxia. In dealing with this subject it will be assumed that we will not expose patients to more adverse conditions than those well tolerated by normal healthy passengers. This means a maximum cabin pressure of not to exceed 10,000 feet under ordinary circumstances and 15,000 feet in an emergency situation during which oxygen is employed in all cases. There is, of course, the possibility of explosive decompressions of aircraft pressure cabins and the occasional case that might have to be flown at still higher altitudes, such as would be encountered in crossing the Andes Mountains in unpressurized aircraft. Such occurrences, however, are exceedingly rare and would have to be dealt with on an individual and emergency basis.

Based on the above considerations patients may be divided into three general classes as follows: (1) Those cases whose primary illness is not adversely affected by the conditions peculiar to flight. This group constitutes the great majority of all patients and they all may fly if they are transportable by any other means. Although some of these cases may need special medical preparations prior to, or care during, a flight this will not be discussed here inasmuch as these are problems which are common to the evacuation of patients by any means. (2) Those cases whose primary illness might be adversely affected by the aeromedical evacuation depending upon the seriousness of the illness, the specific conditions to be encountered during the flight and the availability or absence of prophylactic measures. The basic principles of dealing with this group of patients will be discussed in later sections of this chapter but it is to be emphasized that, in any individual case, the attending physician is the only one in a position to make a final decision. (3) The third and last class of patients are those who should not be evacuated even under the most favorable conditions such as: (a) Patients in such poor physical condition that the successful completion of their evacuation is doubtful unless potential life-saving measures are available at the destination hospital which are not available at the point of origin. (b) Patients with a fatal prognosis in a moribund or semimoribund state. (c) Patients in shock. (d) Patients with severe anemia consisting of less than 2.5 million red blood cells or less than 50 per cent hemoglobin. (e) Patients with coronary occlusion or angina pectoris if an attack has occurred within 60 days. This latter class of patients need no further discussion and accordingly we shall now proceed to a consideration of the patients mentioned in (2) above in regard to their transportability by air under various circumstances.

Air Sickness

In aeromedical evacuation air sickness is of major importance or not depending on whether an attack would seriously affect the patient in view of his primary illness. The incidence of air sickness among patients will depend largely on the amount of air turbulence encountered in flight and whether or not recently discovered prophylactic measures are employed. Before these latter were known Downey and Strickland (4) reported that among 1777 patients with cardiac and pulmonary disorders the incidence of air sickness was 4.1 per cent.

There is one specific contraindication to exposing a patient to possible air sickness and that is the individual with his jaws wired shut who, in the event he vomits, might strangle on the vomitus and aspirate it into his lungs. Such cases, however, may be allowed to travel by air if rubber bands are temporarily substituted for the connecting tie-wires during the trip (see chapter 24).

Serious cases of heart disease, hypertension and ulcers or lesions of the gastrointestinal tract which might perforate should be carefully evaluated by the attending physician on an individual basis as well as any other illness which might be aggravated by vomiting. In making such an evaluation consideration should be given to the fact that rather recently three different methods of preventing air sickness have been discovered and when used in combination the incidence of this disease can be expected to approach the vanishing point. These three methods consist of placing the patient in a reclining or semireclining position, maintaining the patient's head in a fixed position and the use of motion sickness drugs prophylactically. Each of these different methods is described in chapter 14 which should be consulted for the essential details concerning their employment as well as other ancillary means of reducing the incidence of air sickness such as, for example, the avoidance of turbulent air where practicable.

In summary, it may be said that the properly prepared patient runs a very small chance of developing air sickness during evacuation by air but, inasmuch as this is not absolute, any primary illnesses that would be seriously affected by vomiting should be evacuated by other means.

Decreased Atmospheric Pressure

The decrease of atmospheric pressure with ascent has been described in earlier chapters of this book as well as its effects on the normal individual. For our purposes here we can eliminate from consideration the higher altitudes inasmuch as it is neither reasonable nor essential that patients be exposed to pressures above 15,000 feet altitude if we take into consideration the use of pressure cabin aircraft in those rare cases where higher levels are mandatory such as in clearing very high mountain ranges. As a matter of actual fact the great majority of flights can normally be expected to be at an altitude or a cabin pressure of somewhere between 5000 and 10,000 feet. However, specific information on this point should be obtained in any case where the welfare of the patient is concerned and not be left to chance.

At these lower altitudes the effects of decreased barometric pressures are limited to those produced by the expansion of gases contained in closed cavities of the body and it is only this effect that needs to be evaluated in terms of the patient's primary illness. With this brief background of information in mind we shall next consider the various disease states that may be adversely influenced by these various atmospheric pressure changes.

Middle Ear and Sinus Diseases

All patients with middle ear and sinus diseases may be flown except where the openings to these cavities are stenosed and the patient is unable to keep the air pressure within these cavities and that of the atmospheric air constantly equalized. This matter is fully discussed in chapter 11 which should be consulted for details regarding the difficulties to be expected and how they should be dealt with. Briefly stated patients whose eustachian tube or sinus orifices are blocked should not fly except through an altitude range not to exceed 2000 to 3000 feet. If the middle ear or sinuses can be readily ventilated then the presence of infection in these cavities does not contraindicate travel by air inasmuch as a spread or aggravation of such infection by flying has never been known to occur.

Pulmonary Disorders

In order to evaluate properly the effect of altitude on gases confined in closed cavities of the body it is necessary to convert altitude to relative gas volumes as has been done in table 88. From this table it can be seen that a unit volume of gas at sea level becomes 1.2, 1.5 and 1.9 volumes of gas at 5000, 10,000 and 15,000 feet, respectively.

The pulmonary disorders directly affected by decreased atmospheric pressures consist of a therapeutic or spontaneous pneumothorax, a traumatic mediastinal emphysema

TABLE 88

The Relationships between Various Flight Altitudes, the Relative Volume of Gas Contained in Closed Body Cavities and the Per Cent O_2 Saturation of the Arterial Blood

Altitude	Relative Body Cavity Gas Volume	Per Cent Arterial O_2 Saturation
Feet		
Sea level	1.0	96.0
5,000	1.2	92.0
10,000	1.5	88.0
15,000	1.9	80.0

and a sucking chest wound. Owing to the large amounts of gas that may be present, pneumothorax is particularly important. As can be seen from table 88, 750 cc. of air in the pleural cavity at sea level would almost double in volume at 15,000 feet. The result of this might be an excessive collapse of the involved lung and a marked shift of the mediastinum and its contents to the opposite side with its consequences. A second factor is that this increased pressure also tends to expand and elevate the thoracic cage to a position of inspiration which may interfere with this latter function to some extent by decreasing the tidal air (5). If adhesions are present tension on them will cause pain and it may cause them to rupture.

The danger of flying patients with a pneumothorax is related to both the amount of air in the pleural cavity and the altitude. Most any of these cases can be safely flown at altitudes up to 5000 feet and all of them up to 15,000 feet if the amount of gas is minimal. Certain of these patients can be prepared for flight by removing some or all of the air just prior to the trip. Dowd (6) has reported one death as a result of a pneumothorax patient flying at an altitude of 16,000 feet. On the other hand, hundreds of such patients have been flown at or below 10,000 feet altitude with few or no ill effects such as the 19 cases reported on by Downey and Strickland (4).

Cases of mediastinal emphysema and sucking wounds of the chest should be evaluated in the same manner as described above for pneumothorax.

Gastrointestinal Disorders

At the higher altitudes, large unsupported hernias may become distended and strangulate. Patients with colostomies should be advised that their colostomy bag will tend to fill rapidly during ascent and that it ought to be emptied just before departure time or disposable bags utilized. Patients with appendicitis or with deeply eroded peptic ulcers or other serious weaknesses of the gastrointestinal wall may be endangered by expansion of the contained gases, especially if the latter are present initially in more than normal amounts.

In patients who have penetrating wounds

of the gastrointestinal tract or perforated ulcers of the stomach or intestines the expansion of any contained gas may have serious results inasmuch as part of the gas will be forced out of the gastrointestinal tract and carry fecal material into the peritoneal cavity. Likewise, the expanded gas could place tension upon recently sutured wounds or incisions which might cause rupture with resulting peritonitis. A rectal tube and suction by the Wangensteen method may be used to an advantage in these cases to keep the intestines decompressed during flight. This type of suction can operate from a Venturi tube attached to the window of air evacuation aircraft.

Patients who, at ground level, are slightly uncomfortable from gas distension will generally begin to suffer actual pain after a few thousand feet of ascent and this becomes progressively worse if the ascent is continued. Certain of these patients may obtain relief by passing flatus but the very fact that they are suffering from distension makes it unlikely that this can be accomplished. Accordingly, such patients should not be subjected to altitude changes of more than a few thousand feet unless the distension can be relieved prior to flight. An individual with a diaphragmatic hernia may suffer pain as a result of ascent but no other complications in such cases have been reported.

Just as in the case of pulmonary disorders, the gastrointestinal cases described above have to be evaluated on an individual basis as to whether or not they can be evacuated by air which is true also for the entities to be described in the section to follow.

Miscellaneous

Air may be introduced into or around the tissues of the central nervous system as a result of therapeutic procedures or from injury or operative procedures. Such patients should not fly until all such gas has been absorbed since to do so would subject the patient to possible severe headache and nausea and vomiting.

Individuals who have collections of air or other gases in the muscles or subcutaneous tissues must be evaluated in terms of the individual situation. Where the gas is the result of disease, such as, for example, gas gangrene, then we must think not only of the increased mechanical pressure that will result with ascent but also consider the possibility of spreading the disease to the adjacent tissues.

Hypoxia

In dealing with both normal individuals and with patients it is important to remember that the oxygen dissociation curve of blood is not a straight line but a peculiar "S" shaped curve which is fairly flat along its first portion (see chapter 9). It is not until about 10,000 feet altitude that this curve begins turning downward rather rapidly and this explains why there is so little hypoxia in the normal individual at rest at 10,000 feet and why hypoxia develops at a much greater rate above that level as shown in table 88. A mild hypoxia that produces no obvious effects at rest may produce marked symptoms during mild or moderate activity so that patients should be cautioned in this regard. It should also be kept in mind that the body is normally capable of making certain limited physiologic adjustments to hypoxia, after a short period of time, which tends to offset the effects that would otherwise be produced. It is for these reasons that we are not overly concerned about hypoxia in the average patient up to 10,000 feet but are concerned above that level and recommend oxygen. This, however, does not solve our aeromedical problem in all cases owing to the fact that certain cardiovascular, pulmonary and other diseases alter this normal tolerance in an unfavorable way and it is these cases that require special consideration.

In administering oxygen to patients a tube should never be used, as it is not only highly inefficient and wasteful of oxygen but is extremely uncomfortable to hold in the mouth. In using a mask it should not only be well fitting but should cover both the nose and mouth so that either of these channels can be used for breathing. Another precaution is that patients should never be given oxygen intermittently. The reason for this is that it takes several minutes for the body to adjust to hypoxia and if oxygen is suddenly discontinued the hypoxic effect is temporarily much worse than if oxygen had not been used at all. Generally speaking it is not neces-

sary to give 100 per cent oxygen but only
enough to make up the deficit which at 18,000
feet means breathing enriched air with an
oxygen content of 42 per cent. On the other
hand higher percentages of oxygen than
necessary are harmless and it is best to err
on the high side. In addition, certain conditions would be benefited by a higher than
normal oxygen intake.

That hypoxia is not a frequent problem
among patients is indicated by the studies
of Strickland and Rafferty (7) and Downey
and Strickland (4). The former studied
16,020 military patients transported by air
and found that only 0.9 per cent of them
were given oxygen en route and that in many
cases it was administered as a prophylactic
measure rather than being a specific requirement. Seventy-nine per cent of all these
patients were flown at altitudes between
5000 and 10,000 feet and 3.5 per cent above
10,000 feet. The cases were mixed in type
and represented almost 1000 different diag-
noses.

The study by Downey and Strickland is
even more interesting and significant in that
their report deals exclusively with cardiac
and pulmonary patients' flights numbering
1777. All of these patients were flown at an
altitude of 10,000 feet or less except 84 of
them who flew above that level. In this series
there were 464 flights of patients with cardiac
disease only 4 of whom, or less than 1 per
cent, had symptoms related to his primary
disease. There were 568 flights of patients
with pulmonary disorders, other than tuberculosis, of whom 2.4 per cent had mild symptoms related to their disorder. The cases of
tuberculosis and its complications numbered
745 patient flights with mild or moderate
related symptoms in 2.7 per cent of these
cases. In neither of the series mentioned
above was there a death, the great majority
of the relatively few symptoms exhibited
were mild and in no case was there any deleterious after effects. A point of major significance in the tuberculosis series was that
those flown above 10,000 feet altitude had
over twice the incidence of symptoms when
compared to those flown below that level.

Pulmonary Disorders

Patients with poliomyelitis, neurotoric gas
poisoning, meningitis, encephalitis, Guillain-
Barre syndrome, head injury, tetanus or
botulism may have an acute or residual
respiratory insufficiency as one of their complications. The task of moving such patients
by any means is a formidable procedure (8)
and this will not be described here except
to say a word concerning the use of oxygen
in such cases. The point to be made is that
if, through the use of a respirator or other
means, the ventilation of these patients is
normal then their reaction to altitude will
be normal. On the other hand, at any altitude, including sea level, oxygen is never a
substitute for respiratory insufficiency for as
long as the ventilation remains inadequate
the patient's condition will deteriorate and
he will eventually suffer irreversible central
nervous tissue damage, pulmonary complications or both. Respiratory patients with
greatly reduced vital capacities may show
varying degrees of hypoxia at fairly low altitudes or even at sea level. These include
pneumothorax, empyema, lobectomies, thoracic tumors or injuries, partial obstructions
of the air passages, emphysema, fibrosis,
bronchospasm, atelectasis and consolidation
of the lung from pneumonia or other causes.
These patients will, of course, have a lowered
tolerance to the hypoxia of altitude and accordingly must be given oxygen at whatever
altitude is indicated in the individual case.
In this connection it should be remembered
that hypoxia at 12,000 feet altitude normally
produces little or no increase in respiratory
rate but does increase the depth of respiration by 20 to 100 per cent. Patients with
acute pulmonary edema or in status asth-
maticus should not be transported and bronchial asthma cases should be evacuated between and not during attacks. Inasmuch as
apprehension may be a factor in inducing an
attack in the latter these patients should be
sedated.

Cardiovascular Disorders

Over the years a number of crew members
and passengers have had heart attacks during flight but in none of these cases has there
been any evidence that flying was either the
immediate or remote cause of the attack.
In addition, those who first studied the effects of altitude on cardiac cases were greatly
surprised at the amount of tolerance exhibited by these patients. Although these find-

ings make it possible for most all cardiovascular patients to travel, or be evacuated, by air each case must be evaluated on an individual basis.

As has been stated previously patients with severe angina pectoris or coronary occlusion should not be evacuated by air until 60 or more days following the last attack. Milder cases of angina pectoris may fly between attacks but oxygen should be available and used if symptoms develop. Mild to moderate congestive failure cases are transportable on a stretcher and the same applies to patients with decompensated valvular heart disease with oxygen being administered as necessary. Hypertension cases have a normal tolerance to hypoxia but at from 4000 to 10,000 feet altitude may exhibit the normal response of an initial moderate increase in pulse rate and blood pressure which soon tends to return to normal. Accordingly, such patients tolerate flying very well except that if prodromal symptoms of stroke are present they should not fly.

In addition to hypoxia, moderate to severe cardiac cases should be protected against an attack of air sickness, insofar as that is possible, and if they are apprehensive they should be sedated. As a rule of thumb it is generally considered safe for a cardiac patient to fly on the commercial airlines if he is ambulatory and does not have dyspnea on mild exertion.

Patients with severe anemia should not fly but if it is moderate or mild they may do so if oxygen is used as necessary. This applies not only to the primary anemias but also to those produced by such things as shock, head injury and recent hemorrhage. Leukemia cases may be flown but in the more serious cases a preflight transfusion may be advisable and oxygen should be available.

Miscellaneous Conditions

Congenital heart conditions and lung atresias are not ordinarily contraindications to flight. Infants below 10 days of age have an unstable respiratory mechanism and should not be exposed to more than mild degrees of hypoxia and it must be remembered that to supply oxygen to these cases requires a special oxygen mask. Although older persons have as good or a better tolerance to hypoxia

than younger ones this is generally not true of those suffering from the general debility of old age. There is a tendency for epilepsy to manifest itself at altitude but there are no other adverse effects in these cases.

Pregnant women may fly without question, the only problem being the possibility that they may go into labor during the journey. The commercial airlines usually accept all such cases within the first 8 months of pregnancy provided there is no history of premature birth or habitual abortion in multiparous passengers. Some airlines will accept pregnancy cases during the ninth month if furnished a statement from the attending obstetrician that the patient is not due to deliver within 72 hours of the scheduled arrival time.

Discussion

In many cases the question of whether a patient should travel by air or by other means is far from being a purely academic matter. Air evacuation can be life saving and in almost all cases the patient can be expected to arrive at his destination by air in better condition than would otherwise be the case. Inasmuch as this is so the attending physician has just as much responsibility for prescribing any such benefits to a patient as he does to prescribe antibiotics where necessary. Also, just as is the case of antibiotics, the physician has to know the limitations and potential hazards involved in air evacuation and be prepared to advise the patient accordingly, either as to the prophylactic procedures and precautions to be employed or to forbid such travel if indicated. In brief, air evacuation should be looked upon as a therapeutic measure and a thorough understanding of its employment should be a part of the armamentarium of every practicing physician in this air age.

REFERENCES

(1) Guilford, F. R., and Soboroff, B. J.: Air evacuation: an historical review. J. Aviation Med., 18: 601–616, 1947.
(2) May, S. H.: Air travel and the cardiac patient. Am. Heart J., 40: 363–368, 1950.
(3) Friedberg, C. K.: Diseases of the Heart. Philadelphia, W. B. Saunders Co., 1949, p. 392.
(4) Downey, V. M., and Strickland, B. A.: Air transportation of cardiac and pulmonary patients. Ann. Int. Med., 36: 525, 1951.

(5) SMEDAL, H. A.: Air transportation of persons
    with cardio-respiratory disease and/or in-
    jury. J. Aviation Med., 23: 33–37, 1952.
(6) DOWD, K. E.: Report of death of passen-
    ger under treatment by pneumothorax. J.
    Aviation Med., 16: 346–349, 1945.
(7) STRICKLAND, B. A., JR., AND RAFFERTY, J. A.:

    Effects of air transportation on clinical con-
    ditions, an analysis of 16,020 cases reported
    in 1949. J. A. M. A., 145: 129–133, 1951.
(8) WILSON, H. T.: Air transportation of patients
    with poliomyelitis, experience with 193
    respirator cases. J. Aviation Med., 29: 27–32,
    1958.

29

AERIAL HYGIENE AND SANITATION

Hugh W. Randel, M.D.

Keeping pace with the expansion of aviation in all its phases, military and civilian passenger aircraft have undergone dramatic increases in the number of persons transported and the proportion of the earth's surface covered by their operations. With this greatly expanded service, air travel to most parts of the world has now become commonplace. In the 20 year period from 1937 to 1957 the annual number of air travelers on scheduled flights throughout the world increased from 2,500,000 to 90,000,000 persons (1). In the course of this expansion the location of airports has been determined primarily by technical and operational considerations, such as weather and terrain, with health and medical factors considered only secondarily or overlooked entirely. Whereas surface transportation has usually developed along well established routes with stops at larger ports or inland cities, airports have often been built at remote sites in sparsely populated areas lacking facilities conducive to health. In international civilian and military flying operations, therefore, many areas are transited where facilities and standards of sanitation are primitive or at least substandard. Functioning under these less than optimal conditions, the professional flyer must nevertheless maintain a maximum level of personal health and fitness to guarantee the efficient and safe operation of the air-

craft. With the annual increase of man hours in the air for both passengers and crew, more and more attention must be given to the protection of human health in flight and at route stops. To this end this chapter is concerned with the application of the principles of preventive medicine to safeguard man in this new dimension of his environment.

GLOBAL DISSEMINATION OF DISEASE BY AIRCRAFT

Travel has always been a major factor in the propagation of disease and disease vectors throughout the world. Mass migrations have invariably disturbed the ecology of disease to produce epidemics and invasion of new geographic areas. The world's trade lanes have been the traditional invasion routes of smallpox, cholera, plague and yellow fever for centuries. The coming of the airplane as a major means of transportation has threatened to accelerate this phenomenon. The primary difference between the threat of disease dissemination by aviation and the risk from surface transport is in the speed of travel. An air passenger, having been exposed to any of the world's diseases, may travel to many major cities of the world within a few hours. Not only is the rate of person to person contacts vastly increased but mixing of people from different geographic areas and different cultures presents a new threat for those living in the more highly developed parts of the world.

Such persons, having been shielded from their environment by modern preventive medicine, have thus been protected from infectious diseases so prevalent elsewhere. In this way the process of natural selection wherein man develops immunity through exposure has been disturbed. Persons from these protected environments, lacking the natural immunity developed by populations in less sanitary areas, are brought rapidly into contact with infection by air travel. In surface travel, because of the time involved, incubating illness is often revealed before the end of the voyage, whereas aircraft can travel vast distances within the incubation periods of the major epidemic diseases. Countries far from the source of exotic infections, and, hence, having a susceptible population, may become infected by apparently healthy persons entering during the incubation period. Thus, the movement of people and their goods rapidly and frequently from widely separated parts of the world has produced new potentials for disease dissemination with corresponding demands for new methods of control.

Dissemination via Infected Persons

Known instances of the transmission of disease by infected persons on international flights are shown in table 89. Of the international quarantinable diseases only smallpox has been definitely documented as being spread by air traffic. Considering the current number of air travelers, transmission of infection from person to person as a result of international flights would be expected in proportion to the incidence of each particular disease in the traveling public. Therefore, transmission by air travelers of such ubiquitous infections as those of the respiratory and gastrointestinal systems must be exceedingly common. The exact source of infection of diseases with long and variable incubation periods is rarely determined. When persons who have recently traveled by air succumb to such infections the relationship of the disease to the trip is usually not recognized. In 1957, however, during the investigation of an explosive epidemic of infectious hepatitis, dissemination of the

disease by air to five different geographic areas was demonstrated. Military personnel from an air base in northern France carried the disease to such widely separated points as Izmir, Turkey, Sculthorpe, England, Brooklyn, New York, Fort Leavenworth, Kansas and Clovis, New Mexico after exposure in France.

Dissemination via Arthropods

Arthropods are constantly being dispersed to various parts of the world by surface transportation and many instances are known in which the distribution range of species has been extended in this way. Such accidental transportation of arthropods may affect the international spread of disease either by introducing new diseases via infected vectors or by introducing new vectors which become implanted in a territory thus accelerating the transmission of a disease already present. Before the advent of air travel a significant obstacle to the introduction of arthropods was the relatively long time required for international voyages. The short life cycle of many species did not permit them to survive long ocean voyages. With air transportation, however, great distances are now crossed in brief periods so that even short lived species can easily survive the journey. One of the earliest records of insects being accidentally transported from one country to another by aircraft was in flowers carried by passengers aboard the dirigible "Graf Zeppelin" which crossed the Atlantic from Germany to the United States in 1928 (11). Since then large numbers of arthropods have been collected from aircraft arriving at airports all over the world. Table 90 shows the per cent of aircraft on which arthropods were found by four different investigators in different countries (12).

Authenticated instances of insects becoming established in new areas as a result of their transportation by surface vessels are numerous. Most of these species implantations have concerned pests or species of economic rather than medical importance. A striking example of implantation of a medically important species is that of *Anopheles gambiae*, a highly efficient malaria vector of Africa. In 1930 this mosquito was accidentally introduced into South America by ship traffic from West Africa, multiplied rapidly and spread over a vast area of Brazil. This mosquito, with its preference for human blood, was a much more dangerous carrier than the anophelines indigenous to Brazil. This stimulus to transmission of the disease resulted in thousands of malaria deaths before *Anopheles gambiae* was eradicated from Brazil. Thus, arthropods with special capacity as disease vectors may be introduced and become established in territories where only relatively feeble vectors had previously existed. Despite the recognized hazard of introduction of vectors by aircraft few such instances have actually been reported.

Although the effect of the aircraft environment on arthropods is considerably less than optimal, many species, rendered temporarily inactive on long flights owing to cold, vibration and diminished atmospheric pressure, quickly become active and capable of reproduction after landing. By placing marked specimens aboard aircraft traveling from Latin America to the United States, Griffitts has shown that *Aedes aegypti* survived and remained aboard aircraft for almost 80 hours during which multiple stops were made and a peak altitude of 14,000 feet was reached (13). Specimens of *Anopheles gambiae* in test tubes sent by air from French Sudan to Marseilles deposited eggs in France which subsequently produced at least two more generations (14). Representative specimens of most of the important families of insects as well as spiders and ticks have been recovered in the course of aircraft inspections. Approximately 20 different species of anopheline mosquitoes, as well as vectors of yellow fever, dengue, Bancroft's filariasis, Brazilian spotted fever, Kenya tick typhus, Boutonneuse fever, Japanese B encephalitis, St. Louis encephalitis, Gambian trypanosomiasis and onchocerciasis have been taken from aircraft.

Much attention has been given to the possible aircraft introduction of yellow fever infected mosquitoes into areas such as India and Pakistan where the disease does not occur. Although this possibility must be recognized, the habits of *Aedes aegypti* do not favor its frequent entrance into aircraft. With its limited flight range and tendency to remain in and near houses it does not often find its way into aircraft at large international airports. Very few specimens of this insect have been found in thousands of aircraft inspections in the United States and elsewhere. Another apparent threat of introduction of a dangerous vector exists in many islands of the Pacific region where no anopheline mosquitoes now occur. Although highly endemic in Indonesia, the Philippine Islands and the Southwest Pacific, malaria is not known throughout a vast area of the Central and South Pacific because of the absence of the anopheline vector. No explanation for the lack of anophelines in these apparently favorable areas has been found.

Dissemination via Rodents

Dissemination of diseases such as plague, tularemia, salmonellosis and leptospirosis by the transportation of infected rodents aboard aircraft does not appear to be a hazard of great magnitude although ships are well known to have played a major role in the world-wide dissemination of plague *via* infected rats. Aircraft, under the usual conditions of their operation, offer relatively little attraction or harborage to rodents. As a rule rats which enter parked aircraft are soon discovered because of the relatively small space and lack of opportunity for concealment. The most immediate concern in such rodent infestations is for flying safety, as rats may endanger the structure and operation of the aircraft by gnawing the insulation of wire and cables.

Notwithstanding the favorable past record of aviation in international quarantine it is obvious that adequate disease control measures must continue to be devised and applied to keep pace with the rapid increase in air transportation. For certain diseases, such as smallpox and yellow fever, the problem has been partially solved by immunization whereas for other diseases reliance is placed on medical inspection, disinsectization and deratting. The present world-wide standard for quarantine practices is contained in the International Sanitary Regulations which came into effect in 1952.

THE INTERNATIONAL SANITARY REGULATIONS

The International Sanitary Regulations in force today are the result of an evolutionary

TABLE 89

Dissemination of Disease via Infected Persons on International Flights

Disease	Date	Place of Origin	Place of Arrival	Secondary Cases	Remarks	References
1. Smallpox	February, 1946	Morocco	Marseilles, France	8 at Arras, France; 1 death	A French soldier became ill en route by air from Morocco to France. On arrival he was treated for malaria and continued his journey by rail. At his home in Arras, France, his illness was mistakenly diagnosed as varicella	(2)
2. Smallpox	1947	Japan and Korea	Seattle and San Francisco, U. S. A.	81; 20 deaths	The disease was introduced by military personnel returning to the U. S. A. by both aircraft and ship	(3)
3. Smallpox	1951	Karachi, Pakistan	England	28; 10 deaths	Introduced by an R.A.F. officer returning from Karachi. Because of the mildness of the disease in this previously vaccinated patient the correct diagnosis was not made until many persons had been exposed. Three cases occurred among employees of a laundry where the officer's clothes were sent	(4)
4. Smallpox	1952	Cambodia	Brunehamel (Aisne), France	30; 2 deaths		(5)
5. Smallpox	March 1957	West Africa	London, England	6; 2 deaths		(6)
6. Smallpox	April 1957	New Delhi, India	Naples, Italy	6; 1 death	The primary case occurred in a traveller with a valid international certificate of smallpox vaccination. The attending physician who recognized the disease was vaccinated but died of smallpox before immunity could develop. Approximately 1,200,000 persons in the vicinity of Naples were vaccinated	(7)

7. Influenza (Asian strain, A/Singapore/1/57)	May 1957	Singapore, Malaya	Victoria, Australia	Undetermined	Influenza appeared among air passengers who arrived in Australia from Singapore. This was followed by a fairly sharp outbreak in the state of Victoria	(8)
8. Influenza (Asian strain, A/Singapore/1/57)	June 1957	Djakarta, Indonesia	The Hague, Netherlands	Undetermined	As this strain of influenza was introduced into Europe from multiple sources it was not possible to determine the number of secondary cases resulting from this particular introduction	(8)
9. Typhoid	1947	Anchorage, Alaska	Seattle, Washington, U. S. A.	4	Four cases in air travellers resulted from contaminated food eaten aboard a commercial aircraft. Source of infection was a typhoid carrier employed in a restaurant where meals were prepared for the flight	(9)
10. Bacillary dysentery (Shigella paradysenteriae) Flexner type II	1948	Okinawa	Honolulu, Hawaii, and Spokane, Washington, U. S. A.	5 in military personnel at Spokane	An outbreak of bacillary dysentery as the result of contaminated water and ice began in a U. S. Air Force Bombardment Group just as the unit departed from Okinawa in B-29 aircraft for the United States. One-hundred and twenty aircrew members were hospitalized in Honolulu and Spokane. Although most of the patients were infected in Okinawa, Shigella organisms were also isolated from the drinking water supply of one of the aircraft	(10)

TABLE 90

Insects Collected from Aircraft Completing
International Flights

Country of Arrival	Number of Aircraft Searched	Number of Aircraft with Insects	Percentage of Aircraft with Insects	Authority
Kenya	196	57	29.6	Symes, 1935
U. S. A.	398	187	47.0	Welch, 1939
U. S. A.	80,716	28,752	35.6	Hughes, 1949
New Zealand	246	88	35.8	Laird, 1951
New Zealand	343	111	32.4	Laird, 1952

process which began several hundred years ago with the earliest efforts to control the spread of communicable diseases among travelers. For many years these control measures, based on the prevailing beliefs of the time regarding the epidemiology of disease were unscientific, unreasonable and generally ineffective. Since the first international conference on quarantine in Paris in 1851 the steady increase in world commerce and expanding knowledge of disease transmission have led to numerous international sanitary conventions. Most of these were convened to deal with specific problems of the moment involving cholera, plague or yellow fever. As such, each one involved relatively few countries and none entirely replaced the preceding conventions. This resulted in multiple, complicated and overlapping agreements causing great difficulty and confusion in international traffic.

The growth of commercial aviation created a further need for special regulations applicable to aircraft. The International Sanitary Convention for Aerial Navigation, signed at the Hague in 1933, was specifically designed to apply to the conditions of air travel. Although amended in Montreal in 1944, this convention became increasingly inadequate for its purpose as the volume and extent of air travel increased.

The present International Sanitary Regulations, adopted by the Fourth World Health Assembly on 25 May 1951, revised and consolidated the provisions of all previous international sanitary conventions and arrangements. These regulations, becoming effective on 1 October 1952, replaced all of the 13 treaties and similar international agreements

then in force except the Pan-American Sanitary Code. Based on all the earlier conventions as well as current knowledge of disease control these regulations were drafted to give all countries the maximum protection against the introduction of disease with the least interference with world traffic. They have now been accepted by 160 states and territories. The following basic principles of international quarantine practice were taken into account in framing the provisions of the regulations:

1. Every quarantine control measure, no matter how slight, constitutes some interference with the free flow of traffic.

2. Even the most severe quarantine restrictions do not offer complete security against disease introduction and if unusually severe may only lead to subterfuge or evasion by travelers.

3. An effective public health service with prompt reporting of disease and a high level of environmental sanitation provides much better protection for a country or territory than a mass of quarantine restrictions.

Besides protecting the health of international travelers the regulations prevent their being subjected to unnecessary and unreasonable restrictions. The term *medical examination* as used in the regulations refers to visits or inspections of aircraft or preliminary examination of persons on board. Health authorities may perform medical examinations of any person or aircraft on an international voyage, making any inquiries necessary to ascertain the state of health of persons or the sanitary condition of aircraft. The regulations apply specifically to persons and aircraft in transit and refer only to the six international quarantinable diseases—smallpox, plague, cholera, yellow fever, typhus and relapsing fever. Immigrants or travelers remaining in a country are, of course, subject to the national laws of the country. Sanitary measures which may be carried out by health authorities under the regulations with respect to each of these six diseases are summarized in table 91. Although it is recognized that many other diseases may be spread by air travel, the regulations limit the sanitary measures to be taken against them because they do not presently lend themselves to effective international quarantine procedures.

TABLE 91

Control of the Quarantinable Diseases in International Air Traffic
(Provisions of the International Sanitary Regulations)*

Disease	Immunizations Required	Control Measures Applicable by Health Authorities to Persons	Control Measures Applicable by Health Authorities to Aircraft, Baggage and Cargo
Smallpox	Valid vaccination, certificate or sufficient evidence of protection by a previous attack of smallpox, Revaccination every 3 years	1. On arrival from any area: a. *Vaccination* of persons lacking a valid vaccination certificate or sufficient evidence of protection by a previous attack of smallpox b. *Surveillance* for 14 days (incubation period) of such persons who refuse vaccination 2. On arrival from an infected local area or aboard an infected aircraft: a. *Vaccination* followed by *surveillance* of 14 days of persons lacking a valid vaccination certificate or sufficient evidence of protection, by a previous attack of smallpox b. *Isolation* for maximum of 14 days of persons who refuse vaccination	1. On arrival of an infected aircraft: *Disinfection of baggage*, equipment or any part of the aircraft
Cholera	Valid vaccination certificate for persons arriving from infected local areas. Revaccination every 6 months	1. On arrival from an infected local area: a. *Surveillance* for 5 days (incubation period) of persons with valid vaccination certificates b. *Isolation* for 5 days of persons without valid vaccination certificates c. *Stool examination* of any person having symptoms of cholera 2. On arrival of an infected aircraft: a. *Surveillance* for 5 days of persons with valid vaccination certificates b. *Isolation* for 5 days of persons without valid vaccination certificates	1. On arrival of an infected aircraft: a. *Disinfection* of baggage of suspects or any part of the aircraft b. *Disinfection* and *removal* of aircraft drinking water, waste water or human dejecta on board the aircraft 2. On arrival of an infected or suspected aircraft: a. *Removal* and *disposal* of beverages and fish, shellfish, fruit or vegetables to be consumed raw unless such are in sealed containers, *or* b. *Prohibition of unloading* of such fruits or vegetables
Plague	None required	1. On arrival of an infected aircraft: *Disinfecting* followed by *surveillance* for 6 days (incubation period) of any suspect 2. On arrival of a healthy aircraft from an infected local area: *Surveillance* of suspects for 6 days	1. On arrival of an infected aircraft: *Disinsecting* and *Disinfection* of baggage, equipment or any part of the aircraft 2. *Deratting* of aircraft under exceptional circumstances when the presence of rodents is suspected

TABLE 91—*Continued*

Disease	Immunizations Required	Control Measures Applicable by Health Authorities to Persons	Control Measures Applicable by Health Authorities to Aircraft, Baggage and Cargo
		3. Prior to departure from a local area where there is an epidemic of *pulmonary* plague: *Isolation* of suspects for 6 days	
Yellow fever	Valid vaccination certificate prior to departure for persons leaving an infected local area for a yellow fever receptive area. Revaccination every 6 years	1. When proceeding from an infected local area to a yellow fever receptive area: a. Prior to departure—*vaccination* b. On arrival—*vaccination*, if not already accomplished, followed by *isolation* for a maximum of 6 days (incubation period)	1. When proceeding from an infected local area to a yellow fever receptive area: a. Prior to departure—*disinsecting* 2. When proceeding from an airport where *Aedes aegypti* exists to an airport where *Aedes aegypti* has been eradicated: a. Prior to departure—*disinsecting* 3. On arrival of an infected or suspected aircraft—*disinsecting* 4. On arrival of a healthy aircraft from an infected local area—*disinsecting*
Typhus	None required	1. Prior to departure from an infected local area—*disinsecting* 2. On arrival from an infected local area—*disinsecting* followed by *surveillance* for 14 days (incubation period)	1. Prior to departure from an infected local area—*disinsecting* and *disinfection* 2. On arrival from an infected local area—*disinsecting* and *disinfection*
Relapsing fever	None required	Same measures as for typhus except that the period of *surveillance* shall be 8 days (incubation period)	Same measures as for typhus

* This table is a general summary only. For detailed provisions the reader is referred to the *International Sanitary Regulations*, Geneva, World Health Organization, 1957.

Sanitary Airports and Direct Transit Areas

Under the regulations the health administration of each country or territory designates certain of its airports as *sanitary airports*. Each airport so designated will have at its disposal the following personnel, equipment and facilities:

1. A supply of pure drinking water.
2. An organized medical service with adequate staff, equipment and premises.
3. Facilities for transport, isolation and care of infected persons or suspects.
4. Facilities for efficient disinfection and disinsectization, for the destruction of rodents and for any other appropriate measure provided for by the regulations.
5. A bacteriologic laboratory or facilities for dispatching suspected material to such a laboratory.
6. Facilities for vaccination against cholera, yellow fever and smallpox.

Besides these provisions further specific measures are outlined for control of *Aedes aegypti*, the mosquito vector of urban yellow fever. In order that the area within the perimeter of every airport is kept free of this mosquito in its larval and adult stages, active mosquito control measures must be maintained within a protective area extending for at least 400 meters around the perimeter. Throughout the world 199 airports have been designated as sanitary airports.

Special direct transit areas with accommodations for segregating transient travelers are established in connection with international airports. These areas, approved and directly supervised by the health authority concerned, are for the use of passengers and aircrews who are passing through the airport without leaving the vicinity. Their primary purpose is to avoid the health hazards associated with the mingling of transients with the local population. Mosquito proofing of all buildings used for direct transit personnel accommodations in yellow fever infected areas is mandatory. In addition, buildings should have facilities for serving food and have toilets and washrooms. As of 1957, 30 airports in 19 countries were provided with direct transit areas.

Sanitary Documents

With respect to sanitary documents several important improvements in the facilitation of international air traffic were made with the adoption of the International Sanitary Regulations. Requirements for Bills of Health and Personal Declarations of Origin and Health were eliminated and provision was made for the International Certificates of Vaccination. No sanitary documents other than the following are to be required in international traffic.

THE HEALTH PART OF THE AIRCRAFT GENERAL DECLARATION. The pilot of an aircraft landing at an international airport is required to give information in the Health Part of the Aircraft General Declaration concerning details of disinsectization or sanitary treatment performed, illness of passengers or crew and any condition occurring during the flight which may lead to the spread of disease.

PRATIQUE. A plane arriving at an international airport is considered to be in quarantine until a pratique or permission to communicate has been issued by the airport authorities. A free pratique admits the aircraft to the airport where passengers and freight are discharged without further quarantine restrictions. A radio pratique is usually granted to scheduled transport aircraft giving them advance clearance by radio to proceed directly in to the airport.

INTERNATIONAL CERTIFICATES OF VACCINATION. One of the major advances of the regulations was the adoption of the International Certificates of Vaccination (figs. 148 to 151) as a standardized form for recording immunizations. This document is designed primarily for recording smallpox, cholera and yellow fever immunizations with additional space for other vaccinations which may be administered to the traveler. These certificates are used to document all inoculations and other local forms or private physicians' certificates are not acceptable. International certificates must be signed personally by a physician although actual vaccination may be performed by properly qualified nurses or technicians under the supervision of the physician. Certificates must be completed in English or French and each entry must be stamped with an official stamp prescribed by the health authority of the country where vaccination is performed. If a physician considers vaccination to be medically contraindicated he should furnish the traveler with a written statement to this effect outlining the pertinent medical facts. This does not, however, guarantee excusal from the requirements of the regulations. The final decision as to waiver of an immunization requirement is the prerogative of local health authorities.

THE INTERNATIONAL QUARANTINABLE DISEASES

Plague

The plague bacillus, *Pasteurella pestis*, is primarily a pathogen of rodents, producing epidemics in the latter which serve as the reservoir for the human outbreaks that occur accidentally under circumstances favorable to transmission. Two ecologic types of the disease are known in rodents. In urban plague the rodent hosts are species of commensal rats and the usual vector is the Oriental rat flea, *Xenopsylla cheopis*. In sylvatic

OTHER IMMUNIZATIONS (Typhus, Typhoid-Paratyphoid, Plague, Tetanus, etc.)
AUTRES IMMUNISATIONS (Typhus, Fièvre typhoïde et paratyphoïde, Peste, Tétanos, etc.)

Vaccine

Date

Dose

Physician's signature—Signature du médecin

INTERNATIONAL CERTIFICATES OF
VACCINATION

AS APPROVED BY

THE WORLD HEALTH ORGANIZATION

CERTIFICATS INTERNATIONAUX DE VACCINATION
APPROUVES PAR
L'ORGANISATION MONDIALE DE LA SANTE

TRAVELER'S NAME—Nom du voyageur

ADDRESS   (Number—Numéro)   (Street—Rue)
ADRESSE

(City—Ville)

(County—Département)   (State—État)

U. S. DEPARTMENT OF
HEALTH, EDUCATION, AND WELFARE
PUBLIC HEALTH SERVICE

FOR SALE BY SUPERINTENDENT OF DOCUMENTS
GOVERNMENT PRINTING OFFICE—WASHINGTON 25, D. C.
$2.50 PER 100

PHS 731
Rev. 1–57

FIG. 148

plague the hosts are a wide variety of wild rodents with the infection being transmitted by their fleas. Infection results from the bite of infected fleas or less commonly from contamination of the broken skin by infected flea feces. Under normal circumstances man has little contact with wild rodents so that human outbreaks of sylvatic plague are not usually extensive. Even though infection in wild rodents is widespread, the greatest threat to man occurs when the disease spreads from the wild rodent population to domestic rats. Spread of plague from one geographic area to another has occurred most often by infected rats aboard ships. The world incidence of plague has declined dramatically from 15,399 cases in 1951 to only 514 cases in 1957 (15).

The threat of aircraft importation by infected rodents, persons or fleas, although considerably less than for surface transportation, must still be recognized in considering international quarantine measures. The primary antiplague measures in international air travel are directed at control of the disease in rodents and their fleas and at preventing them from infesting airports and boarding aircraft. Measures which may be applied by health authorities against plague are summarized in table 91. *Pulmonary plague*, being highly infectious and readily transmitted from person to person by the respiratory route, requires special preventive measures. Plague vaccination, although worth-while in protecting individuals from the effects of the disease, is not effective in international control and has been given no importance as a quarantine measure. The regulations specify that vaccination shall not be required as a condition of admission of any person to a territory.

INTERNATIONAL CERTIFICATE OF VACCINATION OR REVACCINATION AGAINST SMALLPOX
CERTIFICAT INTERNATIONAL DE VACCINATION OU DE REVACCINATION CONTRE LA VARIOLE

This is to certify that   sex

Je soussigné(e) certifie que _____ sexe _____

whose signature follows   date of birth

dont la signature suit _____ né(e) le _____

has on the date indicated been vaccinated or revaccinated against smallpox.

a été vacciné(e) ou revacciné(e) contre la variole à la date indiquée.

Date	Indicate by "X" whether Indiquer par "X" s'il s'agit de	Signature, professional status, and address of vaccinator Signature, qualité professionnelle, et adresse du vaccinateur	Approved stamp Cachet d'authentification
	1a Primary vaccination performed Primovaccination effectuée }☐		1a
	1b Read as successful }☐ Prise Unsuccessful }*☐ Pas de prise		1b
	2 ☐ Revaccination		2
	3 ☐ Revaccination		3

THE VALIDITY OF THIS CERTIFICATE shall extend for a period of 3 years, beginning 8 days after the date of a successful primary vaccination or, in the event of a revaccination, on the date of that revaccination.

The approved stamp mentioned above must be in a form prescribed by the health administration of the country in which the vaccination is performed. **(In the United States, the stamp is that of the local or State health department of the area in which the immunizing physician practices,** the Department of Defense, a designated yellow fever vaccination center, the seal of the Public Health Service, or the special "S–C" stamp approved by the latter service.)

Any amendment of this certificate, or erasure, or failure to complete any part of it, may render it invalid.

LA VALIDITÉ DE CE CERTIFICAT couvre une période de trois ans commençant huit jours après la date de la primovaccination effectuée avec succès (prise) ou, dans le cas d'une revaccination, le jour de cette revaccination.

Le cachet d'authentification doit être conforme au modèle prescrit par l'administration sanitaire du territoire où la vaccination est effectuée. (Aux États Unis ce cachet doit être celui du Service d'Hygiène, de l'état, de la ville ou du comté où le vaccinateur exerce la médecine du Département de la Défense, d'un centre désigné de vaccination contre la fièvre jaune, le sceau du Service de la Santé Publique des États Unis, ou le timbre spécial "S–C" approuvé par ce service.)

Toute correction ou rature sur le certificat ou l'omission d'une quelconque des mentions qu'il comporte peut affecter sa validité.

*If unsuccessful, vaccination must be repeated and a new certificate executed.

Si la vaccination n'a pas prise, il faudra recommencer et un nouveau certificat devra être établi.

FIG. 149

INTERNATIONAL CERTIFICATE OF VACCINATION OR REVACCINATION AGAINST YELLOW FEVER

CERTIFICAT INTERNATIONAL DE VACCINATION OU DE REVACCINATION CONTRE LA FIÈVRE JAUNE

This is to certify that   sex
Je soussigné(e) certifie que _____ sexe _____

whose signature follows   date of birth
dont la signature suit ⋅_____ né(e) le _____

has on the date indicated been vaccinated or revaccinated against yellow fever.
a été vacciné(e) ou revacciné(e) contre la fièvre jaune à la date indiquée.

Date	Signature and professional status of vaccinator / Signature et qualité professionnelle du vaccinateur	Origin and batch number of vaccine / Origine du vaccin employé et numéro du lot	Official stamp of vaccinating center / Cachet officiel du centre de vaccination

VACCINATING CENTER
CENTRE DE VACCINATION

ADDRESS   (CITY—VILLE)   (STATE—ÉTAT)
ADRESSE

THIS CERTIFICATE IS VALID only if the vaccine used has been approved by the World Health Organization and if the vaccinating center has been designated by the health administration for the country in which that center is situated.

THE VALIDITY OF THIS CERTIFICATE shall extend for a period of 6 years, beginning 10 days after the date of vaccination **(for India, Pakistan, and Ceylon 12 days)** or, in the event of a revaccination, within such period of 6 years, from the date of that revaccination.

Any amendment of this certificate, or erasure, or failure to complete any part of it, may render it invalid.

CE CERTIFICAT N'EST VALABLE que si le vaccin employé a été approuvé par l'Organisation Mondiale de la Santé et si le centre de vaccination a été habilité par l'administration sanitaire du territoire dans lequel ce centre est situe.

LA VALIDITÉ DE CE CERTIFICAT couvre une période de six ans commençant dix jours après la date de la vaccination (pour l'Inde, Pakistan et Ceylan 12 jours) ou, dans le cas d'une revaccination au cours de cette période de six ans, le jour de cette revaccination.

Toute correction ou rature sur le certificat ou l'omission d'une quelconque des mentions qu'il comporte peut affecter sa validité.

U. S. GOVERNMENT PRINTING OFFICE : 1956—O—404968

FIG. 150

Cholera

Cholera provides a classic example of the spread of disease by international travel. Repeatedly during the 19th century this disease migrated along travel routes from its traditional home in India and Pakistan to North and South America, Africa, Asia and Europe. Since then, except for a spectacular epidemic in Egypt in 1947, the disease has been largely confined to Asia where it is steadily diminishing in importance.

Only about 60,000 cases of cholera were officially reported for the world in 1957, virtually all from India and East Pakistan. The improvement in standards of sanitation generally throughout the world is the major cause of this favorable trend. In the Egyptian epidemic, cholera failed to become established in any towns with adequate water and sewage systems even though the disease was repeatedly introduced into these towns from the surrounding villages. Although it

INTERNATIONAL CERTIFICATE OF VACCINATION OR REVACCINATION AGAINST CHOLERA
CERTIFICAT INTERNATIONAL DE VACCINATION OU DE REVACCINATION CONTRE LE CHOLÉRA

This is to certify that
Je soussigné(e) certifie que _____ sexe _____

whose signature follows
dont la signature suit _____ né(e) le _____

has on the date indicated been vaccinated or revaccinated against cholera.
a été vacciné(e) ou revacciné(e) contre le choléra à la date indiquée.

Date	Signature, professional status, and address of vaccinator / Signature, qualité professionnelle, et adresse du vaccinateur	Approved stamp / Cachet d'authentification

THE VALIDITY OF THIS CERTIFICATE shall extend for a period of 6 months, beginning 6 days after the first injection of the vaccine or, in the event of a revaccination within such period of 6 months on the date of that revaccination. (In the United States two injections are given for the initial series.)

The approved stamp mentioned above must be in a form prescribed by the health administration of the country in which the vaccination is performed. **(In the United States, the stamp is that of the local or State health department of the area in which the immunizing physician practices,** the Department of Defense, a designated yellow fever vaccination center, the seal of the Public Health Service, or the special "S-C" stamp approved by the latter service.)

Any amendment of this certificate, or erasure, or failure to complete any part of it, may render it invalid.

LA VALIDITÉ DE CE CERTIFICAT couvre une période de six mois commençant six jours après la première injection du vaccin ou, dans le cas d'une revaccination au cours de cette période de six mois, le jour de cette revaccination. (Aux États Unis deux injections sont données aux séries initiales.)

Le cachet d'authentification doit être conforme au modèle prescrit par l'administration sanitaire du territoire où la vaccination est effectuée. (Aux États Unis ce cachet doit être celui du Service d'Hygiène, de l'état, de la ville ou du comté où le vaccinateur exerce la médecine, du Département de la Défense, d'un centre désigné de vaccination contre la fièvre jaune, le sceau du Service de la Santé Publique des États Unis, ou le timbre spécial "S-C" approuvé par ce service.)

Toute correction ou rature sur le certificat ou l'omission d'une quelconque des mentions qu'il comporte peut affecter sa validité.

FIG. 151

seems unlikely that cholera will ever repeat its performance as a global epidemic disease, the lessons of the past are not to be disregarded. Some authorities in Egypt considered the 1947 epidemic to have been started by cholera infected troops returning by air from India. In the history of international quarantine, measures taken against cholera have been notably severe. Frontier stations manned by armed guards for washing, airing, fumigating and quarantining of travelers were not uncommon. Such drastic measures are not only unnecessary but tend to defeat the purpose of international quarantine agreements and to stimulate surreptitious border crossings with no sanitary control.

The provisions of the regulations for the

control of cholera are directed at the prevention of infection transmitted by means of water, food or infected excreta and vomitus. In addition to the anticholera measures summarized in Table 91, the regulations specify that certain useless and harassing anticholera procedures may not be invoked. For example, travelers are no longer required to submit to the taking of rectal swabs and the stopping or disinfecting of mail or newspapers is specifically prohibited. Although not as effective in cholera control as are environmental sanitation measures, vaccination is useful in preventing infection in exposed persons and so is taken into account in applying other preventive measures of the regulations.

Yellow Fever

For 200 years yellow fever was a constant scourge of West Africa, South America and the ports of the Caribbean. At frequent intervals during the 18th and 19th centuries it spread from these tropical regions along shipping routes from port to port as far as the southern United States and Europe. It was gradually eliminated from the western hemisphere by intensive anti-*Aedes aegypti* measures and it appeared that there would be no more yellow fever in the Americas as long as this vector was kept under control. By 1933, however, unexplained outbreaks had occurred in portions of South America where the *Aedes* mosquito did not exist and it was subsequently shown that yellow fever was being transmitted by mosquitoes other than *Aedes aegypti*. This was the first recognition of jungle yellow fever in which the virus is transmitted from wild monkeys to man by the bite of jungle mosquitoes of the genus *Haemagogus*. Although clinically and pathologically a single disease, yellow fever is now known to occur in two epidemiologically distinct forms. The designation of urban yellow fever refers to the disease in its classic epidemic form in which the virus is transmitted from man to man by the bite of the domestic mosquito *Aedes aegypti*. In jungle yellow fever, on the other hand, infections occur in persons who come in contact with *Haemagogus* mosquitoes inhabiting the forest canopy. Although it is not a major public health problem comparable to the urban form of the disease, jungle yellow fever is significant as a source of human infection and as a reservoir of the virus. Since 1948 a wave of jungle yellow fever beginning in Panama has spread steadily throughout Central America. By 1957 animal and human epidemics had carried the virus north to Guatemala and British Honduras within 70 miles of Mexico.

The principal importance of outbreaks of jungle yellow fever is the threat that the virus may be introduced into a community having a susceptible population and *Aedes aegypti* mosquitoes. Should this occur, wide spread outbreaks of the disease in its urban epidemic form could result. A puzzling epidemiologic phenomenon of significance in international quarantine is the continued absence of yellow fever from certain large areas of the world where climate and the biologic environment appear to be entirely suited to introduction of the virus. The fact that tropical Asia, which is well supplied with *Aedes* mosquitoes and millions of susceptible persons, has so far remained free of yellow fever, is still unexplained.

The preventive measures of the regulations against yellow fever, aside from immunization, are primarily directed at its transmission by *Aedes aegypti*. Specific precautions taken to prevent the entry of the virus in infected persons or infected mosquitoes are to be applied only upon entry into yellow fever receptive areas, *i.e.*, areas where the presence of vectors would permit the disease to develop if introduced. *Aedes aegypti* is found throughout the tropics and during the summer in many parts of the temperate zone including the southern third of the United States. Although all such areas must be regarded as receptive for yellow fever if the virus were introduced, the tropics are more vulnerable because of their favorable temperature ranges and the presence of large numbers of susceptible primates. This apparent vulnerability of tropical Asia has led to unusually strict enforcement of quarantine measures by such countries as India and Pakistan. Owing to the solidity and duration of immunity which follows immunization, travelers with valid vaccination certificates are exempt from all restrictions with reference to yellow fever. Inasmuch as the vaccine is not generally available to private physicians, yellow fever immunizations are given at specified centers designated by the health authority of each country.

Smallpox

The universal susceptibility of man to smallpox and its ease of transmission from person to person have made epidemics of this disease frequent sequelae of transportation and commerce. In addition to classic smallpox a clinically mild form of the disease known as variola minor is also recognized. From a public health standpoint and under the International Sanitary Regulations no distinction is made between these two clinical forms of the disease inasmuch as they are epidemiologically identical. Transmission is usually from person to person by direct contact or by respiratory discharges. A less frequent but important means of transmission is *via* articles such as clothing or bedding which have been used by infected persons. Articles contaminated by dried discharges or crusts may remain infectious for long periods while being transported from place to place. In 1954 the disease was introduced into France by an air traveler from Indochina who inadvertently imported the virus in contaminated pajamas which he had purchased in a market in Saigon (16). Ninety-four cases and 15 deaths occurred before the outbreak was controlled. Smallpox survives as an endemic disease in many parts of South America, Asia and Africa. Its rarity in recent years in many other parts of the world has sometimes led to a false sense of security. Because of lack of suspicion and unfamiliarity with the disease physicians frequently fail to diagnose smallpox in its early stages. Cases are especially likely to go unrecognized when seen in modified form in the partially immune patient. Table 89 lists several occasions on which smallpox has been spread from one country to another by air travel.

The only individual protective measure is revaccination periodically with full strength vaccine correctly administered to insure lasting immunity. Adults in the general population frequently fail to repeat vaccination under the misconception that they are still immune as a result of a childhood vaccina-

tion. Even though such partially immune persons may have only a mild attack they are capable of transmitting the disease in its most serious form. In countries where vaccination is widely practiced, smallpox epidemics may still occur as evidenced by the outbreak in 1947 in New York. Of the several million persons vaccinated at that time, thousands were shown to be susceptible to the disease as indicated by their reactions to immunization. Under the International Sanitary Regulations a valid certificate of smallpox vaccination may be required of all travelers entering any country. No international traveler should be without a valid certificate regardless of his origin or destination inasmuch as at any time a given country may be declared an infected area if cases occur. Properly accomplished, vaccination is a simple, inexpensive and highly effective preventive measure. Because of failures in vaccination technique, however, possession of an apparently valid certificate does not always signify complete immunity. In 1946, for example, 121 cases of smallpox were reported among vaccinated United States troops in Korea and Japan (3).

Typhus

The antityphus provisions of the International Sanitary Regulations refer only to the classic louse borne disease caused by *Rickettsia prowazeki* var. *prowazeki*. Transmission from man to man is by the infected human body louse which excretes rickettsiae in its feces. Infection results from rubbing feces or the crushed louse into openings in the skin caused by the bite and other abrasions. A less common means of transmission is by contact with dried louse feces in contaminated clothing or bedding. Endemic foci of the disease exist in Asia, Central Europe, North Africa and Latin America. Because of its invariable association with lousiness, epidemic typhus is a disease of crowding, cold weather and poor sanitation. Movements of large groups of people such as troops or refugees under conditions of poor personal hygiene favor typhus transmission. It has a long history of association with wars, disasters and mass migrations but to date no proven instance of dissemination by aircraft is known. Typhus control measures in international quarantine are directed almost entirely at the arthropod vector, the important prophylactic measure being disinsectization of persons and their clothing with an insecticide such as DDT (see table 91). In recent years other insecticides have been used in some geographic areas where lice have shown resistance to DDT. A secondary precaution is disinfection of persons and their clothing to insure against transmission *via* infected louse feces. Vaccination, although useful as an individual protective procedure, is not justified as a mandatory quarantine measure as disinsectization and disinfection are adequate insurance against introduction of the disease. For this reason the regulations specify that typhus vaccination shall not be required as a condition of admission to any country. Although immunity following typhus vaccination is not complete its efficacy in preventing severe infection is well established. It should be administered annually for the individual protection of persons traveling in endemic areas.

Relapsing Fever

Relapsing fever as referred to in the International Sanitary Regulations is an epidemic, louse borne infection caused by the spirochete *Borrelia recurrentis*. The regulations do not apply to other closely related forms of the disease which are tick borne. Reservoirs of infection exist in Europe, Asia, North Africa and Central America. The epidemiology of relapsing fever is virtually the same as that of typhus in that it is associated with lousiness in populations living under unhygienic and crowded conditions. In 1942 to 1946 epidemics swept North Africa and the Middle East and the disease was subsequently introduced into West Africa and France by troops evacuated from Morocco. Although earlier conventions had not been concerned with control of relapsing fever it was included as a sixth international quarantinable disease in the present regulations because of these extensive epidemics which indicated the necessity for international control. Inasmuch as the vector of relapsing fever is the same as that for typhus the same control measures are provided in the regulations.

DISINSECTIZATION, DERATIZATION, AND DISINFECTION OF AIRCRAFT

Disinsectization

Ideally all international airports would be located, constructed and maintained in such a way as to preclude arthropods from entering aircraft. Inasmuch as many airports and facilities in remote areas have not yet reached this high degree of development some form of disinsectization of aircraft must be carried out. As yet no general agreement has been reached among operators and public health officials as to technique for disinsectization of aircraft because of two somewhat different objectives. Added to the primary public health objective of insuring against the importation of vectors has been the desire of commercial airlines to use disinsectization procedures which did not delay airline operations on the ground and which resulted in a minimum of inconvenience and discomfort to passengers. Current practices thus represent a compromise between maximum effectiveness of the insecticidal process and maximum speed, comfort and efficiency of the airline operation. In-flight disinsectization, although eliminating delay on the ground, is of limited effectiveness because of the difficulty in securing sufficient concentration of insecticide in the aircraft cabin.

The efficiency of insecticide sprays depends to a great extent on the size of the droplets and their diffusibility, the most desirable space sprays being those which are dispersed in the form of aerosols. Because of their small particle size, aerosols penetrate effectively and remain in suspension for relatively long periods. The aerosol bomb, dispersing a spray of DDT, pyrethrum and solvents with a propellant such as Freon gas, is the most common method of aircraft disinsectization presently used. Pyrethrum has an immediate effect in knocking down insects whereas the effect of DDT is slower and more permanent. Manually employed aerosol bombs have the important advantage of simplicity but give a somewhat variable performance in that the dose of the insecticide is not uniform. For several years built in mechanical insecticide dispersal systems have been sought which could be operated from the cockpit or automatically activated with some essential operational procedure of the aircraft such as raising or lowering the landing gear. A permanently installed system of this type would largely eliminate the possibility of human error and insure a measured dose of insecticide to inaccessible spaces of the aircraft. The disadvantages of such installed equipment are those inherent in adding another mechanical system to the already complex and crowded aircraft, *i.e.*, the increase in weight and the added requirement for maintenance. A highly desirable development would be the perfecting of an effective residual insecticide suitable for impregnating fabrics and applying to interior surfaces. Sufficiently developed, this method could be used to complement or replace aerosol spraying. Periodic application of residual DDT to the aircraft interior supplemented by aerosol spraying has been used with some success. More recently field trials of urea formaldehyde resins impregnated with an insecticide have given encouraging results. If complete reliance could be placed on residual insecticides the interference with air traffic and the passenger discomfort occasioned by disinsectization would be eliminated.

In recent years the phenomenon of arthropod resistance to insecticides has been increasing both as to number of resistant species and number of insecticides to which they are resistant. Resistance has been demonstrated in most of the important disease vectors. This trend, which has progressed faster than counter measures to cope with it, is a primary obstacle in control of arthropod borne diseases and must be taken into account in the development of any future system for aircraft disinsectization. An ideal insecticide with high toxicity, prolonged residual effect and not conducive to the development of resistance has not yet been found in a single compound.

The Expert Committee on Insecticides of the World Health Organization has issued the following recommendations concerning disinsectization of aircraft (17):

1. Disinsectization should take place before takeoff with all luggage and freight loaded but without the passengers. Disinsectization during flight by the crew should not be recognized as complying with the requirements of the International Sanitary Regulations.

2. All possible mosquito sheltering places inside the plane should be sprayed.

3. Foods and utensils should be protected from gross contamination with insecticide.

4. All aircraft openings, including the ventilators, must be kept tightly closed during spraying and for 5 minutes thereafter.

5. Recesses for the landing gear and all parts of the aircraft accessible only from the outside are to be disinsectized as nearly as possible to 5 minutes before starting the engines.

6. If the presence on board of live vectors is suspected, additional disinsectization should be carried out at the discretion of the health authority after landing.

7. For disinsectization inside the aircraft an aerosol of at least 0.4 per cent pyrethrins and 3.0 per cent DDT by weight should be dispensed uniformly at the rate of 35 grams of the material per 100 cubic meters of enclosed space.

8. The formulation used should produce an aerosol in air in which the majority of droplets on a weight basis are of a diameter of 5 to 25 microns.

9. When dispersed at the prescribed rate it must be free of fire hazard, toxicity, visible impurities and harmless to fabrics, wood, metal, rubber and plexiglass.

Deratization

Aircraft, being generally clean and parked on open ramps are infrequently boarded by rats or mice but they are occasionally carried aboard during the loading of cargo. Prevention of infestation requires rodent eradication at airports and dependence on the established principles of denying food, harborage and access to aircraft. Loading ramps should be painted white, well lighted and removed when not in use. In the United States fumigation with HCN, poisoning with sodium fluoroacetate (1080) and trapping have been used in deratization of aircraft but none of these methods has proved entirely satisfactory. Trapping is uncertain and slow involving costly delays while aircraft are out of service. Fumigation and poisoning are rapid and effective but have the disadvantage of requiring the handling of highly toxic rodenticides. Anticoagulants such as Warfarin are unsuited for use in aircraft because of their slow action, requiring several days to produce results. Also such rodenticides kill the rodents but not their ectoparasites. When dealing with plague infected rodents it is of course imperative that the infected fleas be destroyed as well as the rodent host.

Disinfection

Not only are passengers who have become ill en route occasionally disembarked from aircraft in the early stages of acute infectious disease, but persons with known communicable disease are sometimes evacuated by air. Elective air evacuation of patients in the acute stages of communicable disease is not a common practice in military or civilian operations however, because of the deleterious effect on the patient. When such persons are transported by air, isolation technique may be carried out aboard the aircraft and standard precautions for handling infectious hospital patients are to be observed. In the close confines of aircraft cabins it is desirable that persons in the infectious stages of respiratory borne diseases wear gauze face masks as masks are of limited effectiveness after 2 or 3 hours of wear. The infectious person should be placed as far as possible away from other occupants of the aircraft and screened from them by means of sheets or blankets. All dishes and cups should be of paper so that they may be discarded. Disposable tissues for nose and throat discharges and soiled linen are discarded into separate bags for burning or autoclaving. After infectious persons have been carried the aircraft interior may require disinfection prior to its being used again. For this purpose washable surfaces may be scrubbed with soap and hot water followed by hot water containing 2.5 per cent of a cresol compound. Blankets, pillows and seat covers should be steam autoclaved and seats and carpets vacuum cleaned. Oxygen masks may be cleaned by washing the face piece with soap and rinsing with warm water. If a microphone is installed, swabs should be used rather than running water. Disinfection of masks may be accomplished by swabbing with a gauze pad soaked in aqueous merthiolate and wiping dry.

SANITATION OF AIRCRAFT WATER SUPPLIES

Aboard aircraft a safe, potable water supply is mandatory to protect the health of passengers and crew. On international flights an added consideration is the possibility of spreading diseases such as cholera, typhoid and viral hepatitis from country to country *via* contaminated water in aircraft. In the United States, Interstate Quarantine Regulations require that water for commercial aircraft be from sources which are entirely safe by United States Public Health Services standards. In many parts of the world, however, water for aircraft is obtained from supplies which vary greatly as to quality and safety. Individual operators must insure that water from uncertain sources is purified prior to its use in flight and that all water supplies taken aboard are handled and dispensed in a sanitary manner. Although the amount of water required is not great, many technical problems must be solved in designing aircraft water systems which meet weight, space and safety standards. When water is from questionable sources, some airlines chlorinate and then pass it through charcoal filters or treat it with sodium thiosulfate to minimize the taste of chlorine before it is put aboard. Filtration equipment carried aboard the aircraft should be readily accessible and designed for easy cleaning and sterilization. The most efficient and sanitary water procurement points for servicing aircraft are water hydrants located on the ramp in the service area, a direct hose connection from hydrants to the aircraft resulting in a minimum of water handling and reducing the chance of contamination by foreign material. The common practice of providing water to aircraft by means of mobile water carts or trucks introduces a further step in the water handling process. This creates an added opportunity for contamination and so demands the highest sanitary standards of operation and maintenance of these carts. Water service carts must be used exclusively for drinking water obtained from specified water hydrants by trained service personnel. An added safeguard is the fitting of carts with special couplings to insure that they can be filled only from the proper water source. The design and materials used in water servicing carts must permit complete draining, flushing and scouring to be carried out at frequent intervals. Carts should be flushed and hyperchlorinated once each week and scoured once each month. The water servicing panel on the aircraft should be located away from sewage and other service panels so that there is no likelihood of contamination when water is being taken aboard.

At present, water supply systems aboard aircraft are of three general types as follows:

1. SINGLE WATER SYSTEM, NONPOTABLE. Water tanks installed in the aircraft contain only nonpotable water for washing and flushing. Drinking water is carried in portable jugs.

2. DUAL WATER SYSTEM. Drinking water and water for other purposes is contained in separate tanks installed in the aircraft.

3. SINGLE WATER SYSTEM, POTABLE. Installed tanks contain water suitable for all purposes including drinking.

The most desirable water supply, as recommended by the United States Public Health Service is the single installed system wherein water drawn from any tap in the aircraft is fit for human consumption. This ideal of a single potable water system is not yet in general use except on some larger aircraft. Most military and commercial aircraft now carry dual water supplies with drinking water in separate containers. When the latter are of the installed type there is an element of risk in that nonpotable water may be accidentally consumed owing to confusion of the taps. Drinking water is often carried in portable tanks or constant temperature containers which are filled at route stops and carried aboard the aircraft. Such containers should be frequently cleaned with soap and hot water followed by air drying. The layout of aircraft water systems should be determined in the early design phases so that the water system can be properly developed with reference to the remainder of the aircraft.

SANITARY FOOD SERVICE IN AIRCRAFT

Although protection of passengers and aircrews against food borne infections and food poisoning is the vital concern of military and civilian air carriers, they usually have little if any direct control over food service facilities at route stops. As the International Sanitary Regulations do not prescribe food service sanitation standards for airports or aircraft local laws and standards are applicable. In the United States the Public Health Service cooperates with State Health Departments in a continuous program of inspection to insure compliance with Interstate Quarantine Regulations relating to the sanitation of water, food and milk. Based on these inspections suppliers are classified as approved, provisionally approved or prohibited for use by interstate carriers and this information is published every 6 months in the Official Classification of Airline Catering and Watering Points. Because of weight and space limitations in aircraft which do not permit full scale cooking and preparation of food in flight, box lunches or precooked meals are used aboard commercial and military transports. Meals may be brought aboard after cooking and kept warm until served or precooked frozen food may be reheated in the aircraft. The latter method is particularly desirable aboard planes making long overseas flights and equipped with electric ovens for rapid rewarming. The most important immediate result of poor food sanitation practices at route stops and in flight is the occurrence of food poisoning among passangers and crew. In military and civilian air transport experience, occasional instances of acute food poisoning occur during or following flight. Although formal reports of such episodes are infrequent, many mild and sporadic cases undoubtedly occur which are not recognized or not reported. At best such episodes cause serious discomfort, inconvenience and delay for the passengers and embarrassment for the operator. Most serious of all, if the crew of the aircraft is involved, flying safety is gravely compromised and a tragic accident may result. Food poisoning is caused chiefly by lapses in sanitary food handling. Even though food is mildly contaminated at its origin, bacteria will not multiply sufficiently to cause food poisoning unless handled in an unsanitary manner and left unrefrigerated. By far the most common food poisoning outbreaks in military flying experience are those caused by staphylococcus enterotoxin from the contents of box lunches consumed several hours after preparation.

Sandwiches of meat, fowl or fish are unusually hazardous for inflight lunches and must be kept refrigerated until shortly before serving. If refrigeration is not available aboard the aircraft they must be kept as cool as possible by packing in insulated food containers and loading aboard the aircraft just before takeoff. Unrefrigerated sandwiches must be consumed within 4 hours after preparation. If storage temperatures aboard aircraft are maintained below 50° F., food will be outside the temperature range favorable for the activity of bacteria. It should be remembered, however, that staphylococcus enterotoxin, once produced in food, is highly resistant to temperature extremes, surviving both refrigeration and boiling. Aircraft galley equipment, particularly food preparation surfaces, must be easily cleaned and free of cracks or corners which provide harborage for dirt and food particles. Food storage spaces must be dirt and insect proof and be designed for thorough cleaning. Tight seams, rounded corners and equipment parts and sections which may be removed for cleaning aid in maintaining a sanitary galley. In the United States the Public Health Service awards a Certificate of Sanitary Construction for aircraft which are designed in compliance with requirements of the Interstate Quarantine Regulations.

Limitations of space, weight and hot water supply have generally precluded the cleaning of eating utensils in flight. A satisfactory practice is the use of paper or plastic utensils which are discarded after use. Alternative methods are the off loading of soiled utensils at route stops for final cleaning and chemical sterilization aboard the aircraft. An entirely satisfactory method of chemical sterilization of utensils, using a solution which is effective, stable, tasteless, noncorrosive and which does not require rinsing, has not yet been developed.

Aircraft Sewage Disposal

The problem of waste disposal common to all forms of transportation is especially complex in aircraft because the United States Interstate Quarantine Regulations as well as the International Sanitary Regulations prohibit the discharge of excrement from aircraft in flight. Weight and space restrictions conflicting with sanitation requirements and passenger comfort have greatly complicated the task of designing the aircraft toilet facilities. Many older aircraft are still equipped with a removable sewage pail which is cleaned and returned by maintenance personnel at service stops. Because of the obvious disadvantages of this simple method it has been replaced on newer aircraft by installed sewage tanks which may be conveniently emptied, flushed and refilled with chemicals from outside the aircraft by means of sewage carts. For ease of cleaning and flushing, such installed tanks must have smooth seams and rounded interior contours. Chemicals used must be noncorrosive, nonflammable, germicidal and stable at diminished atmospheric pressure. The galley should be as widely separated from the toilet as possible and air from the latter should be discharged outside the aircraft rather than into the ventilating system. Modern commercial aircraft have fixed flush toilets over an installed sewage tank which is drained, flushed and recharged with water and chemicals by means of sewage servicing carts. A toilet servicing panel, located on the under surface of the fuselage, has a waste discharge outlet and a clean water inlet for flushing. Sewage from the tank is discharged through a flexible hose into the cart which in turn is emptied into the airport sewage system. Sewage carts are to be maintained and operated by crews which are entirely separate from those handling drinking water carts.

Aerial Shipment of Biologic Material

Whereas the International Sanitary Regulations contain few provisions for regulating aerial transportation of animals and biologic materials comparable to the quarantine measures against human disease, each country has national laws governing the shipment of such items into and through its territory. In addition to these national laws, the regulations, traffic instructions and policies of individual airline companies and of the International Civil Aviation Organization and the International Air Transport

Association are applicable. International aerial transport of animals is subjected to a wide variety of agricultural and veterinary quarantine regulations which apply generally to all forms of transport. Most countries require that live animals meet specific health requirements before shipment and prohibit the transport of animals in passenger aircraft except pets for which proper accommodations are furnished in the cargo compartment. When animals are carried aboard aircraft the details of the shipment are to be included in the appropriate part of the Aircraft General Declaration. Specific restrictions are imposed against animal importation to control psittacosis and rabies. Infected birds displaying no symptoms of psittacosis may nevertheless shed large amounts of virus which is highly communicable to other birds and to man. Although traditionally considered to be a disease of tropical parrots and parakeets this disease is now known to be endemic in many species of birds and fowls in temperate zones as well. Notwithstanding this rather general distribution of the disease, quarantine measures are still largely directed at psittacine birds. Restrictions on the shipping of dogs, cats and monkeys are often imposed as a rabies control measure, some countries virtually prohibiting their importation. Countries in yellow fever receptive areas have strict regulations to preclude the introduction of yellow fever virus *via* infected monkeys. No uniform international policy exists covering the transportation of plants by air. Some countries admit almost all species of plants whereas a few national laws prohibit nearly all live plant material.

Pathogenic Organisms

Air shipments of live pathogenic organisms for special medical purposes are normally accepted only from health agencies, research institutions, universities, hospitals or licensed commercial firms. Material for air shipment should be sealed in glass bottles or vials which will resist pressure differences incident to altitude changes. These bottles in turn are to be packed in sealed metal containers with enough packing material to absorb the entire contents should leakage occur. Finally, the metal container must be securely packed into a sturdy box which is plainly labeled. In the United States a permit from the Secretary of Agriculture is required for importing or transporting from state to state dead or living microorganisms, infected animals, viruses, serums, toxins or vaccines. In addition, the Department of Agriculture may seize, quarantine and dispose of hay, straw, meat or animal products coming from an infected country. Wool, hides, bristles and brushes are particularly suspect in international traffic because of their frequent contamination with viable anthrax spores.

Human Remains

Many countries do not have specific laws regulating the carriage of human remains in aircraft and, therefore, the general regulations covering the transportation of corpses apply to their movement by air. The International Arrangement Regarding the Transport of Corpses, which was signed in Berlin in 1937, is the basic document after which the laws of many countries are patterned. Some national laws permit the carriage of human remains only on cargo or special aircraft. In other countries remains may be carried aboard passenger aircraft if properly embalmed or placed in hermetically sealed containers. The latter requirement, a provision of the Berlin Arrangement, has sometimes led to leakage of sealed containers in flight owing to decreasing atmospheric pressure at altitude. This risk is minimized by cabin pressurization. Human remains to be air lifted should be embalmed and placed in a sealed container which is encased in an outer box of sturdy construction. The death certificate should accompany the casket and shipment aboard cargo or special aircraft is preferred.

Preventive Medical Advice to Air Travelers

Among the growing number of persons transported by air are many with little previous travel experience and no knowledge of air travel. Such persons, embarking with considerable ignorance, misinformation and anxiety concerning the trip, may seek the advice of their physician before departure. This is especially likely if their itinerary includes the tropics or underdeveloped parts of the world. The informed physician will avoid spoiling the anticipated trip by unduly strict advice and excessive admonitions. Instead, as the traveler's medical counselor the flight surgeon or general physician can do much to prepare his patient for a more healthful and enjoyable journey by discussing its medical aspects with him in advance. Travelers from North America and Western Europe in foreign countries will often be unable to find medical care of the type to which they are accustomed. In addition, contacting a physician in a foreign country where one does not speak the language may prove difficult. For these reasons air travelers may at times have to rely to some extent upon their own judgement and resources in meeting medical problems of travel. Some airlines distribute medical brochures alerting their passengers to health hazards and recommending simple precautions. In foreign countries, travelers who become ill can get the names of reputable physicians who speak their language by inquiring at their hotel, airline, travel agency or their own country's consulate. If travelers are overly concerned with the hazard of exotic tropical diseases it should be pointed out to them that they are much more likely to succumb to commonplace diseases, fatigue or overindulgence. By far the most common illnesses of aircrews and passengers are the acute infections of the respiratory and gastrointestinal tract.

Gastroenteritis of Travelers

Even with the considerable advances made in preventive medicine, and improved sanitation, gastroenteritis with diarrhea as the predominant manifestation is still a frequent experience of all travelers and persons newly arrived in areas of poor sanitation. These acute attacks are usually of moderate severity and subside within 2 to 4 days. In each country or local area the syndrome is given a descriptive popular name, assorted explanations are offered as to its etiology and a variety of treatments recommended. Because of the mildness and short duration of the diarrheal episode, patients are not often seen by a physician and a laboratory diagnosis is infrequently made. Investigations at various times and places, however, have incriminated *Shigella* and *Salmonella* organisms,

Endamoeba histolytica and enterotoxin producing staphylococci. Other possible etiologic agents are certain virulent strains of *Escherichia coli* and viral gastroenteritis. Much further study is required before the relative importance of these several etiologic agents can be determined.

Food and Water Precautions

Although the food and water served aboard aircraft can be carefully safeguarded this control is not extended to include eating and drinking establishments at air route stops. For this reason the individual traveler must be sufficiently indoctrinated in basic principles of hygiene to rely upon his own judgement in protecting his health in areas where sanitary standards are low. Inexperienced persons who are unduly apprehensive regarding health hazards outside their own country may undertake their trip with exaggerated notions of the hazards faced and prepared to go to ridiculous lengths to avoid illness. Others, having been convinced that all precautions are useless or too complicated to follow, may adopt an equally foolish, fatalistic attitude giving no heed to simple health rules offered for their protection. Neither of these extreme attitudes is justifiable in the intelligent traveler who understands certain basic principles of hygiene. By observing minimal precautions and exercising reasonable restraint in eating and drinking the traveler can spare himself most of the illness associated with travel.

Contaminated drinking water is a source of possible infection with amebiasis, shigellosis, cholera, viral hepatitis, typhoid and nonspecific diarrhea. Unfortunately, the water supplies of many cities are not entirely safe for consumption at all times. It is difficult for travelers visiting a large and apparently modern city to realize that the water supply may be unreliable. Water which is not from an unquestionably pure source is best purified by boiling for 5 minutes before being used for drinking or brushing teeth. As an alternative to boiling, small quantities of water may be treated by the addition of water purification tablets which liberate free iodine. Globaline (tetraglycine hydroperiodide) tablets for water treatment are readily obtained and easily used by any traveler.

One Globaline tablet will purify a quart of water after a 30 minute contact period, more tablets being required if the water is cloudy or discolored. In the absence of purification tablets, water can be treated by adding 2 or 3 drops of tincture of iodine per quart and waiting for a 30 minute contact period. Where water supplies are of doubtful purity it is ordinarily safer to drink bottled water than tap water, although bottling does not insure purity. It should be remembered that water made into ice or mixed with alcoholic beverages is not purified in the process. Hot coffee and tea without cream are usually safe by virtue of having been boiled. Bottled beer is free of pathogenic bacteria and may be consumed in moderation as a substitute for water.

In addition to the disease hazards already mentioned for water, contaminated food presents the further risks of salmonellosis, brucellosis, tuberculosis and helminth infections. Many food preparation establishments lack the refrigeration, screening and trained food service personnel essential to the sanitary preparation of food. In areas of low sanitary standards luxury hotels and restaurants catering to tourists are pitfalls for the unwary. At such establishments when appetizing food is served in an attractive setting the traveler is prone to let his appetite over-rule his better judgement and so to be led into indiscretion. Travelers are well advised to adhere to the following simple rules for eating and drinking in areas of questionable sanitation.

1. Use no milk that has not been freshly boiled. Canned or powdered milk is safe if pure water is used in preparing it.

2. Avoid ice cream, custard, cream filled pastries, butter and fresh cheese. Little risk is involved in eating properly aged cheese.

3. Eat only meat that has been recently and thoroughly cooked.

4. Eat no raw fruits or vegetables unless they have been peeled or carefully washed in pure water.

5. In general, any food that is thoroughly cooked and served hot may be eaten with safety.

Drug prophylaxis against amebiasis or shigellosis, as sometimes used under controlled conditions in institutions or areas of hyperendemicity, is not recommended as a routine measure for travelers. Inasmuch as these drugs are useless in preventing other diseases, such as tuberculosis, typhoid and viral hepatitis, their use may engender a false sense of security. Other disadvantages in giving prophylactic drugs for long periods are their toxicity and the possibility that the organism will develop drug resistance. Most diarrhea which occurs during a trip will respond to treatment by rest, a liquid diet and the use of a simple antidiarrhea mixture.

Malaria Prevention

In geographic areas where malaria is still prevalent personal preventive measures such as protective clothing, bed nets, mosquito repellent and prophylactic drugs may be necessary to protect aircrews and passengers. Coggeshall has described experience in establishing airline operations in West Africa in which over 40 per cent of the airline personnel were incapacitated by malaria within 8 weeks of their arrival (18). Such highly malarious areas in the vicinity of airports are fast disappearing but precautions must still be observed where malaria is incompletely controlled. Aircrews assigned to such flight routes must be completely indoctrinated in personal protective measures. Passengers should be given a simple printed statement of the hazard and a list of recommended precautions prior to entering endemic areas. An insecticide aerosol bomb which dispenses a pyrethrum and DDT mixture for spraying the interior of rooms or bed nets and a bottle of insect repellent to be used on exposed portions of the body should be carried in malarious regions. Although drug prophylaxis cannot prevent malaria infection it may be advisable under conditions of heavy exposure where environmental control of the disease is incomplete. A thorough regimen of drug prophylaxis will cure *Plasmodium falciparum* infections without any malarial symptoms being experienced. Infections of *Plasmodium vivax* and *Plasmodium malariae*, on the other hand, are only suppressed and the patient may experience malarial attacks after cessation of prophylaxis. Prophylactic Chloroquine in a dose of 0.5 grams weekly is favored by most authorities in the United States. The drug should be started 10 days before entry into the malarious area and maintained for 2 weeks after exposure. It is important that the aircrew and passengers realize that drugs are not a substitute for personal malaria discipline.

Immunizations

In addition to immunizations for the international quarantinable diseases, certain others may be recommended to travelers who undertake international flights.

TYPHOID-PARATYPHOID. Although of greatly diminished incidence in recent years, typhoid is still prevalent in many parts of the world. All persons traveling to Asia, Africa, South America and Europe should have a basic series or stimulating dose of typhoid-paratyphoid vaccine within 1 year.

TETANUS. Travelers should avail themselves of the excellent protection afforded by active immunization even though the possibility of tetanus infection is relatively slight. Reimmunization is necessary every 4 years.

DIPHTHERIA. Immunization with diphtheria toxoid produces effective immunity and is highly desirable for persons under 35 years of age. Combined tetanus and diphtheria toxoids may be used for the basic series and stimulating doses every 4 years.

INFLUENZA. For persons traveling during the fall and winter months immunization with a polyvalent vaccine prepared against currently prevalent strains is desirable. The patient should understand that this does not protect him against other strains of influenza and other upper respiratory infections.

POLIOMYELITIS. A basic series of three inoculations followed by a stimulating dose in 1 year is recommended for all travelers regardless of age. Although poliomyelitis is uncommon in persons over 40 years of age when infection does occur in this age group it is more likely to be of the severe bulbar type.

Current information on immunizations required and recommended for travel to various countries may be found in the pamphlet "Immunization Information for International Travel" prepared by the United States Public Health Service and available from the Superintendent of Documents, United States Government Printing Office.

Traveler's Medical Kit

Persons planning trips to or through remote areas may seek advice as to the contents of a medical kit to be carried for personal use. Although naturally reluctant to advise self medication, physicians may recommend certain items of a preventive nature which may be safely and effectively used providing the patient is appropriately briefed. The contents of such a kit depends upon the area to be visited, length of the visit and the intelligence and maturity of the patient. The latter should be admonished to seek professional medical advice if he becomes ill during the trip. The following list of suggested items may be decreased or augmented to meet the requirements of each situation:

1. Aspirin tablets, 5 grain.
2. Clinical thermometer.
3. Water purification tablets.
4. Insecticide aerosol bomb, pyrethrum and DDT.
5. Insect repellent (dimethylphthalate or dibutylphthalate).
6. Antidiarrhea mixture (bismuth salts and paregoric or Kaolin-pectate preparation).
7. Chloroquine tablets, 0.5 gram (if traveling in malarious areas).

REFERENCES

(1) World Health Organization Report. J. A. M. A., **167:** 250, 1958.
(2) LE BOURDELLES, B., LESAFFRE, V., AND ROGEZ, C.: A case of smallpox brought into France by air: the Arras epidemic. Bull. Office Internat. Hyg. Publique, **38:** 453–456, 1946.
(3) ELLINGSON, H. V.: Impact of modern aviation on health. Aeronautical Eng. Rev., **12:** 79–81, 1953.
(4) Smallpox in Brighton. Lancet, **260:** 59, 1951.
(5) LE BOURDELLES, B., La variole en France en 1955. Presse méd., **63:** 1247, 1955.
(6) DEUTSCHMAN, Z.: Guard against smallpox. World Health, **11:** 2 No. 1, 1958. Geneva, Switzerland.
(7) The Functioning of the International Sanitary Regulations and Their Effect on International Traffic. Fifth Annual Report by the Director-General. World Health Organization Committee on International Quarantine, 1957.
(8) PAYNE, A. M. M.: Influenza Epidemic in Asia. World Health Organization Reference 12/442/2, 1957. Geneva, Switzerland.

(9) WILLIAMS, R. B., Food-borne typhoid outbreak with rapid dissemination of cases thru air transportation. Northwest Med., 49: 686–689, 1950.

(10) RIZZOLO, J.: Importance and relation of preventive medicine to aviation medicine. J. Aviation Med., 24: 412–422, 1953.

(11) KISLIUK, M.: Air routes, German dirigible "Graf Zeppelin" and plant quarantines. Ent. News, 40: 196–197, 1929.

(12) LAIRD, M.: Insect introduction hazards affecting Singapore and neighbouring territories. M. J. Malaya, 11: 40–62, 1956.

(13) GRIFFITTS, T. H. D.: Air traffic in relation to public health. Am. J. Trop. Med., 13: 283–290, 1933.

(14) SICE, A., SAUTET, J., AND ETHES, Y.: L'un des plus redoubtables vecteurs du paludisme en Afrique, l'Anopheles gambiae Giles, 1902, est-il susceptible d'etre transporté en France par les avions? Rev. méd. hyg. trop. 31: 137–139, 1939.

(15) Plague in 1957. World Health Organization Week. Epidemiological Rec., 33: 47–58, 1958.

(16) LE BOURDELLES, B.: L'epidemie de variole de 1955. Bull. Acad. nat. méd., 139: 417–420, 1955.

(17) Expert Committee on Insecticides. World Health Organization Technical Report Series No. 125, 7th Report, 1957. Geneva, Switzerland.

(18) COGGESHALL, L. T.: Current and postwar problems associated with human protozoan disease. Ann. New York Acad. Sc., 44: 195–206, 1943.

30

AIRCRAFT ACCIDENTS

H. G. Moseley, M.D

Since the inception of aviation, there have been substantial losses resulting from aircraft accidents. This results in a large number of fatalities in a given year, particularly among flying personnel engaged in hazardous flight occupations. The losses in materiel are also significant. Although great progress had been made in lowering the rate of major accidents in recent years, there has been but little concomitant progress in lowering the number of deaths per hour flown. This is because as the performance of aircraft increases any mishap is more liable to be attended with disastrous results. The majority of aircraft accidents are occasioned by human acts or omissions. In this respect, the predominant effort in prevention of aircraft accidents falls upon those who are familiar with human ability to meet the requirements of flight and upon those who are acquainted with the adversities to human tolerances which may be encountered during flight. To a large degree, this is a responsibility of aviation medicine. Therefore, much of the success of flight is directly dependent upon the effectiveness of this science in engaging the problem of aircraft accidents, exploring its epidemiology and countering its virulence.

DEFINITIONS

1. MAJOR AND MINOR ACCIDENTS. An aircraft accident is a mishap during some stage of flight which results in damage to the aircraft. A major aircraft accident is the term usually applied when such damage is substantial or results in destruction of the aircraft; a minor aircraft accident is the term ordinarily used when such damage is slight and its repair requires only a minor expenditure of funds or energy in consideration of the size and complexity of the aircraft involved.

2. INCIDENTS. Mishaps wherein there is no significant damage to the aircraft but wherein occupants are injured or wherein there is inadvertent loss of aircraft components such as hatches or canopies are ordinarily termed incidents. In military flying where there is damage to the aircraft as a result of deliberate rather than accidental factors, such as damage during some rescue or test missions, the term incident may be applied regardless of degree of damage sustained.

3. ACCIDENT RATES. The rate or frequency of aircraft accidents is gaged by comparing numbers of accidents with the amount of aircraft utilization. In military flying it is customary to establish a rate by the number of accidents during a given number of flying hours, *i.e.*, in the United States Air Force, the rate is the number of accidents occurring per 100,000 hours of flying. In civilian flying the accident rate is usually established on the number of accidents occurring in a given number of plane miles flown or passenger miles flown. Accident rates can thus be established for various type aircraft, various operational missions and for various aircraft operators. Rates can also be established concerning the incidence of injury in relation to various types of flying. This allows a method

by which the accident history of one type aircraft can be compared to another or the accident incidence between various operational procedures or various type pilots can be compared.

MAGNITUDE

The magnitude of aircraft accidents, as judged by their impact upon society, is considerable. There are several consequences of significance:

1. LOSS OF LIFE. Owing to the destructive nature of many aircraft accidents a sizable number of fatalities accrue in any situation or enterprise where there is a large amount of flying or a high accident rate. The number of accidents and the number of fatalities in United States domestic flying are shown in table 92. Because of risk factors described below, military flying is accompanied by loss of life of considerable proportions. Among military personnel on flying status aircraft accidents are the primary cause of death. Table 93 lists all deaths among flying personnel within the United States Air Force by cause factors for the calendar years 1954 and 1955. The percentages of death for the causes shown in this table do not vary significantly from year to year.

2. ECONOMIC LOSS. Aircraft, especially those designed for high performance or for

TABLE 92

*Accidents and Fatalities in United States Civil Flying**

Year	Revenue Operations		Non-Air Carrier	
	Number of accidents	Number of fatalities	Number of accidents	Number of fatalities
1946	33	75	7618	1009
1947	44	222	9253	1352
1948	56	98	7850	1384
1949	35	113	5459	896
1950	39	109	4505	871
1951	45	170	3824	750
1952	44	54	3657	691
1953	37	103	3232	635
1954	49	23	3381	684
1955	45	179	3308	613†

* Source: Bureau of Safety, CAB.

† There has been a steady fall in accident rates from one accident per 114,825 miles flown in 1946 to one per 367,594 in 1955.

TABLE 93

*Causes of Death in U.S.A.F. Personnel on Flying Status**
1954 to 1955

Cause of Death	Number	Per Cent
Neoplasms	16	1
Circulatory disease	26	2
Other disease	15	1
Firearms and violence	61	4
Traffic (land vehicles)	95	7
Aircraft accidents	1176	85
Total	1389	100

* Source: Department of the Air Force: Fourth Annual Report of the U.S.A.F. Medical Service.

carrying large numbers of occupants are extraordinarily expensive. Reciprocating engine airliners may cost in excess of one million dollars and large jet aircraft of all types are in the multimillion dollar category. Thus, any single accident can be a severe economic loss and a large number of accidents will place a severe financial drain upon the supporting enterprise or, in the case of military flying, upon the national economy.

3. LOSS OF COMBAT POTENTIAL. Aircraft are one of the most essential factors in the defense of a nation either as weapons or as transport vehicles for personnel and material. Thus, destruction of aircraft through accidents constitutes a compromise of combat effectiveness in a direct ratio to the rate of such aircraft accidents.

4. OTHER CONSEQUENCES. There are several other deleterious consequences of aircraft accidents. These include property loss where the aircraft damages or destroys objects of material value, the detrimental effects of adverse public opinion and a negation of aeronautical progress which is inherent in the setbacks of aeronautical disasters.

AIRCRAFT ACCIDENTS IN RELATION TO RISK FACTORS

The magnitude of aircraft accidents as determined by their rates varies in almost direct proportion to the degree of hazard involved in flying. In this respect the greatest risks are encountered in testing new or modi-

fied aircraft where the flying characteristics
of the machine are relatively unknown and
where mechanical reliability is unproven; in
hazardous operations such as some rescue
missions; and in any type flying wherein new
and inexperienced pilots are learning the art
of flying. Contrariwise the least risk is involved in flying aircraft whose performance
and reliability have been well established and
where the aircraft operators are thoroughly
familiar with the operational and emergency
procedures of the aircraft involved. The
military services by virtue of their mission of
training pilots and operating new and advanced weapons face an aircraft accident
potential of considerable magnitude. In commercial and civilian flying this potential is
much smaller.

There is also a distinct correlation between
risk factors and type of aircraft being flown.
Table 94 lists the accident rate for various
aircraft types in the Air Force during the
calendar years 1956 and 1957. It will be
noted that the accident rate is highest among
jet fighters. The most significant reasons for
this are the high velocities, the high wing
loadings and the reliance (usually) upon a
single engine. As a result, exact handling
techniques are required and a thorough
knowledge of emergency procedures is essential. In flying such aircraft, there is very

TABLE 94

*Major U.S.A.F. Accidents by Type of Aircraft**

Type Aircraft	Rate per 100,000 Hours	
	1956	1957
Jet fighter	41.4	38.1
Jet trainer	20.9	19.2
Jet bomber	9.0	8.9
Nonjet bomber	5.7	5.6
Nonjet trainer	7.2	6.8
Cargo/transport	3.6	2.8
Helicopter, liaison, and miscellaneous	25.2	21.9
Average rate, all air- craft	14.7	13.6

* Source: Statement of Major General J. D. C.
Caldara, U.S.A.F. before the Military Operations
Subcommittee of the Committee on Government
Operations of the House of Representatives, 85th
Congress, 2nd Session, 5 February 1958.

little margin for error and any of the cause
factors mentioned elsewhere in this chapter
carry a higher accident potential when the
operator is flying this type aircraft.

The relatively high accident rate of helicopters, liaison and miscellaneous type aircraft is explained partially on the mission of
many of these aircraft. They are frequently
used in land and sea rescue operations and
may be damaged in the process. In this respect, most accidents involving these aircraft are in the landing phase and are not
serious in nature. One of the enigmas, however, of accidents involving liaison aircraft
is that the operators frequently are highly
experienced in other type aircraft. Due to the
fact that flying light aircraft appears relatively simple, such operators may attempt
flight without adequate transition training
and subsequently make mistakes owing to
their unfamiliarity with the aircraft.

The lowest accident rate is experienced
among cargo and transport type aircraft. In
these machines, handling requirements are
less critical and multiple engines allow continued flight even though there may be some
power plant failure. Of further interest in
the accident rates involving cargo or transport aircraft is the extremely low rate of
scheduled commercial aircraft. During the
five year period 1951 through 1955 such
flights within the United States averaged
only 0.209 fatalities per million miles flown.
Within the military service, flights devoted
solely to passenger transport such as those
conducted by the Military Air Transport
Service have a similar low accident rate.
The fatalities per passenger mile traveled
are considerably lower in such domestic air
operations than those encountered in automobile travel (table 95).

TYPE OF AIRCRAFT ACCIDENTS AND
PHASE OF FLIGHT

Types of aircraft accidents are usually
categorized by the term or terms which
most clearly describe the event or circumstances affecting the aircraft and precipitating the accident. These descriptions also
indicate the phase of flight wherein the accident happens. Table 96 presents the relative
frequency of various types of accidents in
both civilian and Air Force flying which

occurred in the United States during the calendar year 1956. It will be noted that the greatest number under any single type accident are listed under "other collision with object." This category includes all accidents wherein an in-flight aircraft accidentally collided with the ground or water or objects incident to the terrain such as trees and poles. However, in spite of the relatively high number of in-flight collisions the greatest accumulative total of accidents occur during the landing phase. This includes the first six categories listed in table 96. Percentagewise approximately 50 per cent of all major accidents occur in the landing phase, 30 per cent during the in-flight phase, 15 per cent in the takeoff phase and the remaining 5 per cent in go-around or taxiing.

There is a distinct correlation between phases of flight and resultant injury of occupants. Accidents in the landing phase, although frequent, are characterized by a high survival rate because the majority of such accidents involve relatively low velocities and complete destruction of the aircraft is unusual. Accidents occurring in flight, on

TABLE 95

Comparative Accident Data*

1944 to 1955

Calendar Year	Passenger Fatalities per 100,000,000 Passenger Miles			
	Passenger automobiles and taxis	Busses	Railroad passenger trains	Domestic scheduled air transport planes
1944	2.9	0.22	0.26	2.2
1945	2.9	0.17	0.16	2.2
1946	2.5	0.19	0.18	1.2
1947	2.3	0.21	0.16	3.2
1948	2.1	0.18	0.13	1.3
1949	2.7	0.20	0.08	1.3
1950	2.9	0.17	0.58	1.1
1951	3.0	0.20	0.43	1.3
1952	3.0	0.17	0.04	0.4
1953	2.9	0.14	0.16	0.6
1954	2.6	0.11	0.08	0.1
1955	2.7	0.19	0.07	0.8

* Source: Domestic scheduled air transport, CAB. All other data as published in National Safety Council "Accident Facts"; Railroad data from ICC; motor vehicle data approximation by National Safety Council based on data from state traffic authorities, Bureau of Public Roads and *Bus Transportation* magazine.

TABLE 96

Types of Aircraft Accidents of U.S.A.F. and United States Civilian Aircraft*

Calendar Year 1956

Type Accident	Civil Non-Air Carrier	Civil Air Carrier	U.S.A.F.
Ground loop	570	8	79
Wheels up landing	142	6	197
Hard landing	198	8	95
Collapse of retractable landing gear	99	10	71
Undershoot	215	4	66
Overshoot	176	5	55
Nose up or over	183	1	10
Midair collision	14	2	61
Other collision with aircraft	50	1	157
Other collision with object (ground or water)	760	26	205
Spin and stall	606	3	70
Fire in air	9	2	119
Airframe failure on ground or in air	25	7	39
Other	100	22	216†
Total	3147	105	1440

* Source: Civil, CAB Bureau of Safety; U.S.A.F., Directorate of Flight Safety Research, U.S.A.F.

† Of these 120 were abandoned in the air.

the other hand, are characterized by relatively high fatality rate, as high velocities and an abrupt deceleration are frequent. Midair collisions are also attended with a high fatality rate and those cases wherein the aircraft is damaged to the extent that further flight is impossible are almost 100 per cent fatal unless escape by parachuting is possible. Therefore, from the viewpoint of greatest conservation of life and materiel the most productive preventive effort would be directed toward prevention of in-flight accidents.

CAUSE OF AIRCRAFT ACCIDENTS

Aircraft accidents result from unsafe acts, unsafe conditions or miscellaneous adversities. Unsafe acts are errors of commission or omission on the part of the aircraft operator or the individuals who are responsible for support or supervision of the flight. Unsafe conditions are failures or shortcomings of the aircraft and its components or of landing fields and aids to flight. Miscellaneous adversities include weather and other phenomena which may interfere with the successful performance or conclusion of flight. Frequently, an aircraft accident is the result of the inter-relationship or compounding of several causes. For instance, a badly located cockpit instrument, which is an adverse condition, may induce the pilot to mishandle the aircraft and fly it into the ground. Similarly, a cross wind (miscellaneous adversity) may cause a pilot to ground loop (pilot error). Usually the act, condition or adversity which makes the accident most inevitable is denoted as the primary cause of the accident. When all causes are considered, i.e., primary cause (main cause) and secondary cause (contributing cause), there is some shifting of emphasis with errors or oversights on the part of maintenance and supervisory personnel becoming more prevalent as secondary factors. This is because errors or oversights on the part of supporting personnel may not be the direct cause of an accident but may lead to flight conditions which the pilot has difficulty in handling, with resultant unsafe pilot acts and an accident. Table 97 is a listing of all causes of Air Force and civilian aircraft accidents for the periods denoted. The percentages shown

TABLE 97

U.S.A.F. and Civilian Aircraft Accidents; All Causes

Cause Factor	U.S.A.F.	Civilian Aircraft; 1954 to 1955	
	1956	Air carriers	Non-air carriers
	per cent	*per cent*	*per cent*
Unsafe acts	52	51	71
Pilot	32	33	68
Other personnel	20	18	3
Unsafe conditions	35	47	28
Materiel failure	20	16	11
Equipment and accessories		3	1
Airport terrain	7	6	1
Weather	8	22	15
Miscellaneous-undetermined	13	2	1

remain fairly constant from year to year. The following is a more detailed description of the various cause factors.

Unsafe Pilot Acts

Inasmuch as the majority of pilots successfully meet the requirements for flying, it is apparent that the failures which result in an accident are the exception rather than the rule. Thus, pilot factor accidents are the result of inadequacies or adversities affecting *some* aircraft operators. Reviews have revealed that although there are multiple conditions and influences affecting the pilot's actions, those which have an adverse effect on his ability to meet the requirements of flying and lead to an accident usually can be placed in one or more of the following categories (1):

1. CAPACITY DEFICIENCIES. Flying an aircraft requires a certain minimum of physical strength, dexterity, intelligence and emotional stability. When an individual fails to meet one or more of these capacity minimums, an aircraft accident can result. Careful screening requirements make accidents in this category rare.

2. INADEQUATE KNOWLEDGE OR EXPERIENCE. Flying, and particularly the operation of modern, high performance aircraft, requires a high degree of skill, specialized knowledge concerning the operation of the aircraft power plants and familiarity with multitudinous instruments which give information concerning mechanical and physical factors involved or encountered in flight. In addition, flying requires an acquaintance with high velocity, extreme closing speeds and unusual attitudes in space. Inasmuch as these are not natural attributes, the required degree of skill or level of knowledge must be attained through indoctrination and experience. Mistakes made during this learning process, or failure to maintain the required level of skill and knowledge after initial indoctrination, can cause aircraft accidents. Inadequate knowledge or experience can also cause trained pilots to err when they transition into new aircraft or when they fail to remain current.

3. APPLICATION DEFICIENCIES. Flying requires a high degree of mental application. Such application must be sufficiently intense

to guarantee correct interpretation of all things observed and it must be sufficiently broad to encompass multiple sources of vital information. In addition, there is an absolute requirement to preconsider or anticipate adversities and hazards that may be encountered in flight in order that they may be ameliorated or avoided. Failure to give sufficient depth or breadth of attention, or failure of preattention, can lead to an aircraft accident.

4. ATTITUDE DEFICIENCIES. There is a definite requirement for proper mental acceptance of all factors which are essential to flight. Thus, the pilot must have a positive orientation and a willing attitude toward his occupation, as any adversity of attitude is accompanied by a degree of mental rejection of the feared or disliked subject matter. Pronounced cases of attitude deficiency can arise from derelictions of mood or adjustment. In such cases, pilots may not only fail to accept, but may flatly rebel at rules and regulations. Conversely, excessive motivation can also interfere with the pilot's proper acceptance of guidance and information. These are the cases wherein enthusiasm for flying or desire to obtain an objective can cause a pilot to minimize hazardous conditions or take unwarranted chances. In addition, situational apprehension, though usually transitory, can condition the pilot against ready and unprejudiced acceptance of facts or instructions. These are cases wherein excessive concern over such a condition as a short runway can cause the pilot to deviate from recommended approach procedures. Any of such attitude deficiencies may lead to pilot error and result in an aircraft accident.

5. DEFICIENCIES IN AIDS TO FLYING. To fly successfully the pilot is dependent upon many aids. These are both human and mechanical. In almost every phase of flight, from preflight planning to postflight parking, the pilot needs or uses advice and guidance from other human beings. In addition to human assistance, the pilot relies upon multiple mechanical aids which tell him of his position, velocity and attitude in space and which inform him of the functioning or malfunctioning of his machine. In addition to these aids, the pilot is also dependent upon

such structural items as ground approach lights and reliable runways. Deficiencies in such supervision, cockpit instrumentation or structural adjuncts can cause the pilot to err.

6. COMPLICATIONS AND DISTRACTIONS. Even when all other requirements for flying are adequately fulfilled on the part of the pilot, complications or distractions may arise, overwhelm him and cause him to err. These may be entirely beyond his control such as strong and unexpected cross winds or they may be induced by aircraft malfunction, human interference or by compromise of his own physical tolerances (see unexplained accidents).

Unsafe Acts—Supervisors and Maintenance Personnel

In addition to the pilot factor accidents resulting from inadequate assistance mentioned above, errors or omissions on the part of the supervisor and maintenance personnel can be the direct cause of aircraft accidents. The most obvious of these involves maintenance personnel wherein inadequate attention to essential maintenance procedures such as preflight lubrication may result in materiel failure and cause an accident. When the aircraft is subsequently totally destroyed it is frequently difficult or impossible to isolate maintenance oversight as the definitive factor. Thus, the role of inadequate maintenance is deserving of more consideration than afforded by its ordinary identification. Supervisory personnel may likewise lead to an aircraft accident by inadequate supervision or direction of essential aircraft upkeep. However, the most frequent type of supervisory error leading to an aircraft accident lies in the establishment of unsafe flight procedures or failure to properly monitor the flight. In the latter respect instructor pilots or aircraft commanders may be responsible for an aircraft accident even though they were not in control of the aircraft at the time of the accident. These are instances when an inexperienced pilot or crew member commits an unsafe act or omits an essential procedure and the flight supervisor fails to take corrective action.

Unsafe Conditions

Concerning unsafe conditions, failure of the power plant is the most frequent cause of accidents in this category. Also encountered but with less frequency are failures of various aircraft systems and components or inadequacies of runway, runway lighting, etc. Detailed reviews of airframe and power plant problems and their relation to aircraft accidents are presented in various aeronautical engineering publications. In addition, both civilian and government agencies maintain up to date information on facilities, navigational aids, air traffic control and similar fields devoted to support of flight.

Cause of Undetermined Accidents

Accidents in this category are of considerable interest to the Aeromedical profession because many of them are undoubtedly closely associated with human tolerances. In the majority of such cases the reason the mishap can not be determined is because: (1) the accident was highly destructive leaving few clues concerning preceding events or conditions or (2) the aircraft is missing, ordinarily from an over water mission. In both of these conditions there are often no survivors; also in both of these conditions there manifestly has been some deterrent, either mechanical or environmental, to normal human control or guidance of the flight. Inasmuch as investigation of aircraft wreckage usually reveals evidence of mechanical malfunction, it is possible that the majority of cause undetermined accidents are the result of human failure, of which there is little or no tangible evidence. In high altitude flight there is a distinct potential for serious environmental adversity. Whenever pressurization fails or the oxygen system fails the pilot can be quickly incapacitated. In this respect, hypoxia and decompression sickness has emerged as a probable cause in many cause undetermined military accidents. Also, in high performance flight, disorientation or vertigo can cause the pilot to place his aircraft in an attitude wherein recovery is difficult or impossible before it strikes the ground. In addition, toxicants, such as carbon monoxide or noxious fumes, may overwhelm the pilot and lead to a highly destructive accident. All such factors which can lead to partial or total incapacitations are serious accident potentials and the destructive nature of the accident may defy the subsequent identification of its cause. As mentioned under "Accident Investigations" below, careful aeromedical inquiry is essential if the cause factors in this category are to be explained and corrective action taken.

Human Limitations

An additional factor in the cause of aircraft accidents is the basic limitations of the pilot and aircrew. Flying depends upon the pilot's ability to make adequate perceptions, decisions and responses concerning the factors, influences and circumstances affecting flight. Inasmuch as there is a variable time lag in the process of perceiving, deciding and reacting, the rapidity of events may be such that the pilot can not meet the requirements placed upon him. Such human limitations are most obvious in midair collisions. High performance aircraft flying in ordinary cruising speed converge with such rapidity that it is difficult or impossible for the pilot to adequately evade even after perceiving an oncoming aircraft. Therefore, avoidance of such accidents rests upon traffic control or aids which can warn of an oncoming aircraft in time for evasive action. Similarly, the pilot may not be able to react in time to prevent an accident when an emergency arises. For example, when an engine malfunctions on takeoff, an accident may result before the trouble can be diagnosed and proper corrective action taken. Thus, many accidents charged to unsafe pilot acts have their origin in the fact that the aircraft operator is not able to perceive, interpret, decide and react in the brief period of time available during many flight conditions. A full understanding of such limitations is essential to aircraft accident prevention.

INJURIES

Injuries incurred in aircraft accidents are the result of deceleration, fire or miscellaneous adversities such as crushing, falls and asphyxia. The type and degree of injury is directly related to the type and degree of such forces or conditions encountered during the crash or immediately thereafter.

Inasmuch as the majority of aircraft accidents occur during some stage of landing or takeoff where impact forces are not great, survival is the rule (table 98). Also related

TABLE 98
Injuries Incurred in Aircraft Accidents*

Injury	Domestic Air Carriers 1949 through 1955		U.S.A.F. 1951 through 1953	
	Number of cases	Per cent	Number of cases	Per cent
Fatal injury	887	10.7	3,050	16.7
Major or severe injury	240	2.9	907	5.0
Minor or no injury	7191	86.4	14,337	78.3
Total	8318	100	18,294	100

* Source: Domestic, Safety Bureau CAB; U.S.A.F., Moseley, H. G.: Military Medicine, 116: No. 6.

to impact forces are aircraft types. Light aircraft with relatively slow takeoff and landing speeds are less liable to encounter high traumatic forces in their mishaps than heavy, high performance aircraft with their greater velocities. In this respect, the incorporation of larger and faster machines into air carrier systems and military usage carries attendant problems of survival should an accident occur. Although most occupants are not injured in low impact accidents the injuries incurred in high impact accidents are usually severe and often fatal. The most complete records concerning the nature of such injuries are in the United States Military Services (2) and reveal that in fatal cases multiple traumatic lesions are common (table 99). Burns and intracranial injury are also a significant cause of death. Among major nonfatal injuries, fractures, burns and lacerations are common (table 100).

Concerning the causes of injuries, the phenomenon of deceleration is the most frequent offender. This varies from very high impact accidents where there is explosive disintegration of the aircraft to low impact accidents where momentum is negligible. Deceleration acts upon both the occupant and objects within the aircraft and is modified to the degree to which they can be secured. In all cases of deceleration injury the time peak factor is most intimately associated with traumatic results. Dr. De Haven (3), Stapp (4) and others have shown that the human

body can withstand a remarkable degree of deceleration if high rates of onset and high peak loadings are avoided. Most injuries are the result of such deceleration peaks. When the body is unsecured or when the seat tears loose it is carried forward with speed approaching that of the aircraft in flight until its progress is arrested. Usually such arrest is by unresilient obstacles as the earth or previously decelerated aircraft structures. Under such circumstances, high peaks of deceleration are built up and one or more lethal lesions may result. Likewise, when the body is partially secured such as by the lap belt in forward facing seats the head and

TABLE 99
Primary Fatal Injuries Sustained in Major U.S.A.F. Aircraft Accidents
1953 and 1955

Type Fatal Injury	Number of Cases
Multiple traumatic injuries	1180
Burns	105
Intracranial injury	104
Intrathoracic or intra-abdominal injury	13
Transection of spinal cord	9
Hemorrhage (external)	3
Other	8
Missing	150
Total	1572

TABLE 100
Major Nonfatal Injuries, U.S.A.F.
1953 and 1955

Type Injury	Primary	Secondary
Fractures	225	244
Burns	81	165
Intracranial injury	51	12
With skull fracture	15	1
Without skull fracture (concussion)	36	11
Surface wounds	50	359
Sprains and dislocations	16	32
Intra-abdominal or intrathoracic injury	6	5
Other	10	14
Total	439	831

extremities flail during deceleration and build up high peaks of force when they strike the seat or other obstacles in their path. This accounts for many lethal head lesions as well as nonlethal fractures of the extremities.

PROTECTIVE EQUIPMENT

Protection against injuries in aircraft accidents involves the use of clothing, gear or devices which will mitigate against the traumatic factors which may be encountered in an accident. The most frequent adverse condition encountered in aircraft accidents is strong forces of acceleration (deceleration). The most basic consideration in protection against injury is securing of the body. This requires primarily that the seat, litter or object upon which the occupant is placed be firmly moored to the aircraft structures and that it not be dislodged or deformed during deceleration. The second requirement is that the occupant be secured to the seat or structure he occupies. Ideally, the torso, the head and the limbs should all be secured to prevent their flailing and forcibly striking other structures. In forward facing seats, this requirement is partially met by the use of lap belts and shoulder harnesses. Rearward facing seats appear to offer the most adequate total body restraint where use of such seats is practical; *i.e.*, passenger compartments. In addition to torso restraints, significant protection against head injury is offered by a helmet which will withstand relatively high impact forces.

The second most frequent cause of injury is fire. Therefore, protective clothing, including gloves, will reduce the incidence of injury caused by this factor. Other causes of injury, such as falls during escape, drowning, etc., are reduced by use of escape aids such as chutes or ropes and survival gear such as life vests and life rafts.

THE AEROMEDICAL INVESTIGATION OF AIRCRAFT ACCIDENTS

The medical investigation falls into two categories: (1) inquiry into the cause of injury and (2) inquiry into the human factors which may have caused the accident. These are as follows:

Cause of Injury

Ordinarily this phase of inquiry is first pursued. In a typical accident, the following areas need to be explored and are usually engaged more or less in the sequence given.

1. NATURE OF INJURY. The immediate concern of any physician attending an accident is giving professional aid to those who may be injured. Therefore, the first action is to determine the nature and extent of such injury in order that treatment may be given. However, beyond the need for knowing what treatment must be given, there is need to know many details concerning the injury, whether it be serious or trivial, for the injuries sustained are the most fundamental of all exhibits concerning the malevolence of the accident. From this evidence the injurious forces and objects can be measured or traced. On occasions it is possible to reconstruct the entire accident sequence from careful appraisal of injuries and evaluation of their probable cause factors (5).

2. ESCAPE AND SURVIVAL. Coincident with appraisal of injuries, it is necessary to know whether or not such injuries were inevitable under the circumstances encountered or whether they were compounded by inadequate provisions for escape and survival. Examples are burn injuries which would not have occurred had reliable escape mechanisms been provided or sprains and fractures which resulted because escape hatches or exits were so situated that injury was almost inevitable. All such observations form a basis for remedial action. In connection with military accidents, injuries incurred in connection with bailouts and ejections need also be evaluated.

3. FORCES OF DECELERATION. Directly correlated with injury are the forces to which the occupant is subjected. It is apparent that when extremely high or explosive deceleration forces are encountered, the human structure cannot withstand the trauma regardless of protection offered. However, frequently there is injury even though the impact forces were slight or moderate. In these cases, there is an indictment against protective equipment. Without knowing or estimating the force and direction of such force, it is difficult to determine whether or not structural improvements should be made.

4. RESTRAINING EQUIPMENT. As mentioned above, the majority of injuries incurred in aircraft accidents are either owing to the occupant being thrown upon impact or owing to inadequate restraint of head or extremities. There are very fundamental observations to be made in these areas. The first has to do with the effectiveness of torso restraint. In this respect, it is important to determine whether or not lap belts failed, seats failed, seat attachments failed, floors failed or any other restraint or linkage did not meet the requirement of preventing the occupant from becoming a missile. An additional aspect of this investigation is to determine whether or not adequate protection was provided against flailing of the head or extremities. Even though the torso is restrained, unfixed appendages may be whipped about and injured.

5. SHRAPNEL. The traumatic role of hurled objects needs inquiry. Even though the individual is adequately restrained, and in seats which face rearward to prevent flailing or whip lash injury, serious or lethal blows can be caused by flying baggage, tool boxes and other objects. Insofar as possible, these need to be identified in order that their traumatic role may be recognized and corrective action taken.

6. UNYIELDING OBJECTS. In addition to missiles, fixed structures often inflict injury. This may even occur in low impact accidents because of the obtrusive or unyielding nature of such items as gunsights, knobs or metal bars on seat backs. When such items are identified much can be done to eliminate them in future design.

7. OTHER CAUSES. Any other cause of death or injury needs to be traced to its source, and conclusions drawn as to what could be done to prevent it.

Human Factors as Cause of the Accident

By working with other investigators, the medical investigator can help determine whether or not human factors may have contributed or caused the accident. It frequently becomes apparent that some unsafe act on the part of the pilot (or crew) led to the mishap. The reason why, then becomes a matter of concern. It is essential for the aeromedical investigator to consider all of human factors discussed in the section on causes in this chapter and in fatal accidents to carefully consider conditions or events which may have adversely affected the pilot. In this respect, the medical investigator should consider the three major areas where adversities or inadequacies may induce the pilot to err and lead to an accident. These are: (1) environmental adversities, (2) behavior factors and (3) the pilot's physical condition.

1. ENVIRONMENTAL ADVERSITIES. Inasmuch as high altitudes, high velocities and space are hostile to life and well being, an aircraft operator is quickly overwhelmed if the artificial environment of his cabin fails or if there is a disruption of supplementary aids such as oxygen. In addition, any failure of, or distraction from attitude gyros and similar aids to spatial orientation can result in the pilot accidentally placing the aircraft into a flight course wherein the ground is struck before recovery can be effected. In accidents wherein the pilot is overwhelmed or where his perception is compromised, the aircraft usually plunges to earth with little or no effective human guidance. Usually these are vertical disasters (fig. 152). Investigation of the wreckage probably will reveal no evidence of mechanical malfunction and few, if any, clues to such irregularities as improper pressurization or faulty attitude gyros. However, whenever an aircraft accident cannot be explained by any other reason, and when it is of the vertical disaster type, the possibility of physical or physiologic compromise exists. Identification or implication of the basic cause rests upon review of the aircraft altitude and attitude at the time of the onset of the emergency, postulating the various environmental or operational irregularities to which the pilot might have been subjected and then determining the most probable adversity in view of the accident sequence. Supporting clues may be found in the history of the pilot's personal equipment, such as evidence of an ill fitting mask, or in the history of the aircraft's maintenance, such as records of pressurization failures. Relevant information can be obtained from review of the pilot's actions immediately prior to the accident sequence, such as when he announces that he is attending certain controls

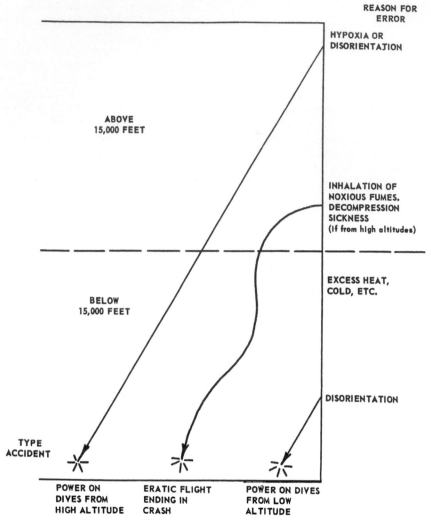

REASON FOR
ERROR

HYPOXIA OR
DISORIENTATION

ABOVE
15,000 FEET

INHALATION OF
NOXIOUS FUMES.
DECOMPRESSION
SICKNESS
(If from high altitudes)

EXCESS HEAT,
COLD, ETC.

BELOW
15,000 FEET

DISORIENTATION

TYPE
ACCIDENT

POWER ON
DIVES FROM
HIGH ALTITUDE

ERATIC FLIGHT
ENDING IN
CRASH

POWER ON DIVES
FROM LOW
ALTITUDE

FIG. 152. Vertical disasters

and where it is probable that such procedures would divert him from monitoring his instruments or maintaining level flight. Also laboratory procedures such as blood and tissue analyses may give evidence of such conditions as hypoxia or poisoning with toxic gases.

2. BEHAVIORAL FACTORS. The majority of pilot error accidents occur as a result of normal human variables such as inexperience, oversights, apprehensions and distractions as discussed in the section on "Unsafe Pilot Acts" above. These accidents are almost always characterized by evidence of conscious control of the aircraft prior to the accident and thus lead to what may be

termed horizontal disasters (fig. 153). In these cases, the pilot is flying straight and level or he is coming in for a landing or he is engaged in a takeoff when, as a result of some inadequacy, the accident occurs. Whenever an accident cannot be explained by other reasons and it is of the horizontal disaster type, the human factors discussed in the section "Cause of Aircraft Accidents" need to be carefully considered.

3. THE PILOT'S PHYSICAL CONDITION. Flying requires that the pilot have certain minimums of physical strength and endurance and that he be physically able to give continuous application to his occupation during the expected conditions experienced

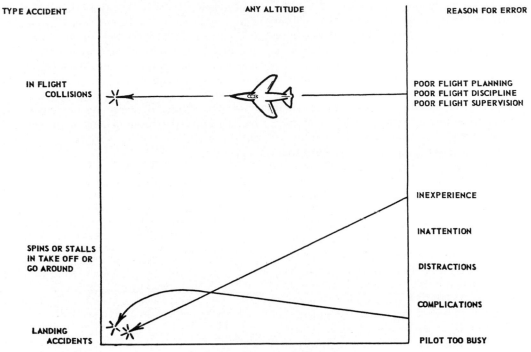

FIG. 153. Horizontal disasters

in flight. Occasionally, pilots are unable to meet these physical requirements because of fatigue, illness or physical disaster. Such inadequacies or infirmities are usually unpredictable and there is no particular pattern as to the type of accident which may result. In addition, there will be no evidence of mechanical malfunction as the aircraft was not at fault. Implication of the role of physical disability, if any, will rest upon exclusion of other causes, a review of the pilot's medical history and a postmortem examination. Concerning the medical history, clues may be found in the individual's size and weight, *i.e.*, was he able to adequately reach the aircraft controls; consideration of recent temporary illness and medication; and an appraisal of the potential decrements of fatigue in view of the length of the flight. In all but extremely disintegrating accidents a postmortem examination should give evidence as to whether or not degenerative disease could have been a factor.

AEROMEDICAL ASPECTS OF AIRCRAFT ACCIDENT PREVENTION

Aeromedical activities in the prevention of aircraft accidents fall into three broad categories: The first of these is care of the aircrew. This embraces all those activities concerned with establishment of physical standards for aircrew selection and with the continued surveillance of aircrew health and welfare including the monitoring of their behavioral variances. The medical phases of this activity are direct and unequivocal. Insofar as the standards of health are maintained, accidents caused by physical incapacities and poor health will be minimized. The behavioral variances of maintaining aircrew effectiveness are more complex. Such factors as the flyer's aptitude and attitude or his ability to meet the flying requirements placed upon him must be weighed against the responsibilities of his organization and the concepts of his society. Isolation of accident potentials lies in understanding the flyer's adjustments and proficiencies. Remedial action may be found in counseling with the flyer or may rest with the education of his supervisors.

An equally important phase of accident prevention is the development of understanding of the machine itself. The aircraft is a highly specialized environment that deserves the full attention of aeromedical personnel. Not only must it preserve the bio-physical requirements of life but its cockpit arrangements and instrumentation must be in equilibrium with the aircrew's ability to perceive, interpret, decide and react. Insofar as instruments replace the more familiar physical senses, preservation of life and avoidance of disaster depend upon their effectiveness and integrity. In accident prevention efforts it is valid to consider accident causes as being endemic in the cockpit area.

The last aeromedical requirement in accident prevention is the necessity for research. One of the most fundamental types of such research is aircraft accident investigation and preventive measures will lie in almost direct proportion to the thoroughness with which such investigations are conducted. However, the greatest contributions will lie in the lessons learned in the entire field of basic and applied aeromedical research. Here, the most important requirement is to recognize the application of observations which may arise. Many observations on human limitations, both physiologic and psychologic, receive little notice until it is somehow proven that an aircraft accident resulted from these same limitations. It then becomes necessary to make after the fact application of observations which could have been used to prevent the accident had they been properly recognized. In this respect, one of the greatest aeromedical requirements in accident prevention lies in the evaluation of research observations and determining how they can be best applied for the benefit of the organization or the society concerned.

REFERENCES

(1) MOSELEY, H. G.: An Analysis of 2400 Pilot Error Accidents. USAF Publication M-40-56. Office of the Inspector General, 1957.

(2) MOSELEY, H. G.: Aircraft accident injuries in the U. S. Air Force. J. Aviation Med., 29: 271–282, 1958.

(3) DeHAVEN, H.: Mechanical analysis of survival in falls from heights of 50 to 150 feet. War Med., 2: 586–596, 1942.

(4) STAPP, J. P.: Effects of mechanical force on living tissues. J. Aviation Med., 26: 268–288, 1955.

(5) ARMSTRONG, J. A., FRYER, D. I., STEWART, W. K., AND WHITTINGHAM, H. E.: Interpretation of injuries in the Comet aircraft disasters; an experimental approach. Lancet, 1: 1135–1144, 1955.

31

SPACE MEDICINE

Hubertus Strughold, M.D.

Human flight as we have seen it now for nearly 50 years according to its nature must be defined as atmospheric flight or transportation by air. The pertinent craft are wing supported and they are equipped with air breathing engines. The operational range of these propeller and jet driven airplanes, therefore, is confined to the denser regions of the atmosphere. But there is one developmental line of engine, based on the jet propulsion principle, that is independent of atmospheric oxygen for fuel combustion: the rocket. This propulsion engine, therefore, enables a vehicle to penetrate the regions beyond the atmosphere or the almost perfect vacuum of space. Furthermore, the potential, powerful thrust of the rocket exceeds by far all other propulsion methods and makes it even possible to reach distances of astronomical dimensions, such as those of the neighboring celestial bodies. Finally, the vehicle itself with regard to motion behaves, during the larger part of the trajectory, like a celestial body in terms of celestial mechanics. All of this represents a revolution in the development of flight and a unique challenge to medicine and biology as far as manned space operations are concerned.

Space Medicine is the name of that branch of medical science which studies the human factors involved in manned space flight. It is actually a logical extension of aviation medicine inasmuch as there are many interrelations between the two. As we will see later in detail there is, for instance, a transitional stage between atmospheric flight and space flight in the form of space equivalent flight.

In the climatization of the space cabin we can benefit from aeromedical experiences. Futhermore, our knowledge about the tolerability of g forces, gained on centrifuges during the past 20 years, can be applied to rocket-flight. It is no accident that Space Medical studies originated in aeromedical institutions (1–4). A special Department of Space Medicine, the first of its kind, for instance, was founded at the School of Aviation Medicine, Randolph Air Force Base, Texas in 1949 (5). This close relationship between aeromedical and space medical problems is aptly expressed by the term "Aerospace Medicine," the title of this book. The specific designation, Space Medicine, the title of this chapter, on the other hand, too, is justified or even necessary for various reasons. In atmospheric flight the flyer always remains to a certain degree under the protection of the atmosphere and is able to reach in a few minutes its safer lower regions. In space flight there is no surrounding atmospheric environment at all; it is a new medium for movement, in addition to land, sea and air. Furthermore, re-entry into the atmosphere is a complicated maneuver and even poses the most serious medical problem by itself. And, some completely novel, exotic conditions, such as weightlessness and radiations in their primary (cosmic) form, are encountered in space flight. The use of the term space medicine also emphasizes that a medical complement to space technology exists. Whereas aeromedicine, or aviation medicine, deals with the human factors involved in aeronautics, space medicine has to do with those involved in astronautics. It is, by and large, identical with bioastronautics, a term frequently found in the astronautic literature.

Space medicine must also include the study of the conditions found on other celestial bodies as to their suitability for terrestrial explorers, *i.e.*, from the viewpoint of human physiology. In this respect, it overlaps with astrobiology, a term used for that extra-terrestrial branch of biology which studies the question of possible indigenous life on other celestial bodies (chapter 32). Both aspects, the medical and the biologic, are covered by the term planetary ecology. So much about the definition of the areas of scientific medical and biologic interest in this beginning space age.

Scope of the Problems

Space medicine—as its parent discipline, aviation medicine—belongs into the categories of industrial medicine and environmental medicine.

Its industrial medical character is indicated by its consultative role in the design and engineering phase of space vehicles. It is not less manifested in the many medical problems faced at the launching sites which pose all the industrial hazards found in big factories, such as hazards connected with a great variety of toxic fuels stored in large quantities, working of the crew with extremely high and low temperatures, exposure to high levels of noise and other industrial hazards, to mention them only briefly. Certain factors of an industrial environment are encountered even in the space cabin itself, such as heat generation, and production of toxic material by the radio and power equipment, paint and other material. A detailed discussion of these items of space medicine as an industrial medicine goes beyond the scope of this chapter. It is essentially space medicine as an environmental medicine that will be the topic of the following discussion. There are several research areas in this respect which deserve special attention and are sufficiently progressed to be discussed in a publication such as a textbook and only these will be treated in the following paragraphs. They are:

1. Biophysics of the environment of space (ecology of space).

2. Gravity and motion in space flight.

3. Classification and medical characterization of the various conceivable kinds of space operations.

4. The space cabin.

5. Weightlessness as the outstanding novel environmental biogravitational factor.

6. Medical aspect of the prospects and limitations of space flight.

The important field of selection, training and physical conditioning will be touched upon only occasionally inasmuch as practical experience in these areas is not yet available. The reader is reminded that certain problems in the border area between aviation medicine and space medicine, such as tolerability of high *g* forces, rapid decompression and others, have already been discussed in previous chapters. As to certain other problems, such as rescue operations, nutrition and certain psychologic problems, as they are related to space medicine, the reader is referred elsewhere (6–9).

Biophysics in Space

The Basic Interplanetary Medium. Space is essentially an environment of radiations both of the electromagnetic and corpuscular kind which may be of solar and galactic origin. The solar electromagnetic rays include the wave lengths from 10 angstroms to radio waves of more than 10 meters. They all move with the speed of light. The corpuscular rays or particle rays consist of electrons and protons which are nuclei of hydrogen, nuclei of helium or alpha particles and nuclei of heavier atoms up to the iron group. They move with various speeds, some approaching that of light. Above a certain kinetic energy level they are called cosmic particle rays. Space also contains very thinly dispersed gaseous matter (about 1 to 10 gas particles, mainly hydrogen, in 1 cu. cm.). In the region of the inner planets these gas particles are mostly ionized by photochemical action of ultraviolet radiation; for this reason and others (emission from the Sun) electrons (about 10 to 100 per cu. cm.) are also found in these regions. The pressure exerted by this extremely rarified gaseous medium is not measurable and exceeds in this respect by far any vacuum that can be artificially produced in the laboratory. In addition to atomic and molecular particles, space contains dust particles (about 1 dust particle in 10 cu. m.). Furthermore, it is criss-crossed by meteorites of all sizes from micrometeorites as small as white blood cells to large lumps of matter. They move with an average velocity of about 40 km. per second or 25 miles per second. In this near vacuum environment scatter of solar light is minimal with the result that the sky is dark despite a bright shining sun (darkness of space). And, of course, this is no medium for sound propagation (silence of space). Such is the basic pattern of the physical—or with reference to life—the ecologic environment of interplanetary space (6, 7). This is in extreme contrast to our atmosphere, which is—near the earth's surface —an environment of dense gaseous matter permeated by relatively mild radiations and practically free of meteorites.

The knowledge of the basic properties and ingredients of the interplanetary medium is not enough for manned flight. There are enormous regional differences in the various parts of the solar system. They impose definite spatial limitations to astronautics. This requires a topographic approach to space ecology after the fashion of geography and can be called spatiography.

THE TRANSITIONAL ZONE FROM ATMOS-PHERE TO SPACE. The first spatiographic question that interests us from a medical point of view is, "Where above the earth's surface does Space begin?" According to theories in astrophysics, the atmosphere as a material continuum extends to about 1000 km. or 600 miles. In this region collisions between air molecules or atoms become very rare and the atmosphere thins out in the form of a spray zone (exosphere) into the nearly perfect vacuum of space. But this astrophysical aspect is not relevant to astronautics and especially not to manned space flight. In this respect, the cessation of the atmospheric functions and effects determine the border between atmosphere and space (10).

Atmospheric functions can, by and large, be divided into three principal categories: (1) life sustaining pressure functions, (2) life protecting filter functions and (3) mechanical effects and functions. By subdividing them more into detail we arrive at the following series of functional borders:

a. As low as 15 km. (about 10 miles) the influx of atmospheric oxygen into the lungs comes to an end because the alveoli are filled with water vapor and carbon dioxide, issuing from the body itself, to the full barometric pressure of 87 mm. of Hg found at that altitude.

b. At nearly 20 km. (12 miles) the corresponding total air pressure of 47 mm. of Hg is no longer effective to keep the body fluids in the liquid state (Armstrong, 1936).

c. At about 25 km. (16 miles) the air, owing to its low density, can no longer be utilized for cabin pressurization; instead, we need a sealed cabin; the same type as is required in space.

d. At 40 km. (24 miles) we are beyond the region of atmospheric absorption of cosmic rays and encounter them in their original primary form.

e. The same is true at 45 km. (28 miles) concerning the sunburn producing ultraviolet of solar radiation which is absorbed within the altitude range of the ozonosphere (20 to 45 km.).

f. The 50 km. (30 mile) level is the limit for aerodynamic lift and navigation even for the fastest winged craft.

g. At about 100 km. (60 miles) the rarified air ceases to scatter light which in the lower, denser atmospheric region produces indirect sunlight or the blue sky light. The absence of indirect sunlight results in a dark sky despite a bright, shining sun (darkness of space).

h. At about the same altitude propagation of sound terminates (silence of space).

i. At 120 km. (75 miles) we are beyond the meteor absorbing region of the atmosphere.

j. This is practically also the aerodynamic heat limit even for the fastest moving vehicle; from here on the temperature of the cabin's wall is determined exclusively by solar radiation.

k. Finally, at about 200 km. (120 miles) air resistance approaches zero. This mechanical border of the atmosphere (Haber (11)) is its final functional limit. At this altitude the "appreciable" or effective atmosphere terminates. If atmospheric interference of this kind is absent the vehicle and its crew are weightless.

For the whole atmospheric range within which the various atmospheric functions for manned flight cease, the term "aeropause" has been suggested (K. Buettner).

We can also explain the environmental situation in this whole region by saying that with the vanishing of its functions the atmosphere becomes partially space equivalent at 15 km. and progresses step by step to total space equivalence at 200 km., as far as the effectiveness of the atmospheric functions is concerned (12).

Three levels in the intra-atmospheric space equivalent region, where atmosphere and space overlap, deserve special attention because of their physiologic and technologic significance.

1. The physiologic zero line of effective air pressure at about 20 km. (12 miles) at which the environment for the unprotected human body attains the equivalent of a vacuum.

2. The aeronavigational zero line at 50 km. (30 miles) (von Karman). Above this line we deal exclusively with ballistics, and navigation by control surfaces has to be replaced by reaction control.

3. The mechanical zero line of air resistance at about 200 km. (120 miles). Here we enter the region of the "Kepler Regime" where the laws of celestial mechanics, unhindered by air resistance, are fully effective. It is here where space in its connotation, "outer space" actually begins.

Such is the picture of the border between atmosphere and space based on a physiologic and technologic analysis.

REGIONAL VARIATIONS OF THE ENVIRONMENT OF SPACE. In the space beyond the final (mechanical) border of the atmosphere, we do not encounter immediately the ultimate environmental medium of interplanetary space as described before; rather, up to considerable altitudes we find distinct regional differences in several respects. These peculiarities are caused by the earth's solid body, by the radiative properties of its surface and cloud cover, and by its magnetic field.

In the vicinity of the earth, for instance, on one side we are always protected from cosmic rays and meteorites by the solid body of our globe itself—just as we are protected on one side of a house against rain, hail or wind. Other peculiarities of the space environment near the earth are its shadow, its

own heat radiation and reflected solar radiation which influence the heat balance of a space vehicle and pose special visual problems.

In the polar regions the charged particles, essentially electrons and protons, are channeled into the atmosphere and produce via photoexcitation the Northern and Southern Lights which extend from 1000 km. (600 miles) down to 85 km. (60 miles). Over the equatorial region up to 45 degrees latitude north and south charged particles are trapped in the earth's magnetic field forming a huge radiation belt consisting of two zones. They were discovered by J. Van Allen by means of the Explorer satellites in 1958 (13). The inner zone extends from about 800 km. (500 miles) to 6500 km. (4000 miles) altitude. It is formed by trapped electrons and protons which are produced by beta decay of cosmic ray neutrons reflected from the fringe region of the atmosphere. The outer zone consists of electrons and protons directly coming from the sun (and stars) and trapped by the magnetic field lines. This zone extends from 12,000 km. (8000 miles) to about 180,000 km. (50,000 miles).

For all these reasons, space in the vicinity of the earth is distinctly different from open interplanetary space. If we wish to emphasize this fact, we might use for that region in which the earth's influence upon the environmental ecologic qualities of space is distinctly recognizable the designation "nearby space." For this nearby space, we might assume an extension up to 14 earth radii, depending on the outer boundary of the great radiation belt. Beyond this region we may speak of deep space which blends with interplanetary space in the region where the earth's gravitational predominance comes to an end (see below).

This deep interplanetary space again shows tremendous regional differences; they are observed in electromagnetic radiation of the sun as a function of the distance from this central source of radiant energy. These variations involve all sections of the electromagnetic spectrum, heat rays, visible, ultraviolet and x-rays. Heat rays include infrared and the neighboring wave lengths of visible rays. Their intensity outside of the earth's atmosphere is expressed by the solar constant which amounts to 2 gram calories per sq. cm. per minute. Owing to heat absorption within the atmosphere, at the earth's surface solar thermal irradiance drops to 1 gram calorie per sq. cm. per minute and less. In the following we choose the solar constant at the earth's mean solar distance as base line and departure point for considering heat radiation throughout the solar system. According to the inverse square law, the solar "constants" for the various planetary distances show tremendous differences (table 101). Heat radiation is, at the distance of Venus, about twice as high, and at the distance of Jupiter, 27 times less than the terrestrial value. That these variations pose problems concerning the climatization of the space cabin and set even definite spatial limitations to space flight will be discussed later.

Similar variations within the solar system are found in the visible portion of the radiation spectrum. The pertinent values for solar illuminance, expressed in lumen per square meter or lux, vary from nearly one million lux at the distance of Mercury to roughly 100 lux in the region of Pluto. At the mean solar distance of the earth solar illuminance amounts to about 140,000 lux. For comparison, on a sunny day at noon at the earth's surface light intensity is never higher than 108,000 lux. Light in space, too, is an important ecologic factor for space flight with regard to vision and as a possible source of energy for photosynthesis.

Concerning ultraviolet rays in space, our knowledge is still insufficient but that they,

too, should show tremendous variations within the solar system can be concluded from their photochemical effect upon the planetary atmospheres. These are manifested in the transformation of the primordial reducing (hydrogen) atmospheres to oxydized atmospheres in the realm of the inner planets (see chapter 32).

Considering all these tremendous regional ecologic differences as a function of the distance from the sun we immediately recognize a zone in which the conditions of interplanetary space and on the planets are not too different from those found at the earth's orbital distance and are relatively less hostile to manned space operations. It may, therefore, be justifiable to speak of a euthermal zone adjoined by a hyperthermal and hypothermal zone and of a euphotic zone adjoined by a hyperphotic and a hypophotic zone.

Heat radiation has, of course, some influence upon the occurrence of water on the planets in its biologically useable, namely liquid, form (liquid water belt in the planetary system) (14). And with regard to the chemistry of the planetary atmospheres we can speak of an oxygen belt.

All of these life favoring zones lie in about the same distance range from the sun—from the region of Venus to Mars—and are, therefore, parts of a general life supporting zone or ecosphere in the solar system. This is the region ecologically most acceptable for space operations.

TEMPORAL VARIATIONS. Most of the regional variations in the radiation "climate"

TABLE 101

Solar, Thermal Irradiance and Illuminance at the Mean Distances of Planets

Planet	Mean Solar Distance		Mean Solar Distance in Astronomical Units (A.U.)	Solar Thermal Irradiance	Solar Illuminance Lux
	10^6 km.	10^6 miles			
				gm. cal./sq. cm./min.	
Mercury	57.8	35.9	0.38	13.3	935,000
Venus	108.1	67.2	0.72	3.8	268,000
Earth	149.5	92.9	1.00	2.0	140,000
Mars	227.7	141.5	1.52	0.86	60,000
Jupiter	777.8	483.3	5.20	0.74	5,200
Saturn	1426.2	886.2	9.54	0.022	1,500
Uranus	2869.1	1728.8	19.19	0.0054	380
Neptune	4495.7	2793.5	30.07	0.0022	150
Pluto	5900.0	3670.0	39.50	0.0013	90

in our solar system are not in a steady state; rather, they show temporal variations as the result of fluctuations in the activity of the sun (solar flares and eruptions associated with sunspots) (15). During the time of a disturbed sun we observe tremendous intensifications in the ultraviolet section of electromagnetic radiations and sudden ejections of huge amounts of particle rays (protons and electrons). These jets of solar plasma may become especially noticeable in the outer zone of the aforedescribed great radiation belt of the earth. Such events represent times of increased radiation hazards (16). Increased solar activity repeats itself in an 11-year sunspot cycle; the resulting temporal pattern in the ecologic variations of space must be considered in scheduling manned space operations.

In the discussions about hazards in space, meteorites play an important role (17). However, the average basic meteoric density distribution seems to be lower than it formerly has been assumed. This has been confirmed by recordings in satellites. But besides these sporadic meteorites we have to consider regions and periods of increased danger in the form of meteor streams and swarms, which are remnants of disintegrated comets and still move in their former orbits. These meteor concentrations cannot be ignored in the topographic ecologic picture of space.

All these regional and temporal variations in the environment of space demonstrate the necessity of an ecologic spatiography or space map for selecting the safest routes and times for manned satellite flight and expeditions to other celestial bodies.

Gravity and Motion in Space

GRAVITY. So far we have discussed space as a material environment of radiant energy. We must add a few remarks about the gravitational forces effective in space which give us a better understanding of the process of motion in space and a basis for a subdivision of space useful for a classification of space operations from a navigational point of view. The underlying basic concept in this respect is that of the gravitational field. This concept is generally used to explain the mutual gravitational attraction of celestial bodies, pertur-

bations of their motions and tidal effects like ebb and flood. But the astronaut is additionally interested in the region within which the gravitational force of a specific celestial body is predominant. This zone is called sphere of gravitational influence in the astronautical literature. More precisely, it is the sphere of predominant gravitational influence and we might call it briefly gravisphere. Actually, we must differentiate between an inner gravisphere and outer gravisphere. The inner gravisphere represents the region within which the gravitational attraction of a large celestial body is able to hold a satellite in orbit (potential satellite sphere). The outer gravisphere determines the distance beyond the potential satellite sphere within which the gravitational force of a celestial body is still strong enough to cause considerable disturbances of the trajectory of a space vehicle.

The inner gravisphere, or potential satellite sphere, of the earth reaches as far as 1.5 million km. (one million miles). Beyond this distance the gravitational attraction of the sun becomes predominant and a space vehicle now moves in a heliocentric orbit as a planetoid. At the border of the earth's gravisphere the vehicle leaves the earth's gravitational domain and enters interplanetary space.

According to O. L. Ritter (18) the radii of the (inner) gravispheres are for Venus one million km. (0.6 million miles), for Mars 0.5 million km. (0.3 million miles), for Jupiter 52 million km. (31 million miles), for Saturn 55 million km. (33 million miles), for Uranus 70 million km. (42 million miles), for Neptune 116 million km. (70 million miles) and for Pluto 57 million km. (34 million miles). They vary considerably in size as a function of the planets' masses and of their distances from the sun because the solar gravitational field becomes weaker.

The Moon's gravisphere extends to 60,000 km. (36,000 miles) from its center. When a rocket crosses this gravitational divide it can, if properly guided, become a satellite of the Moon.

This spatial approach to the gravitational situation encountered in space flight gives us a basis for a subdivision of space into gravitational "territories," useful for a better understanding of satellite flight and interplanetary flight, etc., and of the velocities involved.

MOTION. To escape from the earth's gravisphere requires 7 miles per second, or 25,000 m.p.h. This so-called escape velocity represents a basic astronautical velocity and the above figure is only one example of this category. The respective values concerning other celestial bodies are found in table 102.

Escape velocity has to be attained within minutes after launching. This involves high accelerations up to 10 g with presently known propulsion systems. This active (power on) phase is followed by a passive period of coasting associated with zero g, until the vehicle enters again the atmosphere of a celestial body. During this latter period of deceleration, high g loads are again encountered. A similar pattern of motion dynamics is observed in satellite flight except that the velocities required and the g loads involved are somewhat lower. To orbit around the earth near its surface (if there were no atmosphere) requires 5 miles per second, or nearly 18,000 m.p.h. With increasing altitude the orbital velocities decrease according to table 103. The orbital velocity near the earth's surface, or circular velocity, represents an example of another important category of astronautical velocities. The circular orbital velocity around the moon is 1.1 miles per second and on Mars it is 2.2 miles per second. Since from the standpoint of propulsion the terrestrial orbital velocity is easier to achieve and has actually first been reached (1957), it is called the first astronautic or cosmic velocity. Escape velocity correspondingly is called the second astronautic or cosmic velocity. It was reached in 1959 with unmanned vehicles.

What we have discussed in the last two portions of this chapter about the environment of and motion dynamics in space may seem to be, at first glance, somewhat too much on the astronomic and astronautic side for a medical book; however, knowledge of these data is necessary in order to comprehend the full extent of the enormous task of medicine in the conquest of space.

CLASSIFICATION OF SPACE OPERATIONS

We can now proceed to classify the various space operations, based on the ecologic and

TABLE 102
Planets, Gravity and Escape Velocity

Planets	Gravity	Escape Velocity
	g	*miles per second*
Mercury	0.27	2.2
Venus	0.85	6.3
Earth	1.0	7.0
Mars	0.38	3.1
Jupiter	2.64	37.0
Saturn	1.17	22.0
Uranus	0.92	13.0
Neptune	1.12	14.0
Pluto		6.0?
Moon	0.16	1.5

TABLE 103
Orbital Velocity and Periods of Revolution of Satellites at Varying Altitudes (the Values near Sea Level are Theoretic Because of the Presence of an Atmosphere)

Altitude	Orbital Velocity	Periods of Revolution
miles	*m.p.h.*	*minutes*
1000	15,788	118.5
800	16,116	111.3
600	16,466	104.5
500	16,649	101.1
400	16,839	97.7
300	17,035	94.4
200	17,238	91.1
120	17,449	87.8
Near sea level	17,668	84.6

gravitational properties of the environment, the destination of the flight and on the pertinent motion characteristics and astronautic velocities. We see then developmental phases in the evolution of human flight as we observe them today, may see them tomorrow or in a more or less remote future as shown in table 104.

For the past 50 years we have been in the phase of atmospheric flight. Its very well known characteristics are listed in table 104. The second phase of human flight, and the first one with some space flight characteristics, is space equivalent flight. Its features are: jet and rocket propulsion, the partially space equivalent regions of the atmosphere possibly with ballistic dips beyond the effective atmosphere into nearby space, sealed

TABLE 104

Present and Future Basic Stages of Human Flight

Characteristics	Classification of Flight and Status of Vehicle			
	Atmospheric (Airplane)	Space equivalent (Airplane, rocket glider)	Satellite (Satellite)	Lunar, interplanetary, planetary expeditions (Space ship)
Environment	Troposphere, lower stratosphere	Space equivalent regions of the atmosphere	Nearby space	Deep space, interplanetary space
Dynamics	Aerodynamics	Aerothermodynamics, ballistics	Celestial mechanics	Celestial mechanics
Speed or velocity	Subsonic super-sonic speeds	Supersonic, hypersonic speeds	Orbital velocities	Escape velocities
Gravitational condition	Normal gravity	Subgravity, zero gravity	Zero gravity	Zero gravity

cabin, supersonic and hypersonic speed, multi-*g*'s, reduced *g* and brief periods of zero *g*; operational range, geographic dimensions; duration, fractions of hours; and status of craft, airplane and rocket-glider. High performance jet planes and rocket powered craft like the Bell X-2 and North American X-15 and Dyna Soar types are examples of the space equivalent flight category. When a manned vehicle is launched with orbital velocity, which is the first type of cosmic velocities, into an orbit around the earth we deal with manned orbital or satellite flight. The characteristics are: nearby space as the operational range, a geocentric orbit, sealed cabin, multi-*g*'s, long durations of zero *g* and satellite status of the vehicle.

The next and final basic phase of flight within our solar system will follow as soon as the terrestrial escape velocity of about 25,000 m.p.h. (second cosmic velocity) has been reached. The characteristics of such gravispheric escape operations are similar to those in satellite operations except that the vehicle now enters the gravispheres of other celestial bodies and may be prepared for circumnavigations of the Moon and the other planets, or it may even land there. This category would, therefore, include: lunar operations of several varieties, interplanetary space operations and planetary operations of several varieties.

Correspondingly, we shall have a whole family of rockets and space vehicles. Just as the zoologist speaks of a family tree of fish, or of amphibians and saurians, we can speak

of a family tree based on the jet propulsion principle.

The first descendant of the genealogic tree of jet propulsion is the air breathing jet engine used in jet planes; its maximum altitude ceiling is about 20 miles. The rocket—independent of the presence of air—is the spacebound descendant of the jet propulsion principle.

The first rockets, as designed by R. Goddard and W. von Braun, can be considered the protorockets. Their descendants are the intermediate and intercontinental ballistic missiles. The manned counterpart of the intercontinental ballistic missile will be an intercontinental rocket glider for long distance space equivalent flights. A logical development of the small research satellite will be larger manned satellites and space ships designed for lunar, interplanetary and planetary operations will be the final descendants on the family tree of the primordial rocket.

This general survey of the various kinds of space operations and vehicles, required to carry out these operations, reveals the multitude and diversities of the medical problems involved. Some of them are encountered to a greater or lesser degree in the preliminary stages. The spectrum of the problems widens with more advanced operations. The emphasis may shift from one problem to another. Finally, the time factor or the duration of the flight will move from the background into the focus of all our medical thinking. This becomes especially evident when we discuss the problem of keeping man alive in the environment of space, *i.e.*, the medical problems centered around the space cabin.

SPACE CABIN

The central task of space medicine is human engineering of the space cabin—the astronaut's temporary home. Almost all space medical problems have some relation to this objective which, of course, requires the closest cooperation with space technology. It is the purpose of the space cabin to keep the occupants healthy, well and efficient for days, weeks or many months in the environmental medium of space, thousands or maybe millions of miles away from the earth. By and large this function of the space cabin is two-fold:

1. To protect the astronauts from external factors such as meteorites and radiations.

2. To provide them with all vital necessities for survival and comfort as far as possible.

If the first function cannot be achieved, the efforts concerned with the second one would be futile.

That in a near vacuum, such as that of space, a manned cabin has to be a completely closed or hermetically sealed compartment does not need explanation. And that this is a requirement even in altitudes as low as 75,000 feet has been explained in chapters 12 and 13.

Protection from External Factors

METEORITES. The protective function of the space cabin against dangers from the outside medium of space has a direct bearing upon the structure and material of the cabin's hull. The most discussed factor in this respect is a collision with a meteorite. Most of the meteorites are of cometary origin and have a low density, much lower than ordinary stone and are, therefore, very fragile. Those of asteroidal origin (between Mars and Jupiter) are both stony and metallic. The average velocity is about 40 km. per second (25 miles per second) and at the edge of the earth's atmosphere the velocity can never be less than 11 km. per second (7 miles per second) because of the Earth's gravitational pull. An extensive visual, photographic and radio meteor research program has been under way for about 10 years (17, 19, 20) and

has recently taken advantage of the recording possibilities in research satellites and space probes. The kinetic energy and the density distribution of meteorites and the resulting collision probability are of special interest to space medicine. Generally, the hit frequency decreases with increasing size of the meteorites.

Two types of effects upon a space vehicle can be differentiated: *i.e.*, punctures and surface erosion.

Estimations of hit frequency resulting in a puncture caused by a meteorite, weighing 1 gram or less, range from 1 in 2 months to 1 in 2 years. A puncture can lead to rapid decompression of the cabin's air with all the physiologic consequences for the astronaut: hypoxia, aeroembolism and boiling of body fluids (ebullism) (chapter 13). In such an emergency the time of useful consciousness (H. G. Armstrong) may offer a chance to seal the leak. Also, suggestions have been made for protection in the form of self-sealing devices and of a secondary hull (meteor bumper) (F. Whipple) surrounding the cabin to absorb the kinetic energy of the colliding meteoric body.

Erosive effects of fine meteoric material on surfaces exposed to space may affect the transparency of windows, the maintenance of radiative heat balance of the cabin and the utilization of electronic equipment. Surface erosion may be negligible beyond the belt of the asteroids. But within and near this belt (between Mars and Jupiter) possibly puncturing may be more frequent. The ideal protection would be if the above mentioned protective measures would reduce this meteoritic hazard to the level found on the earth's surface provided by the shielding mantle of the atmosphere.

RADIATION. The same holds true for another, perhaps even more acute, environmental hazard in space; radiation. In the center of medical concern in this respect are the cosmic particle rays which are essentially of extrasolar origin but contain also a solar component. Their biologic effect has been studied in the altitude regions of 30 km. in balloons where they are encountered in the primary form, especially beyond the 55 degree latitudes (16, 20, 21). Primary cosmic particle rays, especially the heavy components, produce in tissue at the end of their tracts a "microbeam" of ions and electrons, destroying thousands of cells. It has been found that when such hits involve pigment cells within the hair follicles they produce streaks of gray hairs on black rats (23). But our knowledge is still far from being sufficient and we need more data from biologic experiments in satellites and deep space probes which have to be supplemented by experiments with accelerated ions in the laboratory (24). Nevertheless, there is no question that some kind of shielding is required especially since we have knowledge of the existence of a two zonal radiation belt surrounding the earth and the occurrence of solar plasma jets after solar flares (15). Basically, the radiation situation of the occupants of a space vehicle is this: The primary particle rays will penetrate, unchanged, the hull of the cabin or they will be transformed within the material of the hull into secondary rays, penetrating the cabin's interior just the same as the primary cosmic rays are transformed into secondary rays by the earth's atmosphere. It then is the purpose of shielding to block the primary cosmic rays and to reduce the secondary rays to tolerable levels. As a rule, the shielding devices must be effective enough to keep the total radiation inside the cabin below the maximum permissible level, which is determined by a significant health and performance decrement. The protective range of shielding must be such that it also can cope with the unpredictable radiation intensifications during increased solar activities (25). At this point it should be mentioned that there are some parallels between shielding from all of this natural radiation and that from radiation artificially produced in nuclear propulsion (26).

Our knowledge about the gamma ray and x-ray component of cosmic rays and x-rays from the sun is still spurious.

Special protection from ultraviolet of solar radiation will be unnecessary because practically all the material of the devices that keep a man alive in a vacuum (cabin hull and pressure suit) absorb these rays sufficiently.

Visible radiation or light in space poses problems. The bright, shining sun on a dark sky which is caused by the absence of in-direct sunlight, leads to a magic illumination inside the cabin in that everything exposed to direct sunlight appears extremely bright and everything in the shadow is dark. This requires light scattering glass in the windows to diffuse the solar light before it enters the cabin if this light source for intracabin illumination should be used (27, 28). At this point it should be mentioned that looking into the sun may lead to retinal damage, such as retinitis solaris and retinal burns (helioscotoma). Eye protection from solar irradiation by means of automatically functioning light absorbing glasses is necessary. Retinal lesions of this kind to be anticipated are actually heat effects by visible rays and the neighboring near infrared rays focused by the eye's lens upon a small area in the fovea centralis retinae. Heat radiation plays an important role as an external factor influencing—in combination with internal factors—the intracabin temperature. Because of this combination we shall discuss this subject matter within the frame of the intracabin environment and not in this portion, which is devoted to the protective function of the cabin from external hazardous agents effective in space.

Provision of Vital Necessities in the Space Cabin

TEMPERATURE. A general vital ecologic factor in any environment is a physiologic range of temperature. The temperature within a space cabin is determined by the difference in heat gain and heat loss. The heat gain involves various sources inside the cabin, such as body heat of the occupants, lighting and other auxiliary equipment. The heat production of one man is roughly equivalent to that of one 100-watt electric light bulb. Heat sources outside the cabin include aerodynamic heating during launching and atmospheric entry and solar radiation. Aerodynamic heating is enormous but lasts only a few minutes and to provide protection against it is the task of technology. Above the effective atmosphere, solar thermal irradiance amounts to 2 gram calories per sq. cm. per minute at the earth's orbital distance but varies considerably with the distance from the sun within the range from Mercury to Pluto (table 101).

The heat loss of a space vehicle—during actual space flight—is essentially effected by radiation (29, 30). Inasmuch as radiation is involved in both heat gain and heat loss this factor determines the heat balance inside a space vehicle. Human engineering in this respect has to aim at an intracabin temperature in the comfort range which is 70 to 80° F. This can be achieved by a suitable surface variation concerning reflection and absorption of solar heat radiation (29).

HUMIDITY. The tolerability of temperature is closely related to relative humidity. This factor in the sealed cabin is essentially determined by the moisture given off—in amounts of from 50 to 80 grams per man per hour—through respiration and perspiration under normal temperature conditions. The relative humidity should be kept within the comfort limits of between 30 and 50 per cent for which various chemical absorbents are available (30, 31).

After the discussion of these general ecologic factors we must consider the cabin's atmosphere, its pressure, composition and the respiratory gases.

AIR PRESSURE AND COMPOSITION. An air pressure must be chosen which conforms with physiologic requirements and technologic considerations. Principally, the barometric pressure should be kept as close as possible to the sea level value. However, the physiologist could make concessions in this respect to the engineer who, for structural reasons, might desire a lower pressure difference between the cabin's air and the surrounding near vacuum. From the physiologic point of view a minimal barometric pressure of half an atmosphere—380 mm. of Hg, corresponding to an altitude of 5.5 km. (3.5 miles) would be acceptable. The pressure difference between cabin and vacuum would then amount to ½ kg. per sq. cm. or about 7 p.s.i. But heavy shielding against cosmic rays and meteorites may make the engineer's concern irrelevant.

The chemical composition of the artificial atmosphere should include nitrogen; there is no compelling reason for replacing this constituent of our natural atmosphere by helium as has been occasionally suggested. If an air pressure of half an atmosphere is chosen, 40 volume per cent oxygen would maintain the oxygen partial pressure in the cabin near sea level values.

METABOLIC DATA. Before we discuss the respiratory and nutritional requirements we first shall consider the fundamental data in this respect for a "standard man" of 70 kg. (154 American pounds), as shown in figure 154 (30).

The assumption of a relatively low meta-

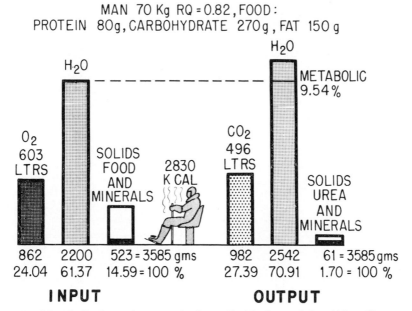

FIG. 154. Metabolic data of a "standard man" of 70 kg. weight. (After Clamann.)

bolic rate of 2800 kg. calories per day, on which all data in this figure are based, may be justified, inasmuch as in the confinement of the space cabin heavy physical exercise cannot be expected, and the weightless state *per se* will tend to tone down metabolism. Assuming a respiratory quotient R Qu $\frac{CO_2}{O_2} = 0.85$, which is the value for a well balanced diet, and assuming light to moderate work for a period of 8 hours during 24 hours, this metabolic level involves: Consumption of roughly 600 liters or 0.85 kg. of oxygen per day and correspondingly production of about 500 liters or 0.96 kg. of carbon dioxide per day.

RESPIRATORY GASES. In a sealed compartment of 50 cubic feet the normal oxygen content of the air would, by the respiratory process of our "standard man," drop in about 4 hours to 14 volumes per cent, the threshold of hypoxia and during the same time carbon dioxide would accumulate to 6 volumes per cent, far beyond its toxic threshold if no means for the regeneration of the air were provided. It is, therefore, a prerequisite for every kind of space flight, except for some short ballistic trajectories, to control the respiratory environment in this respect. That this control must be extended to other environmental factors such as humidity and temperature has been mentioned before.

Two fundamental methods or stages of regeneration of the environment or of environmental control must be differentiated: (1) control by replacement and storing and/or elimination and (2) control by recycling.

Stage 1 is the method of regeneration for short time space operations and is based on physical and chemical procedures. It includes replacement of the consumed oxygen from tanks, elimination of carbon dioxide and water vapor by chemical absorbents and storing or elimination of liquid and semi-liquid waste products.

The two respiratory gases must be controlled in such a way that oxygen pressure does not exceed the permissible maximum, which is about 350 mm. of Hg and that it does not drop below the permissible minimum level of 100 mm. of Hg. And, carbon dioxide pressure should be kept below 10 mm. of Hg, which is the permissible limit for extended periods of time (fig. 155).

Conventional absorbers for carbon dioxide are sodium hydroxide and potassium hydroxide, baralyme (a mixture of calcium hydroxide and barium hydroxide) and soda lime (a mixture of calcium hydroxide and sodium hydroxide) and lithium hydroxide. In addition to chemical absorption of carbon dioxide physical methods such as "freeze out" and others have been considered (30–32).

All of these methods for the regeneration of the breathing air (oxygen supply from stores and removal of carbon dioxide by chemical and physical means) which have a long tradition in U-Boat or submarine medicine (33) can be developed to a stage that they are adequate for space flight operations up to maximally 2 months. Beyond this duration these measures will pose problems in terms of economic logistics when we consider that for such a period an oxygen supply of 50 kg. per man would be required and more than that amount of chemicals for the absorption of carbon dioxide and water vapor. The solution to this is recycling. This leads

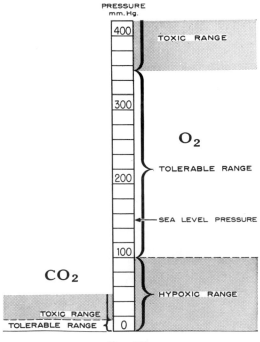

FIG. 155

us to the discussion of the "closed ecologic system."

CLOSED ECOLOGIC SYSTEM. First we can employ physicochemical means for recycling to supply the respiratory and, to a certain extent, other metabolic requirements. This method might be logistically acceptable for a duration of one year. Beyond this time reconstitution of *all* vital necessities, air, water and food, is necessary, if we wish to stay in the payload capabilities of rockets. The method of choice, then, is biologic recycling as we find this in free nature in the biotic relationship between the animal and plant kingdoms, namely in the process of photosynthesis found in all chlorophyl bearing plants.

Photosynthesis is the reverse process of respiration as a comparison of their reaction formulae shows:

Respiration: $C_6H_{12}O_6 + 6O_2 \rightarrow$

$$6CO_2 + 6H_2O + \text{heat energy}$$

Photosynthesis: $6CO_2 + 6H_2O +$

$$\text{radiant energy} \rightarrow C_6H_{12}O_6 + 6O_2$$

In the early pioneer studies it was found that about $2\frac{1}{2}$ kg. of fresh weight of the alga *Chlorella pyrenoidosa* are capable of meeting the respiratory requirements of one man (34). Recently at the School of Aviation Medicine, Randolph Air Force Base, other green microorganisms have been found to be three times as effective under conditions of light saturation. Mice could easily be kept alive in a small closed ecologic system equipped with such a photosynthetic gas exchanger for a month (35–37).

Research in this field goes on in the direction of finding still better strains of green microorganisms and of attaining higher rates of light saturation under operational conditions. An interesting but hazardous by-product of photosynthesis has been discovered in the appearance of small amounts of carbon monoxide which, after some time, accumulate to toxic quantities (38). This was not known in botany, but a solution has already been found to counteract this danger by eliminating this hemoglobin blocking gas.

Biologic cycling will be the method for the regeneration of the breathing air in extended space operations, such as planetary expeditions. As the reaction formula for photosynthesis shows, apart from the liberation of oxygen, carbohydrates are built up. Actually this is generally considered the main function of photosynthesis. Accordingly, research is being conducted to take advantage of this fact in order to use photosynthesis as a method of food production. Ultimately, recycling must include not only the carbon cycle (as in photosynthesis) but also the nitrogen cycle, phosphorcycle and so on (39). It will require some time of intensive research until a well functioning closed ecologic system will be achieved for use in extended space flight and at temporary inhabited bases on the Moon or Mars. A rigid economy in human logistics, dictated by the vertical pay load capabilities of space vehicles and anthropometric considerations, has to be the guiding principle in these efforts of bioastronautics (40–43).

SPACE CABIN SIMULATOR AND MEDICAL ASTROINSTRUMENTATION. The groundwork to attain successful space flight has to be done in the laboratory. A new type of experimental chamber, a completely closed or sealed cabin, has been developed for the purpose of testing air regeneration devices and the behavior of the occupants in a sealed off compartment. The first one-man chamber of this type was developed in 1954 in the Department of Space Medicine, at the School of Aviation Medicine, Randolph Air Force Base, Texas (44) (fig. 156). The objectives of the experiments in such space cabin simulators include the study of the best kind of artificial atmosphere with regard to composition and pressure and the achievement of a maximum efficiency of the air regenerating and controlling devices combined with a minimum of their volume and weight (45). Miniaturization and minimization has to be the rule in the field of astroinstrumentation. This refers also to recording equipment concerning the physical conditions in the space cabin (oxygen sensors, carbon dioxide sensors, etc.) and concerning physiologic reactions (electrocardiogram, electroencephalogram, respiratory movements, body temperature, etc.). That all data recording must include telemetry, is novel in this medical astroinstrumentation. Considerable progress has been made in this respect in the development

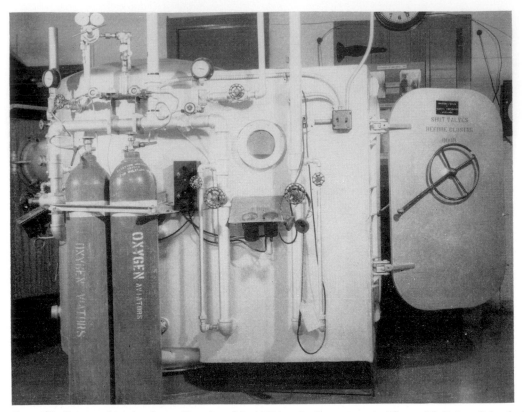

FIG. 156. Space cabin simulator. Developed in 1954 by the Department of Space Medicine, School of Aviation Medicine, U. S. Air Force.

of so-called "biopaks" for animal experiments in rockets (46) (fig. 157). Parallel with this went the development of capsules for man which led to successful flights in balloons such as that of D. G. Simons (47), M. D. Ross and M. L. Lewis (48) who penetrated deep into the atmospheric space equivalent regions which require a sealed compartment. Actually sealed capsule flights in a balloon up to 42,000 feet were made by A. Piccard as early as 1930, and by A. W. Steven and O. A. Anderson up to 72,000 feet in 1934.

Returning to laboratory experimentation, the studies in space cabin simulators include also the search for the best pattern for the alternation of work, rest and sleep, generally referred to as day-night cycling. No less important are the psychologic reactions of man to confinement, sensory deprivation and isolation (49, 50). Their study comprises a large part of the experimental program in space cabin simulators and will have some bearing upon the selection of astronauts.

Space cabin simulator experiments in the order of a month's duration are a matter of routine. A further temporal extension and the inclusion of more than one occupant in a multiseat space cabin simulator surrounded by a vacuum (space simulator) are the objectives of present and future space medical research.

Space cabin simulators also can serve as training devices (51, 52) to indoctrinate future astronauts in the medical problems involved in a closed ecologic system and to familiarize them with the procedures necessary to cope with emergency situations such as failure of the automatic controls and a leak in the cabin. We cannot, of course, simulate in such space cabin simulators all the conditions encountered in space flight such as, for instance, zero gravity or weightlessness. This condition affects considerably human engineering of and life in the space cabin and demands, therefore, special attention of both technology and medicine.

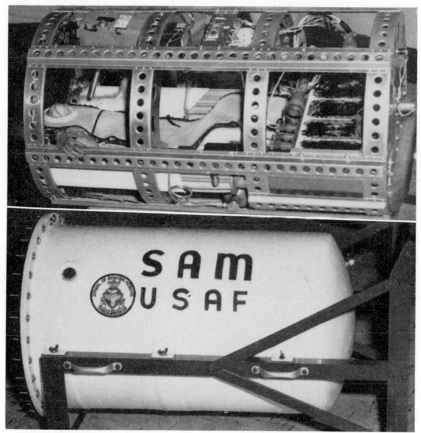

Fig. 157. Biopak: upper picture, animal container; lower picture, shell. Developed by the School of Aviation Medicine, U. S. Air Force.

WEIGHTLESSNESS

The basic dynamic pattern of a space flight trajectory consists of an active (power on) phase, a passive (power off) phase of coasting, and atmospheric re-entry. The first and last of these phases are associated with high accelerations and decelerations, respectively, resulting in multiples of g as high as 10; the phase between the two, which represents the actual motion situation in space, is characterized by zero g or weightlessness. The physiologic effect of the increased g pattern in flight has previously been discussed in chapter 17 (53–56). Only the effects of zero g, therefore, will be the topic of the following paragraphs.

Occurrence of zero gravity or weightlessness can be imagined in two ways: First, it could be established if we build a giant tower over the North Pole many thousand miles high. Inasmuch as gravitational attraction

decreases with increasing altitude according to the inverse square law, the weight of everything in and on the tower would decrease to one-fourth of its earth's surface value at 4000 miles (twice the earth's radius from its center); at 8000 miles it would drop to one-ninth, and so on. At 36,000 miles or 10 times the earth's radius from its center it would be reduced to one-hundredth. From a physiologic point of view this would be practically weightlessness. In this sense, reduced weight and weightlessness would depend on the distance from the earth's gravitational center but this interpretation of weightlessness would be valid only for a supported body at rest as in the above hypothetical example (we might call it static weightlessness), and is by no means applicable to a moving body in space. In space, flight weightlessness is not a function of the distance from the earth's gravitational center, rather it is a matter of motion dynamics and can be produced everywhere (57–59). It occurs when the gravitational pull of the earth is balanced by inertial (usually called centrifugal) forces originating in the vehicle by its motion. This is dynamic weightlessness. This state is maintained as long as no external forces such as atmospheric friction or motive power interfere with this balanced condition.

Above the mechanical border of the atmosphere (120 miles), therefore, dynamic weightlessness can be observed for any length of time. Within the atmosphere it can be produced in so-called parabolic flight maneuvers or semiballistic and ballistic trajectories in jet or rocket powered planes and rockets for periods in the order of seconds and minutes.

With regard to the effect of weightlessness upon the human body we are essentially concerned with two questions: (1) What is the effect of zero gravity or weightlessness upon the somatic nervous system which is responsible for spatial orientation and sensomotoric control of position and movement of the body and body parts? That is, what is the effect on performance? (2) What is the effect upon the autonomic nervous system and vegetative processes controlled by it, such as respiration, circulation, digestion, and on the general well being?

A number of theoretic papers have been written and numerous experiments testing the effects in both respects have been carried out in aircraft on man and animals, in rockets and satellites (60–66).

The study of human performance has been concentrated upon neuromuscular coordination and on orientation in space during parabolic trajectories in aircraft. The subjects had to perform certain tests such as cross-marking and stylus aiming with open and closed eyes. After some initial deviations neuromuscular coordination became satisfactory, especially when supported by visual control. It has also been shown that spatial disorientation rarely takes place as long as the subject retains visual reference. The feeling of falling is generally absent in the weightless state, especially if the subject has the mental set that he is weightless and therefore cannot fall (67).

In the transitional phase from one or several g's to zero g, optical illusions have been described which consisted of upward and downward movements of the after-image (61, 68).

In the weightless state proper, then, performance seems to be not markedly disturbed, at least not for periods of reduced and zero g of below 1 minute. This has been supported by experiments on animals which were trained to perform certain tasks during ballistic trajectories in aircraft and rockets. For an explanation of this whole sensory motoric behavior in the gravity free state, we must briefly analyze the sense organs involved.

The human body possesses several sense organs equipped with specific nerve endings that serve as "mechanoreceptors," such as the very well known centrally located otolith organ in the inner ear, and the (not so well known) group of peripheral mechanoreceptors, such as the pressure sense receptors distributed over the entire skin—Meissner's corpuscles and nerve endings on hairs—specific nerve endings in the muscles—the so-called "muscle spindles"—and finally nerve endings in the connective tissue surrounding the muscles—the Pacinian corpuscles (posture sense). All of these receptors have an exteroceptive function, insofar as they react to external forces and inform us about the outer world such as manifestations of the gravitational pull of the earth in the form of weight. They also have an enteroceptive or proprioceptive function insofar as they inform us of the tension conditions of the skin, the muscles and the connective tissue. They play, therefore, an important role in the sensomotor control of the movement of the whole body as well as its parts. In the otolith organ and the pressoreceptors in the skin the exteroceptive function is more pronounced. In the other mechanoreceptors, the proprioceptive function is dominant. But all of these functions are in more or less degree related to the effect of the earth's gravity. The whole group of these mechanoreceptors is, therefore, called "gravireceptors," although we cannot of course sense gravitational forces as such.

In the gravity free state the exteroceptive function of the mechanoreceptors is eliminated; the proprioreceptive function, however, is not. This explains why after some familiarization, performance of neuromuscular tasks is not particularly impaired. For orientation in the weightless state (69), the absence of the exteroceptive function of the mechanoreceptors must be compensated by the eye, the only sense organ that can furnish information in this respect in space flight. That there are certain sensory parallels between the condition of weightlessness and submersion in water can be mentioned only briefly (70).

Some of the gravireceptors, namely, the otolith organ in the inner ear and those mechanoreceptors found in great numbers in the peritoneum of the abdomen (Pacinian corpuslces), have strong reflex connections with the autonomic nervous system which controls circulation, motion of the stomach and intestines, etc. The most conspicuous and discomforting manifestation of such reflexes are those producing the symptom complex of motion sickness.

This brings us to the second problem, vegetative processes under the condition of weightlessness.

Motion sickness and nausea have been actually observed in about one-third of 50 subjects during and after parabolic flights in jet planes. The majority were indifferent in this respect, and some of them even felt elated and enjoyed the weightless state, which of course lasted never longer than 40 seconds. Inasmuch as this phase was preceded and followed by a brief period of increased g, we cannot conclude from these experiments that weightlessness was the cause of the observed nausea; rather, it might have been the result of the fast sequence of variations of g as this is also the case in sea sickness and air sickness.

The behavior of respiration and circulation during the weightless state, lasting 3 to 8 minutes, has been recorded in animals (dogs and monkeys) during ballistic trajectories in rockets, with the result that there was a general tendency to a decrease in the activity of these functions (66). This, too, was found in the several days long orbital flight of the Russian dog, Laika (71). There are some noteworthy effects associated with the transition from increased g to zero g. It took the dog Laika three times longer to

return to normal (zero g) circulation rate and blood pressure following the ascent into orbit than it did after simulated rocket launching accelerations on a centrifuge which, of course, ended at 1 g.

Similarly, it was found that blackouts of human subjects during brief periods of high accelerations up to 6.5 g lasted longer when they were followed by zero gravity (72). These transition symptoms, namely, effects of increased g upon the physiologic zero g conditions and, of course, *vice versa*, effects of prolonged zero g upon the tolerance of increased g (during atmospheric re-entry), will demand special medical attention in the future.

As soon as space flight over longer durations can be made, other vegetative factors have to be considered such as nutrition and elimination of the body wastes and all vegetative processes connected therewith. Drinking of fluids is, of course, not possible from an open container and requires a squeeze bottle. Concerning swallowing we must consider potential hazards by aspiration. Micturition has been found to be possible under weightless conditions although the familiar urge sensation is not experienced (73).

All of these examples and results in psychologic and physiologic research demonstrate the necessity of a kind of human engineering in this respect. In more spacious vehicles, movement of the occupants will require hand rails, magnetic shoes and other special equipment. All of this will be necessary if weightlessness can be tolerated without too great discomfort over longer periods of time. Certain questions are still completely open, such as sleep under weightless conditions. The answer in this and other respects can be found only in experiments in orbital space flight. If the answer is negative, then artificial gravitation must be provided by rotating the space vehicle. In this case two questions will arise: (1) how much of a fraction of 1 g is required to reach a sort of normalization in the gravitational life of the astronaut, and (2) will Coriolis effects influence his well being?

So far, medical zero gravity experimentation seems to indicate that artificial gravitation will not be required. Whether or not it is, a careful indoctrination and training of the astronaut will be necessary.

MEDICAL ASPECTS OF THE PROSPECTS AND LIMITATIONS OF MANNED SPACE FLIGHT

Plans and projects for manned space flight, offered in the astronautical literature, are numerous. The potentialities in the space age seem to be limitless and the velocities appear to have become meaningless. From a medical point of view this is not so! Some of the projects are sound and are indeed a unique challenge for space technology and space medicine but there are also definite limitations from the viewpoint of the physician. After more than 10 years of theoretic and experimental studies, space medicine can and is obliged to make definite statements in this respect. The following remarks will concentrate upon the limitations which reflect also the medically conceivable possibilities.

The limitations to manned space flight are determined by two factors: (1) the extreme regional variations of the physical environment of space itself and the degree of hostility of the environment found on the celestial bodies and (2) the time involved, or the duration of the flight; this is closely related to velocity which by itself can become a limiting factor.

Regional limitations to space flight are found immediately in the vicinity of the earth. The factor in question is Van Allen's great radiation belt with its inner and outer zone, as described before. Although at this time the exact topographic intensity pattern is not known, this much can be said—that both of these zones will be prohibitive for manned satellite flight; the relatively safe region for this type of space flight will probably not extend beyond 800 km. (500 miles) above the earth's surface. Whether or not repeated satellite passage through the "slot" between the two belts (from about 6500 to 13,000 km. (4000 to 8000 miles) is medically permissible, requires further exploration. In all other more extended space operations into deep space, protective measures must be considered. They are: avoiding the danger zones by choosing the polar regions as exit and re-entry routes, higher velocities to shorten the time of exposure and shielding, or a combination of them. This is the problem that will occupy astrophysics, space technology and space medicine in the coming years. The same is true concerning the possible occurrence of similar radiation belts surrounding other celestial bodies, such as Venus and Mars. These localized corpuscular radiation concentrations seem to be more important from the standpoint of radiation hazards than the more or less evenly distributed omnidirectional cosmic rays including their heavy components.

With this we have already touched upon interplanetary space. Here, too, we recognize spatial limitations to manned space flight as the result of the extreme regional variations in solar electromagnetic radiation within the range from Mercury to Pluto, as described before and shown in table 101.

With regard to the temperature control of a space cabin, for instance, it makes a great difference whether a space vehicle stays in the earth-moon region or whether an excursion is intended into the border regions of the ecosphere beyond Venus or into the sparsely irradiated space beyond Mars. The temperatures measured within the shell of the Explorer satellites were well within the physiologically tolerable range, around 25° C. But a space ship penetrating the intravenusian space would run into a kind of solar heat barrier and it would be impossible to aircondition the cabin. On the other hand, an expedition into the remote, sparsely irradiated regions of the outer planets would require extraordinary cabin temperature control measures in the reverse sense.

Solar illuminance—it is suggested—might be utilized in the space cabin for photosynthetic recycling of metabolic respiratory and nutritional body wastes. Table 101 shows quantitatively the decrease of this ecologic factor as a function of solar distance, and indicates that it may fall below the light minimum for photosynthesis somewhere beyond the belt of the asteroids. The utilization of solar light in this respect is then out of the question. If solar radiation is of no value at all in this respect and for temperature control and illumination, this would make the closed ecologic system a completely isolated one. For this case a nuclear power plant would have to replace solar power. Then we would deal with a completely autonomous or autark closed ecologic system. This would be a prerequisite for interstellar flight.

The interplanetary space projects, based on present propulsion systems, involve considerable durations. These methods permit essentially only minimum energy trajectories to other celestial bodies. This fact finds its expression in the term "coasting" or "passive phase" of the trajectory. A flight to the Moon and return in this way is a matter of less than a week. This would not pose difficult medical and supply problems. A flight to Mars, based on minimum velocity requirements, however, would take more than 8 months. Experiments made in space cabin simulators indicate that flights of such durations in a sealed cabin under the conditions of confinement and isolation might meet with the greatest difficulties. These arise essentially from the necessity to recycle the environment and from the psychophysiologic nature of the human creature. It seems to be necessary to shorten the duration of planetary missions. This, of course, would mean a change from a minimum energy orbit to an optimum time orbit which would require more effective propulsion methods, possibly continuous slight acceleration. In this way a compromise concerning the flight duration may be found—feasible from the standpoint of space technology and acceptable from the viewpoint of space medicine.

Constant slight accelerations, of course, lead to very high speed, ultimately approaching that of light. But not every speed the engineer likes to choose is permissible from a medical point of view because extreme speeds change the environment for the vehicle and the crew. The collision energy of meteorites and dust particles will be higher; rushing through the omnidirectional flux of cosmic rays increases their energy level at impact upon the vehicle. At very high velocities we would observe the Doppler effect in the electromagnetic spectrum insofar as in the direction to a star infrared will become visible and visible light will turn into ultraviolet and x-rays for the space traveller. Looking back to a star, we would experience the reverse. This shows that velocity in higher fractions of the speed of light becomes a limiting factor by its effect upon the environment related to

the fast moving space vehicle and its occupants. Time dilation (74) associated with near light speed is often discussed as a phenomenon favorable to extended space flight, such as interstellar flight. However, flights of interstellar dimensions are presently for all the aforementioned reasons not conceivable and the operational range will almost with certainty—at least for a century or so—be confined to the celestial bodies of our home solar system. What the astronaut will find there will be discussed in the next chapter.

REFERENCES

(1) Armstrong, H., Haber, H., and Strughold, H.: Aeromedical problems of space travel. J. Aviation Med., 20: 383–417, 1949.

(2) Marberger, G. P.: Space Medicine; the Human Factors in flights Beyond the Earth. Urbana Illinois, University of Illinois Press, 1951 (with contributions of Armstrong, H. G., von Braun, W., Strughold, H., Haber, H., Campbell, P. A., and Buettner, K.

(3) Gantz, K. F. Man in Space. New York, Duell, Sloan and Pearce, 1959.

(4) Hanrahan, I. S.: The Beginnings of Research in Space Biology at the A. F. Missile Development Center. Holloman Air Force Base, New Mexico, 1946-1952. Historical Report, 1958.

(5) Tenth anniversary of space medicine. Research in the U. S. Air Force. U. S. Armed Forces M. J., 10: 389–440, 1959.

(6) White, C. S., and Benson, O. O., Jr.: Physics and Medicine of the Upper Atmosphere. Albuquerque, University of New Mexico Press, 1952.

(7) Benson, O. O., Jr., and Strughold, H. (Editors): Physics and Medicine of the Atmosphere and Space. New York, John Wiley & Sons, Inc., 1960.

(8) Oshima, M.: Space Medicine. Tokyo, 1959.

(9) Lansberg, M. P.: Ruimtefart Geneeskunde. Amsterdam, 1958.

(10) Strughold, H., Haber, H., Buettner, K., and Haber, F.: Where does space begin? J. Aviation Med., 22: 342–349, 1951.

(11) Haber, H.: The Physical Environment of the Flyer. Randolph Air Force Base, Texas, School of Aviation Medicine, USAF, 1954.

(12) Strughold, H.: Space equivalent conditions within the earth's atmosphere: physiologic aspects. Astronautica acta, 1: 32–40, 1955.

(13) Van Allen, J. A.: Radiation hazards in space. Chapter 1 in Reference 7.

(14) Shapley, H.: Climatic Change, Evidence, Causes and Effects. Cambridge, Harvard University Press, 1953.

(15) Roberts, O.: The Sun. Chapter 37 in Reference 7.

(16) Schaefer, H. J.: Appraisal of cosmic ray

hazards in extra-atmospheric flight. In ALPERN, M., STERN, M., AND WOOSTER, H.: Vistas in Astronautics. New York, Pergamon Press, Inc., 1958, pp. 291–297.

(17) WHIPPLE, F.: Meteoric phenomenon and meteorites. In WHITE, C. S., AND BENSON, O. O., JR.: Physics and Medicine of the Upper Atmosphere. Albuquerque, University of New Mexico Press, 1952, chapter 10; and Chapter 3 in Reference 7.

(18) STRUGHOLD, H., AND RITTER, O. L.: The gravitational environment in space. Chapter 8 in Reference 7.

(19) GRIMMINGER, G.: Analysis of Temperature, Pressure and Density of the Atmosphere Extending to Extreme Altitudes. Santa Monica, California, The RAND Corporation, 1948.

(20) WATSON, F. G.: Between the planets. Cambridge, Harvard University Press, 1956.

(21) SIMONS, D. G., AND STEINMETZ, C. H.: The 1954 Aeromedical Field Laboratory balloon flights: physiological and radiobiological aspects. J. Aviation Med., 27: 100–110, 1956.

(22) YAGODA, H.: Frequency of thindown hits by heavy primary nuclei in emulsion and tissue. J. Aviation Med., 27: 522–532, 1956.

(23) CHASE, H. B.: Cutaneous effects of primary cosmic radiation. J. Aviation Med., 25: 388, 1954.

(24) TOBIAS, C. A.: Radiobiological studies with accelerated heavy ions. Chapter 12 in Reference 7.

(25) SCHAEFER, H. J.: Solar influences on the extra-atmospheric radiation field and their radiobiologic implications. Chapter 10 in Reference 7.

(26) PICKERING, J. E.: Biological aspects of nuclear propulsion. Chapter 27 in Reference 7.

(27) CIBIS, P.: Retinal adaptation applicable to visual problems in flight at increasing altitudes. In WHITE, C. S., AND BENSON, O. O., JR.: Physics and Medicine of the Upper Atmosphere. Albuquerque, University of New Mexico Press, 1952, pp. 562–566.

(28) ROSE, H. W.: Perception and reaction times. Chapter 30 in Reference 7.

(29) BUETTNER, K.: Bioclimatology of manned rocket flight. In MARBERGER, G. P.: Space Medicine; the Human Factors in Flights Beyond the Earth. Urbana, Illinois, University of Illinois Press, 1951, pp. 70–79.

(30) CLAMANN, H. G.: The engineered environment of the space vehicle. In GANTZ, K. F.: Man in Space. New York, Duell, Sloan and Pearce, 1959, chapter 6.

(31) FENNO, R. M.: Man's milieu in space. J. Aviation Med., 25: 612–622, 1954.

(32) LUFT, U. C.: Physiological limitations in cabin environment and human adaptations. In WHITE, C. S., AND BENSON, O. O., JR.: Physics and Medicine of the Upper Atmosphere. Albuquerque, University of New Mexico Press, 1952, chapter 21.

(33) SCHAEFER, E. K.: Experiences with submarine atmospheres. J. Aviation Med., 30: 350–359, 1959.

(34) MYERS, J.: Basic remarks on the use of plants as biological gas exchangers in a closed system. J. Aviation Med., 25: 407–411, 1954.

(35) GAUME, J. G.: Plants as a means of balancing a closed ecological system. J. Astronautics, 4: 72–75, 1957.

(36) GAFFORD, R. D., AND CRAFT, C. E.: A Photosynthetic Gas Exchanger for Small Animals. Research Report No. 58-124. Randolph Air Force Base, Texas, School of Aviation Medicine, USAF, 1959.

(37) BATES, J. H.: Recent Advances in the Development of a Closed Ecological System. Research Report Brooks Air Force Base, Texas, Aerospace Medical Center, 1959, in press.

(38) WILKS, R. S.: Carbon monoxide in green plants. Science, 129: 964–966, 1959.

(39) TISCHER, R. G.: Nutrition on long space voyages. Chapter 24 in Reference 7.

(40) CAMPBELL, P. A.: Human logistics from the viewpoint of space travel. In ALPERN, M., STERN, M., AND WOOSTER, H.: Vistas in Astronautics. New York, Pergamon Press, Inc., 1958, pp. 285–287.

(41) FLICKINGER, D.: Biomedical aspects of space flight. In GANTZ, K. F.: Man in Space. Urbana, Illinois, University of Illinois Press, 1959, chapter 4.

(42) KONNECI, E. B.: Human factors and space cabins. Astronautics, 3: 42–43, 71–73, 1958.

(43) HOOVER, G. W.: The man-machine system in space vehicles. In Space Medicine Symposium. London, British Interplanetary Society, 1958.

(44) STRUGHOLD, H.: The U. S. Air Force experimental sealed cabin. J. Aviation Med., 27: 50–52, 1956.

(45) STEINKAMP, G. R., AND HAWKINS, W. R.: Experimental use of a sealed cabin simulator. Chapter 22 in Reference 7.

(46) CLARK, R. T., FULTON, J. D., CLAMANN, H. G., GRAYBIEL, A., AND VOGEL, J.: Basic research problems in space medicine. Presented at the 21st International Congress of Physiological Sciences, Symposia and Special Lectures, Buenos Aires, 9–15 August 1959.

(47) SIMONS, D. G.: The "Manhigh" sealed cabin atmosphere. J. Aviation Med., 30: 314–325, 1959.

(48) ROSS, M. D., AND LEWIS, M. L. The Stratolab balloon system for high altitude research. J. Aviation Med., 29: 375, 1958.

(49) HAUTY, G. T.: Chapter 7 in Reference 7.

(50) RUFF, G. E. Isolation. Astronautics, 4: 22–23, 1959.

(51) BALKE, B.: Experimental studies on the conditioning of man for space crews. In GANTZ, K. F.: Man in Space. New York, Duell, Sloan and Pearce, 1959, chapter 11.

(52) CLARK, C. C., AND HARDY, J. D. Preparing man for space flight. Astronautics, **4**: 18–21, 1959.

(53) STAPP, J. P.: Biodynamics of space flight. In GANTZ, K. F.: Man in Space. New York, Duell, Sloan and Pearce, 1959, chapter 5.

(54) LAMB, L. E.: Medical aspects of interdynamic adaptation in space flight. J. Aviation Med., **30**: 158–161, 1959.

(55) LOVELACE, W. R., II, AND CROSSFIELD, S.: Atmospheric reentry, biomedical aspect. In BENSON, O. O., JR., AND STRUGHOLD, H.: Physics and Medicine of the Atmosphere and Space. New York, John Wiley & Sons, Inc., 1959, chapter 28.

(56) HESSBERG, R. R., JR.: Accelerative forces associated with leaving and re-entering the earth's gravitation field. J. Astronautics, **4**: 6–8, 1957.

(57) GAUER, O. H., AND HABER, H.: Man under gravity free conditions. In German Aviation Medicine, World War II, Vol. I. Washington, D. C., Government Printing Office, 1950, pp. 641–644.

(58) HABER, F., AND HABER, H.: Possible methods of producing the gravity free state for medical research. J. Aviation Med., **21**: 395–400, 1950.

(59) RITTER, O. L., AND GERATHEWOHL, S. J.: The concept of weight and stress in human flight. Research Report 58-154. Randolph Air Force Base, Texas, School of Aviation Medicine, USAF, 1959.

(60) BALLINGER, E. R.: Human experiments in subgravity and prolonged acceleration. J. Aviation Med., **23**: 319, 1952.

(61) GERATHEWOHL, S. J.: Weightlessness. In GANTZ, K. F.: Man in Space. New York, Duell, Sloan and Pearce, 1959, chapter 8.

(62) VON BECKH, H.: Fisiologic der volo. Buenos Aires, Alfa, 1955.

(63) DIRINGSHOFEN, V. H.: In GARTMAN, H.: Medicinische Probleme der Raumfahrt in Rammfahrtforschung. München, Oldenburg, 1952.

(64) LOMONACO, T., ET AL. Alcuni dati sperimentali fisiopsichici sugli effetti delle accelerazioni e della sub-gravita previsti nell'uomo lanciato nello spazio. Riv. med. aeronaut., **20**: 363–390, 1957.

(65) BERGERET, P.: Problemes physiologiques de la vie a bord des satellites artificiels. Med. aeronaut, **6**: 249–252, 5951.

(66) HENRY, J. P., BALLINGER, E. R., MAHER, P. J., AND SIMONS, D. G.: Animal studies of the subgravity state during rocket flight. J. Aviation Med., **23**: 420–432 1952.

(67) SIMONS, D. G.: Review of biological effects of subgravity and weightlessness. Jet Propulsion, **25**: 209–211, 1955.

(68) SCHOCK, G. J. D.: Apparent motion of a fixed luminous target during subgravity trajectories. Research Report AFMDC, TN-58-3. Holloman Air Force Base, New Mexico, Missile Development Command, USAF, 1958.

(69) CAMPBELL, P.: Orientation in space. In MARBERGER, G. P.: Space Medicine; the Human Factors in Flights Beyond the Earth. Urbana, Illinois, University of Illinois Press, 1959.

(70) KNIGHT, L. A.: An approach to the physiologic simulation of the null-gravity state. J. Aviation Med., **29**: 283–286, 1958.

(71) KOUSNETZOV, A. G.: Some results of biological experiments on rockets and Sputnik II. J. Aviation Med., **29**: 781–784, 1958.

(72) VON BECKH, H.: Weightlessness and space flight. Astronautics, **4**: 26, 1959.

(73) WARD, J. E., HAWKINS, W. R., AND STALLINGS, H.: Physiologic responses to subgravity. J. Aviation Med., **30**: 151, 1959.

(74) GOLTRA, E. R. Time dilation and the astronaut. Chapter 31 in Reference 7.

32

PLANETARY ATMOSPHERES

Hubertus Strughold, M. D.

As indicated in the foregoing chapter the rocket has brought about the possibilities of reaching other celestial bodies, first by instrumented research probes and later by manned space vehicles. This immediately brings the study of the conditions of the neighboring planets, especially of their atmospheres, into the focus of our interest. But, in addition to this, a comparative study of the atmospheres of all the planets is necessary for a better understanding of our own atmosphere, particularly its chemistry. But we cannot understand the planetary atmospheres in their present state completely if we do not examine the past, *i.e.*, the original atmospheres and their historic development up to the present time. In this respect we have to refer to the earth's atmosphere which has always been in the center of respective astrophysical studies (1, 2). In the following pages we shall, therefore, discuss the evolution of the earth's atmosphere as a background for the main topic of this chapter, "the atmospheres of the other planets," with biologic, or more precisely, ecologic remarks on the side.

The Evolution of the Earth's Atmosphere

The chemical composition of the earth's primordial atmosphere, or protoatmosphere, some $2\frac{1}{2} \times 10^9$ years ago, was very different from the present day atmosphere or neoatmosphere. The present day atmosphere contains essentially nitrogen, oxygen and the oxygen compound carbon dioxide and water vapor (see chapter 8). It is an oxidized atmosphere with oxidizing power. In contrast the protoatmosphere consisted mainly of hydrogen and hydrogen compounds, such as methane and ammonia, with some helium and water vapor (table 105). It was a reduced and reducing atmosphere. It had no actual oxidizing power. In brief, chemically, the present atmosphere is essentially an oxygen atmosphere; the protoatmosphere was essentially a hydrogen atmosphere.

But gradually a change in the primordial atmosphere took place. According to recent astrophysical theories (3, 4), water vapor molecules in the higher regions of the protoatmosphere were split into hydrogen and oxygen by the ultraviolet of solar radiation (photodissociation). The lighter hydrogen disappeared into space; the heavier oxygen, however, remained. With the appearance of this initial oxygen the protoatmosphere attained oxidizing power. This started a decisive development in its chemical composition. Ammonia (NH_3) was oxidized to free nitrogen (N_2) and water, and methane (CH_4) to carbon dioxide (CO_2) and water.

In this way, in the course of millions of years, the protoatmosphere became more and more oxidized. With the appearance of chlorophyl bearing primitive plants, such as algae, this process of oxidation was accelerated by photosynthetic activity. Oxygen produced in this biologic way oxidized the remaining bulk of the hydrogen compounds and even an excess of free oxygen accumulated in rather large amounts such as are found in the present day atmosphere. This stock of atmospheric free oxygen (O_2) is estimated to be around 1.2 quadrillion (10^{15}) metric tons. The effectiveness of photosynthesis in the oxidation and oxygenation of our atmosphere has, without a doubt, exceeded by far the oxygen production by photodissociation.

In this whole oxygen complex and that of carbon dioxide we must not only consider the atmosphere alone. The atmosphere is in a continuous gas exchange with the hydrosphere, i.e., the oceans, lakes and rivers, with the lithosphere, i.e., the solid earth's crust and the biosphere, i.e., the whole living world. It would be a difficult task to estimate the losses and gains in the oxygen balance of our atmosphere as the result of these interrelations. Since the first chemical analysis of the air was accomplished some 150 years ago the oxygen content of the earth's atmosphere has remained constant and drastic, or even measurable, changes cannot be expected to have occurred in this relatively short period of historic time.

Summarizing, we find in the historic development of the terrestrial atmosphere two basic types of atmospheres with pronounced chemical reaction tendencies, a hydrogen atmosphere, an oxygen atmosphere and a transition phase between these two.

In the anoxic hydrogen atmosphere, which existed in the early part of the protoatmosphere, organisms are hardly conceivable. If, however, organic compounds like amino acids, etc., were produced from methane and ammonia by solar radiation with some CO_2 available, anoxibionts could have existed in this primitive atmosphere. Also, in the transitional atmosphere, chemoautotrophs (iron, sulfur, ammonia and hydrogen bacteria) and photoautotrophs (chlorophyl bearing organisms of lower order) could

TABLE 105

Main Components of the Terrestrial Protoatmosphere and Atmosphere in Order of Abundance

	Components
Protoatmosphere	H_2 He Ne H_2O NH_3 CH_4 A
Present atmosphere	N_2 O_2 H_2O A CO_2

exist. The oxygen atmosphere of today, or neoatmosphere, provided the basis for the development of higher plants, animals and of man.

So much for the origin and historic evolution of the earth's atmosphere. We must keep in mind that behind this chemical atmospheric transformation, the effective agent was and is the radiation of the sun. We can now proceed to our main topic.

THE ATMOSPHERES OF THE OTHER PLANETS

It can be assumed that the protoatmospheres of all the other planets (2, 5, 6), about $2\frac{1}{2}$ billion (10^9) years ago, had the same chemical composition as the protoatmosphere of the earth. Then they must have very different chemical properties now inasmuch as they have been exposed to different intensities of solar radiation corresponding to their respective distances from the sun.

In the following, we shall consider the planets, not with increasing distance as is usually done, but rather with decreasing distance from the Sun, because this sequence conforms to the foregoing discussion of the chemical evolution of the terrestrial atmosphere. Table 106 shows the mean solar distances of the planets and the main chemical components of their atmospheres in order of their abundance.

Approaching the solar system from the outside, we first encounter Pluto, the outermost planet. It is assumed that its atmosphere consists of hydrogen, helium and methane in a frozen state.

The other outer, but larger planets, Neptune, Uranus, Saturn and Jupiter, can be considered here as a group. Their atmospheres consist mainly of hydrogen, methane,

TABLE 106

*Chemical Components of the Planetary Atmospheres**

Planets	Solar Distance in Million Miles	Most Important Atmospheric Chemical Components in Order of Abundance
Pluto	3675	H_2 He CH_4†
Neptune	2797	H_2 He CH_4 NH_3† H_2O†
Uranus	1785	H_2 He CH_4 NH_3† H_2O†
Saturn	887.2	H_2 He CH_4 NH_3 H_2O†
Jupiter	483.9	H_2 He CH_4 NH_3 H_2O†
Asteroids	—	— — — — —
Mars	141.7	N_2 A CO_2 H_2O‡ O_2‡
Earth	93.0	N_2 O_2 H_2O A CO_2
Venus	67.3	N_2 CO_2 H_2O‡ O_2‡ —
Mercury	36.0	— — — — —

* After Hess, S. (5), Kuiper, G. (2), Urey, H. (1), DeVaucouleurs, G. (7) and Whipple, F. L. (6).

† Probably in frozen state only.

‡ In traces only.

ammonia, helium and probably frozen water. The similarity of this composition to that of the protoatmosphere of the earth is striking. Apparently, escape of these light components has been prevented by the strong gravitational forces of these giant planets. Furthermore, they seem to be preserved in a frozen state because of their greater distance from the Sun. They are still protoatmospheres.

The main constituents in the Martian atmosphere are probably nitrogen, argon and carbon dioxide (7). The amount of carbon dioxide is about twice as high as that on earth. Water is present in very small amounts, mainly in the form of ice and vapor. This atmosphere is an oxidized, very thin atmosphere and qualitatively similar to that of the earth, except that it contains only traces of free oxygen. During its evolution this planet lost most of its atmosphere because of its low gravitational force (37 per cent of that of the earth). Not only hydrogen but also oxygen might have escaped from proto-Mars.

The Venusian atmosphere is also a completely oxidized atmosphere. It probably contains nitrogen and carbon dioxide, the latter in large amounts. The presence of free oxygen is still a matter of astronomical dispute. Water seems to be present.

Mercury has no atmosphere at all. It probably could not hold an atmosphere because of its low gravitational force and its high temperature owing to its nearness to the Sun.

Summarizing, in the solar planetary system in its present state of development, we find two basic types of atmospheres:

1. Hydrogen and hydrogen compounds containing atmospheres found on the outer planets.

2. Oxygen and/or oxidized compounds containing atmospheres on the inner planets with three varieties: (a) The atmosphere of the earth—a dense oxidized atmosphere with a high content of free oxygen, (b) the Venusian variety—a dense oxidized atmosphere with only a small amount of free oxygen and (c) the Martian variety—a thin oxidized atmosphere, also with only traces of free oxygen.

The group of the oxygen dominated atmospheres of the inner planets forms a kind of oxygen belt in the planetary system and the earth is the specific oxygen planet in this belt; the group of the hydrogen dominated atmospheres represents a hydrogen belt. These two belts correspond exactly with the two basic phases in the historic development of the earth's atmosphere: the hydrogen phase, some 2½ billion years ago and the present oxygen phase. Indeed, we notice the same sequence when we travel through the planetary system beginning at its remote outer regions into those of the vicinity of the Sun: a change from hydrogen and hydrogen compounds containing atmospheres to oxygen and/or oxidized compounds containing atmospheres. The atmospheres of the outer planets, orbiting beyond the effective range of solar radiation, apparently have preserved their hydrogen atmospheres of the protoatmospheric stage up to the present time. Chronologically, they are all of about the same age as those of the inner planets, but younger with regard to their chemical structure which, unaffected by the Sun's radiation, still shows the primordial features.

But we do not find a transitional phase as we should logically assume. This can be explained by the large spatial gap between Mars and Jupiter which is criss-crossed by minor planets or asteroids. If this region were occupied by a planet today it might show the postulated transitional phase of atmosphere. But it should be mentioned that the next planet beyond the belt of asteroids, Jupiter, shows some signs of photochemical reactions in its atmosphere as manifested by red, green and yellow colorations which are caused by free radicals of ammonia and methane produced by photodissociation (8).

This survey shows the usefulness of a comparative study of the planetary atmospheres; we recognize better the unique qualities of the earth's atmosphere by comparing them with the atmospheres of those celestial bodies which belong to the same family of planets but revolve around the Sun at different distances.

So far I have hardly touched upon the possibility of life on the other planets. This field of science which studies their ecologic qualification as an abode of life is called planetary ecology, or more generally, astrobiology (9–11). Such studies must consider a number of ecologic factors such as mass, period of rotation of the planet, light intensity, temperature, chemical composition of soil, atmosphere, presence of water, etc. The atmospheres are, of course, always in the center of such astrobiologic studies.

Two questions are of interest to us:

1. Is there indigenous life on the other planets? This is a question of general biologic interest.

2. What are the conditions with regard to the physiology of a terrestrial explorer? This is essentially an aeromedical and space medical problem.

In conformity with the subject matter of this textbook we shall concentrate mainly on the latter question and touch only slightly upon the first.

Beginning again with the outer planets, anoxibionts and hydrogen, methane and ammonia bacteria could exist in their atmospheres provided that the temperatures at the surfaces are in the biologically required range. This latter does not seem to be doubtful because the temperatures of their upper atmospheric layers range from $-150°$ to $-250°$ C. These superarctic temperatures would pose great difficulties for man's penetration, not to mention the highly toxic ammonia component in the atmosphere.

There is more than one indication for the possibility of life on Mars in the form of vegetation. Whether this is true or not can probably be answered only by an expedition to this planet. Such manned space operations to Mars are conceivable provided the necessary protective measures are taken. Inasmuch as the air pressure on its surface only amounts to about 70 mm. of Hg, a full pressure suit will be required when the astronaut leaves the sealed compartment of the space ship. For comparison, this barometric pressure corresponds to 55,000 feet in our atmosphere. The 47 mm. of Hg pressure level which is found in our atmosphere at 63,000 feet and is the threshold for "boiling of body fluids" or ebullism, is encountered at 13,000 feet above the Mars' surface. Generally, therefore, on Mars the atmospheric pressure conditions at ground level are of terrestrial stratospheric character. The temperature conditions during the day are better ($+ 25°$ C). During the night, however, they may exceed the cold in our stratosphere.

All of this shows that Mars is not a second Earth; its climatic conditions are too severe inasmuch as they lie around or below the minimum that is required from the standpoint of human physiology.

In certain aspects the ecologic conditions on Venus go in the other direction to the maximum. The air pressure may be in physiologic range, but the carbon dioxide content is rather high. This probably leads to very high atmospheric temperatures owing to a greenhouse effect. Venus, therefore, is not very inviting for a space operation and the direction in astronautics probably will go away from the Sun toward Mars and, of course, to the Moon. But an expedition to the airless Moon will always be like that to Mars, of a temporary nature and requiring all of the protection necessary for survival in a vacuum. Nevertheless, there is no question that lunar and Martian expeditions will be attempted in the interest of broadening our knowledge about the Universe. Aeromedical and space medical research will play an important role in the preparations for and conduction of these astronautical operations.

REFERENCES

(1) UREY, H. O.: The Planets, Their Origin and Development. New Haven, Yale University Press, 1952.

(2) KUIPER, G. P.: The Atmosphere of the Earth and Planets. Chicago, University of Chicago Press, 1951.

(3) POOLE, G. H. Y.: The evolution of the atmosphere. Proc. Roy. Soc. Dublin, 22: 345, 1951.

(4) WILD, L.: Photochemistry of planetary atmospheres. Astrophys. J., 86: 321, 1937.

(5) SLIPHER, E. C., HESS, S. L., ET AL.: The Study of Planetary Atmospheres. Flagstaff, Arizona, Lowell Observatory, 1952.

(6) WHIPPLE, F. L.: Earth, Moon and Planets. Philadelphia, Blakiston Co., 1958.

(7) DEVAUCOULEURS, G.: Physics of the Planet Mars. London, Faber & Faber, Ltd., 1953.

(8) RICE, F. O.: The Chemistry of Jupiter. Scientific American, 194: 119, 1956.

(9) JONES, S.: Life on Other Worlds. New York, The Macmillan Co., 1940.

(10) STRUGHOLD, H.: The Green and Red Planet. Albuquerque, University of New Mexico Press, 1953.

(11) TIKHOV, G. A.: Astrobiology. Moscow, 1953.

AUTHOR INDEX

This index lists the authors or senior authors of reference material who are cited by name in the body of the text. The names of the contributing authors to this work and the page numbers at the beginning of their respective chapters appear in bold face type.

SUBJECT INDEX

A

A-14 oxygen mask, 153
Abdomen, examination of, 28, 29
Acapnia, 124
Accelerations, 238
  definitions, 238
    negative, 239
    positive, 239
    transverse, 239
  terminology, 238
  types of,
    angular, 238, 254
    linear, 263
    radial, 239
Accelerations, angular, *see also* vertigo
  definition of, 238
  spinning, effects of, 254
  tumbling, effects of, 254
Accelerations, combined
  effects of, 258
  tolerances to, 258
Accelerations, linear, 263, *see also* decelerations,
    linear
  equations pertaining to, 264
  Newton's law, 263–265
  in orbital escape, 281
  in space flight, 280, 282
  units of, 265
  visual effects of, 406
Accelerations, radial, 239
  definition, 239
  general considerations, 240–242
  magnitude of, 239, 240
  negative g, 250
    objective symptoms, 251
    subjective symptoms, 250
  positive, *see* positive g
  protective devices, 254–261, *see also* anti-g de-
    vices
  terminology, 239
  transverse, 252
    objective symptoms, 253, 254
    subjective symptoms, 253
Acceleration-time patterns in aircraft, 240
Accidents, aircraft, 582–594
  causes of, 585
    human limitations, 588
    pilot error, 586
    supervisor and maintenance personnel error,
      587
    undetermined, 588
    unsafe conditions, 587
  definition of, 582
    incidents, 582
    major, 582
    minor, 582
  fatalities, number of, 583
  flight phase and, 584, 585
  injuries in, 588
    fatal, 588
    major, 588
    minor, 588
    types of, 588
  investigation of, aeromedical, 590
    human factors, 591
    injury, cause of, 591

losses from,
    combat potential, 583
    economic, 583
    other, 583
  prevention, aeromedical aspects of, 593
  rates, computation of, 582
  rates by type aircraft, 584
  risk factors, relation to, 583
  travel fatality rates, comparative data, 585
Acclimatization to altitude, 138, 160
Acclimatization, temperature, 331
Accommodation, visual,
  in depth perception, 36
  measurement of, 49, 50
Acoustic energy, effects of, 284
  measurement of, 285–287
Acoustic measurement relationships, 290, 291
Acoustic power level, 289
Acoustic principles, application of, 292–294
Acoustic zone, 114
Adaptability rating for military aeronautics,
    development of, 91
  validity of, 91
Aerial hygiene and sanitation, 557–581
Aerial perspective, in depth perception, 36
Aero Medical Association, founding of, 9
Aero Medical Research Laboratory, establish-
    ment of, 10
Aerodontalgia, 468
Aerodynamic heating, 326
Aeroembolism, 175, *see also* decompression sickness
Aeromedical evacuation, 548–556
  advantages of, 548, 550, 555
  air sickness in, 551
  aircraft available for,
    airline, 548, 549
    chartered, 549
    military, 548
  arrangements for, 549
  contraindications for, 550–555
  decreased atmospheric pressure in, 551
  general considerations, 550
  hypoxia in, 553, 554
  prohibitions against, 548, 549
  special precautions in,
    cardiovascualar diseases, 554, 555
    gastrointestinal diseases, 552, 553
    maxillofacial patients, 472
    middle ear diseases, 552
    miscellaneous diseases, 552, 554
    pulmonary diseases, 552, 554
    sinus diseases, 552
Aeromedical indoctrination of aircrews, 513–516
Aeromedical Research Laboratory, C.A.A., 16
Aeropause, the, 598
Aerosinusitis, 173
Aerospace medicine, definition of, 1
Aerotitis media, 162
  chronic, 166, 168
  complications, 170
  definition of, 164
  dental aspects of, 472
  diagnosis, 168
  differential diagnosis, 169
  etiology, 164

623